IAP Specialty Series on
PEDIATRIC INTENSIVE CARE

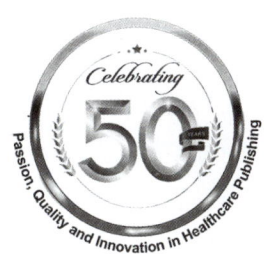

IAP Specialty Series on
PEDIATRIC INTENSIVE CARE

IAP Specialty Series on
PEDIATRIC INTENSIVE CARE

THIRD EDITION

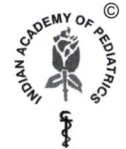

Founder Editor
Nitin K Shah
Section Coordinator (Pediatrics)
PD Hinduja Hospital, Mumbai
Hon Hematologist Oncologist
BJ Wadia Hospital for Children
Mumbai, Maharashtra, India

Editors-in-Chief

Soonu Udani
Medical Director and Head
Department of Critical Care and
Emergency Services
SRCC Children's Hospital
(Managed by Narayana Health)
Mumbai, Maharashtra, India

Jayashree Muralidharan
Professor and In-charge
Pediatric Emergency and PICU
Department of Pediatrics
Advanced Pediatric Centre
Postgraduate Institute of Medical
Education and Research
Chandigarh, India

Co-Editor and Foreword
Santosh T Soans

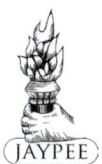

JAYPEE BROTHERS MEDICAL PUBLISHERS
The Health Sciences Publisher
New Delhi | London | Panama

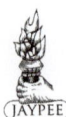

Jaypee Brothers Medical Publishers (P) Ltd

Headquarters

Jaypee Brothers Medical Publishers (P) Ltd
4838/24, Ansari Road, Daryaganj
New Delhi 110 002, India
Phone: +91-11-43574357
Fax: +91-11-43574314
E-mail: jaypee@jaypeebrothers.com

Overseas Offices

J P Medical Ltd
83 Victoria Street, London
SW1H 0HW (UK)
Phone: +44 20 3170 8910
Fax: +44 (0)20 3008 6180
E-mail: info@jpmedpub.com

Jaypee-Highlights Medical Publishers Inc
City of Knowledge, Bld. 235, 2nd Floor, Clayton
Panama City, Panama
Phone: +1 507-301-0496
Fax: +1 507-301-0499
E-mail: cservice@jphmedical.com

Jaypee Brothers Medical Publishers (P) Ltd
Bhotahity, Kathmandu, Nepal
Phone: +977-9741283608
E-mail: kathmandu@jaypeebrothers.com

Website: www.jaypeebrothers.com
Website: www.jaypeedigital.com

© 2019, Jaypee Brothers Medical Publishers

The views and opinions expressed in this book are solely those of the original contributor(s)/author(s) and do not necessarily represent those of editor(s) of the book.

All rights reserved. No part of this publication may be reproduced, stored or transmitted in any form or by any means, electronic, mechanical, photocopying, recording or otherwise, without the prior permission in writing of the publishers.

All brand names and product names used in this book are trade names, service marks, trademarks or registered trademarks of their respective owners. The publisher is not associated with any product or vendor mentioned in this book.

Medical knowledge and practice change constantly. This book is designed to provide accurate, authoritative information about the subject matter in question. However, readers are advised to check the most current information available on procedures included and check information from the manufacturer of each product to be administered, to verify the recommended dose, formula, method and duration of administration, adverse effects and contraindications. It is the responsibility of the practitioner to take all appropriate safety precautions. Neither the publisher nor the author(s)/editor(s) assume any liability for any injury and/or damage to persons or property arising from or related to use of material in this book.

This book is sold on the understanding that the publisher is not engaged in providing professional medical services. If such advice or services are required, the services of a competent medical professional should be sought.

Every effort has been made where necessary to contact holders of copyright to obtain permission to reproduce copyright material. If any have been inadvertently overlooked, the publisher will be pleased to make the necessary arrangements at the first opportunity. The **CD/DVD-ROM** (if any) provided in the sealed envelope with this book is complimentary and free of cost. **Not meant for sale.**

Inquiries for bulk sales may be solicited at: jaypee@jaypeebrothers.com

IAP Specialty Series on Pediatric Intensive Care

First Edition: 2008

Second Edition: 2013

Third Edition: **2019**

ISBN: 978-93-5270-938-0

Printed at: Samrat Offset Pvt. Ltd.

Dedicated to

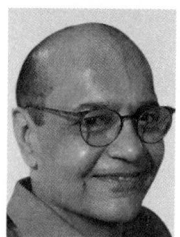

Anand Shandilya
(21.07.1962–01.01.2019)

*Our dear friend and colleague Anand Shandilya,
whose untimely death on New Year's day
left the Pediatric community in deep mourning.
Anand has contributed a chapter to every edition of this book and
this one will be a worthy addition to his legacy of education and
teaching, to which he devoted his professional life.*

Contributors

Abdul Rauf
Fellow
Division of Pediatric Emergency
and Critical Care
Sir Ganga Ram Hospital
New Delhi, India

Abhishek Bansal
Consultant Pediatric Intensivist
and Neonatologist
Apple Children Hospital
Ahmedabad, Gujarat, India

Amish Vora
Senior Intensivist and
Neonatologist
SRCC Children's Hospital
(Managed by Narayan Health)
Mumbai, Maharashtra, India

Anand Bhutada
Pediatric Intensivist
Department of Pediatric
Intensive Care
Director
Nelson's Mother and Child
Hospital
Nagpur, Maharashtra, India

Anand Shandilya
Senior Consultant
Department of Pediatrics
SRCC Children's Hospital
(Managed by Narayan Health)
Mumbai, Maharashtra, India

Aoyon Sengupta
Consultant Pediatric Intensivist
SRCC Children's Hospital
(Managed by Narayana Health)
Mumbai, Maharashtra, India

Arun Bansal
Professor
Division of Pediatric Critical Care
Department of Pediatrics
Advanced Pediatrics Centre
Postgraduate Institute of Medical
Education and Research
Chandigarh, India

Arun Kumar Baranwal
Professor
Pediatric Emergency and
Intensive Care Unit
Head, Pediatric Cardiology Unit
Advanced Pediatric Centre
Postgraduate Institute of Medical
Education and Research
Chandigarh, India

Ashwath Ram RN
Consultant Pediatric
Intensivist and Pediatric
Emergency Medicine
Manipal Hospitals
Bengaluru, Karnataka, India

Azeem Khan
Senior Intensivist
SRCC Children's Hospital
(Managed by Narayana Health)
Mumbai, Maharashtra, India

Bala Ramachandran
Consultant and Head
Department of Intensive Care and
Emergency Medicine
Kanchi Kamakoti CHILDS Trust
Hospital
Chennai, Tamil Nadu, India

Bharat Mehra
Fellowship in Pediatric
Emergency Medicine
Fellow, Pediatric Critical Care
Sir Ganga Ram Hospital
New Delhi, India

Deepali Wankhade
Fellow and Consultant
SRCC Children's Hospital
Managed by Narayana Health
Mumbai, Maharashtra, India

Dilip Jain
Fellow PICU (IDPCCM)
Lotus Hospitals for Women and
Children
Hyderabad, Telangana, India

Gaurang Upadhyay
Critical Care Fellow
Great Ormond Street Hospital
London, UK

Indira Jayakumar
Senior Consultant
Department of Pediatric and
Emergency Unit
Apollo Children's Hospital
Chennai, Tamil Nadu, India

Isha Bhagat
Consultant Pediatric
Intensive Care
Surya Hospital, Mumbai
Maharashtra, India

Javed Ismail
Consultant
Department of Pediatric
Critical Care
Apollo KH Hospitals
Vellore, Tamil Nadu, India

Jayashree Muralidharan
Professor and In-charge
Pediatric Emergency and PICU
Department of Pediatrics
Advanced Pediatric Centre
Postgraduate Institute of
Medical Education and Research
Chandigarh, India

Jhuma Sankar
Assistant Professor
Department of Pediatrics
All India Institute of Medical Sciences
New Delhi, India

Kundan Mittal
Senior Professor
In-charge (Pediatric Intensive Care, Respiratory Services and Genetic Clinic and Molecular Diagnostics)
Department of Pediatrics
Fellowship in Pediatric Critical Care and Clinical Genetics
Pandit Bhagwat Dayal Sharma Postgraduate Institute of Medical Sciences
Rohtak, Haryana, India

Lalitha AV
Professor and Head
Division of Pediatric Critical Care
Department of Pediatrics
St John's Medical College and Hospital
Bengaluru, Karnataka, India

Madhumati Otiv
Consultant Pediatric Intensivist
KEM Hospital
Pune, Maharashtra, India

Mahesh A Mohite
Pediatric and Neonatal Intensivist
Sai Child Care Clinic
Navi Mumbai, Maharashtra
Bai Jerbai Wadia Hospital for Children
Mumbai, Maharashtra, India

Maninder Dhaliwal
Associate Director
Intensive Care
Medanta—The Medicity
Gurugram, Haryana, India

Manish Sharma
Senior Specialist Pediatrics
In-charge Accident/Emergency
Pediatric Intensivist
State Nodal Officer
Organ Donation Programme
Department of Pediatrics
Sawai Man Singh Medical College
Jaipur, Rajasthan, India

Manisha Patil
Senior Project Coordinator
Division of Pediatric Critical Care
Department of Pediatrics
Advanced Pediatrics Centre
Postgraduate Institute of Medical Education and Research
Chandigarh, India

Manu Sundaram
Consultant Pediatric Intensivist
Sidra Medicine
Doha Qatar, UAE

Manvinder Singh Sachdev
Senior Consultant
Department of Pediatric Cardiology
Medanta—The Medicity
Gurugram, Haryana, India

Mounika Reddy
Assistant Professor
Division of Pediatric Critical Care
St John's Medical College and Hospital
Bengaluru, Karnataka, India

Namita Ravikumar
Senior Resident
Division of Pediatric Critical Care
Advanced Pediatrics Centre
Postgraduate Institute of Medical Education and Research
Chandigarh, India

Nayani Sridevi
FNB Postgraduate
Pediatric Intensive Care Unit
Mehta Multispeciality Hospital
Chennai, Tamil Nadu, India

Neeraj Gupta
Consultant
Division of Pediatric Emergency and Critical Care
Sir Ganga Ram Hospital
New Delhi, India

Nirmal Chorari
Pediatric Intensivist
Nirmal Hospital Pvt Ltd
Surat, Gujarat, India

Nisha Krishnamurthy
Junior Consultant
Department of Pediatric Nephrology
SRCC Children's Hospital
Mumbai, Maharashtra, India

Nitin K Shah
Section Coordinator
Department of Pediatrics
PD Hinduja Hospital and Medical Research Centre
Hon. Hematologist Oncologist
BJ Wadia Hospital for Children
Mumbai, Maharashtra, India

Praveen Khilnani
Clinical Director and Senior Consultant
Pediatric Critical Care and Pulmonology
Rainbow Children's Hospital
New Delhi, India

Preetha Joshi
Consultant
Department of Pediatric Intensive Care, Cardiac Intensive Care and Neonatology
Kokilaben Dhirubhai Ambani Hospital and Medical Research Institute
Mumbai, Maharashtra, India

Contributors

Puneet A Pooni
Professor and Head
Department of Pediatrics
Dayanand Medical College and Hospital
Ludhiana, Punjab, India

Rachna Sharma
In-Charge
Pediatric Critical Care
BLK Superspecialty Hospital
New Delhi, India

Rajappan Pillai
Consultant and Pediatric Intensivist
Aster Medcity
Kochi, Kerala, India

Rekha Solomon
Pediatric Intensivist
Bai Jerbai Wadia Hospital for Children
Mumbai, Maharashtra, India

S Thangavelu
Pediatric Consultant and Director
Department of Pediatrics
Mehta Multispeciality Hospital
Chennai, Tamil Nadu, India

Sahana P
Resident
Department of Pediatric Intensive Care Unit
AJ Institute of Medical Sciences
Mangaluru, Karnataka, India

Sanah Merchant-Soomar
Pediatric Cardiologist
Mumbai, Maharashtra, India

Santosh T Soans
Pediatrician and Intensivist
Professor and Head
Department of Pediatrics
AJ Institute of Medical Sciences
Mangaluru, Karnataka, India

Siddharth Bhargav
Associate Professor
Department of Pediatrics
Dayanand Medical College and Hospital
Ludhiana, Punjab, India

Soonu Udani
Medical Director and Head
Department of Critical Care and Emergency Services
SRCC Children's Hospital (Managed by Narayana Health)
Mumbai, Maharashtra, India

Suchitra Ranjit
Consultant
Department of Pediatric ICU
Apollo Children's Hospital
Chennai, Tamil Nadu, India

Suneel K Pooboni
Divisional Chief
Pediatric Critical Care
Professor of Pediatrics
Mafraq Hospital
Abu Dhabi, UAE

Suresh Gupta
Senior Consultant and In-charge
Department of Pediatric Emergency
Sir Ganga Ram Hospital
New Delhi, India

Suresh Kumar Angurana
Assistant Professor
Division of Pediatric Critical Care
Department of Pediatrics
Advanced Pediatrics Centre
Postgraduate Institute of Medical Education and Research
Chandigarh, India

U Sridhurga
Assistant Professor
Velammal Medical College Hospital and Research Institute
Madurai, Tamil Nadu, India

Uma Ali
Consultant Pediatric Nephrologist and Section Head
SRCC Children's Hospital, Mumbai
Consultant Pediatric Nephrologist
Lilavati Hospital and Research Centre, Mumbai
Jupiter Hospital, Mumbai
Maharashtra, India

Umesh Vaidya
Chief Neonatologist
KEM Hospital
Pune, Maharashtra
Regional Medical Director
Cloudnine Hospital
Pune, Maharashtra, India

Vasanth Kumar
Consultant
Department of Pediatric ICU
Apollo Children's Hospital
Chennai, Tamil Nadu, India

Veena Raghunathan
Senior Consultant
Department of Pediatric Intensive Care
Medanta—The Medicity
Gurugram, Haryana, India

Vijai Williams
Senior Resident
Division of Pediatric Critical Care
Advanced Pediatrics Centre
Postgraduate Institute of Medical Education and Research
Chandigarh, India

Vikas Taneja
Senior Consultant and Head
Manipal Hospitals
New Delhi, India

Vinay Joshi
Senior Intensivist
SRCC Children's Hospital
Mumbai, Maharashtra, India

Vinay Munikoty
Assistant Professor
Division of Pediatric Hematology
and Oncology
St John's Medical College and
Hospital
Bengaluru, Karnataka, India

Vinayak Patki
Chief Consultant
Advanced Pediatric Critical Care
Centre and Head
Wanless Hospital
Miraj, Maharashtra, India

Vishal Baldua
Consultant
Department of Pediatric
Intensive Care Unit
SRCC Children's Hospital
Mumbai, Maharashtra, India

Vishram Buche
Pediatric Intensivist
Department of Pediatric
Intensive Care
Director
Nelson's Mother and Child
Hospital
Nagpur, Maharashtra, India

VSV Prasad
Chief Consultant, Neonatologist
and Pediatric Intensivist
Chief Executive Officer
Lotus Hospitals for Women and
Children
Hyderabad, Telangana, India

Foreword

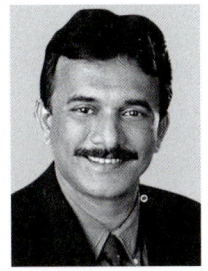

I am delighted to know that *IAP Specialty Series on Pediatric Intensive Care* has been revised under the editorial stewardship of Soonu Udani. This, the third edition, continues the tradition of excellence with thorough revisions that bring you fully up-to-date with all that's new in the field of intensive care. Few new chapters and a reconfigured format make this a comprehensive and clearly written resource for the experienced clinician as well as the physician-in-training. As Critical Care Fellowships are getting popular, I am sure that this is going to be an excellent ready reference for the would-be pediatric intensivists. This is a remarkable and commendable achievement. I am astonished that they have brought out this edition in record time. I wish to congratulate all colleagues involved in this monumental effort.

Critical care has proved to be one of the great successes of modern medicine. Thanks to this discipline today that we are in a position to achieve life-saving feats which would have been considered impossible in medical science few decades back.

In the early 1990s, having just completed my postgraduation, I was at a crossroads as to what subspecialty to pursue. Those days, pediatric and neonatal critical care were just beginning to make their appearance and my heart gravitated towards this new field. As there were only a handful of pediatric intensive care specialists in my entire state, I felt that this field would give me ample opportunities to explore and grow. Rather than reinvent the wheel, here was a field which tested my competence on a daily basis and let me try out new ideas and approaches. That our efforts had a life-saving impact was a greater point of satisfaction too. The passion has stayed with me to this day and I am grateful to the Pediatric Intensive Care Chapter for giving me an outlet to share it with other like-minded colleagues.

The intensive care unit (ICU) is a place where we are expected to deliver miracles. Not a day passes when we are not confronted with extraordinary challenges. As the famous doctor-author Atul Gawande says, "This is the reality of intensive care: at any point, we are as apt to harm as we are to heal." Talent is one of the essence in a critical care facility. As intensivists, our clinical knowledge should be backed with sharp observation, perceptiveness, keen insight, shrewd decision making and other cognitive resources.

I wish the readers an enlightening academic experience. I am sure this book is going to be favorite of IAPians and hope to see next edition as soon as possible.

Santosh T Soans
President
Indian Academy of Pediatrics, 2018

Preface to the Third Edition

Pediatric critical care has run a double marathon since it started in India in the early 1980s. The Academy entrusted us with the task of putting together the second edition of the book and now we have another. We may have overstepped our brief in some areas where we have gone beyond presenting the subject in a compact form as is needed for this series, but put it down to the enthusiasm of the authors to deliver the complete goods. We have, till now, mostly relied upon textbooks from the Western world. This edition is a huge leap forward towards this purpose. We attempted to involve everyone in the Pediatric Critical Care Community in India in order that the topics would be covered by the very people who deal with and are experts in these problems. Old and experienced, young and enthusiastic—all were involved in preparing this comprehensive book on Pediatric Intensive Care. Many of the contributors are researchers in the subjects of their contribution. We hope that the book will be of use to residents, academic institutions and private practitioners alike as the chapters are detailed, yet have clarity and important key messages. We have incorporated the latest guidelines on most topics while keeping in mind the various levels of care available in the country. Management has been discussed with alternatives for resource poor situations as well as for tertiary care institutions. A few chapters have been retained from the old edition as there was no update needed. The Indian Pediatric Critical Care Community is making huge strides in India and this book is one more milestone in our path to deliver quality care to each and every child in India. We do hope you will find the book useful towards the care of your sickest patients.

Nitin K Shah
Soonu Udani
Jayashree Muralidharan
Santosh T Soans

Preface to the First Edition

No other subspecialty in pediatrics in India has seen as much of a growth and interest in the last decade as has critical care. This is akin to the growth seen in neonatology in the 1970s and 1980s. Our specialty was seen as being technology dependent and out of the reach of the average practitioner and patient. Additionally, there was little exposure in most medical schools at both the undergraduate and postgraduate levels. Graduates who sought training abroad rarely returned as they perceived that our country would not afford them the opportunities, both professional and financial, in this field.

As the gap between the new world and the developing world narrows, many of these young well-trained individuals are now seeking careers at home. Corporate hospitals have well-staffed and well-equipped units and several teaching hospitals have equally equipped, excellently staffed units that are fertile training grounds for new generations of intensivists.

The origins of formal training in Pediatric Critical Care was born from the initiative of a group who recognized the need for standardized training across the country. A course was designed and offered; first for a few days, then for a few weeks and finally for one year at 5 institutions. Many fresh students and practitioners enrolled for these courses. Today, there are several parallel courses, catering to various needs. There is also National Board recognition for the specialty on a two years fellowship.

No doubt there are many excellent textbooks on the subject. Many in much more detail and by much more eminent people who are internationally recognized as doyens in the field. Why then are we bringing out this book? Across the length and breadth of the country, pediatricians look after very sick children and all of them do not have the luxury of critical care units at their disposal, neither can they all complete fellowships in the subject. Yet they cannot turn away the critically ill child in the remote areas where they practice. The majority of our critically ill children do not go to the PICUs of the metros, they go to pediatricians in their towns and villages. This book is aimed at giving the practicing pediatrician knowledge of the subject in as comprehensive a manner as he/she needs. It is a book by our own IAP for us, by us—many of us. It is the collective effort of many. Certain issues such as infections that have been covered in other recent IAP series are omitted here.

We thank all our contributors and hope that this book fulfills the needs of all our fellow IAP members. Feedback would help us improve the next edition.

Soonu Udani
Deepak Ugra
Krishan Chugh
Praveen Khilnani

Acknowledgments

We acknowledge the day-to-day contribution of our students and fellows who constantly challenge us and teach us so much more than we teach them. To all our contributors, we are grateful for the excellent work delivered, albeit by making us sweat the deadlines. We would not have any knowledge and skills without our very dear patients who are our greatest heroes; both for lessons in life as well as in medicine. Last but not least, we must acknowledge our spouses and children who continue to love and support us despite being ignored and neglected by our obsessive compulsive behavior towards our work.

We are thankful to Shri Jitendar P Vij (Group Chairman), Mr Ankit Vij (Managing Director), Mr MS Mani (Group President), Ms Chetna Malhotra Vohra (Associate Director—Content Strategy), Ms Pooja Bhandari (Production Head) and Dr Savleen Kaur (Development Editor) of M/s Jaypee Brothers Medical Publishers (P) Ltd, New Delhi, India, for giving a go-ahead at the very beginning and helping us in every way possible to bring out this book.

Contents

1. **Critical Care Scenario in India** 1
   Santosh T Soans, Sahana P

2. **Recognition and Stabilization of the Critically Ill Child** 4
   Puneet A Pooni, Siddharth Bhargav

3. **Resuscitation** 19
   Anand Shandilya

4. **Fluid and Electrolytes in the Critically Ill Child** 32
   Preetha Joshi, Vinay Joshi

5. **Oxygen Therapy in the Emergency Room and PICU** 50
   Suresh Kumar Angurana, Vijai Williams

6. **Lung Mechanics with Ventilation: Physiology and Monitoring** 62
   Abdul Rauf, Neeraj Gupta

7. **Basics of Mechanical Ventilation** 73
   Arun Kumar Baranwal, Namita Ravikumar

8. **Noninvasive Ventilation** 86
   Ashwath Ram RN, Manu Sundaram

9. **Respiratory Monitoring in Pediatric Intensive Care Unit** 117
   Vishram Buche, Anand Bhutada

10. **Acute Respiratory Distress Syndrome** 136
    Vinay Joshi, Gaurang Upadhyay

11. **Hemodynamic Monitoring** 153
    Vasanth Kumar, Suchitra Ranjit

12. **Acute Heart Failure** 164
    Vikas Taneja, Manvinder Singh Sachdev

13. **Cardiac Arrhythmias** 183
    Sanah Merchant-Soomar, Vishal Baldua

14. **Vasoactive Agents** 205
    Rekha Solomon, Isha Bhagat

15. **Hypertensive Crises** 219
    Indira Jayakumar, U Sridhurga

16. **Sepsis and Septic Shock** 226
    Soonu Udani

17. **Approach to a Comatose Child** 241
    Manisha Patil, Arun Bansal

18. **Head Injury in Children** 249
    Soonu Udani

19. **Status Epilepticus** 268
    Soonu Udani

20. **End-of-life Care in the Pediatric Intensive Care Unit** 280
    Bala Ramachandran

21. **Diabetic Ketoacidosis in Children** 288
    Vijai Williams, Jayashree Muralidharan

22. **Basics of Renal Replacement Therapy** 299
    Nisha Krishnamurthy, Uma Ali

23. **Gastrointestinal Tract Bleed** 310
    Abhishek Bansal

24. **Acute Liver Failure** 324
    Maninder Dhaliwal, Veena Raghunathan

25. **Pre- and Postoperative Management of a Liver Transplant Patient** 341
    Aoyon Sengupta, Rajappan Pillai

26. **Nutrition in Critically Ill Children** 357
    Madhumati Otiv, Umesh Vaidya

27. **Dengue in Pediatric Intensive Care Unit** 362
    Javed Ismail, Jhuma Sankar

28. **Management of a Child with Polytrauma** 380
    Bharat Mehra, Suresh Gupta

29. **Drowning** 391
    Kundan Mittal, Vinayak Patki

30. **Pediatric Emergency Care: Poisoning and Toxidromes** 395
    S Thangavelu, Nayani Sridevi

31. **Envenomation (Snake Envenomation and Scorpion Sting)** 449
    Mahesh A Mohite

32. **Oncological Emergencies** 463
    Lalitha AV, Mounika Reddy, Vinay Munikoty

33. **Blood Components in Intensive Care Practice** 480
    Nitin K Shah

34. **Ventilator-associated Pneumonia and Hospital-acquired Pneumonia** 491
    VSV Prasad, Dilip Jain

35. **Catheter-related Bloodstream Infection** 509
    Azeem Khan

36. **Catheter-associated Urinary Tract Infection** 515
    Vishal Baldua, Deepali Wankhade

37. **Antimicrobial Stewardship in PICU** 521
    Rachna Sharma

38. **Pain and Sedation** 532
    Arun Bansal, Amish Vora

39. **Nursing Issues in the PICU** 546
    Nirmal Chorari

40. **Extracorporeal Membrane Oxygenation** 555
    Amish Vora, Praveen Khilnani, Suneel K Pooboni

41. **Pediatric Organ Donation and Donor Maintenance** 563
    Manish Sharma

Index 575

Critical Care Scenario in India

Santosh T Soans, Sahana P

Every year about 5 million patients are admitted to the intensive care units (ICUs) in India. Pediatric intensive care in India started in the early 1990s. It simultaneously initiated at four centers in the north, south, and west by individual efforts. The pioneering institutions were the Postgraduate Institute of Medical Education and Research (PGIMER), Chandigarh; Sir Ganga Ram Hospital, Delhi; Hinduja Hospital, Mumbai; and Child Trust Hospital, Chennai. Pioneers who were trained abroad returned to India to set up pediatric ICUs (PICUs). Soon the specialty became popular with pediatricians; and in 1996, there were already 21 centers offering pediatric intensive care and the number grew steadily. In 2004, the number of ICUs in the country had surpassed 100. During the early period, intensivists worked with limited gadgets and encouraged indigenous manufactured equipment.

The tremendous growth in pediatric intensive care (PIC) was due to the continuous emphasis on training programs. The Indian Academy of Pediatrics (IAP) was quick in realizing the importance of critical care training. IAP introduced Pediatric Advanced Life Support (PALS) courses in the early 1990s with the help of Dr N Janaki Raman. In 1995, a formal IAP-PALS course was launched. By the year 2000, almost 200 courses were conducted and more than 7,000 pediatricians had been trained. The IAP—Intensive Care Chapter was established in 1998 to provide satisfactory critical care to the needy children across the country. And in the year 2000, the Indian Society of Critical Care Medicine—Pediatric Section was founded. The first National Conference of PIC was held at Nagpur in the year 1999. It was followed next year at Chandigarh. Since then the conference is conducted every year with faculties from India and abroad. From national to international conference was not a long journey. In 2007, the International Advanced Course in PIC was organized, and in 2009, the First Asian Congress of PIC was conducted at Chandigarh. The later was attended by delegates from 21 countries and regional leaders from Asia, and the faculty included giants of PIC.

In the past decade, pediatric critical care has rapidly grown, but still remains a developing branch as far as our country is concerned. Throughout modern science, and increasingly within the fields of medicine, new hybrid disciplines have emerged from division and recombination of mature specialties. Pediatric critical care is one such permutation and combination in evolving medicine. Subspecialty chapters were identified to promote research, to impart specialized training in pediatric subspecialties, and to organize scientific meetings on pediatric subspecialties. Pediatric critical care medicine is a relatively new but a rapidly growing pediatric specialty in resource-limited countries.

Since then we have come a long way with more than 1,500 members, 17 state branches, 3 city branches, around 300 fellows, and an index journal. The intensive care chapter of the IAP started a formal fellowship program in 2002, and it is now being run through 22 accredited centers in India. A well-organized, multi-layered, training program has evolved—we are one of the few countries with a well-organized training program in pediatric critical care.

Because of its lack of ionizing radiation, as well as its availability and its ability to be performed without sedation, ultrasound is an ideal imaging modality for children, and numerous pediatric-specific point-of-care ultrasound (POCUS), echocardiography (ECHO) applications are clinically relevant and is being introduced in the fellowship training curriculum. An adequate dose of subspecializing training cannot be defined as it is not known whether "bolus" doses of focused subspecialty care of 3–6 months or steady infusion of caring for similar patients over 1–2 years results in a better retention of knowledge and skills.

The role of pediatric critical care nursing is complex. First, the nurse has to continually examine physiologic monitors and treatment devices, along with the child's body. Second, in the event of any irregularity, the nurse has to instantly judge the significance of the event and initiate an appropriate response. Third, the nurse has a primary responsibility for ensuring patient safety. Fourth, the nurse is also responsible for maintaining a bedside environment that fosters the psychosocial adaptation of the child and family. Fifth, the nurse also functions as an "integrator" of patient information. The strength of a PICU's service is directly tied to the quality and rigor of care that the nursing team can provide, in collaboration with the entire pediatric critical care team.

Many of the PICUs in metropolitan cities have state-of-the-art facilities, including extracorporeal membrane oxygenation (ECMO). In large cities, the transportation of a critically ill child has moved on from a hand–ventilated child in a basic ambulance to the state-of-the-art transport which includes a trained team, transport ventilators, oximetry, and end-tidal CO_2 ($ETCO_2$). Children previously thought to be too unstable for transport can now be safely transported from one center to a higher one. Needless to say, large proportions of children in rural and remote parts of India are still deprived of timely critical care services and succumb to the illness. Simulation is now a well-accepted and practiced method of training.

India is a fast-growing emerging market, with a great potential for research, especially in pediatrics given the young population and disease burden. As the Pediatric Critical Care Medicine specialty continues to grow, more research is likely to occur at both government-run teaching institutions and corporate hospitals. Multidisciplinary, interdisciplinary, and transdisciplinary are the ways forward in pediatric critical care. Sharing knowledge and research bring multiple perspectives and help avoid some of the blind spots of a single discipline. Patient care shared by a local regular pediatrician and the superspecialist known as "shared care" is an appropriate model for our country.

The biggest question is whether specialization is a boon or a bane? Do we need people who know more and more about less and less until they know everything about nothing? Subsubspecialists should develop new knowledge in their areas of critical care, identify best practices and at the same time—keep in touch with basics and other systems. The contributions of national societies and quality of standards of Pediatric Critical Care Medicine Fellowship programs will define the future of pediatric critical care training in India.

In short, since the beginning of the new century, the Pediatric Critical Care Medicine training in India has grown by leaps and bounds and is still growing. About 30–40 years from now, will there still be an ICU? There will be a department of intensive care for sure, but a dedicated unit for that maybe obsolete. Experts suggest that rather than having a separate ICU, if a patient needs intensive care, the regular hospital bed itself can be transformed into a critical care bed by bringing in equipment like the respirators and other sophisticated monitors.

SUGGESTED READING

1. Bhalala US, Sadawarte J, Sadawarte S, et al. Development and Implementation of Pediatric Critical Care Focused Simulation Workshop and Program in India. J Paediatr Critical Care. 2014;1(4):240-4.
2. Bhalal U, Khilnani P. Pediatric Critical Care Medicine Training in India: Past, present and future. Front Pediatr. 2018;6:34.
3. Carnevale FA, Dagenais M. Nursing care in the paediatric intensive care unit. In: Wheeler D, Wong H, Shanley T (Eds). Paediatric Critical Care Medicine. London: Springer; 2014.
4. Good R, Orsborn J, Stidham T. Point-of-care ultrasound education for pediatric residents in the pediatric intensive care unit. MedEdPORTAL. 2018;14:10683.
5. IAP-Intensive Care Chapter. Available from: http://www.piccindia.com.
6. World Federation of Pediatric Intensive and Critical Care Societies. Available from: http://www.wfpiccs.org/history-of-picu-in-india.
7. Yeolekar ME, Mehta S. ICU Care in India - status and challenges. April 2008;56:221-2.

Recognition and Stabilization of the Critically Ill Child

2

Puneet A Pooni, Siddharth Bhargav

LEARNING OBJECTIVES

- Proper, systematic, and structured evaluation of a child helps in early recognition of severity of illness, which helps in proper and timely intervention, thus decreasing morbidity and mortality.
- In this chapter, reader will be able to evaluate any child coming to emergency in an organized way thus classifying the severity of illness and hence intervening in timely manner, and saving precious lives.

INTRODUCTION

"Critically ill child" is a child who is in a clinical state which may result in respiratory or cardiac arrest or severe neurological complications if not recognized and promptly treated. Many diseases can lead to this "critically ill state." Whether a child presents with a primary cardiovascular, respiratory, neurological, infectious, or metabolic disorder, the goal of initial evaluation should be early recognition of respiratory and circulatory insufficiency or compromise. Timely intervention in seriously ill or injured children is the key in preventing progression toward cardiac arrest and in saving lives. Early recognition and treatment of a patient with deficiencies in oxygenation, ventilation, or perfusion frequently prevents deterioration to respiratory or cardiac arrest. Outcomes for children who develop cardiopulmonary arrest are poor.

An experienced clinician finds it easy to recognize a critically ill child. It is essential for the clinician to assess and classify the degree of illness. It is also important to identify a child with physiological derangement in its early stages when signs are subtle. The "golden hour" concept applies to all children with illnesses presenting as emergencies. Early recognition of a "critically ill child" requires a systematic, structured approach and rapid clinical assessment, with background knowledge of age appropriate physical signs and level of development. This process of examining a child in short time is known as "rapid cardiopulmonary assessment". With practice, it should take the clinician about 30 seconds to complete this assessment.

For this reason, we would like to endorse and quickly summarize the methodology followed in the Advanced Life Support (ALS) course. Kindly refer to the Indian Academy of Pediatrics (IAP)-ALS provider manual for details.

The management of a critically ill child follows the loop of "Evaluate–Identify–Intervene" (EII).

EVALUATION

The components of evaluation include:
- Initial impression [pediatric assessment triangle (PAT)]
- Primary assessment
- Secondary assessment
- Diagnostic tests.

Initial Impression

Pediatric assessment triangle (PAT) is a rapid assessment which relies primarily on three observations—(i) appearance, (ii) breathing, and (iii) color; in short, "ABC" to quickly identify a child with respiratory or circulatory compromise, and is highly reliable.

In addition to recognizing children who require stabilization with respiratory or cardiovascular interventions, the PAT also identifies most children with serious illnesses who should receive prompt evaluation.

Appearance: Infants and young children in hospital may be agitated or crying because of unfamiliar environment. Such patients must be distinguished from children who are restless or anxious due to hypoxia. The following characteristics of a child's appearance [the tone, interactiveness, consolability, look or gaze, and speech or cry (TICLS) mnemonic] help the clinician identify normal from abnormal appearance.
- *Tone*: Sick children have decreased tone and appear limp whereas normal movements are reassuring.
- *Interactiveness*: If the child is looking around or has appropriate stranger anxiety, then it is not that worrying but if the child is not responding or looking around, that is a serious concern.
- *Consolability*: Can the infant be consoled or distracted by a parent or caregiver? Crying may be a nonspecific symptom but if the child can be consoled or distracted, rather than let it inconsolably cry or just whimpering, that is reassuring.
- *Look/gaze*: Does the infant or child focus on the examiner or objects or has an unfocused gaze? An unresponsive stare suggests an altered mental status.
- *Speech/cry*: Loud and strong crying is normal but if the cry is weak or if the voice is hoarse or muffled that is abnormal.

To summarize, any child who is alert, easily consolable when crying, has good muscle tone, and responding to a caregiver is unlikely to be critically ill. On the other hand, the clinician should be very concerned about an infant who is limp, noninteractive, listless, and has a weak cry.

Work of breathing: Deficiencies in oxygenation and/or ventilation may be indicated by either increased work of breathing or decreased work of breathing or apnea. Assessment of airway sounds, the child's position of comfort, and use of accessory muscles provides information regarding the patient's work of breathing.

Color: Pallor or cyanosis is a worrisome finding that may indicate hypoxemia or inadequate perfusion to the skin.

Monitoring: Children who are critically ill require frequent assessment and continuous monitoring of vital signs, particularly heart rate and pulse oximetry. All patients should be on a multichannel monitor. This is essential to evaluate the effectiveness of interventions and to identify clinical deterioration.

Physical examination: Following the rapid initial assessment (PAT) and initiation of appropriate supportive care as mentioned in stabilization of a sick child, a thorough physical examination should be performed, which includes the following.

Primary Assessment Using the ABCDE Model

- *Airway*: To check for secretions, any abnormal sound like stridor and impression is made regarding the status of airway like clear or maintainable by simple positioning and suctioning or not maintainable, which needs further assistance like with invasive devices.
- *Breathing*: The respiratory rate and effort should be noted, including any retractions. Auscultation provides essential information regarding air entry, tidal volume, abnormal sounds, i.e., upper versus lower airway sounds, crepitations in case of lung parenchymal disease. Pulse oximetry should be done in all sick children. It should be monitored continuously for measurements at or below 94%. Within the range of partial pressure of oxygen (PaO_2) that represents clinically significant hypoxemia, small changes at the level of saturated hemoglobin reflect much larger decreases in PaO_2. As an example, a normal blood oxygen saturation level (SpO_2) of 98% correlates with a PaO_2 of approximately 100 mm Hg, 95% with 80 mm Hg, and 90% with 60 mm Hg; the latter value is the level that represents clinically significant hypoxia. In addition, low perfusion states, the presence of abnormal hemoglobin (such as carboxyhemoglobin or methemoglobin), and anemia can also result in inaccurate pulse oximetry readings.
- *Circulation*: It includes heart rate and rhythm, peripheral and central pulses, skin color and temperature to touch, capillary refill time, and blood pressure (BP). In addition, abnormal heart sounds (such as a gallop rhythm or a murmur) may indicate a cardiac etiology.
- *Disability*: Pertains to neurologic assessment—consciousness level provides an important indication of brain perfusion. The AVPU scale can be used, where A is alert, V responds to verbal commands, P responds to painful stimuli, and U is unresponsive. Abnormal mental status may result from a non-neurologic cause (such as hypoxia or hypovolemic shock) or from a primary neurologic disorder. Focal findings consistent with a neurologic process include abnormalities in pupillary light response, extraocular movements, or motor activity.
- *Exposure*: Examination of the skin may provide information regarding the patient's circulatory status, as well as clues to a specific underlying condition. For instance, petechiae or purpura indicates an infectious process, such as meningococcemia, while urticaria suggests anaphylaxis. Bleeding, burns, bruises, deformities, etc., need to be observed which could explain the condition of the patient.

This information may identify the underlying condition and guide-specific treatment. In addition, it establishes a baseline from which changes in the child's condition can be recognized and supportive care and specific treatment modified. As an example, the condition of a child who was initially in severe respiratory distress with an anxious appearance and now has decreased work of breathing and lethargy has deteriorated from respiratory distress to respiratory failure. The patient may now require assisted ventilation, as well as supplemental oxygen.

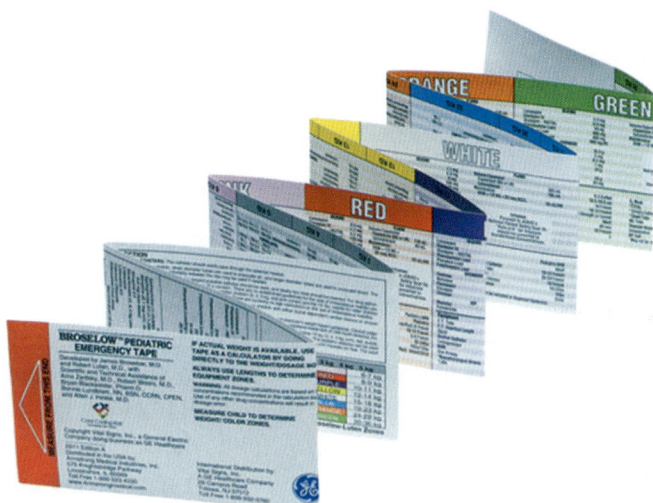

Fig. 1: Broselow tape, length-based dosages of drugs.

Vital signs should be obtained, particularly respiratory rate, heart rate, blood pressure (BP), and pulse oximetry. Weight in kilograms should also be recorded whenever possible.

Estimation of weight: Medications and fluid resuscitation need accurate weight of the child. Healthcare provider weight estimates can be inaccurate. While parent estimation is most accurate (within 10% of actual body weight approximately 80% of the time); parents frequently are not available during pediatric resuscitation.

When parent estimation is not available, length-based measurements using Broselow tape, as shown in Figure 1, can be used. The Broselow pediatric emergency tape is a color-coded length-based tape. It can be used to check a child's height as measured by the tape to his/her weight to provide medical instructions including medication dosages, the size of the equipment that should be used, and the amount of shock when using a defibrillator.

Most resuscitation drugs have a volume of distribution associated with lean weight; length-based methods provide reasonable estimates when weights cannot be measured.

If neither parent estimation nor length-based methods are available, age-based methods can be used but will often be inaccurate. Of the age-based formulas, the modified European Paediatric Life Support formula appears to perform best:
- 1–10 years of age: weight (kg) = 2 × (age in years + 4)

Secondary Assessment

After completing the primary assessment and appropriate interventions to stabilize the child, the next priority is a focused history and physical examination.

The SAMPLE mnemonic may be useful:
- S—signs and symptoms
- A—allergies

- M—medications
- P—past medical history
- L—last meal
- E—events

Diagnostic Tests

It consists of ancillary studies to detect and identify the presence and severity of respiratory and circulatory abnormalities.

Investigations like arterial/venous blood gas, blood sugar, hemoglobin concentration, arterial lactate, chest X-ray, electrocardiography (ECG), echocardiogram, etc., would help in assessing the abnormalities. Further investigations would depend on the findings and working diagnosis from the initial assessment. They may entail anything from electrolytes to sophisticated imaging.

Arterial blood gas/venous blood gas: Accurate information regarding a critically ill patient's oxygenation, ventilation, and acid–base status is an essential determinant of optimum management. Sampling of arterial blood should be performed in the following circumstances:
- To assess ventilation when end-tidal carbon dioxide ($ETCO_2$) or total carbon dioxide (TCO_2) measurements are not available
- To correlate with trends in noninvasive monitoring
- To measure PaO_2 and partial pressure of carbon dioxide ($PaCO_2$) when noninvasive measurements may be inaccurate.

An arterial sample that is properly handled provides the most accurate information regarding a patient's oxygenation, ventilation, and acid–base status.

Venous pH generally correlates well with arterial pH. However, the correlation between venous and arterial $PaCO_2$ and PaO_2 is not sufficient to provide an accurate assessment of ventilation and oxygenation in critically ill patients.

Identification: Units should have charts of normal heart rate and BP for ages for ready referral.

INTERPRETING ABNORMAL VITAL SIGNS

Pulse Rate/Heart Rate

In a child with tachycardia, consider the following:

Ask yourself if the heart rate is appropriate to the age, physiological state of the child and explainable by the level of physical activity. Tachycardia is expected due to pain, fever, exercise, anemia, anxiety, crying, thyrotoxicosis, as well as with tachypnea.

Tachycardia in an afebrile child who is sleeping/resting is generally abnormal and may be a subtle sign of myocardial dysfunction, or may indicate nonconvulsive seizures in an unconscious child. Tachycardia is often associated with abnormal pulse volume and other signs of compromised peripheral perfusion.

Look for beat-to-beat variability of heart rate with changing level of activity to distinguish sinus tachycardia from supraventricular tachycardia (SVT).

Rapid changes of heart rate and BP in high and low extremes may suggest autonomic instability.

In a child with bradycardia, consider the following:
Assess if bradycardia is associated with adequate perfusion, or does the patient have symptomatic bradycardia with cardiopulmonary compromise. Individuals into active sports may have a relatively lower heart rate due increased vagal tone. Also differentiate sinus bradycardia from bradyarrhythmia with the help of an ECG. Do not forget the 5 Hs [hypoxia, H ions (acidosis), hypovolemia, hypo/hyperkalemia, head injury] and 5 Ts [trauma, toxins, tension pneumothotax, tamponade (cardiac), thromboembolism] to find the cause of bradycardia.

Respiratory Rate

Check if respiratory rate is appropriate for the age and physiological status. See if tachypnea is occurring alone or accompanied by signs of respiratory distress (nasal flaring, chest wall retractions, grunting, head bobbing, etc.). Reduction in respiratory rate in an alert and playful child is a sign of improvement, while reducing respiratory rate with worsening sensorium and shallow breathing is a sign of respiratory failure.

Look for any abnormal breathing pattern and listen for abnormal respiratory sounds (snoring, stridor, wheeze, expiratory grunt, etc.).

Blood Pressure

Signs of adequate peripheral perfusion are as important as having normal BP. One may not necessarily chase a low BP record if a child is otherwise well with good peripheral perfusion, especially in the context of malnutrition or myocardial dysfunction.

The mean arterial pressure (MAP) is more important than individual systolic and diastolic BP because it is the most important determinant of tissue perfusion.

STABILIZATION

Children who have any abnormalities found using the PAT are critically ill and require immediate intervention. A detailed primary assessment from the physical examination and/or ancillary studies may also provide indications for respiratory or circulatory support.

Follow the key elements of effective team dynamics to achieve stabilization in the shortest possible time. These elements include clear roles and responsibilities, clear messages, closed loop communication, constructive intervention, knowing limitations, knowledge sharing, mutual respect, re-evaluation, and summarizing.

After every stage of evaluation, starting from the initial impression, one needs to follow the cycle of EII. Re-assessment is important after every intervention. If a life-threatening condition is identified at any stage of evaluation, urgent lifesaving interventions should be started before proceeding with any further evaluation.

The priorities during stabilization follow the same order as in assessment, i.e., ABC, except during cardiopulmonary resuscitation (CPR), when the sequence is compression, airway, and breathing (CAB).

The following interventions should be done in a patient with any abnormality of appearance, breathing or color on initial impression followed by primary assessment.

For the sake of discussion, we would like to divide the process of stabilization into (i) general measures and (ii) specific measures.

General measures include interventions that are common to most emergency situations, like (i) calling for help as appropriate (activating the emergency response system, code blue team or the rapid response team) depending on the patient's location; (ii) providing oxygen; (iii) achieving vascular access [intravenous (IV)/intraosseous (IO)]; and (iv) connecting the patient to vital signs monitor, including ECG monitoring.

Specific measures entail disease or problem-specific interventions. Details of management of individual illnesses are beyond the scope of this chapter. Depending on the physiologic status of the child, the following stabilization measures can be undertaken.

Airway

Airway can be maintained by simple measures like allowing the child to assume a position of comfort. Avoid unnecessary agitation. Head-tilt/chin-lift maneuver can be used to open the airway unless cervical spine injury is suspected in which case jaw thrust without neck extension should be done.

- *If the airway is open and clear*: No immediate intervention is needed.
- *Maintainable*: Simple measures like head-tilt/chin-lift, jaw thrust (in suspected cervical spine injury), suctioning of secretions, insertion of oropharyngeal or nasopharyngeal airway, nebulization with adrenaline (croup, postextubation stridor).
- *Not maintainable*: Advanced interventions like endotracheal intubation, laryngeal mask airway insertion, cricothyrotomy, tracheostomy, or foreign body airway obstruction relief techniques (in severe choking).

Breathing

Any child who appears seriously ill by the PAT should be put on oxygen. In general, patients with two or more abnormalities in the PAT require oxygen therapy. In addition, most patients with an oxygen saturation ≤94% should receive supplemental oxygen.

One hundred percent humidified oxygen should be provided to any critically ill child irrespective of the physiologic status. Use a high concentration nonrebreathing system if available. Monitor oxygen saturation continuously.

In respiratory distress, the child is kept with the caregiver, is allowed to maintain a position of comfort, and oxygen is provided in a non-threatening manner. Turbulent airflow leads to increased airway resistance; hence, the child should be kept calm.

Anticipate respiratory failure if the following features are found:
- An increased respiratory rate, particularly with signs of distress (e.g., increased respiratory effort including nasal flaring, retractions, seesaw breathing, or grunting)
- An inadequate respiratory rate, effort, or chest excursion (e.g., diminished breath sounds or gasping), especially if mental status is depressed
- Cyanosis with abnormal breathing despite supplementary oxygen.

If the child has *respiratory failure*, the approach is more aggressive. In case of inadequate chest expansion or respiratory arrest, bag and mask ventilation should be given with 100% oxygen. Tracheal intubation may be required.

Tracheostomy or cricothyrotomy may be required in cases of complete upper airway obstruction caused by diphtheria, severe orofacial injuries or laryngeal fractures.

In addition to disease specific interventions, a child may be provided respiratory support by one of the following means, depending upon the extent of respiratory compromise:

If a child has respiratory distress, s/he should be provided supplemental oxygen by an appropriate oxygen delivery device. The basic prerequisites for using an oxygen delivery device are that the child should be breathing spontaneously with an intact airway, conscious enough not to aspirate and not in respiratory fatigue. If these prerequisites are not met in a child with abnormal breathing, s/he needs of an advanced airway with or without positive pressure ventilation.

Oxygen delivery devices are broadly classified as low-flow systems (nasal prongs, simple face mask) and high-flow systems (venturi mask, oxygen hood, partial rebreathing, and nonrebreathing mask). The concentration of oxygen delivered is unpredictable through a low-flow system and more reliable through a high-flow system. The concentration of oxygen delivered to the patient can be increased by (i) use of a high flow system; (ii) preventing rebreathing of exhaled air by increasing the oxygen flow rate beyond patient's own minute ventilation and use of an assembly with an inbuilt expiratory valve; (iii) use of an oxygen reservoir; and (iv) ensuring a tight seal between the face and the mask to prevent mixing of room air.

The choice of oxygen delivery device depends on (i) the age and acceptance of the child and (ii) the severity of respiratory distress/hypoxia, and hence the need for supplemental oxygen. At times, one may have to settle for free flow oxygen provided by the parents through simple oxygen tubing in an anxious and agitated infant or toddler, provided the distress is mild without significant hypoxia.

Recent years have witnessed an increasing utilization of noninvasive ventilation (NIV) and high flow nasal cannula (HFNC) with rewarding results. Many children with moderate-to-severe respiratory distress who would have received invasive ventilation in the past are being successfully managed with early and judicious use of these modalities.

Circulation

Patients with inadequate perfusion as indicated by decreased mental status, poor skin perfusion, and/or abnormal vital signs are in shock. Vascular access should be established, and they should receive fluid resuscitation. Vascular access and the initial management of shock are discussed elsewhere.

The focus of brief discussion under this heading would be some basic aspects of management of a child in shock. The first step in the management of a child in shock is to administer 100% oxygen through a nonrebreathing mask, or a higher level of breathing support if needed. The second objective is to achieve a reliable vascular access (IV or IO, if IV access not possible) to begin with and a central venous access (femoral, internal jugular, or subclavian) in many situation where shock is refractory to initial management.

The subsequent management depends on the type and severity of shock. Hence, it is very important to identify the type of shock correctly. The treatment includes crystalloid (occasionally colloid) boluses, inotropes, vasopressors, inodilators, either alone or in combination. The treatment is guided by ongoing multimodal hemodynamic monitoring, including clinical assessment, intra-arterial BP, functional echocardiography, and noninvasive cardiac output monitoring as per the availability of equipment. The quantity and rapidity of fluid boluses also depend on the type of shock. Boluses are large volume and rapid in hypovolemic and septic shock, and much more restricted in cardiogenic shock.

A stable, normotensive child should be allowed to remain with the caregiver while an unstable child should be put in the Trendelenburg position.

High-flow oxygen is indicated in all children with shock.

Once airway and breathing have been stabilized, vascular access is to be secured. IO route may be used in case of collapsed veins. *No child should die due to a lack of vascular access.* Any drug can be infused using this route provided it is followed by a flush of fluid to get the drug in the central circulation.

Fluid resuscitation should be given. Isotonic crystalloids like normal saline or ringer lactate is preferred over colloids. Administer fluids as a 20 mL/kg bolus over 5–20 min. The child needs to be monitored after administration of each fluid bolus. The rate of administration and the number of boluses depend on the type of shock. Repeat boluses should be given till the BP and tissue perfusion is restored. Blood products should be administered only when specifically indicated for replacement of blood loss or for correction of coagulopathies.

The SpO_2, heart rate, BP, pulse pressure, mental status, temperature, and urine output should be monitored frequently to evaluate trends and determine response to therapy.

Conduct ancillary laboratory and nonlaboratory studies to help in identification of the etiology and severity of shock, evaluation for organ dysfunction, identification of metabolic derangements, and evaluation of the response to therapeutic interventions.

When the circulation does not improve with fluid boluses alone, inotropes, phosphodiesterase inhibitors, vasodilators, and vasopressors are used.

The goal of therapy is to improve the perfusion and correct the hypotension.

Arrhythmias if present need to be corrected.

Disability

The most common neurological problems encountered in an emergency setting are altered level of consciousness, seizures, and raised intracranial pressure (ICP), irrespective of the basic disease process. The emergency treatment begins with the maintenance of ABCs. Any unconscious child should be actively monitored for signs of raised ICP and managed accordingly, until proved otherwise. Details of management are discussed elsewhere.

DO'S AND DONT'S OF EMERGENCY MANAGEMENT

Airway and breathing: Do not interfere with the child's own spontaneous efforts to maintain his airway in suspected upper airway obstruction as long as the child is alert and not in respiratory fatigue. Let the child remain with his caregivers and administer oxygen in a nonthreatening manner by an age appropriate device. Agitation worsens upper airway obstruction.

Never use respiratory depressants.

Use standardized scoring systems available for respiratory illnesses (e.g., asthma, croup) to make assessment more objective and decision making streamlined.

Do not sedate an agitated or crying child without knowing the cause. Try to identify and treat the cause of agitation (e.g., hypoxia, raised intracranial pressure, intussuception, etc.)

Recognition, categorization, and initial stabilization based on PAT are shown in Table 1.

Initial recognition and management as per physiological status can be documented in triage form in the emergency [used in the Postgraduate Institute (PGI) and Dayanand Medical College (DMC)], as shown below.

Recognition and Stabilization of the Critically Ill Child

Table 1: Categorization and initial stabilization based on PAT.

Appearance	Breathing	Circulation	Interpretation	Initial stabilization
Normal	Normal	Normal	Stable	None
Normal	Abnormal	Normal	Respiratory distress	Allow position of comfort (mother's lap) Oxygen in a nonthreatening manner
Abnormal	Abnormal	Normal	Respiratory failure	Stabilize airway Start on 100% oxygen Provide bag and mask ventilation if required
Normal	Normal	Abnormal	Compensated shock	Start on 100% oxygen Establish vascular access Connect to cardiac monitor Check glucose values
Abnormal	Normal	Abnormal	Decompensated shock	Start on 100% oxygen Establish vascular/intraosseous access Connect to cardiac monitor Check glucose values
Abnormal	Normal	Normal	Primary brain dysfunction/systemic dysfunction	Start on 100% oxygen Establish vascular access Connect to cardiac monitor Check glucose values
Abnormal	Abnormal	Abnormal	Cardiorespiratory failure/cardiac arrest	CPR if HR <60/min despite adequate ventilation or absent central pulses

Adapted from AHA-PALS provider manual 2015.

PEDIATRIC EMERGENCY ROOM

Date .... Time ....AM/PM

Weight........ kg   Ht: ....   Informant................

Chief complaints:

Name
Age
Gender

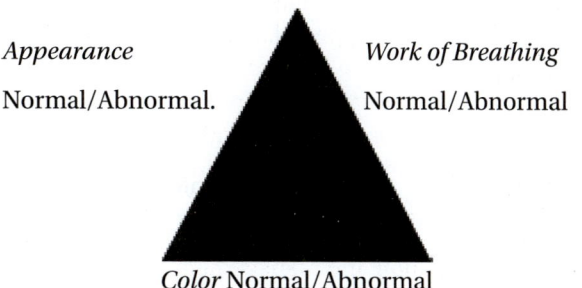

Pediatric assessment triangle (PAT)

Appearance Normal/Abnormal.

Work of Breathing Normal/Abnormal

Color Normal/Abnormal

Detailed clinical assessment (ABCDE)

AIRWAY	BREATHING RR;............. /min	CIRCULATION HR........./min
• Open and stable • Open but unstable • Obstruction	Efforts: Normal poor increased acidotic Air Entry: Normal poor differential Auscultation: None stidor wheeze crackles SpO₂ (room air)................. SpO₂ (on oxygen)..................	Central pulse: Good/Poor Peripheral pulse: Good/Poor CFT ....BP................ Skin Temp Warm Cool ECG: Rhythm..................... T-wave........Others..........
DISABILITY A V P U GCS E V M Pupil size.............Reaction.......... Motor activity Normal and symmetrical Asymmetrical seizures Posturing flaccidity Extrapyramidal movements Blood sugar................. mg/dL		EXPOSURE Temp.........°F Color: Normal pallor cyanosis Ashen gray skin Surface findings: Rash abscess pustules Cellulitis Patechie Purpura ecchymosis Hemorrhagic nodules Mucosal ulcers Dermatosis Desquamation edema Trauma/others (specify.........................

Final physiological impression	*Triangle classification*
• Stable • Respiratory distress • Respiratory failure • Compensated shock • Hypotensive shock • Cardiopulmonary failure • Primary brain/metabolic dysfunction	• Level 1 (Resuscitation) • Level 2 (Emergent) • Level 3 (Urgent) • Level 4 (Less urgent) • Level 5 (Nonurgent)

Any other important gross clinical finding:

EXAMINATION

Pallor icterus cyanosis clubbing Edema neck veins lymphadenopathy

Head and neck

Cardiovascular system (CVS)

Chest

Abdomen

Central nervous system (CNS)

Extremities

PROVISIONAL DIAGNOSIS:

Investigations sent	Emergency treatment administered
Plan	

Staff nurse   Junior resident
Reviewed by senior resident/consultant
Emergency room outcome   *Transfer*: PICU/ward/ nursery/Pvt room no-/OT/other....
                                        Discharge Death DAMA

Pediatric emergency triage classification system should be employed and used in every first encounter area, be it the emergency room or a clinic. This could be the five-level or color-coded system that the unit chooses.

Level 1 (resuscitation): Patients requiring continuous assessment and intervention to maintain physiological stability; e.g.,
- Severe respiratory distress
- Respiratory failure
- Shock
- Cardiopulmonary arrest
- Seizures
- Unconsciousness
- Coma
- Major bums
- Significant bleeding
- Severe trauma.

Level 2 (emergent): Any physiologically unstable patient and those who requires comprehensive assessment and multiple interventions to prevent further deterioration like
- Moderate respiratory distress
- Altered consciousness [Glasgow Coma Scale (GCS) <13]
- Severe dehydration
- Fever (age <3 months and temperature >102°F),
- Sepsis
- Toxic ingestion/overdose
- Severe asthma
- Seizure (postictal)
- Diabetic ketoacidosis (DKA)
- Child abuse with ongoing risk
- Purpuric rash
- Violent patients
- Severe testicular pain
- Lacerations
- Open fractures
- Other orthopedic injuries with neurovascular compromise or dental injury with an avulsed permanent tooth.
- Dehydration may be difficult to accurately assess.
- Any suspicion (or evidence) should cause concern.
  Temperature is may not always be a reliable indicator of the severity of illness.
  Younger patients can have significant infections and serious problems even though the signs and symptoms may be subtle.

Level 3 (urgent): Patient who is alert, oriented, well hydrated, but minor alterations in vital signs, Level 3 patients need carefully planned reassessment while awaiting care since critical illness in children may present with common symptoms and evolve rapidly, e.g.,
- Fever (age >3 months and temperature >101°F)
- Mild respiration distress

- Minor head injuries
- Simple burns
- Fractures
- Dental injuries
- Pneumonia without distress
- History of seizure
- Suicide ideation
- Ingestion requiring observation only
- Head trauma with GCS 14 or 15 and alert/vomiting.

Level 4 (less urgent): Patient who is alert, oriented, and may have a condition that causes distress and may progress with development of complications, e.g.,
- Vomiting/diarrhea and no dehydration in a child >2 years
- Simple lacerations/sprains/strains
- Fever and simple complaints such as ear pain, sore throat, or nasal congestion, or
- Head trauma with no symptoms.

Level 5 (nonurgent): Patient who is afebrile, alert, oriented, well hydrated, with normal vital signs. Interventions are not usually required other than assessment/discharge instruction. These patients may be referred to outpatient department (OPD) or transferred to ward for management.

Flowchart 1 can be used in emergency room to recognize and stabilize critically ill or injured children.

SUMMARY AND RECOMMENDATIONS

- Rapid identification and stabilization of critically ill children with respiratory or circulatory compromise are essential components of evaluation and management. Critically ill children who require immediate stabilization of respiratory and circulatory function can generally be identified through the following evaluation:
    - PAT—The three components of the PAT are appearance, breathing, and color denoting circulation.
    - A thorough physical examination, with primary assessment including airway, breathing, circulation, disability, and exposure, which provide additional information to guide assessment and treatment.
    - Parent estimation of weight or use of Broselow tape or measured height when an actual weight is not available.
    - Pulse oximetry and end-tidal CO_2 measurement often provide a rapid noninvasive evaluation of oxygenation and ventilation.
- The initial stabilization of the critically ill child must occur concurrently with evaluation and treatment of the underlying condition.
    - Most children with two or more abnormalities in the PAT or an oxygen saturation ≤94% should receive oxygen therapy.
    - Oxygen should be provided at the highest concentration available through whatever device the child tolerates.

Flowchart 1: JumpSTART pediatric multiple casualty incidents triage.

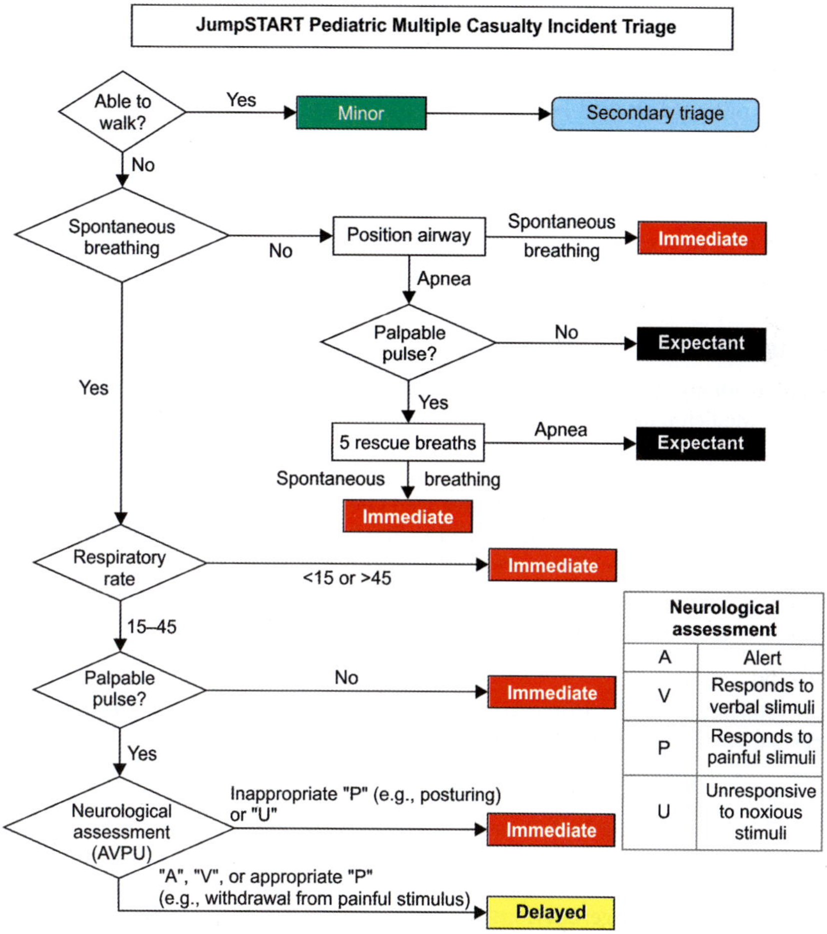

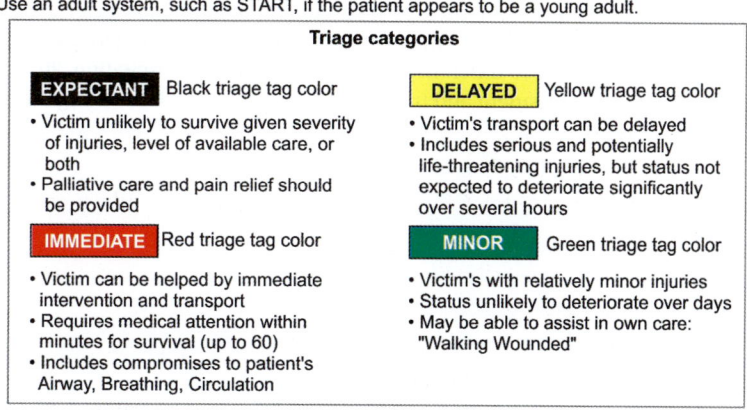

Use jumpSTART if the patient appears to be a child.
Use an adult system, such as START, if the patient appears to be a young adult.

Triage categories

EXPECTANT — Black triage tag color
- Victim unlikely to survive given severity of injuries, level of available care, or both
- Palliative care and pain relief should be provided

IMMEDIATE — Red triage tag color
- Victim can be helped by immediate intervention and transport
- Requires medical attention within minutes for survival (up to 60)
- Includes compromises to patient's Airway, Breathing, Circulation

DELAYED — Yellow triage tag color
- Victim's transport can be delayed
- Includes serious and potentially life-threatening injuries, but status not expected to deteriorate significantly over several hours

MINOR — Green triage tag color
- Victim's with relatively minor injuries
- Status unlikely to deteriorate over days
- May be able to assist in own care: "Walking Wounded"

Adapted from: http://www.jumpstarttriage.com

- Children with respiratory failure or impending respiratory arrest (as suggested by apnea, bradypnea, or an irregular respiratory pattern) should initially receive bag-mask ventilation. Further airway management, including endotracheal intubation, may be required.
- All shock patients should be started on oxygen and early vascular access, followed by 20 mL/kg of crystalloids bolus, expect if patient is suspected to have cardiogenic shock when smaller bolus is given and response assessed. Use of inotropes and vasopressors as indicated.
- Critically ill children should be closely monitored with frequent vital signs and pulse oximetry to evaluate the effectiveness of interventions and to identify clinical deterioration.

SUGGESTED READING

1. American Academy of Pediatrics, American College of Emergency Physicians. APLS: The Pediatric Emergency Medicine Resource, 5th edition. In: Fuchs S, Yamamoto L (Eds). Burlington: Jones and Bartlett Learning; 2012.
2. American Heart Association and American Academy of Pediatrics. Systematic approach to seriously ill or injured child. In: Pediatrics Advanced Life Support Provider Manual; 2015.
3. Dieckmann RA, Brownstein D, Gausche-Hill M. The pediatric assessment triangle: a novel approach for the rapid evaluation of children. Pediatr Emerg Care. 2010;26:312.
4. DuBois D, Baldwin S, King WD. Accuracy of weight estimation methods for children. Pediatr Emerg Care. 2007; 23:227.
5. Fuchs S. Initial assessment and stabilization of children with respiratory or circulatory compromise. Uptodate. Aug 2018.
6. Gausche-Hill M, Eckstein M, Horeczko T, et al. Paramedics accurately apply the pediatric assessment triangle to drive management. Prehosp Emerg Care. 2014;18:520.
7. Horeczko T, Enriquez B, McGrath NE, et al. The Pediatric Assessment Triangle: accuracy of its application by nurses in the triage of children. J Emerg Nurs. 2013;39:182.
8. IAP ALS Handbook - Bring Back Breaths and Beats. Jayashree M, Kulgod V, Sharma AK (Eds). 1st Edition; 2018.
9. Jayashree M, Singhi S. Initial assessment and triage in ER. Indian J Pediatr. 2011;78(9):1100-8.
10. JumpSTART and MCI Triage; 2017.
11. Mary EH, Ira MC. Pediatric emergencies and resuscitation. In: Kliegan R, Stanton B, St Geme JW, et al. (Eds). Nelson Textbook of Pediatrics, 20th edition. Philadelphia: Elsevier; 2016. pp. 498-506.
12. Wells M, Goldstein LN, Bentley A. It is time to abandon age-based emergency weight estimation in children! A failed validation of 20 different age-based formulas. Resuscitation. 2017;116:73.
13. WHO. Emergency triage assessment and treatment. Geneva: World Health Organization; 2005.

3
Resuscitation

Anand Shandilya

LEARNING OBJECTIVES

- To learn the importance of cardiopulmonary resuscitation
- To learn the steps involved in resuscitation
- To be able to administer high quality CPR.

INTRODUCTION

Cardiopulmonary resuscitation (CPR) is vital in cases of cardiopulmonary arrest and may make the difference between intact survival versus neurological impairment or death. Pediatric emergencies are of various types—respiratory, cardiac, endocrine, traumatic, and infectious. However, most pediatric arrests are respiratory (asphyxia) and not cardiac in nature. Sudden, unanticipated, nontraumatic cardiac arrests are uncommon in children in contrast to the primary nature of cardiac arrest in adults due to ischemic heart disease and subsequent ventricular fibrillation (VF) or ventricular tachycardia.

It is important for all pediatric clinicians to know the fundamental steps in resuscitation and be prepared to implement resuscitation immediately. The goal in pediatric resuscitation is to maintain adequate oxygenation and perfusion of blood throughout the body while steps are taken to stabilize a child. In a hospital setting, the need for CPR should be anticipated and trained personnel, equipments and resuscitation drugs should be available round the clock. Immediate CPR is associated with early return of circulation and neurologically intact survival. Good quality CPR improves a victim's chances of survival.

BASIC LIFE SUPPORT

Respiratory failure or arrest is a common cause of cardiac arrest during infancy and childhood. Basic life support (BLS) emphasizes immediate bystander CPR before activation of any local emergency provider system. BLS should be part of a community effort that includes prevention, early CPR, prompt access to the emergency response system, and rapid pediatric advanced life support (PALS), followed by integrated postcardiac arrest care. These five links form the

Flowchart 1: BLS Healthcare Provider. Pediatric cardiac arrest algorithm for the single rescuer—2015 update.

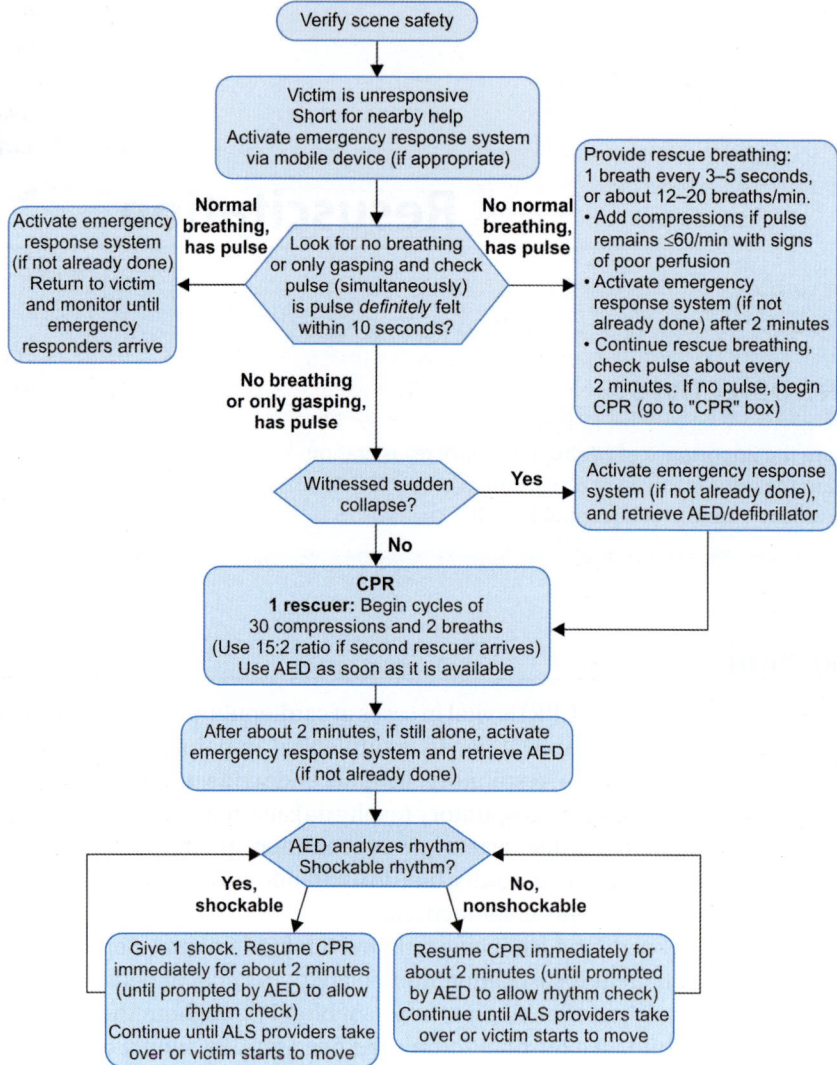

American Heart Association (AHA) pediatric Chain of Survival; the first three links constitute pediatric BLS. In BLS, CPR requires skills with no devices or with bag-mask ventilation or barrier devices and can be performed even outside the hospital. Though the links in the chain of survival follow different paths depending on whether the arrest was in hospital or out of hospital, all converge in the intensive care unit (ICU) for a common sequence. For providing BLS all that is needed are two hands, a mouth, and a sincere desire to save a life! Flowchart 1 outlines the sequence to be followed for BLS with a sigle rescuer.

The recommended sequence of CPR has previously been known by the initials "ABC": airway, breathing/ventilation, and chest compressions (or circulation). The *2010 AHA Guidelines for CPR and emergency cardiovascular care (ECC)* recommend a compression, airway, and breathing/ventilations (CAB) sequence. The CAB sequence for infants and children excluding newborns is recommended in order to simplify training with the hope that more victims of sudden cardiac arrest will receive bystander CPR. It offers the advantage of consistency in teaching rescuers, whether their patients are infants, children, or adults. This sequence has been retained in the guidelines issued in 2015 as well.

The following is the explanation for using the CAB sequence.

In the majority of cardiac arrests, the critical initial elements of CPR are chest compressions and early defibrillation.

In the CAB sequence, chest compressions will be initiated sooner and ventilation only minimally delayed until completion of the first cycle of chest compressions. Ventilation is started 18 seconds after initiation of chest compressions with single rescuer CPR and after 9 seconds in two rescuer CPR in infants and children.

The ABC sequence could be a reason why less than a third of people in cardiac arrest receive bystander CPR. ABC starts with the most difficult procedures: opening the airway and delivering rescue breaths.

It is better to do chest compressions alone in case the lay provider is reluctant to give rescue breaths rather than give no CPR.

CARDIOPULMONARY RESUSCITATION

Cardiopulmonary resuscitation is intended to externally support the circulation and ventilation in a child with respiratory or cardiopulmonary arrest. The sequence of resuscitation may be remembered as A-B-C-D-E for airway, breathing circulation, drug delivery, and electricity.

Good quality CPR improves a victim's chances of survival. The critical concepts for quality CPR include:
- Push hard, push fast: compress at a rate of 100–120 compressions/min.
- Allow full chest recoil after each compression—do not lean on the patient's chest in between compressions so as to allow full chest recoil.
- Minimize interruptions in chest compressions; try to keep them to <10 s.
- Avoid hyperventilation.

POSITIONING THE CHILD

The child should be in the supine position and on a hard surface before you begin CPR.

RAPID ASSESSMENT (BEGINNING CARDIOPULMONARY RESUSCITATION)

The rescuer arriving at the side of the child must be sure that the scene is safe. The initial step of CPR includes establishing the unresponsiveness of the patient by gently shaking, tapping or shouting at the child. The rescuer should position himself at the victim's side so that he can open the airway and start giving breaths to the child. Ideally, in unwitnessed collapse, 1 min of CPR is given before help is activated. In witnessed collapse help is activated before CPR.

The use of mobile phones to activate an emergency team is encouraged. Using the mobile device with speaker mode also enables the provider to get guidance and instructions during CPR (remote assistant guided CPR).

OPENING THE AIRWAY

The first step in CPR is to open the airway and restore breathing by positioning (supine) and opening the airway by head-tilt/chin-lift or by jaw thrust. The jaw thrust without head tilt is the safest technique in opening the airway of a patient with suspected neck injury. If no obstruction by a foreign body is found and if the child has no spontaneous respirations, steps should be immediately taken to breathe for the child. A common cause of airway obstruction in an unresponsive child is the tongue occluding the airway.

Method

Head tilt/chin lift: The rescuer's hand is placed on the patient's forehead and with gentle backward pressure the head is brought to the sniffing position. The fingertips of one hand are placed under the mandible near the protuberance of the chin, bringing the chin forward and supporting the jaw, which results in tilting the head back. The things to avoid with the head-tilt/chin-lift maneuver are—not to press deeply into the soft tissue under the chin as this might obstruct the airway, not to use the thumb to lift the chin and not to close the child' mouth completely.

Jaw thrust: To perform a jaw thrust, the rescuer holds the angle of the mandible and lifts with both hands, one on each side, displacing the mandible forward while tilting the head back ward.

Inspect the mouth briefly; if secretions, vomitus, blood, dental fragments, or foreign body is visible, it should be removed. If the patient resumes adequate spontaneous ventilation, the patient is turned on his side in the recovery position.

BREATHING

If the healthcare provider does not detect adequate breathing within 10 s, the rescuer should give two breaths.

"Look, Listen, and Feel" has been removed from the BLS algorithm as performance of "Look, Listen, and Feel," is inconsistent and time consuming.

The provider should look for unresponsiveness, apnea, or agonal respirations and if present start rescue breathing. If on the mobile with the remote assistant, the rescuer can be guided to recognize agonal gasps.

RESCUE BREATHS

If the patient is not breathing spontaneously, use a barrier device to give two breaths (duration of each breath being 1 s) while watching for chest rise. In children, make sure you give only enough air to make the child's chest rise. For very small children, you may use less air than for larger children or adults.

Rescue breathing is established by mouth-to-mouth, mouth-to-nose, or mouth-to-mouth and nose ventilation if bag and mask is not available.

In the infant, the rescuer makes a seal covering the infant's mouth and nose with his mouth. In the older child, the nose is pinched and mouth of the patient is covered by the rescuer's mouth. When an airtight seal has been established by either of above methods, two breaths are delivered. An appropriate breath is one that allows the patient's chest to rise.

Rescuers may need to try a couple of times to give a total of two breaths that make the patient's chest rise. If either breath does not make the chest rise, the rescuer should try again to open the child's airway and give a breath that makes the chest rise.

Mouth-to-nose ventilation is recommended when it is impossible to ventilate through the mouth because of facial injuries or an anatomic abnormality, or when it is difficult to achieve tight seal around the mouth. To perform this maneuver, the rescuer maintains the head tilt while lifting the mandible to close the mouth if it is open. During exhalation with this technique, it may be necessary to open the patient's mouth or separate the child's lips to allow the air to escape.

When a patient has a tracheostomy tube *in situ*, mouth to stoma artificial ventilation should be used. Cricoid pressure should not be used routinely in cardiac arrest.

In the hospital setting, if there is no spontaneous respiration, then assisted ventilation should be provided by bag and mask. In a patient who is comatose or who has stopped breathing, use of an oropharyngeal airway is often sufficient to prevent the tongue from obstructing the hypopharynx.

BAG AND MASK TECHNIQUE AND RESCUE BREATHING

Bag-mask devices consist of a bag attached to a face mask. They may also include a non-rebreathing valve. To provide effective ventilation, perform a head tilt and then press the mask against the face while lifting the jaw. A proper-sized mask should provide an airtight seal around the nose and mouth extending from the bridge of the nose to the cleft of the chin and then a tidal volume is delivered by compressing the bag to make the chest rise. The technique of opening the airway and sealing the mask to the face is called the E–C clamp technique.

One Rescuer Using the Bag Mask

- Position yourself directly above the child's head.
- Place the mask on the child's face, using the bridge of the nose as a guide for the correct position.
- Use the E–C clamp technique to hold the mask in place while you lift the jaw to hold the airway open: Perform a head tilt.

Use the thumb and index finger of one hand to make "C" pressing the edges of the mask to the face. Use the remaining fingers to lift the angles of the jaw (three fingers form an "E") and open the airway.

Squeeze the bag to give breaths (1 s each) while watching for chest rise. The delivery of breaths is the same whether you use supplementary oxygen or not.

Give one breath every 6 s (10 breaths/min). Give each breath in 1 s. Each breath should result in visible chest rise. Check the pulse about every 2 min.

Table 1: Two-rescuer cardiopulmonary resuscitation.		
Rescuer	Location	Actions
Rescuer 1	At the victim's side	• Performs chest compressions • Counts out loud • Switches duties with rescuer 2 every 10 cycles (for 2 min), taking less than 10 s to switch
Rescuer 2	At the victim's head	• Maintains an open airway • Give breaths, watching for chest rise and avoiding hyperventilation • Encourages rescuer 1 to perform compressions that are fast and deep and to allow full chest recoil between compressions • Switches duties with rescuer 1 every 10 cycles (for 2 min) taking less than 10 s to switch

Two Rescuers Using Bag Mask

When two rescuers use the bag mask system, one rescuer opens the airway with a head tilt and jaw lift and holds the mask to the face while the other rescuer squeezes the bag.

Bag and mask ventilation provided by two rescuers is more effective than that given by a single rescuer when there is poor lung compliance or in cases of airway obstruction.

The self inflating ventilation bags for resuscitation are available in sizes suitable for tall pediatric age groups. Ventilation is carried out at the recommended rate.

Successful rescue breathing will provide good chest rise and relief of deep cyanosis. Health care providers should be able to identify respiratory arrest and should be able to determine when respirations are inadequate to maintain effective oxygenation or ventilation.

In two-rescuer CPR, each rescuer has specific role. Each "cycle" consists of 15 compressions and two rescue breaths (Table 1).

Switching of rescuer roles about every 10 cycles (2 min) helps decrease rescuer fatigue which may cause the chest compressions to be too shallow or too slow.

If a third rescuer arrives, she can help with bag mask and also rotate into position to give compressions.

PULSE CHECK

After giving two breaths, healthcare providers should take at least 5 s and no more than 10 s to check for a pulse.

If there is no pulse or if the heart rate is less than 60 beats/min with signs of poor perfusion, chest compressions must be given. If you are not sure whether the victim has a pulse, you should start the steps of CPR.

CHEST COMPRESSIONS

Chest compressions must always be accompanied by ventilation at the recommended compression ventilation ratio (Table 2).

Table 2: Chest compression and ventilation ratio.

Age	Compression method	Sternal depression	Compression rate	Landmark	Compression ventilation ratio
Newborn	Two thumbs encircling hands for two trained person or two finger technique	Approx 1/3rd depth of chest	120/min 1/3rd depth of chest	Lower 1/2 of sternum (one finger width below inter mammary line)	3:1
Infants	Two thumbs encircling hands for two trained persons or two finger technique	1/3rd to 1/2 depth of chest (1.5 in)	100–120/min	Lower ½ of sternum (one finger width below inter-mammary line)	15:2 for two rescuers or 30:2 for single rescuer
Child <8 years	Heel of one hand	1/3rd to 1/2 depth of chest (2 in)	100–120/min	Lower half of sternum	Same as above
Child >8 years	Heel of one hand, other hand on top	2 in	100–120/min	Lower half of sternum	Same as above

When an advanced airway is in place during two person CPR for victim's of all ages, give breaths at a rate of one breath every 6 s (10 breaths/min), without attempting to synchronize breaths between compressions. There should be no pause in chest compressions for delivery of breaths.

Flowchart 2 outlines the steps when two or more rescuers are present.

The following are characteristics of *high-quality CPR*:
- Chest compressions of appropriate rate and depth.
- "Push fast": Push at a rate of 100–120 compressions/min.
- "Push hard": Push with sufficient force to depress at least one-third the anterior–posterior (AP) diameter of the chest or approximately 1½ in (4 cm) in infants and 2 in (5 cm) in children [Class I, level of evidence (LOE) C].
- Allow complete chest recoil after each compression to allow the heart to refill with blood. Do not lean on chest between compressions to ensure complete chest recoil.
- Minimize interruptions of chest compressions.
- Avoid excessive ventilation.

Table 3 shows the difference in compressions for victims with and without advanced airway in place.

The effectiveness of chest compressions is determined by the presence of a palpable pulse. Perform cycles of compressions and ventilation at a rate of 100–120 compressions per minute (30:2 ratio for one rescuer CPR and 15:2 ratio for two rescuer CPR). The rationale for maintaining age specific differences in compression ventilation ratios during resuscitation is for the following reasons:
- Respiratory problem emergency response system is the most common cause of arrest in the pediatric age group; therefore, effective ventilation should be emphasized.

Flowchart 2: BLS Healthcare Provider. Pediatric cardiac arrest algorithm for two or more rescuers—2015 update.

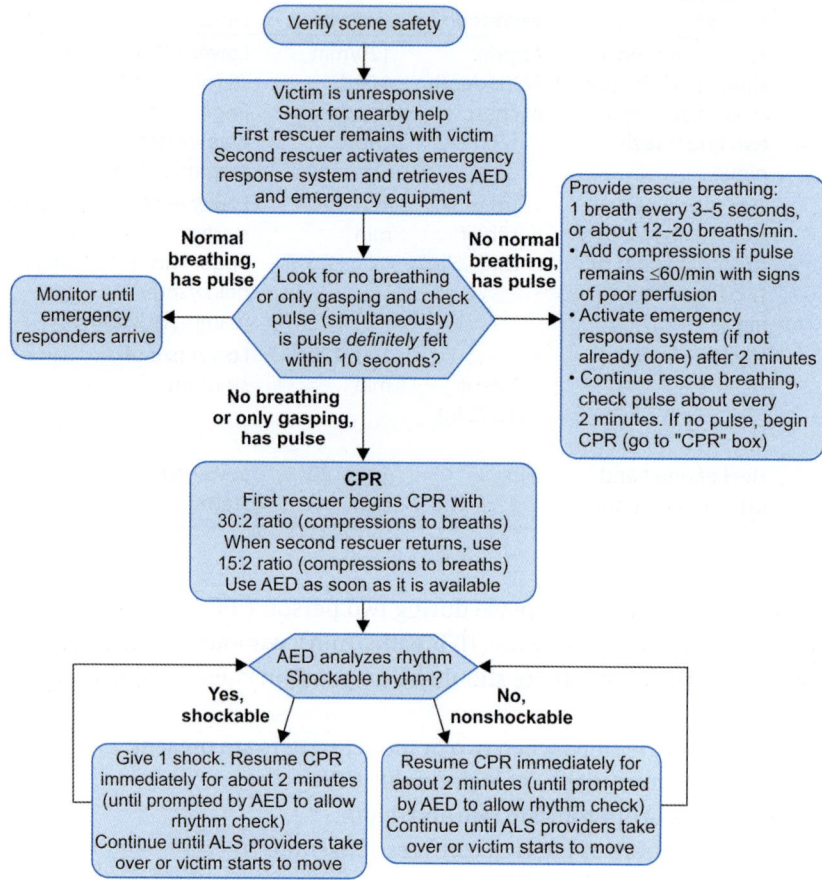

Table 3: Difference in compressions for victims with and without advanced airway in place.		
	No advanced airway in place	*Advanced airway in place*
Compression rate	100–120/min	100–120/min
Ventilation rate	Two breaths following 30 compressions	One breath every 6 s (10 breaths/min)
Pause compressions	Pause compressions to give two breaths. The first exhalation occurs between the two breaths and the second during the first chest compression of the next cycle of CPR	Do not pause chest to provide breaths

- Physiological respiratory rates in infants and children are higher than those in adults.
- In adults, the primary cause for arrest is cardiac in nature and hence sustained compressions are required to improve coronary perfusion.

The resuscitation effort should pause periodically to make an assessment of the possible return of spontaneous heart rate, pulse, and respirations. Try to keep the interruptions to less than 10 s. It is recommended that the patient should be monitored by an electrocardiogram.

WHEN TO ACTIVATE THE EMERGENCY RESPONSE SYSTEM

For unresponsive children, the lone rescuer should provide about five cycles of CPR before leaving the child to activate the emergency response system and use the automated external defibrillator (AED). For a witnessed sudden collapse, activate the emergency response system and then start CPR. With availability of mobile phones, activation of emergency response system can be done immediately.

CARDIOPULMONARY RESUSCITATION FOR INFANTS

The term infant includes the neonatal period outside the delivery room setting and extends to 1 year of age.

The infant BLS sequence is airway, breathing, and circulation.

Airway: After checking the infant for response, the airway should be opened by the head-tilt or chin-lift maneuver. Make sure that you tilt the head back only to the neutral or sniffing position. In case the tongue is obstructing the airway, lift the tongue away from the back of the throat.

Breathing: Once apnea or agonal respirations are identified, using a barrier device (if available), give two breaths (one second each) while watching for the infant's chest rise. The volume of each breath should be sufficient to cause the chest to visibly rise. Mouth-to-mouth or mouth-to-nose breathing techniques can be used for giving breaths to infants.

Pulse check: After delivering two breaths, check for the brachial pulse taking at least 5 s and not more than 10 s.

Chest compressions: It should be started if the heart rate is less than 60 s/min or the infant is pulseless and not breathing. The lone rescuer should use a compression ventilation ratio of 30 compressions to 2 breaths and two rescuers should use a 15:2 compression ventilation ratio until an advanced airway is in place. The depth of compressions for infants is approximately one-third to one-half of the anteroposterior diameter of the chest. The two thumbs-encircling hands technique or two-finger technique can be used for giving chest compressions. After five cycles, if alone, activate the emergency response system. Then return to the infant and provide CPR. Frequent assessment should be done to check for the return of circulation and spontaneous breathing taking not more than 10 s.

Bag and mask technique and rescue breathing: After selecting an appropriate-sized mask and bag, open the infant's airway with a head-tilt and chin-lift method and press the mask to the face while lifting the infant's jaw, creating a seal between the infant's face and the mask. Use the E–C clamp technique to hold the mask in place. Connect to an oxygen supply when available. Effective ventilation is more likely to occur if two rescuers use the bag-mask system; one rescuer holds the mask against the infant's face while lifting the jaw and the other squeezes the bag. Both rescuers should watch for chest rise.

AVOIDING HYPERVENTILATION DURING CARDIOPULMONARY RESUSCITATION

Avoid delivering too many breaths/min (hyperventilation) during CPR, particularly once an advanced airway is in place [such as laryngeal mask airway, or endotracheal (ET) tube]. Hyperventilation may worsen the outcome of cardiac arrest. It can decrease venous return to the heart and reduce blood flow during chest compressions.

ADVANCED AIRWAY CONSIDERATIONS

When an advanced airway [laryngeal mask airway (LMA), ET] is in place during CPR, give breaths at a rate of one breath every 6 s, without attempting to synchronize breaths between compressions. There should be no pause in chest compressions for delivery of breaths.

AUTOMATED EXTERNAL DEFIBRILLATORS

Ventricular fibrillation or pulseless ventricular tachycardia (pVT) can be the cause of sudden collapse or may develop during resuscitation attempts. Children with sudden witnessed collapse (e.g., a child collapsing during an athletic event) are likely to have VF or pVT and need immediate CPR and rapid defibrillation. VF and pVT are referred to as "shockable rhythms" because they respond to electric shocks (defibrillation).

Automated external defibrillators are computerized devices that are reliable, simple to operate, allowing health care providers to attempt defibrillation safely. Use AEDs only when victims have the following three clinical findings—(i) no response, (ii) no breathing, and (iii) no pulse.

Early defibrillation is critical for patients of sudden cardiac arrest for the following reasons:
- The most common initial rhythm in witnessed sudden cardiac arrest is VF. When VF is present, the heart quivers and does not pump blood.
- The most effective treatment for VF is electrical defibrillation along with high-quality CPR.
- The probability of successful defibrillation decreases quickly over time.
- Ventricular fibrillation deteriorates to asystole if not treated.

If one is available, the rescuer should use a pediatric dose-attenuator system for attempted defibrillation of children 1–8 years of age with an AED.

If the rescuer does not have an AED with a pediatric dose attenuator system, the rescuer should use a standard AED.

For infants (<1 year of age), a manual defibrillator is preferred. If a manual defibrillator is not available, an AED with pediatric dose attenuation is desirable.

If neither is available, an AED without a dose attenuator may be used.

The earlier defibrillation occurs, the higher is the survival rate. In an arrest, defibrillation is carried out for VF or ventricular tachycardia without pulse. The recommended dose is 2 J/kg initially. The lowest energy dose for effective defibrillation in infants and children is not known.

The upper limit for safe defibrillation is also not known, but doses >4 J/kg (as high as 10 J/kg) have effectively defibrillated children and animal models of pediatric arrest with no significant adverse effects. AEDs with relatively high-energy doses have been used successfully in infants in cardiac arrest, with no clear adverse effects.

As soon as the AED gives the shock, CPR should be restarted beginning with chest compressions. Do not delay CPR to check the patient's pulse even if a displayed rhythm looks normal. After 5 cycles of CPR, allow the AED to analyze the heart rhythm. If a shock is not advised, resume CPR for 5 more cycles. Continue until advanced care providers take over or the victim starts to move. Drugs that can be administered are epinephrine and antiarrhythmic drugs like amiodarone, or lidocaine. AEDs can be used in children of all age groups. Child pads and circuits if available should be used for children from 1 to 8 years of age.

As of now mechanical chest compression devices and impedance threshold devices are not recommended.

Extracorporeal techniques and invasive perfusion devices may be used where the etiology is potentially reversible. Such situations would include hypothermia, drug overdose, myocarditis (transplant), and myocardial infarction (adults—revascularization).

A feedback device for monitoring the depth of compressions has been found to be useful.

Using an end-tidal CO_2 ($ETCO_2$) probe to monitor the quality of CPR is useful. Absence of CO_2 suggests poor circulation and or inadequate compressions or a displaced ET tube. An $ETCO_2$ of over 20 mm Hg suggests good quality CPR.

RELIEF OF CHOKING IN CHILDREN AND INFANTS

Foreign body aspiration should always be suspected if respiratory distress has a sudden onset or if the chest does not rise when ventilation is first attempted in an unconscious, apneic infant or child. Foreign bodies may cause either mild or severe airway obstruction. In a suspected foreign body obstruction or in witnessed cases of foreign body aspiration, if the child is conscious and coughing actively or breathing spontaneously, he or she should be encouraged to cough spontaneously until coughing is not effective or aphonic, respiratory distress and stridor increase or the child becomes unconscious. Intervention is needed only in cases of complete airway obstruction or when the child becomes unconscious. The airway is then opened by the head-tilt/chin-lift maneuver and ventilation is attempted. If unsuccessful, the airway is repositioned and ventilation again attempted. If there is still no chest rise, attempts to remove a foreign body are indicated.

A conscious child older than 1 year is administered a series of 5 abdominal thrusts known as the Heimlich's maneuver with the child sitting or standing. If unconscious, resume CPR in the usual manner with a check for a visible foreign body in the mouth or pharynx before rescue breaths. If the foreign body is visible, it is removed.

Clearing an object from an infant's airway requires a combination of 5 back blows and 5 chest thrusts if the child is conscious. If unconscious, resume CPR in the usual manner with a check for a visible foreign body in the mouth or pharynx before rescue breaths. If the foreign body is visible, it is removed.

POSTCARDIAC ARREST CARE

To improve survival for victims of cardiac arrest who are admitted to a hospital after return of spontaneous circulation, a comprehensive, structured, integrated, multidisciplinary system of postcardiac arrest care should be implemented in a consistent manner. Treatment should include cardiopulmonary and neurologic support, as well as therapeutic hypothermia, renal support, and management of hematologic derangements. An electroencephalogram for the diagnosis of seizures should be performed with prompt interpretation and should be monitored frequently or continuously in comatose patients after return of spontaneous circulation.

DISCONTINUATION OF LIFE SUPPORT

In an emergency department, the decision to terminate resuscitation is usually based on the patient's response to advanced life support. In children, the failure to respond to two standard doses of epinephrine is highly correlated with death. Cold water drowning is perhaps the most common clinical situation in which long resuscitation attempts have occasionally produced variable survivors. In the absence of recurrent or refractory VF or VT, history of toxic drug exposure or hypothermia, the resuscitation team should discontinue resuscitative efforts after approximately 30 min especially if there is no return of spontaneous circulation. If the $ETCO_2$ fails to show a rise in spite of good CPR, recovery is unlikely. When resuscitation fails and the patient dies, attention should be focused on comforting the grieving family and also the medical team should analyze the course of events and understand how and why their efforts did not succeed. This is the time to identify potential organ donors and take steps accordingly if feasible. The legal and procedural duties if any should be completed.

SUGGESTED READING

1. American Heart Association. (2015). Highlights of the 2015 American Heart Association. Guidelines Update for CPR and ECC. Available from: https://eccguidelines.heart.org/wp-content/uploads/2015/10/2015-AHA-Guidelines-Highlights-English.pdf.
2. Behrman RE, Kleigman RM, Jenson HB. Stabilization of the critically ill child, chapter 57, 17th edition, Nelson Textbook of Pediatrics; 2003. pp. 279-96.
3. BLS for Health Care Providers Manual. American Heart Association. Hazinski MF, Gonzales L, O'Neill L (Eds); 2006. pp. 17-65.
4. Cummins RO. From concept to standard of care. Review of the clinical experience with automated external defibrillators. Ann Emerg Med. 1989;18:1269-75.
5. Emergency Cardiac Care Committee and Subcommittee. American Heart Association. Guidelines for cardiopulmonary resuscitation and emergency cardiac care. VI; Pediatric advanced life support. JAMA. 1992;2262-75.
6. Kern KB, Hilwig RW, Berg RA, et al. Efficacy of chest compression only BLS CPR in the presence of an occluded airway. Resuscitation. 1998;39:179-88.
7. Kern KB, Sanders AB, Raife J, et al. A study of chest compression rates during cardiopulmonary resuscitation in humans. The importance of rate directed chest compression. Arch Intrn Med. 1992;152:145-9.
8. Larsen MP, Eisenberg MS, Cummins RO, et al. Predicting survival from out of hospital cardiac arrest: A graphic model. ANN Emerg Med. 1993;22:1652-8.

9. Nadkarni V, Hazinski MF, Zideman D, et al. Pediatric resuscitation: An advisory statement from the pediatric working group of the international Liason committee on resuscitation. Circulation. 1997;95:2185-95.
10. O'Rourke PP. Out of hospital cardiac arrest in pediatric patient; Outcome. Crit care Med. 12:283,1984.
11. Ornato JP, Hallagen LF, Reesewa Clark RF, et al. Treatment of paroxysmal supraventricular tachycardia in the emergency department by clinical decision analysis. Am J Emerg Med. 1998;6:555-60.
12. PALS Provider Manual, American Academy of Pediatrics. In: Hazinski MF (Ed) American Heart Association; 2002. pp. 46-63.
13. Perry JC, Fenrich AL, Hulse JE, et al. Pediatric use of intravenous amiodarone. Efficacy and safety in critically ill patients from a multicenter protocol. J Am Coll Cardiol. 1996;27:1246-50.
14. Roger MC. Textbook of pediatric intensive care, 3rd edition, chapter 1, In: Charles, L. Schleien, John W. Kuluz, D. Hal Schaffner (Eds). Cardiopulmonary Resuscitation; 1996.
15. Sirbaugh PE, Pepe PE, Shook JE, et al. A prospective population based study of the demographics, epidemiology, management and outcome of out of hospital pediatric cardiopulmonary arrest. Ann Emerg Med. 1999;33:174-84.
16. Whyte SD, Sinha AK, Wyllie JP. Pediatric basic life support: A practical assessment. Resuscitation. 1999; 41:153-57.
17. Zartsky A, Nadkarni V, Geston P, et al. CPR in children. Ann Emerg Med. 1987;16:1107-10.

Fluid and Electrolytes in the Critically Ill Child

4

Preetha Joshi, Vinay Joshi

LEARNING OBJECTIVES

- To learn the principles of fluid balance in children
- To apply these principles to critically ill children.

INTRODUCTION

The main principles that govern fluid and electrolyte physiology and therapy in older children are similar to adults. There are however some important differences with regard to smaller children, infants, and neonates. Special consideration needs to be used when prescribing fluids in this population.

Many of the principles used to estimate fluid replacement therapy, come from limited studies published over 60 years ago, when the pathophysiology of critical illness in children was not yet fully understood as it is in the present time.

BODY WATER DISTRIBUTION IN CHILDREN

The total body water in the human ranges from 40 to 70%, with a number of influencing factors like age, sex, and body fat content. During fetal life, this water represents 90% of the body weight, 75% at birth, 65% at 6 months, and 60% at 1 year. In contrast, the intracellular fluid (ICF) volume remains relatively constant during childhood.

Approximately two-third of this total body water is located intracellularly and remaining one-third is in the extracellular space. The extracellular fluid (ECF) is further divided between interstitial space (three-fourths) and intravascular (one-fourth). The solute content differs between the spaces, K^+ being the primary intracellular cation and Na^+ being the predominant extracellular cation.

The Na^+–K^+ ATPase pump plays an important role in maintaining the respective solute concentrations in both compartments which then helps in maintaining the blood osmolality within the normal narrow range between 280 mOsm/kg H_2O and 290 mOsm/kg H_2O. When

Table 1: Water content of body compartments in children.

Age	TBW (% body weight)	ECF (% body weight)	ICF (% body weight)
Premature	80	45	35
Term newborn	75	40	35
1 month–1 year	65	30	35
1–12 years	60	20	40
Adolescent			
Male	60	20	40–45
Female	55	18	40

(ECF: extracellular fluid; ICF: intracellular fluid; TBW: total body water)

a concentration gradient develops, water moves passively across the easily permeable cell membranes, from the compartment with the lower to the higher gradient, and thus restores this osmolality. Most other solutes in either compartment freely diffuse between each other; therefore, Na^+ remains the most important solute that drives the water homeostasis (Table 1).

WATER HOMEOSTASIS

For homeostasis to occur, fluid intake must balance fluid losses.

In the normal child, the total solute concentration of ICF is the same as that of extracellular fluid. Thus, changes in the latter (more common) result in passive osmotic shift of water with alteration of intracellular volume. On the other hand, extracellular fluid volume is controlled by a number of mechanisms. First, the presence of volume receptors controlling the ECF volume and secondly, the concentration of extracellular solute which stimulates the release of antidiuretic hormone (ADH) from the pituitary and hence the volume is reabsorbed by the renal tubules (Fig. 1).

Renal function in infants and smaller children differ from adults in that, they have lower rates of glomerular filtration rate (GFR), excretion of solutes, and concentrating ability, especially so in preterm infants where GFR is lower as the gestation decreases. Hence, physiological renal insufficiency would result primarily in alterations of extracellular solute concentration and thereby changes in intracellular volume.

Fluid losses are in the form of urine output and insensible losses—evaporative loss from skin and respiratory tract, and fluid loss in the stool—which is minimal, in the absence of diarrhea.

Insensible losses from the respiratory tract are calculated to be in the range of 12–15 mL/100 kcal/day and are mostly electrolyte-free water. With humidification and warming used in mechanical ventilation, this is eliminated. Sweat contains mostly water with a small amount of sodium (except in cystic fibrosis). Evaporative losses increase in situations of fever and thermal stress.

Water excretion in the urine is dependent on solute load and ability to concentrate and dilute urine. Infants are not able to maximally dilute urine (infants—200 mOsm/L vs. adults—

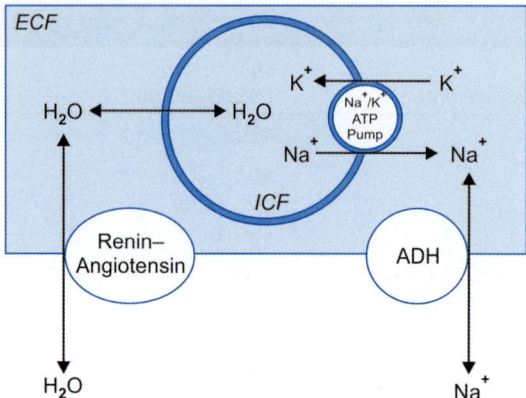

Fig. 1: Model depicting total body water, factors influencing sodium concentration and osmolality.
Source: Adapted from Heymsfield SB, Wang Z, Deurenberg P, et al. Hydration of fat-free body mass: new physiological modeling approach. Am J Phys End Met. 1999;276(6):E995-E1003.

80 mOsm/L) or concentrate urine (infants—800 mOsm/L vs. adults—1,200 mOsm/L). Therefore, the high solute load and the limited urine concentrating ability make them prone to significant extracellular fluid contraction (dehydration) when water loss is excessive (seen in very preterm babies in the first week of life). This is accentuated in situations of gastroenteritis, when decreased oral intake is combined with excessive water and electrolyte loss in stool.

Urine is the major source of electrolyte loss in the body, except when there are fluid losses from gastrointestinal tract (GIT). The commonly used values for sodium (Na^+) and potassium (K^+) requirements in parenteral fluids in children are 2–3 mmol/kg/day and 1–2 mmol/kg/day, respectively. These are based on normal homeostasis, but this may vary greatly in critically ill children, where urinary water loss varies and urinary Na^+ and K^+ concentration may be significantly higher.

In normal healthy people, water intake is largely regulated by thirst, which is stimulated by osmoreceptors in the hypothalamus. Infants and smaller children may not be able to demand, similar to older children with altered levels of consciousness or under sedation in the critical care setting. These patients are therefore placed on parenteral fluids, where the amount of water replaced is calculated based on body weight and energy expenditure (Table 2). Holliday and Segar studied these energy, water, and solute requirements in healthy infants being fed cow's milk or breast milk and extrapolated it to hospitalized children and their need for maintenance of parenteral fluids.

As a result of these calculations, using hypotonic intravenous solutions has been the regular practice for over 60 years. However, it has been increasingly recognized that certain nonphysiological and nonosmotic stimuli for ADH secretion (pain, anxiety, narcotics, positive pressure ventilation), which inhibit the excretion of electrolyte-free water, exist in critically ill children. Therefore, mild to moderate degrees of hyponatremia would be common in children receiving parenteral fluid therapy. In addition, nonosmotic stimulation of ADH is seen in several disease states like pneumonia, bronchiolitis, meningitis, encephalitis, traumatic brain injury, and even gastroenteritis. Also, some of these conditions cause syndrome of

Table 2: Requirements for maintenance parenteral fluids.

Body weight	0–10 kg	10–20 kg	>20 kg
Water requirements	100 mL/kg/day	1,000 mL + 50 mL/kg/day for each kg >10	1,500 mL + 20 mL/kg/day for each kg >20
	4 mL/kg/hour	3 mL/kg/hour	2.3 mL/kg/hour

Sodium requirement 3 mmol/100 kcal/day and potassium requirement 2 mmol/100 kcal/day calculated from sodium and potassium concentration in cow's milk and breast milk.

Source: Based on the formula by Holliday MA, Segar WE. The maintenance need for water in parenteral fluid therapy. Pediatrics. 1957;19:823-32.

inappropriate antidiuretic hormone secretion (SIADH) also, which further worsens the predicament. Mortality directly attributed to hyponatremic encephalopathy in postoperative children is as high as 5–8%.

There is now a lot of evidence to support use of isotonic or near-isotonic fluids in children to avoid administration of electrolyte-free water. Hypotonic fluids like Isolyte P need to be reserved for patients with a need for electrolyte-free water [serum Na$^+$ (S. Na$^+$) >145 mmol/L] and should be prescribed only in justifiable circumstances.

UNDERSTANDING "FLUID" CONCEPTS

- *Osmotic activity*: It is the solute activity in a solution and is expressed as osmoles (osm).
- *Osmolarity*: It is the osmotic activity per volume of solution (solutes + water) and is expressed as mOsm/L.
- *Osmolality*: It is the osmotic activity per volume of water and is expressed as mOsm/kg H$_2$O. It is commonly used to express osmotic activity of body fluids. The volume of water in body fluids is far greater than the volume of solutes. So, there is very little difference between the two and they can be used interchangeably.
- *Tonicity*: When two solutions with different osmotic activity are separated by a membrane that allows the passage of water and not solutes, the relative osmotic activity in the two solutions is called effective osmolality or tonicity. The solution with the higher osmolality is hypertonic and the solution with the lower osmolality is hypotonic. Some solutes, if added to a solution, increase the osmolality of the solution but not the tonicity, as they can pass freely across the membrane [e.g. blood urea nitrogen (BUN)].
- *Calculated plasma osmolality* = 2 × Na + glucose/18 + BUN/2.8

$$= 2 \times 140 + 90/18 + 14/2.8$$
$$= 290 \text{ mOsm/kg H}_2\text{O}$$

- *Measured osmolality*: Since solutes other than Na, Cl, glucose, and urea are present in the ECF, the measured plasma osmolality will be greater than the calculated osmolality.
- *Osmolal gap*: Difference between the measured and calculated osmolality, usually about 10 mOsm/kg H$_2$O. An increase in this gap can occur with certain toxin ingestions (ethanol, methanol, ethylene glycol) or unidentified toxins accumulate in renal failure.

- *Effective osmolality or plasma tonicity*: Since BUN freely crosses cell membranes, effective osmolality/tonicity can be calculated by eliminating BUN from the plasma osmolality equation, the result is 280–285 mOsm/kg H_2O. This reiterates the fact that plasma sodium concentration is the principal determinant of the tonicity and therefore volumes of ECF and ICF.

FLUID THERAPY IN THE INTENSIVE CARE UNIT

There are three different situations where fluid therapy needs to be implemented in the intensive care unit (ICU) setting. It can be used as:
- Maintenance fluid
- Replacement fluid
- Resuscitation fluid.

Maintenance Fluid

While administering intravenous fluids as maintenance, it is important to make all regular considerations as in case of a drug.
- *Patient*: Age, weight, disease
- *Infusion*: Composition, route, rate
- Monitoring for side effects—too much, too less, effects of excessive electrolyte-free water, and desired response to therapy. Serum electrolytes need to be measured in every child on parenteral fluids for more than 12 hours and need to be done once or twice a day especially in postoperative cases.

Patients at risk for nonosmotic ADH stimuli (most critically ill and postoperative patients), requiring more than 12 hours of intravenous fluids, should be started on two-third maintenance fluids of isotonic saline or Ringer lactate. The S. Na^+ can be used as a guide and should be maintained between 135 mEq/L and 140 mEq/L. The National Patient Safety Agency (NPSA) in United Kingdom has mentioned that hypotonic fluids should not be used as postoperative maintenance fluid and hypotonic fluids need to be withdrawn from the market.

Maintenance K^+ can be added at 20 mEq/L or 40 mEq/L once the urine output is optimal and K^+ is in the normal range. Dextrose containing, isotonic saline solutions need to be used in infants less than 3 months of age, malnourished children, and postoperative cases with a total of more than 12 hours fasting. In others, the sugar needs to be monitored closely to prevent hypoglycemia.

Specific Situations

- *Renal failure*: 400 mL/m^2 with previous day's urine output with no added K^+ unless patient is hypokalemic. Hypotonic fluids need to be avoided as the patient has water retention.
- *Dengue shock*: Maintenance fluids to be given at the rate of 5–7 mL/kg/hour to match with ongoing third space losses.
- *Cardiac failure*: Fluids need to be started at half to two-thirds maintenance depending on the clinical status and can be increased as soon as the urine output improves with diuretics. Hypotonic fluids need to be avoided.
- *Patients with raised intracranial pressure*: The aim of fluid therapy in this case involves maintaining a high normal mean arterial pressure in order to maintain the cerebral

Table 3: Guide to fluids in different conditions.

Clinical state	Water mL/kg	Na mmol/kg	K mmol/kg
Average patients receiving only parenteral fluids	100–120	2–4	2–4
Heat stress	120–240	Variable	Variable
Anuria	45	0	0
Acute CNS infections	80–90	2–4	2–4
Diabetes insipidus	Up to 400	Variable	2–4
Hyperventilation	120–210	2–4	2–4

(CNS: central nervous system)

perfusion pressure. Hypotonic fluids need to be strictly avoided aiming for Na⁺ levels between 145 mEq/L and 160 mEq/L with the use of intermittent hypertonic saline (3% saline) boluses (Table 3).

Using Hypotonic Solutions as Maintenance Fluids

These can be used only in specific cases of diabetes insipidus, where Na is more than 150 mEq/L. It is important to remember here that the basic pathology is loss of electrolyte-free water due to the absence of ADH secretion. This can be replaced by two-third saline or half saline. But fluids may need to be changed back to isotonic saline when DDAVP (desmopressin acetate) is used as this will cause a precipitous fall in Na due to free water retention. A useful guide in this situation is paired serum and urine osmolality and electrolytes, at least twice or thrice a day.

Replacement Fluid

Isotonic saline or Ringer lactate is the preferred solution for replacement of intraoperative and postoperative fluid losses, including drains and excessive nasogastric aspirates.

Children have large postoperative third space losses, especially in gastrointestinal surgeries, through a laparotomy. The fluid loss has to be replaced by isotonic fluids.

In cardiac surgery, the postoperative loss is usually blood from the drains (if >5 mL/kg/hour), which needs to be replaced by packed cells and plasma as the situation warrants.

Resuscitation Fluid

Fluids used for resuscitation in children are isotonic or near-isotonic crystalloids.
- *Hypovolemic shock*: Normal saline (NS) is to be used as resuscitation fluid in all cases of gastroenteritis with 10% dehydration—hyponatremic, isonatremic, and hypernatremic dehydration. Following the initial resuscitation, the fluids can be changed based on S. Na⁺ levels and calculation of Na⁺ and water deficit.
  - In cases of trauma, where the hypovolemia is a result of blood loss—this needs to be replaced as soon as possible.

- In postoperative conditions, where ongoing third space losses are anticipated, up to 150–200 mL/kg may be required to maintain intravascular volume in the first 24 hours.
- *Septic shock*: Up to 60–80 mL/kg/day may be required in children with septic shock within 1 hour of admission. Isotonic fluids are the fluid of choice.
- *Anaphylactic shock*: The primary cause for hemodynamic compromise is due to vasodilatation and the child will need isotonic fluids to maintain perfusion pressures in addition to vasoconstrictors.
- *Cardiogenic shock*: Fluids need to be administered judiciously in aliquots of 5 mL/kg over half an hour and repeat fluids given only if there is a positive hemodynamic response.
    - Presence of edema, as in congestive cardiac failure or renal failure does not assure a normovolemic status and the patient hemodynamics might improve significantly with cautious fluid resuscitation if he is hypovolemic.
- *Dengue hemorrhagic shock and dengue shock syndrome*: In cases of hemorrhage, packed red cells and fresh frozen plasma needs to be replaced.

In dengue shock without hemorrhage, isotonic fluid resuscitation with slow rates at 25 mL/kg over an hour, with simultaneous increase of maintenance fluids as mentioned in the previous section may be given. The fluids need to be titrated using hematocrit and S. Na$^+$ as a tool.

CRYSTALLOID VERSUS COLLOIDS IN CRITICALLY ILL CHILDREN

Colloid use is widespread in cases of postcardiopulmonary bypass, burns, postoperative cases, and sometimes in septic shock. Though hypoalbuminemia has been shown to increase mortality in critically ill adults, this has not been proven in children.

Colloids cause greater increase in intravascular fluid volume for much lower volumes infused. However, this is a very expensive resuscitation fluid. Moreover, Cochrane meta-analyses have shown that colloid use was associated with an increased mortality. Studies in dengue shock have shown better hematocrits and pulse pressure among patients who received colloids. Further randomized controlled trials in children are required to recommend the regular use of colloids in resuscitation.

ELECTROLYTE DISORDERS

Sodium

Sodium chloride and bicarbonate are the major solutes (90%) in the ECF that determines the ECF volume. Any disturbance in the ECF Na can have tremendous effects on the intracellular volume.

Hyponatremia

Definition: S. Na$^+$ less than 130 mEq/L

Hyponatremia is the most common electrolyte disorder in the children. Almost *30% of patients treated in the ICU develop hyponatremia*. Acute hyponatremia (developing over 48 hours or less) can lead to severe degrees of cerebral edema and it has been found that mortality can be as high as 50% when serum sodium levels are below *105 mEq/L*.

Table 4: Causes of increased antidiuretic hormone in critical illness.

Physiological stimuli	Nonphysiological stimuli
• Hyperosmolality • Hypovolemia • Hypotension	• Pain (trauma) • Infection • Anxiety • Nausea • Drugs

Altered Na level (osmolality) is the result of disturbances in water homeostasis.

Water gain:
- Excessive free water retention
- Excessive free water administration.

Sodium loss:
- Excessive renal or extrarenal losses of Na
- Very rarely deficient intake.

Kidney plays a significant role in normal water homeostasis and thereby sodium levels, through ADH, along with other mechanisms like thirst and excretion (Table 4).

Approach to hyponatremia: Before embarking on treatment, the etiology of hyponatremia needs to be ascertained and has to be divided into either water gain or sodium loss and then accordingly managed.

History:
- History suggestive of primary illness
- Fluid status and intake/output
- Check IV fluids—composition, rate
- Check diuretic use
- Check other drugs.

Investigations:
- Hematocrit (hydration status)
- Serum electrolytes (trend)
- Serum Na—verify if *truly low*
- BUN and creatinine levels, random blood sugar (RBS)
- Urine Na, specific gravity, osmolality.

Management: It should include answering the following five questions:
- *True hyponatremia (hypotonic)*: True hyponatremia is when both the sodium and the osmolality are low. Pseudohyponatremia is when the sodium concentration is low (<135) but osmolality is normal. Factitious hyponatremia when Na is low but osmolality is high. Hypertonic hyponatremia (translocational): Glucose, mannitol—1.6–2.4 mEq/L decrease of serum Na for 100 mg/dL rise in glucose
- *Symptomatic hyponatremia*:
  - *Mild symptoms*: Headache, nausea, vomiting, confusion, lethargy

Table 5: Causes of hyponatremia.

Euvolemic	Hypovolemic	Hypervolemic
Factitious: • Mannitol infusion • Hyperglycemia • Hyperlipidemia • Hyperproteinemia *Syndrome of inappropriate ADH* • CNS disorders • Respiratory diseases • Malignancy • Medications • Postoperative • Idiopathic—AIDS *Excessive water intake*: • Fresh water drowning • Diluted infant formula	*Loss of sodium*: • GIT loss • Burns • Third space loss • Renal: diuretics, ARF, salt losing nephropathy • Cerebral salt wasting • Mineralocorticoid deficiency • Glycosuria • Ketonuria • Low salt intake • Low sodium diet	*Edema forming states* • CHF • Nephrotic syndrome • Cirrhosis • Acute or chronic renal failure • Excessive free water administration

(AIDS: acquired immunodeficiency syndrome; ARF: acute renal failure; CNS: central nervous system; CHF: congestive heart failure; GIT: gastrointestinal tract)

- *Severe symptoms*: Seizures, altered sensorium, falling *Glasgow coma scale* (GCS), respiratory irregularities, pupillary changes, neurogenic pulmonary edema
- *Hyponatremic encephalopathy*: Seizures, coma, permanent brain damage, respiratory arrest, and brainstem herniation leading to death.
- Volume—hypovolemic, hypervolemic, euvolemic? As given in Table 5
- Is the kidney excreting adequate free water?
- Cause of hyponatremia?

Treatment principles:
- *Pseudohyponatremia*: No correction needed
- Na^+ deficit should be corrected over 48–72 hours.
- Acute hyponatremia can cause significant changes in osmolality and thereby fluid shifts in the brain-cerebral edema.
- Chronic hyponatremia is better tolerated.
- Rate of correction of sodium in asymptomatic children should not be more than 0.5 mEq/L/hour.
- Rapid correction—only in symptomatic patients and only till resolution of symptoms or Na^+ more than 120 mEq/L.
  - Demyelination of pontine and extrapontine neurons is caused by rapid correction of Na^+ deficit. It is manifested by quadriplegia, pseudobulbar palsy, seizure, coma, and death.

Table 6: Differentiating features between syndrome of inappropriate antidiuretic hormone secretion (SIADH) and cerebral salt wasting (CSW).

	SIADH	CSW
Serum Na	↓	↓
ECFV	Normal	↓
Urine Na	↑	↑↑
Urine osmolarity	↑	↑
Urine volume	↓	↑
Serum urate	↓	N or ↓
Urine urate	↑	N or ↑

(ECFV: extracellular fluid volume; N: normal)

Specific situations:
- *SIADH treatment principles*:
  - Fluid restriction—50% of maintenance requirements
  - Monitor serum Na⁺
  - Fluid balance—input/output, daily weight.
- *Hyponatremic seizure/encephalopathy*:
  - Hypertonic saline (3% NaCl) infusion—to increase S. Na⁺ by 5 mEq/L
  - To increase Na⁺ by 5 mEq/L sodium = 0.6 × 30 kg × 5 = 90 mEq
  - 3% NaCl = 0.5 mEq/L, therefore 90 mEq bolus = 180 mL (6 mL/kg).
- *Cerebral salt wasting—e.g. cerebral disease [particularly subarachnoid hemorrhage (SAH)]*:
  - Mimics SIADH with hyponatremia, except primary defect is salt wasting not water retention.
  - Treatment is NS to correct ECF volume contraction (Table 6).
- *Hyponatremic dehydration*:
  - Fluid resuscitation [early goal directed therapy (EGDT)]: NS
  - Fluid replacement-maintenance and deficit over 48 hours (NS/RL)
  - Closed clinical [heart rate (HR), peripheral pulses, perfusion, urine output], weight, serum electrolytes (Na⁺) monitoring.
- *Dilutional hyponatremia*: Excessive free water intake
  - Initial rapid correction with 3% NaCl (1–2 mEq/L/hour) until symptomatic relief or serum Na⁺ more than 120 mEq/L, followed by slow correction, 10–12 mEq/L/day
  - Close monitoring of hydration and serum Na.

Hypernatremia

It is defined as serum more than 145 mEq/L.

Flowchart 1: Approach to hypernatremia.

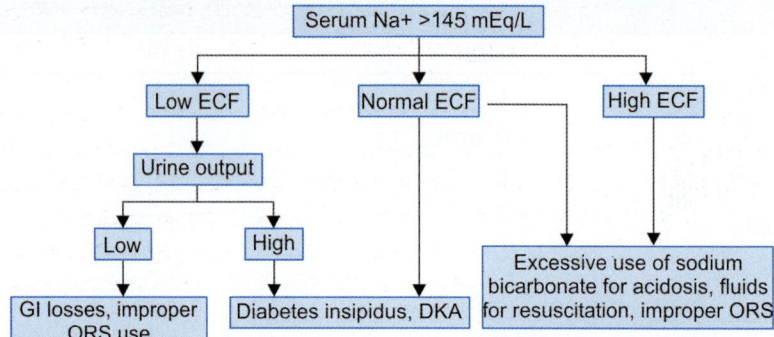

(DKA: diabetic ketoacidosis; ECF: extracellular fluid; GI: gastrointestinal; ORS: oral rehydration solution)

Causes:
- *Unreplaced water losses (associated with impaired thirst or access to water)*:
  - Insensible water losses (sweat)
  - Gastrointestinal water losses
  - Diabetes insipidus (central or nephrogenic)
  - Osmotic diuresis
  - Hypothalamic lesion impairing thirst center.
- *Water loss into cells*:
  - Severe exercise or seizures.
- *Sodium overload*:
  - Administration of hypertonic solutions
  - Excessive intake (Flowchart 1).

Specific situations:

Diabetes insipidus:
- Hypernatremia
- Polyuria
- Inappropriately dilute urine (urine osmolality < serum osmolality)
- May be see with midline defects
- Frequently occurs in brain dead patients.

Two types:
1. Central diabetes insipidus (DI)
   - Idiopathic—autoimmune
   - Neurosurgery, head trauma
   - Cerebral hypoperfusion
   - Tumor (craniopharyngioma, pituitary adenoma, suprasellar meningioma)
   - Infiltration (Fe, sarcoid, Histiocytosis X).
2. Nephrogenic DI
   - X-linked recessive

- Hypokalemia
- Hypercalcemia [secondary *hyperparathyroidism* (HPT) in particular]
- *Renal disease*: After *acute tubular necrosis* (ATN), postobstructive uropathy, renal artery stenosis (RAS), renal transplant, sickle cell anemia
- *Drugs*: Demeclocycline, amphotericin, colchicine.

Management: Hypernatremia causes rise in serum osmolality and due to hypertonicity of ECF, there is intracellular dehydration which produces osmotically active substances called idiogenic osmoles over a period of time. If the fluid resuscitation is done rapidly, these osmoles draw fluids and lead to cellular damage, most prominently seen as cerebral edema. Therefore, rehydration should be done over 48–72 hours, taking care not to drop serum Na by more than 10 mEq/L (serum osmolality by 20 mOsm/L) in 24 hours.

- *Hypernatremic dehydration*: Fluid resuscitation as per guidelines followed by slow correction of hypernatremia over 48–72 hours
- *Treatment of diabetes insipidus*:
  - *Treat dehydration*: Normal saline initially if ECF volume contraction followed by IV 0.45 NS or one-fourth NS to lower serum Na^+ by 1–2 mEq/L/hour if Na^+ more than 160 or symptomatic (coma, seizures), otherwise 0.5–1.0 mEq/L/hour
  - *DDAVP (desmopressin)*: Reduces urine output (U/O) and therefore simplifies fluid therapy
  - *Long half-life*: Duration 8–12 hours, up to 24 hours, use judiciously. Dose: DDAVP 1 µg IV/SC.
  - Only repeat if breaks-through again (i.e. becomes hypernatremic with dilute polyuria)
  - Subsequently, it can be switched to intranasal route.
  - *Caution*: Do *not* replace urine output if giving DDAVP
  - *Arginine vasopressin (AVP), aqueous vasopressin* (Pitressin): only available in parenteral form
  - Dose: 5–10 U SC q2-4h, side effects: hypertension, coronary vasospasm
  - *Indomethacin* 100–150 mg po bid-tid [prostaglandins (PGs) antagonize AVP action].

Potassium

Potassium is the principal intracellular cation with a concentration of 150 mmol/L and helps in regulating the resting membrane potential. Hypokalemia therefore makes the cell membrane more resistant to depolarization and hyperkalemia makes the cell more excitable. The movement of K^+ into the intracellular compartment is increased by insulin, alkalosis, and catecholamines.

Hypokalemia

K^+ is less than 3.5 mEq/L.

Causes:
- *Gastroenteritis*: ECF contraction leads to aldosterone secretion.
- *Diabetic ketoacidosis*: Total body K^+ depletion, although initial levels may be high in the face of ketoacidosis

- Anorexia nervosa
- Prolonged use of diuretics, like furosemide
- Nasogastric suction/aspirates
- Hypomagnesemia
- Metabolic alkalosis
- Bartter syndrome and renal tubular acidosis (RTA)—increased K⁺ output in urine
- Drug-induced—amphotericin, ticarcillin, and steroids
- Iatrogenic—decreased intake—enteral/parenteral.

Clinical features: Muscle weakness, intestinal ileus, and arrhythmias. It increases the potential for digoxin toxicity.

Treatment: Potassium supplementation is usually done with KCl but can also be done with K acetate or phosphate in hyperchloremic metabolic acidosis or diabetic ketoacidosis where phosphate may be low.

Routine correction can be done with addition of KCl in maintenance fluids 10–60 mEq/L, beyond which a neat KCl solution can be started through a central line with rigorous monitoring of K⁺ levels. It is important to correct magnesium levels, in the absence of which hypokalemia may remain resistant to therapy.

Hyperkalemia

K⁺ is more than 5.5 mEq/L.

Causes:
- Failure of potassium excretion—renal failure, adrenal insufficiency, aldosterone deficiency
- Movement of K⁺ from ICF to ECF:
  - Rhabdomyolysis, burns, trauma, and tumor lysis syndrome
  - Malignant hyperthermia, drugs (captopril), and acute metabolic acidosis
  - Use of depolarizing neuromuscular blocker (succinylcholine) can lead to abrupt increase in K⁺ and cardiac arrest.
- *Iatrogenic*: Excessive intravenous K administration, transfusion of stored blood
- *Spurious hyperkalemia*: Very common and due to squeezing during collection or collection from a line infusing K⁺ containing fluids, elevated white blood cell (WBC), or platelet counts.

Clinical features:
- *Arrhythmias*: Electrocardiography (ECG) changes begin with tall T waves, PR prolongation, loss of P waves, QRS widening, ventricular fibrillation, and finally asystole.
- Muscle weakness, paresthesias, tingling, abdominal pain, or distension (Fig. 2).

Treatment: Emergency measures are aimed at *shifting* the K⁺ from the extracellular to the intracellular compartment (temporizing measures):
- Bicarbonate to correct acidosis
- *Beta-agonist therapy*: It helps in movement of K⁺ into the ICF through adrenergic mediated mechanism.
- Glucose and insulin
- *Intravenous calcium chloride or gluconate*: It stabilizes the myocardium—helps prevent arrhythmias.

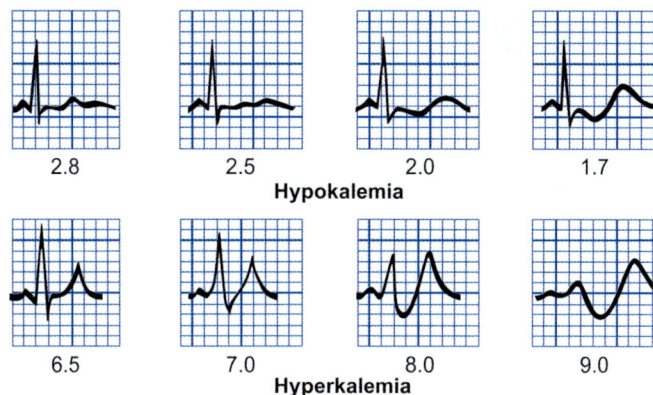

Fig. 2: ECG changes with hypokalemia and hyperkalemia.

Removal of K^+: Increase K^+ removal from the body is the more permanent but slow-acting measure. This can be done with:
- Na-K exchange resins rectally or via nasogastric route
- Loop diuretics—furosemide
- Dialysis.

Calcium

Calcium levels are influenced by vitamin D, parathyroid hormone, and calcitriol. It is the most abundant electrolyte in the body, but 99% is in the bone. Calcium in plasma is present in three forms: 50% bound to proteins (80% to albumin); 5–10% chelated, and the remaining is in the form of functionally active calcium ions. In critically ill children, total calcium levels might be low due to hypoalbuminemia, but this does not affect the ionized calcium levels (Table 7).

Hypocalcemia

Ionized hypocalcemia (<1 mmol/L) is reported in 50–65% of ICU admissions. Predisposing conditions are:
- *Infants*: Low birth weight newborns with less calcium stores, asphyxia, infants of diabetic mothers, DiGeorge syndrome.
- *Magnesium depletion*: Promotes hypocalcemia by inhibition of parathormone and reducing end-organ responsiveness to parathormone. In this case, hypocalcemia remains refractory to calcium replacement therapy in the absence of magnesium supplementation.
- *Critically ill*: Sepsis, cardiopulmonary bypass, burns.
- *Alkalosis*: Promotes binding of calcium to albumin and reduces the ionized fraction. Also seen following a bicarbonate correction due to direct binding of calcium to bicarbonate.
- *Blood transfusions*: 15% of patients receiving blood transfusions due to binding of calcium with citrate in the banked blood and is usually transient.
- *Drugs*: Aminoglycosides, heparin, theophylline, loop diuretics.

Table 7: Normal ranges for calcium and phosphorus in blood.

Serum electrolyte	Traditional units (mg/dL)	Conversion factor	SI units (mmol/L)
Total calcium	8.0–10.2	0.25	2.2–2.5
Ionized calcium	4.0–4.6	0.25	1.0–1.5
Phosphorus	2.5–5.0	0.32	0.8–1.6

- *Tumor lysis syndrome*: Due to hyperphosphatemia.
- *Renal failure*: Ionized hypocalcemia usually noted due to phosphate retention and impaired conversion of vitamin D to its active form in the kidneys.

Clinical features:
- *Neuromuscular excitability*: Hyperreflexia, generalized seizures, and in worse cases tetany.
- *Myocardial dysfunction*: This is mainly seen in neonates and infants, as in this population, calcium works as an inotrope, and it is extremely important to maintain normal ionized calcium levels in this population especially in cases of shock. Patients can present with hypotension and ventricular ectopics—especially ionized Ca^+ 0.8–1 mmol/L. With further drop in levels, less than 0.65 mmol/L, ventricular tachycardia and refractory hypotension may result.

Treatment:
- Correction of calcium levels is an emergency, in cases of symptomatic hypocalcemia. The underlying cause needs to be investigated and treated.
- *Dose*: 0.5 mL/kg of 10% calcium gluconate (9 mg elemental Ca^+/mL) diluted in an equal amount of saline over 10 minutes. Close monitoring is essential for bradycardia (<10% of baseline). This can be followed with Ca replacement of 150–200 mg/kg/day to maintain ionized Ca^+ more than 1 mmol/L.
- *Adjunctive measures*: Correct magnesium, potassium, and pH. Lowering of high phosphorus levels may be of some help. Supplementation with vitamin D in case of low levels is helpful in increasing intestinal absorption of calcium.

Hypercalcemia

Total calcium is more than 10.5 mg/dL or ionized calcium is more than 1.2 mmol/L.

Causes:
- Excessive calcium administration
- Prolonged diuretic therapy—may be associated with nephrocalcinosis
- Neonatal hyperparathyroidism
- Williams syndrome.

Clinical features:
- CNS depression, fatigue, seizures
- Arrhythmias
- GI—nausea, vomiting.

Treatment:
- Stop intake of Ca⁺
- Rehydration with saline will help Ca⁺ excretion in urine
- Drugs—pamidronate, steroids, calcitonin
- Dialysis—in cases with cardiac and renal failure.

Phosphorus

Most phosphorus is present as phospholipids and phosphoproteins and 85% located in the bony skeleton. Unlike calcium, inorganic phosphorus is prominently present in ICF and is responsible for energy production through ATP.

Hypophosphatemia

- S. PO_4 less than 2.5 mg/dL or 0.8 mmol/L
- This is usually seen in malnutrition, vitamin D deficiency, prolonged parenteral nutrition, refeeding syndrome, and DKA.

Clinical features:
Muscle weakness, prolonged ventilator dependency, paresthesias, seizures, cardiac failure.

Treatment:
- Oral phosphorus supplementation
- IV preparations of phosphorus are not easily available and are usually required only in very symptomatic patients, 0.1–1.5 mmol/kg/day as a continuous infusion.

Hyperphosphatemia

Causes: Renal failure, hypoparathyroidism, tumor lysis syndrome, increased phosphate supplementation.

Clinical features:
- Most symptoms are due to associated hypocalcemia
- Seizures, sign of hypocalcemia
- Secondary hyperparathyroidism and renal osteodystrophy in chronic renal failure.

Treatment:
- Good hydration
- IV calcium if there is hypocalcemia
- Phosphate binders
- Tumor lysis syndrome—alkalinization in addition to hydration
- Hemodialysis.

Magnesium

Magnesium is predominantly present in the ICF and like calcium works through its active ionized form.

Hypomagnesemia

- Levels less than 1.5 mEq/L
- Low Mg^+, in association with low K^+ and low Ca^+ levels predisposes to life-threatening arrhythmias especially in postoperative cardiac patients.

Causes:
- Malnutrition
- GI losses—diarrhea, malabsorption
- Renal loss—diuretics.

Clinical features:
- Tetany, tremor, fasciculations
- Refractory hypocalcemia
- Ventricular arrhythmias—ventricular tachycardia, torsade de pointes refractory to other electrolyte replacement, and drugs.

Treatment:
For ventricular arrhythmias: 25–50 mg/kg of 50% magnesium sulfate is given over 30 minutes with close hemodynamic monitoring for ECG response and hypotension. It can also cause respiratory depression. It is equally important to correct the Ca^+ and K^+ levels for maximal response.

Hypermagnesemia

Level more than 4.5 mg/dL.

Causes:
- Renal failure
- Increased administration of Mg—seen very uncommonly.

Clinical features:
Muscle weakness, hypotonia, lethargy.

Management:
- Stop extraneous Mg supplementation
- Calcium—direct antidote in life-threatening cases
- Increasing IV fluid intake
- Diuresis
- Dialysis.

SUGGESTED READING

1. Androgue H, Madias NE. Hyponatremia. NEJM. 2000;342:1581-9.
2. Arieff A, Cosmo F. Hyponatremia and death or permanent damage in healthy children. BMJ. 1992;304:1218-22.
3. Choong K, Bohn D. Hypotonic versus isotonic saline in hospitalised children: a systematic review. Arch Dis Child. 2006;91:828-35.
4. Conley SB. Hypernatremia. Pediatr Clin North Am. 1990;37(2):365-72.
5. Greenbaum LA. Pathophysiology of body fluids and fluid therapy. In: Nelson's Textbook of Pediatrics, 17th edition. Philadelphia: WB Saunders; 2004.

6. Halperin ML. Potassium. Lancet. 1998;352:135-40.
7. Holliday MA, Segar ME. The maintenance need for water in parenteral fluid therapy. Pediatrics. 1957;19:823-32.
8. Maclaurin JC. Changes in body water distribution during the first two weeks of life. Arch Dis Child. 1966;41(217):286-91.
9. Perel P, Roberts I. Colloids versus crystalloids for fluid resuscitation in critically ill patients. Cochrane Database of Syst Rev. The Cochrane Library. 2012;7.
10. Wood EG, Lynch RE. Electrolyte management in Pediatric Critical Illness. In: Zimmerman J, Fuhrman (Ed). Pediatric Critical Care, 3 edition. St. Louis, MO: Mosby Publication; 2006.

Oxygen Therapy in the Emergency Room and PICU

5

Suresh Kumar Angurana, Vijai Williams

LEARNING OBJECTIVES

- Mechanisms of hypoxemia
- Different oxygen delivery devices: Classification and characteristics
- Heated humidified high flow nasal cannula and continuous positive airway pressure
- Hazards of oxygen therapy.

INTRODUCTION

Oxygen is important in emergency rooms and intensive care units to treat hypoxemia. The oxygen delivery devices range from simple facemask to heated humidified high-flow nasal cannula. The use of these devices should be guided by age of the child and tolerability, clinical condition, and familiarity with the device. Though the oxygen is cheap, widely available, and easy to administer, it is a drug and should be used judiciously. Inadequate use may not provide anticipated clinical benefit, whereas continued use for prolonged period and/or higher concentration may be detrimental.

HYPOXEMIA VERSUS HYPOXIA

Arterial hypoxemia is reduced partial pressure of arterial oxygen (PaO_2) and can result from any one or combination of the following: reduced fraction of inspired oxygen (FiO_2), hypoventilation, dead-space ventilation, intrapulmonary shunting, or a diffusion defect.

On the other hand, tissue hypoxia is inadequate tissue utilization of oxygen, low-hemoglobin (Hb) concentration, abnormal Hb or histotoxic hypoxia (e.g. cyanide poisoning).

MECHANISMS OF HYPOXEMIA

As the venous blood from the right side of the heart traverses the lung via pulmonary capillaries, oxygen diffuses from alveolus to blood. In a perfect lung, partial pressure of oxygen (PO_2) in pulmonary venous blood should be equal to PaO_2. But three factors (ventilation/

perfusion mismatch, shunt, and diffusion defects) cause the PO_2 in pulmonary veins to be less than PAO_2.

Ventilation/Perfusion Mismatch

The normal lungs have some degree of ventilation/perfusion (V/Q) mismatch. The upper zones are relatively over ventilated and lower zones are relatively under ventilated and over perfused. The V/Q mismatch is marked on diseased lungs. Some alveoli are relatively over ventilated while others are relatively over perfused. V/Q mismatch decreases the PO_2 in pulmonary capillary blood.

Shunt

Shunt occurs when deoxygenated venous blood passes through nonventilated alveoli and enter pulmonary veins and systemic arterial system leading to unchanged PO_2 (40 mm Hg). Collapsed alveoli, consolidated lung, pulmonary edema, or small airway obstruction are main causes of the shunt.

Diffusion Defects

The diffusion of oxygen from alveolus to pulmonary capillaries is complete by the time blood traverses through one-third of the capillaries. It is rare for the diffusion defects to cause hypoxia except in diseases with pulmonary fibrosis.

OXYGEN DELIVERY AND CONSUMPTION

The quantity of oxygen available to the body in 1 minute is known as the oxygen delivery.

Oxygen delivered (DO_2) = oxygen carrying capacity of blood (CaO_2) × cardiac output

where, CaO_2 = [Hb in g × 1.34 × blood oxygen saturation (SpO_2)] + (PaO_2 × 0.003), and cardiac output = stroke volume × heart rate.

The oxygen delivered to cells is more than they actually use in normal situations. When demand increases (as during exercise), the cardiac output increases to increase the supply. Adequate tissue oxygen delivery depends on adequate ventilation, optimum perfusion across alveolocapillary membrane, proper blood flow across heart and pulmonary vasculature, uninterrupted distribution of blood by cardiovascular system to all tissues, and adequate oxygen carrying capacity of the blood. Failure at any level will decrease oxygen supply to the tissues and demand extra oxygen supplementation. When oxygen supply is less than the consumption, tissues extract more oxygen from Hb leading to a fall in mixed venous oxygen saturation (MVO_2). This compensation acts only till a certain point, beyond which anaerobic metabolism ensues leading to lactic acidosis.

HUMIDIFICATION OF OXYGEN

Normally inhaled gases are humidified up to 100% relative humidity in upper respiratory tract which provides large surface area for humidification and warming of gases. The supplementation with nonhumidified, cold oxygen can lead to impaired mucociliary function, squamous epithelial changes, drying and thickening of secretions, airway obstruction, atelectasis, tracheitis, heat loss leading to hypothermia, and staphylococcal sepsis due to drying and cracking of the mucosa. A simple humidifier without heating capacity can be used in patients without artificial airways and on low-flow oxygen delivery device. Heated humidifiers should be used for patients on high flow of oxygen (>4–6 L/min) and with artificial airways (ventilator). The optimum requirement is 80–100% humidity at 32–37°C temperature.

ADMINISTRATION OF OXYGEN THERAPY

Oxygen is a drug and should be delivered in right dose, right manner (device), and for right duration.

Various devices are used depending upon age and size of the patient, dose of oxygen needed (flow and FiO_2), underlying disease, patient tolerability, and familiarity with the device among physicians.

Oxygen delivery devices are categorized into high flow (fixed concentration devices) and low flow (variable concentration devices) based on their ability to meet the flow requirement or not of the patient respectively (Table 1).

The patient's flow requirements depend on the minute ventilation (MV) of the patient. The flow rate of oxygen should be set 3–4 times the calculated MV in case of low flow devices, e.g. a 5 kg child breathing at rate of 60/min requires a flow rate of 6–7 L/min [considering the average tidal volume (VT) of 6 mL/kg]. Since this flow rate is high and may pass the humidifying surfaces quickly and humidification is required. Humidification must be provided if flow rates are high (>6–8 L/min).

LOW-FLOW OR VARIABLE-CONCENTRATION DEVICES

Devices that are unable to meet the flow requirements of the patient (low-flow device) cause entrainment of the room air in addition to the oxygen he/she is getting through the oxygen delivery device. The FiO_2 delivered through low-flow device will therefore depend on oxygen flow, patient's respiratory efforts (flow requirement), and amount of entrained air and is variable (22–60%). These devices can be used in children with mild-to-moderate distress when the FiO_2 need is less.

Blow-By Oxygen

Blow-by oxygen delivery is the simplest form of oxygen delivery. It is a tubing connected to a simple mask and placed in front of patient's mouth and nose. The delivery of FiO_2 is unreliable and may vary between 30% and 40% at flow of 10 L/min. It is usually indicated in those patients

Table 1: Low-flow and high-flow oxygen delivery devices.	
Low-flow or variable-concentration devices	*High-flow or fixed-concentration devices*
• Blow-by oxygen • Nasal prongs • Intranasal catheter • Simple oxygen masks • Partial rebreathing mask	• Venturi mask • Oxygen hood • Oxygen and face tents • Nonrebreathing mask • High flow nasal cannula

who cannot tolerate other cumbersome oxygen delivery devices and need lower FiO_2 for a short period of time or intermittently.

Nasal Prongs/Cannula (Fig. 1A)

Nasal cannula remains one of the most commonly used delivery devices. It consists of two soft prongs, which rest in patient's anterior nares and a long oxygen tubing that connects to oxygen source. The delivered FiO_2 depends upon set flow, patient's flow demand, and amount of entrained room air and varies from 22% to 60% at flow of 0.25–4 L/min. Though the FiO_2 delivered to the patient is variable, it remains an effective method of providing oxygen in mild-to-moderate distress.

Simple Facemask (Fig. 1B)

It consists of a plastic mask with perforations which act as exhalation as well as entrainment ports. The mask adds 100–200 mL to the capacity of the reservoir. The mask fits the face well and is often loose enough to allow entrainment of room air. The FiO_2 provided by the mask is not very high (33–60% at 6–10 L/min) and therefore facemasks should not be used in presence of moderate to severe hypoxemia. The delivered FiO_2 may decrease if child's respiratory flow increases, mask is ill fitting, or when flow rate into mask is low. Facemask tends to increase agitation in young children, but may be easily used in older children.

Intranasal Catheter (Fig. 1C)

It consists of soft plastic tubing that is inserted into nasopharynx and an oxygen tubing attached to an oxygen source. It will provide low FiO_2 between 25% and 40% depending upon oxygen

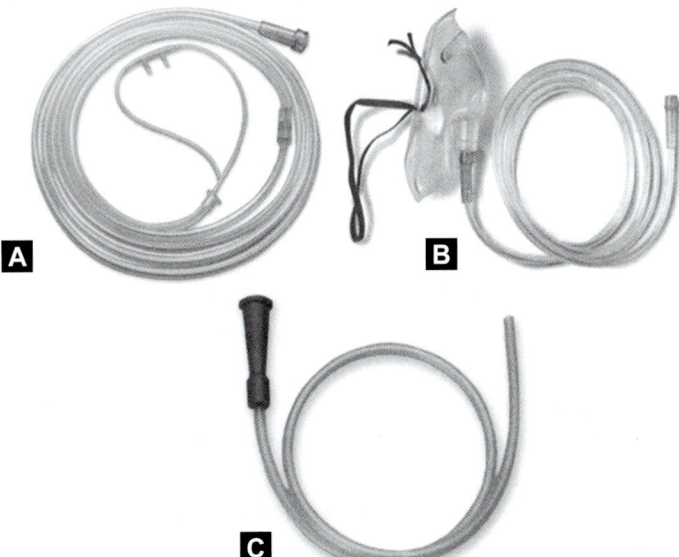

Figs. 1A to C: Low-flow oxygen delivery devices. (A) Nasal prongs/cannula; (B) Simple facemask; (C) Intranasal catheter.

flow rate, inspiratory flow rate of the patient, nasal and oropharyngeal resistance, tidal volume, and nasopharyngeal volume. A high-flow rate more than 4–6 L/min through intranasal catheter irritates the nasopharynx.

Partial Rebreathing Mask

It consists of a facemask, reservoir, two-way valve between mask and reservoir and two-way expiratory valve. The additional reservoir increases the capacity of oxygen by 600–1,000 mL. The two-way valve between reservoir and mask allows the oxygen from source to enter mask as well as initial part of exhaled volume from the anatomical dead space, which is rich in oxygen to enter reservoir. This allows the accumulation of oxygen enriched gas in the reservoir for rebreathing. The two-way expiratory valve allows expiratory gases to exit during expiration and room air to enter during inspiration. Partial rebreathing mask provides up to 60% FiO_2 at flow of 10 L/min. The pitfalls are similar to a simple mask.

HIGH-FLOW OR FIXED-CONCENTRATION DEVICES

The flow though these devices is same or above the patient's flow requirement. Since the flow demand of the patient is met by the device, there will be no entrainment of atmospheric air thus guaranteeing a fixed FiO_2 (low- or high-concentration of oxygen). These devices provide reliable FiO_2 of more than 60% at flow rates of 10 L/min. They are preferred in emergency setting in children with moderate-to-severe distress and shock.

Remember that low-flow devices do not always mean low FiO_2 (e.g. partial rebreathing mask is a low-flow device, but can provide FiO_2 as high as 75%) and high-flow devices do not always mean high FiO_2 (e.g. venturi mask is high-flow device but can provide maximum FiO_2 of 60%). In small infants, low-flow systems can result in high FiO_2.

Air-Entrainment or Venturi Masks (Figs. 2A and B)

Venturi mask is designed to provide a controlled and graded flow and FiO_2 (25–60%) and works on the Bernoulli's principle (Fig. 2B). The oxygen from source is delivered through a narrow orifice (nozzle) at a high flow. This creates a negative lateral wall pressure in the tubing system, which is known as viscous drag. This allows for entrainment of room air through the ports leading to dilution of the oxygen. The desired FiO_2 can be controlled by changing the size of the nozzle, flow rate, and size of the ports. Color-coded venturi masks are available for delivering different FiO_2 based on the size of the nozzle, size of the ports, and flow rate. It is commonly used where gradual weaning of FiO_2 is needed. The advantages of a venturi system include:
- High flow device with guaranteed fixed FiO_2
- Saves oxygen as the high flow comes from the room air.
- It can be used to deliver low FiO_2 also.
- It helps in deciding whether oxygen requirement is increasing or decreasing.
- No need for humidification.
- Fairly cheap and reliable.

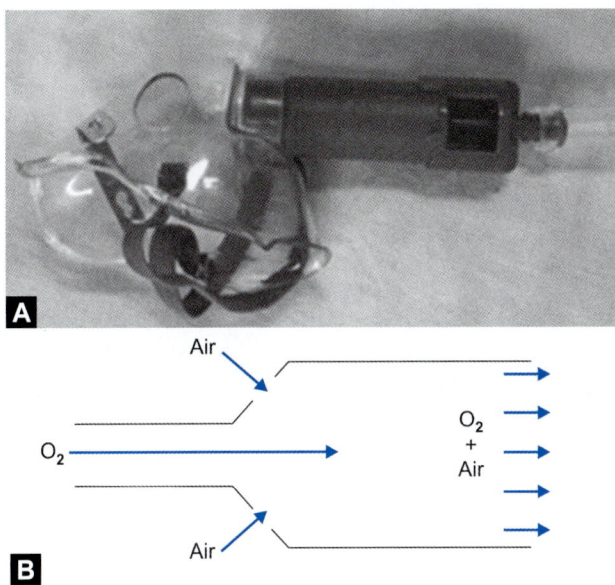

Figs. 2A and B: (A) Venturi mask; (B) Principle of the air-entrainment in venturi mask.

Nonrebreathing Mask (Fig. 3A)

It consists of a facemask, reservoir bag, one-way valve between mask and reservoir, and one-way expiratory valve. One-way expiratory valve prevents entrainment of room air during inspiration. One-way valve between reservoir and mask allows only oxygen from reservoir and not the expired gases to enter the reservoir, thus allowing for inspiring almost pure oxygen. It can deliver FiO_2 of 95% at a flow rate of 10–15 L/min when the mask is well sealed (Table 2). The oxygen flow should be such that the oxygen reservoir remains inflated all the times.

Oxygen Hood (Oxyhood) or Head Box (Fig. 3B)

A clear transparent plastic hood that surrounds the head of the patient. It is commonly used in neonates and small infants. It is available in three to four different sizes. An appropriate size should allow space for the baby's head to fit and free neck and head movement. Bigger hood dilutes the oxygen and too small hood can cause discomfort. The flow of humidified oxygen should be enough to prevent rebreathing of expired gases (usually >10 L/min). It can deliver a fixed oxygen concentration of 80–90% with a flow rate of 10–15 L/min. The oxygen gradients may vary from top to bottom by 20%. Continuous flow at least 6–10 L/min avoids this problem. Oxygen hood is well tolerated by infants; allows easy access to chest, trunk and abdomen; and allows control of concentration, temperature, and humidification of inspired gases. The cold air that condenses on the baby's head can be mistaken for perspiration.

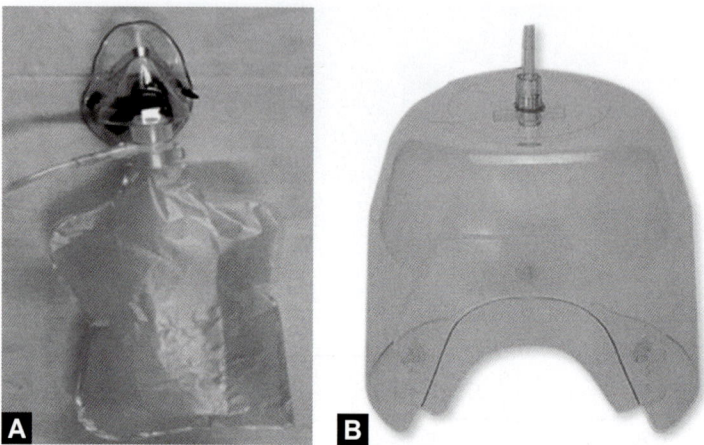
Figs. 3A and B: (A) Nonrebreathing mask; (B) Oxygen hood.

Table 2: Oxygen delivery devices, reservoir capacity, and FiO_2 delivered by them.			
Device	Reservoir capacity	Oxygen flow (L/min)	Approximate FiO_2 (%)
Nasal cannula	50 mL	1	21–24
		2	24–28
		3	28–34
		4	34–38
		5	38–42
		6	42–46
Oxygen facemask	100–300 mL	6	35
		8	45–50
		10	60
Partial rebreathing mask	750–1250 mL	5–7	35–75
Nonrebreathing mask	750–1250 mL	6	55–60
		8	60–80
		10	80–90
		12	90
		15	90–100
Venturi mask		3	24
		3	26
		6	28
		6	30
		9	35
		12	40
		15	50–60
(FiO_2: fraction of inspired oxygen)			

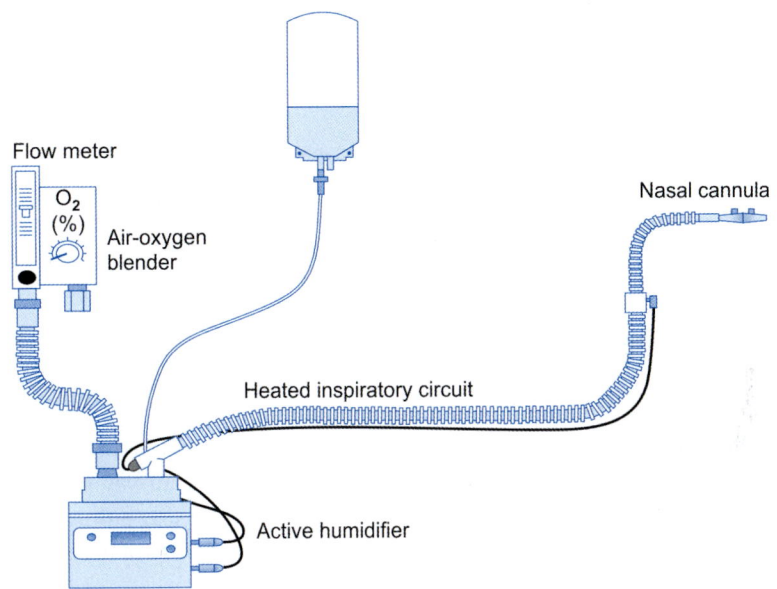

Fig. 4: Setup for high-flow nasal cannula oxygen delivery.

HEATED-HUMIDIFIED HIGH-FLOW NASAL CANNULA (FIG. 4)

Heated-humidified high-flow nasal cannula (HHHFNC) is classified as a high-flow fixed performance oxygen delivery device and provides oxygen at high-flow and high humidity via a nasal cannula.

Before the advent of HHHFNC, the use of flow more than 1 L/min via nasal cannula for newborns and more than 2 L/min in older children was considered uncomfortable primarily because of inadequate humidification. HHHFNC comprises a large bore nasal cannula, a large bore corrugated rubber tubing connected to humidification chamber, humidifier base with controls, oxygen tubing connected to the source, air-oxygen blender, and a stand. The flow delivered by this device can vary from 4 L/min to 70 L/min. The air-oxygen blender allows adjustment of FiO_2. The higher flow, above patient's demand flushes the dead space and prevents entrainment of room air. This ensures delivery of higher flow and FiO_2 in a precise manner that can be hardly achieved by any other devices mentioned above. The FiO_2 delivered ranges from 21–100% and generates flow up to 50–60 L/min. The flow administered is around 2 L/kg/min. The recommended flow rates are less than 2 L/min for premature or term babies, up to 12 L/min for older infants and toddlers, up to 30 L/min for children, and up to 40 L/min for adults. HHHFNC is capable of delivering FiO_2 of 60%, 80%, 90%, and 95% with flow rates of 10, 15, 20, and 30 L/min. It also provides some positive end expiratory pressure (PEEP), depending upon the flow rate and size of the prongs.

Recent evidence suggests that HHHFNC is safe, well-tolerated, and a feasible option for oxygen delivery in infants and young children with moderate-to-severe respiratory distress. Common indications include acute bronchiolitis, pneumonia, congestive cardiac failure,

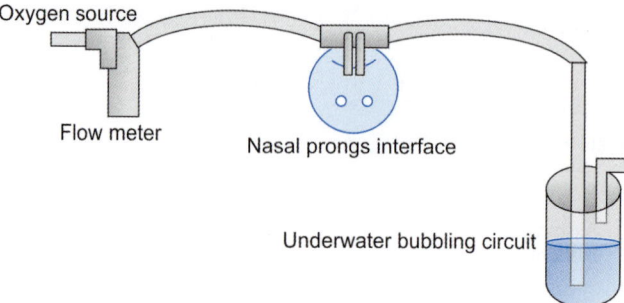

Fig. 5: Bubble continuous positive airway pressure (CPAP) circuit.

apnea of prematurity, and weaning from mechanical ventilation. HHHFNC reduces need for escalation of respiratory support therapy to continuous positive airway pressure (CPAP) or invasive ventilation by decreasing extrathoracic dead space, increasing pulmonary compliance by providing distending pressure, humidification, and reducing work of breathing.

Continuous Positive Airway Pressure (Fig. 5)

Continuous positive airway pressure provides positive airway pressure throughout the respiratory cycle which leads to increase in functional residual capacity (FRC) and improvement in lung compliance and correction of hypoxemia. CPAP is used for providing noninvasive respiratory support for patients with adequate respiratory mechanics and respiratory drive. It also splints and maintains collapsed airways, reduces work of breathing and oxygen consumption, reverses hypoventilation (increasing tidal volume), and improves diaphragmatic activity. CPAP is indicated in bronchial asthma, pulmonary edema, atelectasis, pneumonia, and neuromuscular weakness.

Continuous positive airway pressure can be given using various interfaces like nasal cannula, oronasal mask, nasal mask, full facemask, or endotracheal tube (ET) tube. Indigenous CPAP using underwater seals (made locally with oxygen tubing, nasal cannula, and chest bag or bottle with markings) (Fig. 5) can be used in places where no ventilator driven CPAP is available. The amount of CPAP provided is determined by adjusting the height of water column from tip of the underwater tube to the top of the water level, with 1 cm equals 1 cm H_2O. With oxygen flow of 5–8 L/min, the constant bubbling of gas delivers the CPAP effect. The FiO_2 provided by locally made CPAP systems may however be inaccurate. In standalone CPAP systems, the flow and FiO_2 can be controlled with oxygen blender, but these are expensive.

MONITORING OF A PATIENT ON OXYGEN THERAPY

The patient's response to oxygen therapy should be monitored using clinical parameters (work of breathing and improvement in respiratory distress), pulse oximetry, or arterial blood gases. The monitoring frequency should be individualized and based on severity of hypoxemia, level of FiO_2 required, severity of illness, and oxygen delivery device used.

WEANING FROM OXYGEN THERAPY

With the resolution of the disease process, the flow and FiO_2 can be slowly tapered guided by the clinical parameters and SpO_2. The fixed concentration can be replaced by variable concentration systems. Venturi masks with variable flow and FiO_2 are useful during weaning.

HAZARDS OF OXYGEN

Direct Lung Injury

The lung injury due to oxygen therapy is akin to injury seen in acute respiratory distress syndrome (ARDS) and the severity of injury depends on the concentration and duration of oxygen therapy. Breathing at FiO_2 of 100% for even 3 hours leads to chest pain and for longer period to bronchopneumonia. Exposure to high FiO_2 first damages the capillary endothelium, followed by interstitial edema (0–12 hours), worsening of compliance, and decreased vital capacity (12–30 hours), thickening of alveolar–capillary membrane (30–72 hours), destruction of type I alveolar cells, proliferation of and type II cells, followed by an exudative phase resulting in low V/Q ratio, physiologic shunting, and worsening hypoxemia. Oxygen toxicity has been observed at a FiO_2 more than 60%. When the antioxidant stores in the lungs are depleted, oxygen toxicity may develop even at FiO_2 of less than 60%.

Oxidative Stress

Oxygen increases reactive oxygen species (ROS), such as hydroxyl ion and peroxynitrite, which being unstable react with deoxyribonucleic acid (DNA), lipids, and proteins via oxidative reactions or radical-mediated mechanisms leading to oxidative injury, necrosis, or apoptosis.

The body's antioxidant defense mechanisms (superoxide dismutase, catalase, and glutathione) are either impaired (premature neonates, malnourishment, etc.) or overcome by concentrations of oxygen more than 50%. The former group is at risk for oxygen toxicity even at lower FiO_2 between 25% and 50%. To avoid oxygen toxicity, the best practice is to reduce the FiO_2 to lowest tolerable level, whenever possible.

Injury

Catheters, masks, and dry and nonhumidified gas can cause nasal and oral injuries, thus predisposing to infections.

Absorption Atelectasis (Derecruitment)

High FiO_2 increases risk of absorption atelectasis by depleting alveolar nitrogen levels. The gases within the alveoli rapidly diffuse into the venous blood leading to collapse.

Retinopathy of Prematurity

Babies less than 32 weeks or less than 1,500 g are at higher risk of retinopathy of prematurity (ROP). ROP can be prevented by keeping the desired PaO_2 less than 80 mm Hg and SpO_2 between 88% and 93%. Periodic retinal examination after completion of 32 weeks is mandatory to detect early retinal damage.

Fire

Oxygen supports combustion and hence avoids spark emitting equipments, toys, and near vicinity.

KEYPOINTS

- Oxygen is a drug and it should be used judiciously similar to other drugs.
- Oxygen delivery devices are divided into high and low flow devices based on whether or not they meet the flow demand of the patient.
- Oxygen delivery device should be chosen based on the clinical status of the patient, size of the patient, amount of flow and FiO_2 required, tolerability, and familiarity among clinicians.
- If respiratory distress in not improving on conventional oxygen delivery devices, one can use HHHFNC or CPAP before intubation and mechanical ventilation.
- Oxygen requirement can be decreased by maintaining euthermia, controlling sepsis, optimizing Hb, and cardiac output.
- Oxygen content and cardiac output should be adequate when assessing the effectiveness of oxygen therapy.
- The FiO_2 used should be as minimal as possible and guided by clinical and laboratory parameters.
- The weaning plan should be clear from the beginning and oxygen should be weaned as soon as possible to avoid using oxygen for prolonged period.

SUGGESTED READING

1. Angurana SK, Jayashree M. Know your respiratory crash cart. IAP-ALS Handbook. 1st edition. New Delhi: IAP, National Publication House, Department of Pediatrics, Sir Ganga Ram Hospital. pp. 46-50.
2. Baudin F, Gagnon S, Crulli B, et al. Modalities and complications associated with the use of high-flow nasal cannula: experience in a pediatric ICU. Respir Care. 2016;61:1305-10.
3. Beggs S, Wong ZH, Kaul S, et al. High-flow nasal cannula therapy for infants with bronchiolitis. Cochrane Database Syst Rev. 2014;(1):CD009609.
4. Gilbert-Kawai ET, Mitchell K, Martin D, et al. Permissive hypoxaemia versus normoxaemia for mechanically ventilated critically ill patients. Cochrane Database Syst Rev. 2014;(5): CD009931.
5. Jayashree M, KiranBabu HB, Singhi S, et al. Use of Nasal Bubble CPAP in Children with Hypoxemic Clinical Pneumonia-Report from a Resource Limited Set-Up. J Trop Pediatr. 2016;62:69-74.
6. Kubicka ZJ, Limauro J, Darnall RA. Heated, humidified high-flow nasal cannula therapy: yet another way to deliver continuous positive airway pressure? Pediatrics. 2008;121:82-8.
7. Mikalsen IB, Davis P, Øymar K. High flow nasal cannula in children: a literature review. Scand J Trauma Resusc Emerg Med. 2016;24:93.
8. Milési C, Boubal M, Jacquot A, et al. High-flow nasal cannula: recommendations for daily practice in pediatrics. Ann Intensive Care. 2014;4:29.
9. Myers TR, American Association for Respiratory Care (AARC). AARC clinical practice guideline: selection of an oxygen delivery device for neonatal and pediatric patients: 2002 revision & update. Respir Care. 2002;47(6):707-16.
10. Nishimura M. High-Flow Nasal Cannula Oxygen Therapy in Adults: Physiological Benefits, Indication, Clinical Benefits, and Adverse Effects. Respir Care. 2016;61:529-41.

11. Pham TM, O'Malley L, Mayfield S, et al. The effect of high flow nasal cannula therapy on the work of breathing in infants with bronchiolitis. Pediatr Pulmonol. 2015;50:713-20.
12. Slain KN, Shein SL, Rotta AT. The use of high-flow nasal cannula in the pediatric emergency department. J Pediatr (Rio J). 2017;93 Suppl 1:36-45.
13. ten Brink F, Duke T, Evans J. High-flow nasal prong oxygen therapy or nasopharyngeal continuous positive airway pressure for children with moderate-to-severe respiratory distress? Pediatr Crit Care Med. 2013;14(7):e326-31.
14. Walsh BK, Smallwood CD. Pediatric Oxygen Therapy: A Review and Update. Respir Care. 2017; 62:645-61.

Lung Mechanics with Ventilation: Physiology and Monitoring

6

Abdul Rauf, Neeraj Gupta

LEARNING OBJECTIVES

- To understand the basic physiological aspect of lung mechanics
- To know the important lung mechanics parameters to be monitored during ventilation
- To learn the concepts of airway driving pressure and transpulmonary pressure

INTRODUCTION

Mechanical ventilators have undergone progressive evolution over the past few years. Apart from advanced ventilator modes, other innovations including novel monitoring techniques have come up. The monitoring potential of modern ventilators provides an opportunity to apply and use respiratory physiology at the bedside.

Assessment of respiratory mechanics has a crucial role in the management of critically ill patients undergoing mechanical ventilation. Thus, it may help to:
- Understand the pathophysiology of the underlying disease process
- Assess the progression or improvement of the disease process
- Guide therapeutic measures like positive end-expiratory pressure (PEEP) titration
- Take measures to prevent ventilator-induced lung injury (VILI).

Despite the virtues of monitoring lung mechanics in ventilated patients, these measurements are neither regularly performed nor incorporated into practice in many units. Underuse of these parameters by physicians might be due to the preconception that these measurements are difficult to interpret. It is true that majority of the data and graphs which scroll on the ventilator display screen do not receive the deserved attention.

Selection of the right parameter to monitor and correct data interpretation in the clinical scenario is crucial while monitoring respiratory mechanics. In this chapter, the authors give a simplified description of the physiology and monitoring of lung mechanics in ventilated children, with focus on parameters with practical utility.

PHYSIOLOGY OF RESPIRATORY MECHANICS

Mechanical Properties of the Respiratory System

Ventilation involves movement of the chest wall to produce a pressure gradient that will permit flow and movement of gases. The parameters commonly used to describe the mechanical properties of the respiratory system in relation to elastic and frictional forces opposing lung inflation are compliance and resistance, respectively.

Resistance: Resistance is a measure of the frictional forces that must be overcome during breathing. Predominant frictional force acting is due to the anatomical structure of the airways. The resistance offered by tissues is less in normal conditions. An equation for airway resistance, which describes the relationship between gas flow, pressure, and resistance in the airways, is:

$$R_{aw} = P_{TA}/\text{flow}$$

Or the P_{TA} = Flow resistive pressure = $R_{aw} \times$ flow

[R_{aw}—airway resistance, P_{TA}—transairway pressure (pressure difference between the mouth and the alveolus)]

Compliance: The compliance (C) of any object is the relative ease with which it can be distended. Elastance (e) is the inverse of compliance; it is the tendency of a structure to return to its original form after being stretched.

Thus, $\quad C = 1/e \text{ or } e = 1/C.$

In practice, compliance values are calculated commonly than elastance to describe the elastic forces that oppose lung inflation. The compliance of the respiratory system is determined by measuring the change (Δ) of volume (V) that occurs when pressure (P) is applied to the system:

$$C = \Delta V/\Delta P$$

It is to be noted that compliance of the respiratory system will depend upon compliance of lung and chest wall. The compliance of respiratory system will be lower than the individual values of compliance of the lung and chest wall as the two add in parallel (elastance, the inverse, add in series).

Equation of Motion

Displacement of gases always occurs in response to a pressure gradient, created by positive pressure ventilation in case of a mechanical ventilator. The fundamental theory of respiratory mechanics is explained by the equation of motion. Both ventilator and respiratory muscles can apply pressures to the respiratory system, a total of which should be equal to the sum of opposing pressures in the system. The opposing respiratory system pressures at any time has a resistance component as the air flows through the airway (P_{res}), an elastic component necessary for the distension of the pulmonary parenchyma (P_{el}), and an inertial component (P_{in})

Equation of motion: $\quad P_{vent} + P_{mus} = P_{el} + P_{res} + P_{in}$

(P_{vent}—ventilator pressure, P_{mus}—muscle pressure, P_{res}—flow resistive pressure, and P_{el}—elastic recoil pressure)

In case of controlled ventilation with a patient completely sedated and paralysed, the value of P_{mus} is zero. Also the inertance is usually practically negligible in most clinical conditions. Hence, the equation can be modified in controlled ventilation as:

$$P_{vent} = P_{el} + P_{res}$$

As described earlier, the flow resistive pressure (P_{res}) is calculated as a product of flow and resistance. And the elastic recoil pressure is given as the product of elastance and volume

$$P_{res} = V' \times R_{aw} \ (V'\text{—flow}, R\text{—airway resistance})$$
$$P_{el} = E_{rs} \times V = 1/C_{rs} \times \Delta V$$

(E—elastance of respiratory system, ΔV—tidal volume, and C_{rs}—compliance of respiratory system)

Combining the above three equations,

$$P_{vent} = \text{flow} \times \text{resistance} + \text{elastance} (1/\text{compliance}) \times \Delta\text{volume}$$
$$P_{vent} = V' \times R_{aw} + \Delta V/C_{rs} \ (V'\text{—flow})$$

Ventilator pressure is identical to P_{aw} (airway opening pressure). A component of PEEP also needs to be added to the opposing forces when external PEEP is applied, hence the equation can also be written as:

$$P_{aw} = V' \times R_{aw} + \Delta V/C_{rs} + PEEP_{total} \quad (1)$$
$$(PEEP_{total} = PEEP_{external} + PEEP_{intrinsic})$$

For an easy understanding, the equation of motion is schematically represented in Figure 1.

Principles of the Measurements of Static Respiratory Mechanics

The classic measurements of respiratory mechanics such as compliance, resistance, and $PEEP_{total}$ are performed in paralyzed patients during controlled ventilation with a constant inspiratory flow (volume control mode). For these measurements, it is necessary to interrupt the normal ventilatory pattern with two-airway occlusion maneuvers, one performed at the end inspiration, and the other one at the end expiration.

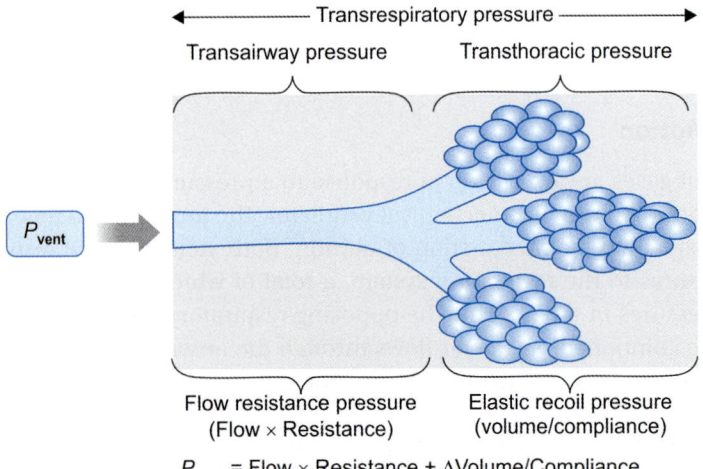

Fig. 1: Schematic model depicting the key elements of the equation of motion.

In the equation of motion, parameters such as P_{aw}, ΔV, and V' are set or directly measured by the ventilator. Other parameters C_{rs}, R_{aw}, and $PEEP_{total}$ need to be calculated by applying different maneuvers.

End-inspiratory Occlusion Maneuver

Application of end-inspiratory hold results in a no-flow state where the pressure measured will depend only upon the elastic recoil pressure, which is called the plateau pressure (P_{plat}).

End-expiratory Occlusion Maneuver

The pressure measured during the end-expiratory hold maneuver (when both flow and ΔV are zero) gives the value of $PEEP_{total}$. Both occlusions are generally performed by means of internal valves of the ventilator operated by specific knobs on the ventilator.

Calculation of Resistance and Static Compliance

As the flow is nil during an inspiratory hold, equation of motion will get modified as:

$$P_{plat} = \Delta V / C_{rs} + PEEP_{total} \quad (2)$$
$$\text{Or} \quad C_{rs} = \Delta V / (P_{plat} - PEEP_{total})$$

This compliance value measured during no flow condition is called static compliance (C_{stat}). P_{aw} measured at maximum inspiration is called peak pressure (P_{peak}) or peak inspiratory pressure (PIP). On subtraction of equation (2) from (1),

$$P_{peak} - P_{plat} = V' \times R_{aw}$$
$$\text{Or} \quad R_{aw} = (P_{peak} - P_{plat})/\text{flow} = P_{transairway}/\text{flow}$$

C_{stat} calculation needs the measurements of the elastic recoil pressures of the respiratory system—P_{plat} by end-inspiratory hold and also the $PEEP_{tot}$ obtained by the end-expiratory occlusion. Resistance measurement needs only P_{plat} measurement by inspiratory hold. A pressure time curve in volume control ventilation depicting the use of inspiratory hold maneuver is shown in Figure 2.

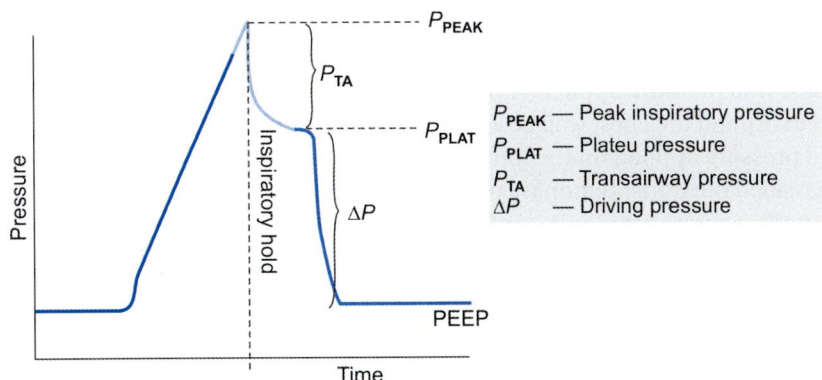

Fig. 2: Pressure–time curve in volume control mode with use of an inspiratory hold maneuver. (PEEP: positive end-expiratory pressure)

Another simplified approach to calculate static mechanics in a paralyzed patient on controlled mode with a constant inspiratory flow, is to apply a small end-inspiratory pause without end-expiratory occlusion. An end-inspiratory pause of 10–20% of the total cycle time corresponds to an end-inspiratory occlusion maneuver, though does not guarantee a real static condition. The advantage of such a short occlusion is that it may be included in the respiratory pattern set in the mechanical ventilator, thus allowing breath-by-breath monitoring of respiratory mechanics. However, the limitation of this simplified approach is the lack of an end-expiratory occlusion and uses the value read for set PEEP as an estimate of the $PEEP_{total}$. With this approach, the measurements of both R and C_{stat} may be underestimated due to insufficient pressure equilibration during the inspiratory pause, resulting in overestimation of P_{plat}. However, the results may be reasonably correct in patients with short respiratory system time constant, such as the acute respiratory distress syndrome (ARDS) patients.

Measurement of Dynamic Respiratory Mechanics

Static methods for measuring respiratory mechanics, though accurate, have some limitations like requirement of ventilator manipulation. Moreover, they are not continuous and the occlusion maneuvers may interfere with the ventilator settings. Advanced ventilators have built-in pressure transducers and pneumotachographs to permit continuous measurement of pressure and flow. By incorporating these data into linear mathematical models, such as the least squares fit method, measurements of respiratory mechanics can potentially be monitored continuously without ventilator manipulation. With a constant understanding of flow, pressure, and volume, other variables (compliance, resistance, and auto-PEEP) respiratory mechanics can be measured. The least square fit method requires no special respiratory pattern and no occlusion maneuver. Hence, it can be applied on a breath-by-breath basis, in any ventilation mode, with any inspiratory flow pattern, only provided that the patient is relaxed. A continuous monitoring enables an early detection of alteration in disease process and can help in rapid therapeutic response. However, patient–ventilator interaction and the mathematical error of "fitting" nonlinear patient breaths into linear mathematical models will always create some degree of fallacy in dynamic measurements.

Dissociation of Lung Mechanics from Chest Wall

As the respiratory system is composed by two elastic structures connected in series, the lung and the chest wall pressure applied at the airway opening is used in part to inflate the lungs and in part to expand the chest wall according to their relative compliances.

The real pressure applied on the lungs is the difference between P_{aw} and pleural pressure (P_{pl}), and is called the transpulmonary pressure (P_L or P_{tp}).

During end-inspiratory hold, $P_{plat} = P_{aw}$

$$P_L = P_{plat} - P_{pl} \ (P_{pl}\text{—pleural pressure})$$

Thus, transpulmonary and plateau pressures can be significantly different in the presence of chest wall abnormalities causing elevated pleural pressure values. In other words, a high P_{plat} value can be non-injurious in a patient with relatively normal lung compliance but with a very stiff chest wall.

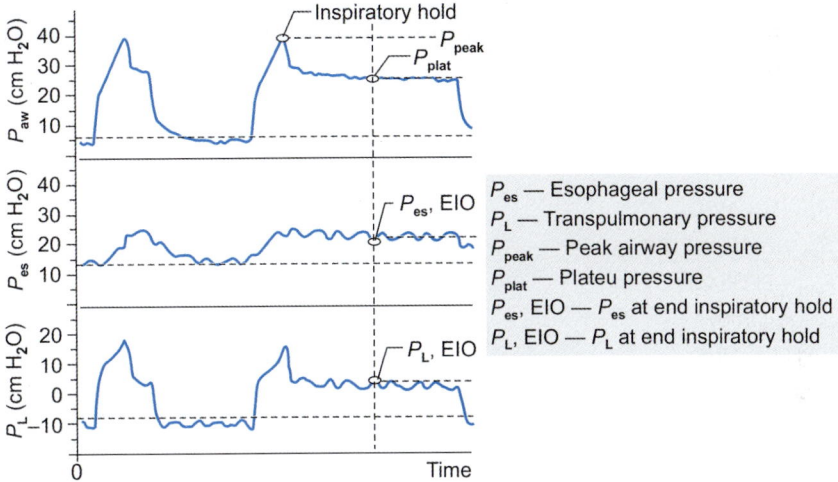

Fig. 3: Determination of transpulmonary pressure using P_{es} ($P_L = P_{aw} - P_{es}$) and application of inspiratory hold.

The most common method used for estimating P_{pl} at the bedside is esophageal manometry. The pressure measured by means of a catheter positioned in the lower third of the esophagus (P_{es}) is considered a reasonable surrogate of the average P_{pl} surrounding the lungs.

When a P_{es} signal is available, classic measurements of respiratory mechanics can provide data concerning the chest wall and lungs separately.

$$P_L = P_{plat} - P_{es}$$

The same maneuvers like end-inspiratory hold used for total respiratory system mechanics can be used for separate chest wall and lung mechanics, provided that a P_{es} signal is available (Fig. 3).

The important mathematical equations related to lung mechanics are summarized in Table 1.

Monitoring of Lung Mechanics

Bedside monitoring of pulmonary mechanics provides important information related to the status of the disease and the impact of mechanical ventilation. It should be an integral component of daily care of ventilated children. The Pediatric Acute Lung Injury consensus conference (PALICC) group strongly recommends to continuously monitor inspiratory pressures (PIP or P_{plat}), exhaled tidal volume, pressure-time, and flow-time scalars during invasive ventilation in children with pediatric acute respiratory distress syndrome (PARDS). Apart from these parameters and pressure–volume (PV) loops, in this section, authors discuss about airway driving pressure and transpulmonary pressures, considering the recent interest and growing literature with these.

Table 1: Summary of key equations—mathematics of lung mechanics.

Rescuer	Actions
$R_{aw} = P_{TA}/\text{flow}$	R_{aw}—airway resistance, V'—flow
$C = 1/e = \Delta V/\Delta P$	C—compliance, e—elastance
$P_{vent} = P_{res} + P_{el}$	C_{rs}—compliance of respiratory system
$P_{res} = V' \times R_{aw}, P_{el} = \Delta V/C_{rs}$	P_{res}—airway resistance pressure
$P_{aw} = V' \times R_{aw} + \Delta V/C_{rs} + PEEP_{total}$	P_{el}—elastic recoil pressure
$C_{rs} = \Delta V/(P_{plat} - PEEP_{total})$	P_{peak}—peak pressure, P_{plat}—plateau pressure
$R_{aw} = (P_{peak} - P_{plat})/\text{flow}$	P_L—transpulmonary pressure
$\Delta P = P_{plat} - PEEP = \Delta V/C_{rs}$	ΔP—driving pressure
$P_L = P_{plat} - P_{pl} = P_{plat} - P_{es}$	P_{pl}—pleural pressure, P_{es}—esophageal pressure

(PEEP: positive end-expiratory pressure)

Inspiratory Pressures (Peak Inspiratory Pressure and Plateau Pressure)

The measurement of inspiratory pressure aims to contemplate the pressure applied to the alveoli at the end of inspiration. This is important as these pressures are one of the prime causes for VILI.

During pressure-regulated ventilation, inspiratory pressure is relatively stable over inspiration, and peak pressure (PIP) is considered to evaluate inspiratory pressure. In volume-controlled ventilator mode, the PIP is much influenced by the resistance of the airways; in those cases, the plateau pressure (P_{plat}) better reflects the lung elastic recoil pressure. As described earlier, plateau pressure is measured with a no flow state produced by an inspiratory pause, in the absence of spontaneous breathing. It is advisable to keep the PIP value <30 cm H_2O and P_{plat} value <25 cm H_2O to minimize the risk of VILI.

Exhaled Tidal Volume

Excess tidal volumes can also contribute to VILI (volutrauma) like excess ventilator pressures (barotrauma). Continuous monitoring of exhaled tidal volume during invasive ventilation in children with PARDS is recommended, to prevent injurious ventilation. Use of low tidal volume set according to the ideal body weight of the patient (4–8 mL/kg) is an important component of lung protective ventilation. Monitoring exhaled tidal volume can also help in identifying leaks (significant difference between inspiratory and expiratory tidal volume in pressure-controlled ventilation).

Compliance

Decreased lung compliance is one of the important features of ARDS In ARDS, compliance measurements are useful in assessing the severity, monitoring improvement, and in adjusting ventilator settings like PEEP titration.

Static compliance calculation in controlled ventilation using constant flow can be done using the formula $C_{rs} = \Delta V/(P_{plat} - PEEP_{total})$. Of course, this requires the child to be paralyzed and application of inspiratory and expiratory hold maneuvers.

As mentioned previously, the dynamic compliance values displayed by modern ventilators should be interpreted with caution, as they can be fallacious. However, they provide some information and may be used to see the trends in improvement. The slope of the quasi-static pressure volume loop is a reference method to evaluate compliance of the respiratory system, but its use in clinical practice is complex as discussed in the section below.

Pressure-time and Flow-time Scalars

Apart from pressure-time scalar, monitoring of the flow-time curves is also recommended by the PALICC group to detect the expiratory flow limitation, patient–ventilator asynchrony and to assess the accuracy of the respiratory times.

Pressure–Volume Loop

The static pressure–volume loops can provide much information on the mechanical properties of the respiratory system. It is obtained using the graphic representation of lung volume for a particular pressure in the absence of airway flow. Hence, the pressure measurement is the true elastic recoil pressure of the lung, which may guide ventilation therapy like estimation of C_{rs} (given by the slope of PV loop) and PEEP adjustment. A static PV loop which shows the characteristic recordings is shown in Figure 4.

The older concepts of identification of lower inflection point (LIP) as an indication of recruitment and PEEP setting above LIP is now challenged. It is now known that alveolar recruitment occurs on a stretch of this loop and optimal PEEP should be evaluated in the expiratory limb. There are many concerns which make the static PV loop not useful in routine clinical practice. The acquisition of static pressure–volume loops requires complex methods like super syringe technique and the interpretation can also be difficult. More importantly, there is little conclusive evidence regarding the clinical benefit of the using them, even in adult population. Hence, they continue to be used more as a research tool.

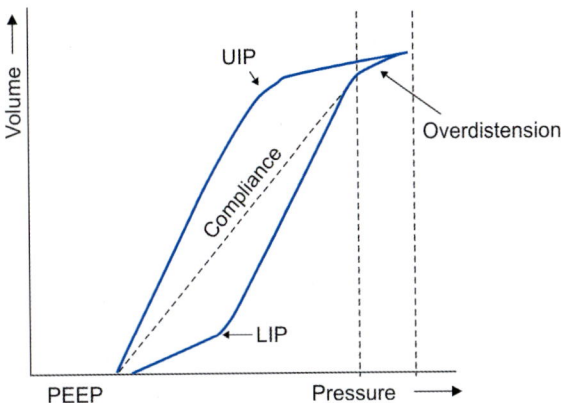

Fig. 4: A static PV loop showing lower inflection point (LIP), upper inflection point (UIP), compliance, and zone of overdistension.
(PV: pressure–volume)

The most present generation ventilators display the dynamic pressure–volume continuously.

In comparison with the static loops, these loops are obtained during airflow and are impacted by the resistance component of the system. Therefore, dynamic pressure–volume loops should be looked at with caution.

Airway Driving Pressure

In ARDS patients, the lung available for ventilation is significantly and not uniformly reduced among different patients (concept of "baby lung"), a similar tidal volume based on ideal body weight can generate different lung stress/strain in different patients.

Airway driving pressure is measured as the airway pressure changes from PEEP to end-inspiratory plateau pressure (Fig. 1) and is equivalent to the ratio between the tidal volume and compliance of respiratory system.

$$\text{Driving pressure } (\Delta P) = P_{\text{plat}} - \text{PEEP} = \Delta V/C_{\text{rs}}$$

Driving pressure represents the cyclic strain to which the lung parenchyma is subjected during each ventilatory cycle and correlates directly with the transpulmonary pressure. It can reflect the lung injury better because it allows adjusting the tidal volume according to the lung compliance in the patient. There is a noteworthy interest in the concept of driving pressure ever since Amato et al. demonstrated that driving pressure, as opposed to tidal volume and PEEP, was the variable that best correlated with survival in patients with ARDS. Though seemingly simple, it is an elegant concept that promises to simplify the optimization of mechanical ventilation in patients with ARDS.

A high-driving pressure is strongly associated with higher mortality and morbidity. However, exact safe limits of the driving pressure have not been identified and the generally accepted cutoff is 15 cm H_2O. As of now, with the available evidence, it seems wise to monitor driving pressure and use ventilation strategies that limit driving pressure below 15 cm H_2O.

Transpulmonary Pressure

Transpulmonary pressure is the actual pressure exerted upon the lung which is responsible for VILI while airway driving pressure represents the pressure change across the entire respiratory system. Hence, transpulmonary driving pressure (ΔP_L) should better reflect lung stress than airway driving pressure. ΔP_L is the difference between the static value of driving airway and pleural pressures, with pleural pressure estimated by esophageal pressure (P_{es}).

$$\Delta P_L = (P_{\text{plat}} - \text{end-inspiratory } P_{\text{es}}) - (\text{PEEP} - \text{end-expiratory } P_{\text{es}})$$

Few studies on use of transpulmonary driving pressure for PEEP titration targeted to achieve positive values of end-expiratory P_L, while maintaining end-inspiratory P_L to less than 25 cm H_2O. In a study by Talmor et al, patients in the intervention group where PEEP titration was done using transpulmonary pressure had significantly higher PEEP levels and improvement in oxygenation and lung compliance (Fig. 5).

Though promising, the exact role of transpulmonary pressure as a therapeutic target for titration of mechanical ventilation settings is still unclear and needs further evaluation in prospective studies. Moreover, the sparse availability of ventilators equipped with the module

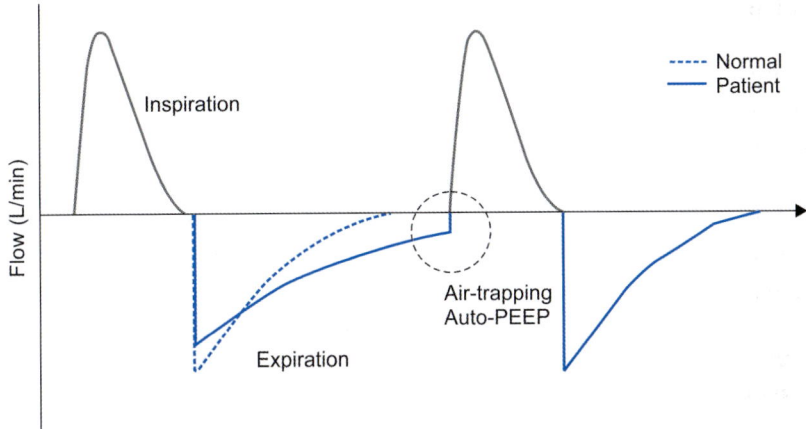

Fig. 5: A flow time curve in pressure control ventilation showing auto-PEEP. (PEEP: positive end-expiratory pressure)

to measure P_L and the questionable reliability of estimating P_L by P_{es}, limit the use of this modality in clinical practice.

Routine monitoring of other parameters of respiratory mechanics like flow–volume loop, stress index, functional residual capacity (FRC), assessment of respiratory muscle activity using airway occlusion pressure (P0.1) is not recommended and hence a detailed description of those parameters are beyond the scope of this chapter. Interested readers can read related excellent reviews.

SUGGESTED READING

1. Akoumianaki E, Maggiore SM, Valenza F, et al. PLUG Working Group (Acute Respiratory Failure Section of the European Society of Intensive Care Medicine). The application of esophageal pressure measurement in patients with respiratory failure. Am J Respir Crit Care Med. 2014;189:520-31.
2. Albaiceta GM, Luyando LH, Parra D, et al. Inspiratory vs. pressure-volume curves to set end-expiratory pressure in acute lung injury. Intensive Care Med. 2005;31:1370-81.
3. Amato MB, Meade MO, Slutsky AS, et al. Driving pressure and survival in the acute respiratory distress syndrome. N Engl J Med. 2015;372:747-55.
4. Bryan AC, Wohl ME. Respiratory mechanics in Children. In: Terjung R (Ed). Comprehensive Physiology; 2011.
5. Bugedo G, Retamal J, Bruhn A. Driving pressure: A marker of severity, a safety limit, or a goal for mechanical ventilation? Crit Care. 2017;21:199.
6. Crotti S, Mascheroni D, Caironi P, et al. Recruitment and derecruitment during acute respiratory failure: A clinical study. Am J Respir Crit Care Med. 2001;164:131-40.
7. Gattinoni L, Pesenti A. The concept of baby lung. Intensive Care Med. 2005;31:776-84.
8. Grinnan DC, Truwit JD. Clinical review: Respiratory mechanics in spontaneous and assisted ventilation. Crit Care. 2005;9:472-84.
9. Henderson WR, Chen L, Amato MBP, et al. Fifty years of research in ARDS. Respiratory mechanics in acute respiratory distress syndrome. Am J Respir Crit Care Med. 2017;196:822-33.
10. Lucangelo U, Bernabè F, Blanch L. Lung mechanics at the bedside: Make it simple. Curr Opin Crit Care. 2007;13:64-72.

11. Pediatric Acute Lung Injury Consensus Conference Group. Pediatric acuterespiratory distress syndrome: Consensus recommendations from the Pediatric AcuteLung Injury Consensus Conference. Pediatr Crit Care Med. 2015;16:428-39.
12. Polese G, Serra A, Rossi A. Respiratory mechanics in the intensive care unit. Eur Respir Monogr. 2005;31:195-206.
13. Rosen WC, Mammel MC, Fisher JB, et al. The effects of bedside pulmonary mechanics testing during infant mechanical ventilation: A retrospective analysis. Pediatr Pulmonol. 1993;16:147-52.
14. Talmor D, Sarge T, Malhotra A, et al. Mechanical ventilation guided by esophageal pressure in acute lung injury. N Engl J Med. 2008;359:2095-104.

Basics of Mechanical Ventilation

7

Arun Kumar Baranwal, Namita Ravikumar

LEARNING OBJECTIVES

- To understand the pathophysiology of respiration and mechanics of ventilation
- To know the various terminologies used in mechanical ventilation
- To get a brief overview of the common modes of invasive mechanical ventilation
- Initial settings in various pathologies and monitoring of a ventilated child.

INTRODUCTION

Mechanical ventilator is a device system that supports or takes over the mechanical function of the body's respiratory system till resolution of the primary disease. It helps in inflating the lung with gas, helps in opening up of alveoli and expiration. The ventilator improves gas exchange in pulmonary parenchymal diseases by opening the alveolar units and by creating a concentration gradient of oxygen across the respiratory membrane. The failing myocardium is supported by provision of positive pressure, which reduces afterload on the left ventricle. It helps in providing controlled ventilation in disorders of central nervous system and raised intracranial pressure, while it acts as a mechanical pump in neuromuscular disorders. In order to deliver disease-specific targets through mechanical ventilation, we need to understand the physiology and mechanics of ventilation.

INDICATIONS

Most common indications for mechanical ventilation include:
- *Respiratory failure*: Clinically, increased work of breathing and fatigue are indications for mechanical ventilation. Although there are no absolute blood gas parameters to initiate the need for mechanical ventilation, generally PaO_2 less than 60 mm Hg, $PaCO_2$ more than 60 mm Hg, and pH less than 7.25 would need ventilation. The target is not to normalize blood gas parameters but to maintain adequate oxygenation and ventilation required for cellular metabolism, without causing damage to the lung till the disease process resolves.
- *Myocardial dysfunction*: Positivet pressure reduces afterload on the left ventricular failure.

- Disordered control of breathing secondary to CNS causes.
- *Raised intracranial pressure*: Controlling minute ventilation to target a narrow range of normocapnia.
- *Neuromuscular disorders*: It takes over the function of the respiratory muscles.
- *Septic shock*: To reduce demand–supply mismatch by decreasing the work of breathing and by improving the cardiac output through reduction in left ventricular afterload.

VENTILATOR HARDWARE

The set-up of a ventilator consists of a gas source, humidification system, energy source, ventilator circuit, control system regulating gas inflow and outflow, display monitor with alarms and finally the interface which attaches to the patient.
- *Gas source:* It consists of a continuous supply of medical air and oxygen to the ventilator as a compressed gas source. The gas source could be from central supply through pipes or oxygen cylinders with compressor.
- *Humidification system:* As the air delivered from the gas source is cold and dry, it needs to be heated to body temperature and humidified before entering the patient.

    A heated humidification system consists of a heating base, humidifying chamber filled with sterile water, and heater wires which heat the gases up to the inspiratory limb connecting to the interface. There are sensor cables which measure and maintain the temperature at beginning and end of heater wire.

Heat moisture exchanger: It is a small device attached closed to the interface which traps the moisture from the patient's expired gas to humidify the inspired gases.
- *Energy source:* Ventilator and humidifier require electrical power source for functioning but most ventilators have backup in case of power supply failure.
- *Display monitors:* Computer monitors display the set and measured variables in both numerical and graphic format.
- *Interface:* Interface in invasive ventilation is appropriate-sized endotracheal tube. Leaks around the tracheal tube can happen if smaller tubes are used.

PHYSIOLOGY

The normal spontaneous respiration is negative pressure ventilation. The respiratory centers located in the pons and medulla control the trigger and rate. Inspiration is initiated by the contraction of intercostal muscles in a bucket handle fashion and the diaphragm. It causes fall in the intrathoracic pressure and creates a negative intrapleural pressure followed by negative intra-alveolar pressure. As air moves from a high pressure region to low pressure region, the air flows from the atmosphere to the alveoli leading to inflation of lung (Fig. 1). The expiration occurs passively due to the natural recoil properties of lung and chest wall.

Mechanical ventilation could be negative or positive pressure ventilation. The early ventilators used during the epidemic of poliomyelitis were negative pressure ventilators. The present-day ventilators are positive pressure ventilators wherein the compressed air is pushed into the lung under positive pressure. The lung and airways function as a unit akin to the balloon and a tube through which air is blown. The equation of motion gives the relationship between the pressure (P), volume (V), and flow (F). The pressure required to inflate the alveoli needs to overcome the resistive property of the airway and the compliance of the lung and chest wall.

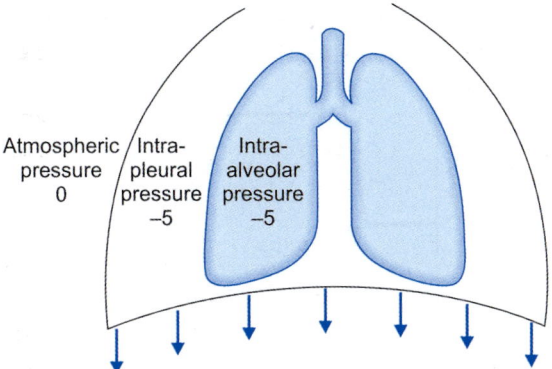

Fig. 1: Negative pressure generated by diaphragmatic and intercostal muscle contraction during spontaneous inspiration.

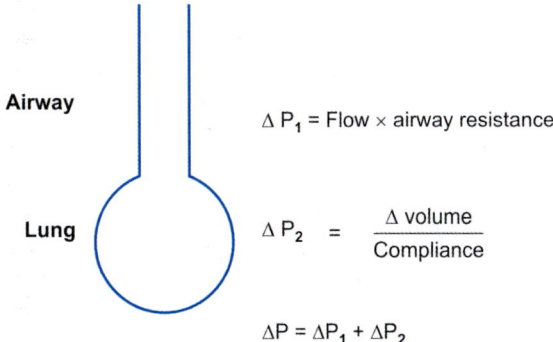

Fig. 2: Pressures required to push gas through airway and lung during positive pressure ventilation.

Resistance across a given tubular structure is the opposition to airflow. Here, it includes the ventilator tubings, the endotracheal tube, and patient's airway. According to Poiseuille's equation, the resistance across the airway would be inversely related to the fourth power of the radius. Any small occlusion or block would markedly increase the resistance across the airway. Pressure needed (ΔP_1) to overcome airway resistance is given by the product of flow (F) and airway resistance (R) (Fig. 2).

$$\Delta P_1 = F \times R$$

Compliance of the lung and chest wall determines the pressure required to inflate the lungs after the airway resistance is overcome. Compliance is the property which determines its ability to undergo a change in terms of volume. High compliance means large change in volume for a given unit change in pressure, while poor compliance is when a higher pressure is required for a small change in volume. Elastance is the reciprocal of compliance and the property by which a substance retains its shape (Fig. 2).

Compliance = $\Delta V / \Delta P_2$

$$\Delta P = \Delta P_1 + \Delta P_2$$

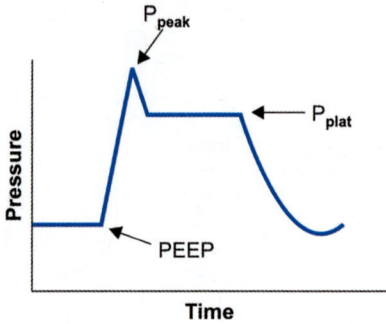

Fig. 3: The baseline pressure (PEEP), peak inspiratory pressure (P_{peak}/PIP) and plateau pressure (P_{plat}) during inspiration.

The total pressure required (ΔP) to push the gas into the lung will thus be a sum of pressure required to overcome the resistance of the airway and the compliance of the lung and the chest wall, and is defined by the equation of motion, obtained by rearranging the formulae for resistance (R) and compliance (C).

$$\Delta P = \Delta V/C + (F \times R)$$

The pressure gradient required to overcome both resistance of the airway as well as the elastic properties of the lung and chest wall is the dynamic component and used to measure dynamic compliance (C_{dyn}) and the maximum pressure attained is known as peak inspiratory pressure (PIP/P_{peak}). When there is no flow in the airway, the resistive property of the airway is eliminated and this pressure, known as Plateau pressure (P_{plat}), is taken for measuring the static compliance (C_{stat}). After a normal tidal expiration, the volume of gas left in the lung constitutes the functional residual capacity. The baseline pressure applied to maintain this functional residual capacity during expiration is known as peak end expiratory pressure (PEEP) (Fig. 3).

$$\text{Static compliance} = \frac{\text{Tidal volume (Vt)}}{P_{plat} - \text{PEEP}} \qquad \text{Dynamic compliance} = \frac{\text{Tidal volume (Vt)}}{P_{peak} - \text{PEEP}}$$

The compliance curve is given by plotting the pressure versus the volume in the P–V loop and airway resistance component is visually analyzed by the expiratory part of the flow–volume loop (Fig. 4).

Time constant is the mathematical product of compliance and resistance, measured in seconds. Some time is required for pressure to equilibrate between the atmosphere and alveoli. It takes three time constants for 95% and five time constants for 99% pressure equilibration to occur.

Parenchymal disease: They usually have decreased compliance and pressure equilibration occurs early and hence, has a small time constant. Both P_{peak} and P_{plat} will be elevated as they require high pressure to generate adequate tidal volume, for example, acute respiratory distress syndrome (ARDS).

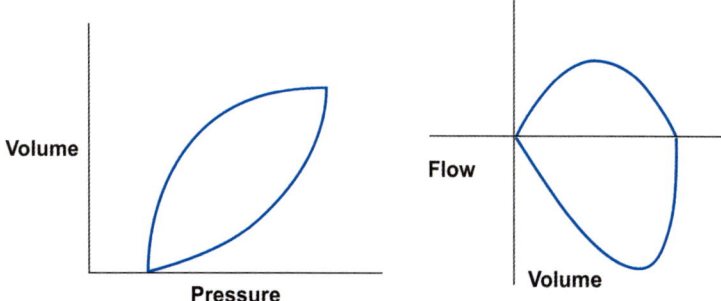

Fig. 4: Pressure–volume loop showing compliance curve and flow–volume loop.

Airway disease: They have high resistance and more time is required for pressure equilibration leading to higher time constant. P_{peak} will be elevated as higher pressure is required to overcome the initial airway resistance, however P_{plat} will be normal as the lung compliance is normal, for example, asthma.

CONTROL VARIABLES IN MECHANICAL VENTILATION

Pressure, volume, and flow are the factors that can be modified during mechanical ventilation. Only one of the variables can be kept constant while the others change depending on the lung compliance and airway resistance. In pressure control ventilation, pressure is set constant and volume varies based on the compliance which needs to be monitored. In volume control ventilation, the volume target limit is set. However, as volume cannot be directly measured by the flow sensors, flow is kept constant and pressure varies with compliance and resistance.

In pressure control mode, flow is of decelerating type wherein maximum flow at the beginning opens the alveoli and then the flow decreases (Fig. 5). It is useful in parenchymal involvement-especially with homogeneous lung disease.

In volume control mode, the flow assumes a plateau after initial rapid rise and remains constant throughout inspiration (Fig. 6). This type of flow is preferred in normal lung ventilation and in heterogeneous lung involvement (e.g. severe ARDS) where decelerating flow (as in pressure-control ventilation) may selectively inflate good compliant alveoli and under-inflate stiff ones worsening the already existent dead-space ventilation and V/Q mismatch.

PHASES OF VENTILATION

Based on the phases of the respiratory cycle, these are as follows (Fig. 7):
- *Trigger:* The initiation of the breath is known as trigger.
  - *Machine trigger*: A breath that is triggered by the machine which usually occurs after a specified time interval based on the set rate (time trigger).
  - *Patient trigger*: Breath triggered by the patient due to lowering of circuit pressure (pressure trigger) or flow change (flow trigger) as a result of the negative pressure generated by the inspiratory effort.

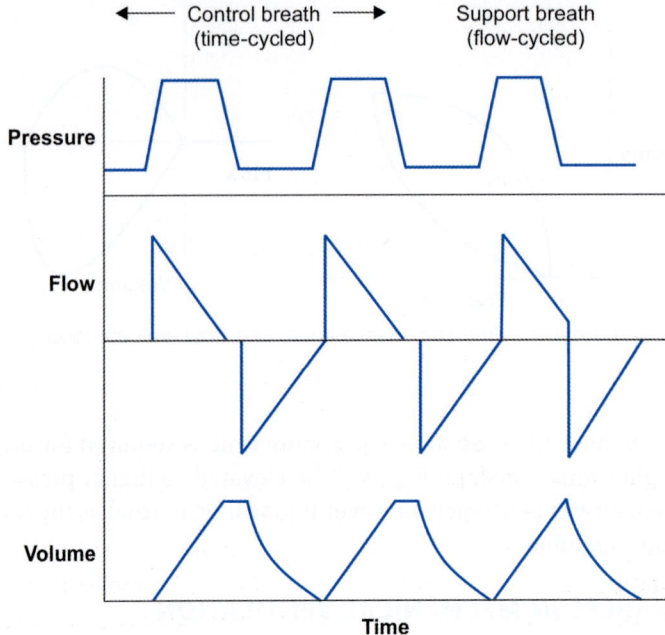

Fig. 5: Scalars in pressure control mode of ventilation.

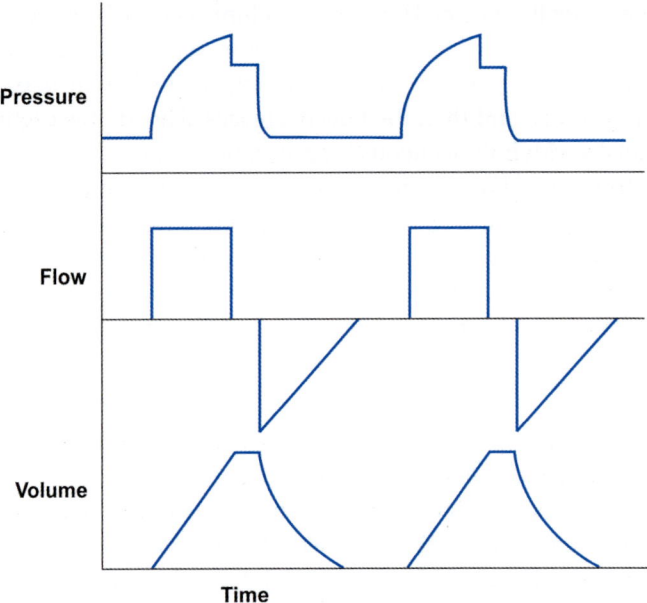

Fig. 6: Scalars in volume control mode of ventilation.

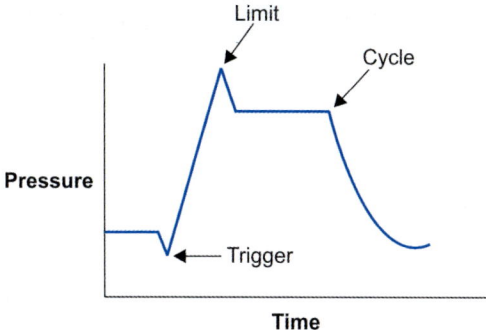

Fig. 7: Phase variables of a mechanical ventilatory cycle.

- *Limit:* The maximum limit to attain the set pressure or volume is the limit variable.
  - Pressure-limited: The peak pressure is the limit set in pressure control ventilation
  - Volume-limited: The tidal volume is set as volume limit in volume control ventilation.
- *Cycle:* The termination of inspiration and start of expiration is the cycling variable.
  - *Time-cycled*: After a set inspiratory time, the inspiratory time ends and expiration starts either after an inspiratory pause with no flow or immediately after end of inspiration.
  - *Flow-cycled*: A percentage of flow is set as expiratory trigger and once the flow is reduced to the set percentage, inspiration stops and expiration starts.
- *Baseline variable:* The PEEP set is sometimes known as the baseline variable which is the pressure during expiration. It is the baseline pressure above which the pressure rises during inspiration.

TYPES OF BREATH

On the the basis of control of various phase variables by the machine or patient, there are four types of breath in patients on mechanical ventilator. The control breath is entirely controlled by the ventilator. The assisted breath differs from control breath only in terms of trigger. It is triggered by patient but gets full support from the machine to the same limit and same inspiratory time as set for a machine breath. But in support breath, although triggered by patient and supported to the limit set for machine breath, the inspiratory time is decided by patient. The spontaneous breath gets no support from the ventilator (Table 1 and Fig. 8).

ASYNCHRONY AND SYNCHRONIZATION

Asynchrony: It is a state of disharmony between the ventilator and patient breath. It can occur during initiation of breath (trigger asynchrony), mismatch of flow during inspiration (flow asynchrony), termination of inspiration (termination asynchrony), and incomplete or prolonged expiration leading to air trapping (expiratory asynchrony).

Synchronization: It is ensuring matching spontaneous and machine breaths during a respiratory cycle. Trigger system used should be reliable, appropriate for the patient and have short response time. Previously used trigger devices include detection of abdominal motion during respiration using Grasby's capsule and measuring thoracic impedance using standard

Table 1: Phase variables in different types of the breaths in patients on mechanical ventilator.

Phase variable	Trigger	Limit	Cycled
Control breath	Machine	Machine	Machine
Assisted breath	Patient	Machine	Machine
Support breath	Patient	Machine	Patient
Spontaneous breath	Patient	Patient	Patient

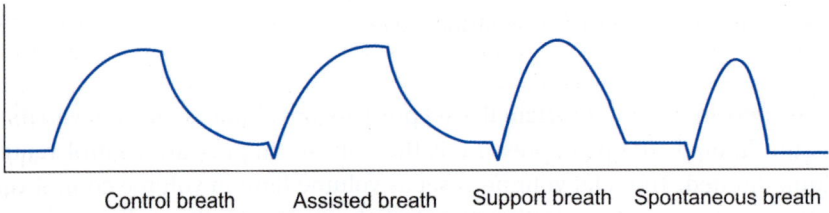

Control breath   Assisted breath   Support breath   Spontaneous breath

Fig. 8: Types of breaths in a patient on mechanical ventilator.

electrodes used for cardiorespiratory monitoring. Contemporary machines use transducers where changes in circuit pressure and/or flow are detected during patient's triggering efforts. Pneumotachographs which detect flow by movement of membrane and heated wire anemometer which sense temperature change due to flow of gas are the commonly used flow transducers.

MODES OF VENTILATION

Control Modes

Intermittent mandatory ventilation (IMV): In this mode, the ventilator delivers breaths at a set rate independent of patient's effort. Spontaneous breaths occur in-between the machine breaths but there is no coordination between the machine and the patient breaths. This leads to ventilator–patient asynchrony as machine may deliver breath when the patient is trying to take an inspiration. Decreasing the ventilator rate as per improvement in patient status is the method of weaning. Currently, this mode is out of practice for its obvious limitations.

Synchronized intermittent mandatory ventilation (SIMV): In order to decrease the patient–ventilator asynchrony, synchronization was instituted between machine breaths and patient effort, where a patient effort is recognized and the ventilator delivers the breath in synchrony with the patient effort. The ventilator has a set backup rate and the time window is given during which any patient effort is recognized and machine breath is delivered during such efforts rather than in a random manner as in IMV. If no breath is recognized during this time window, machine breath is delivered mandatorily. During weaning, as the patient triggers, the mandatory rates may be gradually reduced and finally all breaths may be triggered by the patient. This mode can be used during initiation of ventilation, during maintenance phase, and during the weaning as well.

Assist-control mode: In this mode, machine breaths are delivered as control breaths as well as the patient's efforts are recognized and assisted by delivering the same pressure/volume and inspiratory time as in case of a control breath. So, this mode would include control breaths as well as assisted breaths. Weaning will be achieved by gradual reduction in the pressure/volume support and reduction in the rate of control breaths. Decreasing the machine rates will not alter the assistance of spontaneous efforts by the ventilator.

Assisted Modes

Pressure support ventilation (PSV): The ventilator recognizes the patient effort based on set trigger, and it supports as per pressure limit set and is flow cycled. Inspiratory time is decided by the patient, and not by the machine unlike in assist-control mode. It is more comfortable for the patient as machine is in synchrony with the patient's effort and inspiratory time. It improves patient comfort, reduces sedation needs, prevents disuse atrophy, and facilitates early weaning. A back up rate for mandatory breath is set for inadequate patient effort, if any.

Proportional assist ventilation (PAV): The ventilator delivers with a continuous input of patient's respiratory effort through servo control and also facilitates in respiratory mechanical unloading throughout the respiratory cycle.

Adaptive support ventilation (ASV®): The ventilator adjusts delivery based on the real-time respiratory mechanics with a closed loop feedback system between patient and machine.

Neurally adjusted ventilatory assist (NAVA®): The ventilatory support is triggered by and adjusted according to electrical activity of the diaphragm.

Dual Mode

Pressure-regulated volume control ventilation (PRVC®): It is a mode with decelerating flow and has breath-to-breath dual control wherein it adjusts the pressure in order to deliver a set tidal volume. The initial breaths could be of varying tidal volume during which machine uses patient's compliance curve and learns from it to deliver the target tidal volume within the set pressure limit. Pressure limit of 5 mm Hg more than the required pressure is set. It has automatic weaning of pressures as compliance improves. It is also known as Adaptive Pressure Ventilation SIMV (APV SIMV) in Hamilton®, Autoflow in Draeger®, or Volume Control Plus in Nellcor Puritan Bennett®.

Hybrid modes: These are various combinations of above mentioned modes to facilitate weaning from ventilator.
- *P-SIMV +PSV:* Pressure control SIMV mode can be used along with pressure support (PSV).
- *V-SIMV+PSV:* Volume control SIMV can also be clubbed with PSV to support spontaneous breaths.
- *APV- SIMV+PSV* and PRVC along with pressure support.

Newer mode:
Airway pressure release ventilation (APRV): It is a newer mode in which high pressures are maintained for prolonged periods with brief period of release of pressure. Spontaneous breathing is allowed during all phases of respiratory cycle. It is a form of inverse ratio ventilation where higher pressures (P_{high}) are given during the time equated to inspiration (T_{high}).

This pressure is release to a lower pressure (P_{low}) for a shorter time similar to expiration (T_{low}). Advantages include better oxygenation where conventional modes have failed and high frequency ventilation facilities are unavailable. It predisposes the patient to higher potential of air-leaks and hemodynamic compromise during the P_{high} phase.

INITIAL VENTILATOR SETTINGS

Initial mechanical ventilatory settings include choosing the mode and setting the FiO2, rate, PEEP, PIP or tidal volume, inspiratory time or I:E ratio

Normal lung:
- *Mode*: Volume control or pressure control SIMV
- *Rate*: Set according to normal age—appropriate respiratory rate, i.e., 30 in infants, 20 in children, 15–18 in adolescents.
- FiO_2 less than 0.4
- PEEP 3–5
- PIP of 10–12 or tidal volume of 6–10 mL/kg of ideal body weight
- Inspiratory time based on the natural time constant which depends on age; from 0.45 seconds in infants to 0.8 seconds in older children, or I: E ratio of about 1:2.

Parenchymal lung disease:
- *Mode*: Pressure control SIMV is preferred.
- *Rate*: Slightly higher than the normal age—appropriate respiratory rates may be required, as time constant gets reduced in these situations.
- Limit FiO_2 less than 0.6
- Incremental increase in PEEP to achieve recruitment of alveoli
- PIP to achieve tidal volume of 6 mL/kg of ideal body weight
- Inspiratory time may need to be increased to achieve adequate oxygenation such that I:E ratio of less than 1:2 may be required.

Airway disease:
- *Mode*: Volume control SIMV is preferred.
- *Rate*: Lower than normal respiratory rate is set in order to increase the duration of each respiratory cycle to allow full completion of expiration. It is in accordance to the increased time constant in these patients.
- Limit FiO_2 less than 0.6
- Low PEEP as air trapping creates some auto-PEEP
- PIP to achieve tidal volume of 6–10 mL/kg of ideal body weight
- Higher expiratory time to complete expiration such that I:E ratio of more than 1:3 may be required.

High-frequency Oscillator Ventilation: Brief Overview

General Principles (Table 2 and Fig. 9)

- A continuous positive airway pressure system with piston displacement of gas
- Active exhalation
- Tidal volume less than anatomic dead space (1 to 3 mL/kg)

Basics of Mechanical Ventilation

Table 2: Initial settings on high-frequency oscillator ventilation.

Frequency	8–12 Hz; 1 Hz = 60
I: E ratio	1:2 or 1:3
Bias gas flow	15–20 L/min may have an effect on MAP
Mean arterial pressure (MAP)	Start 2–3 above the MAP as compared to controlled mechanical ventilation settings adjust by 1–2 cm H_2O for desired SpO_2
Amplitude	Adjusted to chest vibrations and CO_2
FiO_2	Adjusted to SpO_2

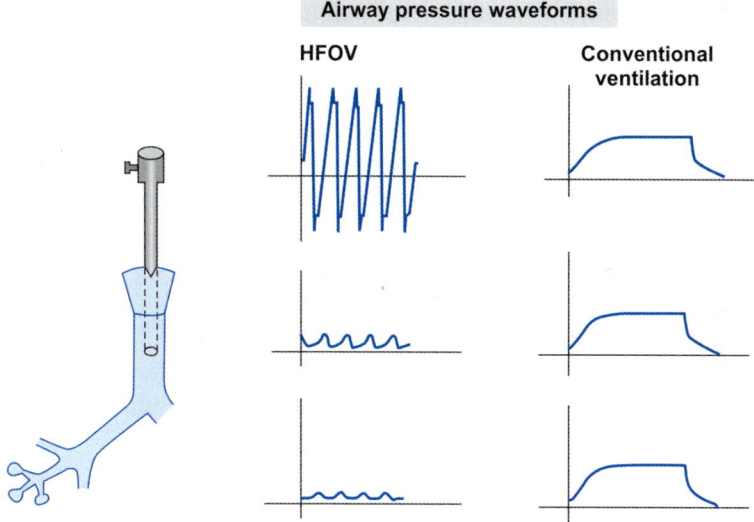

Fig. 9: Change in pressure at different parts of the airway and alveoli as seen in high-frequency oscillator ventilation (HFOV) versus conventional ventilation.

- Rates of 180–900 breaths per minute
- Lower peak inspiratory pressures for a given mean airway pressure as compared to controlled mechanical ventilation (CMV)
- Decoupling of oxygenation and ventilation.

This type of ventilation features active inspiration as well as active expiration delivered by a special ventilator. Low-volume, low-compliance tubing is used to deliver support from a special ventilator. Flow is generated from a piston-driven acoustic speaker cone, or diaphragm. Movement of this diaphragm creates sinusoidal oscillations in the airway pressure relative to the mean airway pressure. The fluctuations in airway pressure higher than the mean airway pressure create an inspiratory force, and pressure less than the mean create a relatively negative or expiratory force. The tidal volumes less than dead space are used, typically 1–3 mL/kg. Rates in frequency set between 1 Hz and 60 Hz (60–3,600 cycles per minute). In practice, mean airway pressure recruits lung volume, prevents atelectasis, and thereby supports oxygenation along with FiO_2. The two main factors determining ventilation are Hz and delta amplitude, also called delta P. There is a close relationship between pressure amplitude and tidal volume.

Tidal volume depends on:
- The volume displaced by the piston or diaphragm
- The resistance of the airways
- The compliance of the ventilator circuit
- The patient's lung mechanics.

Therefore, search for visible chest vibrations, change amplitude to control ventilation ($PaCO_2$).

Mean arterial pressure or continuous distending pressure (CDP) recruits alveoli/airways and maintains alveolar volume ⟶ it is closely related to lung volumes and oxygenation.

Goals for "Typical" Patient with ALI/ARDS

The goals may differ for: other disease states—reactive airway disease, acute chest syndrome, flail chest, congenital diaphragmatic hernia, sepsis, and pulmonary hypertension.
- Reasonable oxygenation to limit oxygen toxicity: SaO_2 86–92%/PaO_2 55–90 mm Hg
- Permissive hypercapnia: Provide "just enough" ventilatory support to maintain normal cellular function.
- Monitor cardiac function, perfusion, lactate, and pH
- Allow $PaCO_2$ to rise but keep arterial pH 7.25–7.30.
- This strategy helps to minimize ventilator-associated lung injury.
- "Normal" pH, $PaCO_2$, and PaO_2 are indicators of OVER ventilation.

Conclusion

High frequency oscillator ventilation is a simple to use technology, if used early (not only as a rescue therapy) alone or in combination with other adjuncts (such as sildenafil, nitric oxide, prone positioning) has been shown to improve the oxygenation, CO_2 removal, and possibly eventual outcomes in severe neonatal and pediatric respiratory failure. It fits well in the concept of lung protective strategies when used early in the course of disease and allows, especially in small children to maintain spontaneous ventilation. However, it has not really proven to be better than CMV in the clinical set-up.

MONITORING OF PARAMETERS

Throughout the duration of ventilation, monitoring of vital clinical parameters, oxygenation and ventilation is necessary. Apart from these, ventilator displays the numerical values of independent and measured variables like tidal volume, minute ventilation, compliance, resistance, peak and plateau pressures. Graphic displays as scalars and loops help in real-time evaluation of pulmonary pathophysiology to fine tune the ventilation support and to identify problems, if any, for timely troubleshooting.

KEY POINTS

- Spontaneous respiration is a negative pressure ventilation while mechanical ventilation is a positive pressure ventilation.
- To propel gases into the lung, a pressure gradient is required to counter the elastic and the restive forces.
- The ventilator settings depend upon the indication and respiratory pathophysiology.
- Selection of ventilator mode is usually as per unit preferences and familiarity. No mode has been proven to be superior over the other.
- Continuous monitoring of the ventilated child and troubleshooting using ventilator graphics is the key to smooth ventilation and weaning.

SUGGESTED READING

1. Kliegman RM, Stanton BF, St Geme III JW, Schor NF (Ed). Mechanical ventilation. Nelson Textbook of Pediatrics, 20th edition. US: Elsevier, Inc; 2016. pp. 536-44.
2. Nichols DG, Shaffner DH (Ed). Mechanical ventilation. Roger's Textbook of Pediatric Intensive Care, 5th edition. Philadelphia: Wolters Kluwer; 2016. pp. 541-64.
3. Rimensberger PC (Ed). Mechanical ventilation. Pediatric and Neonatal Mechanical Ventilation: From Basics to Clinical Practice. Berlin Heidelberg: Springer-Verlag; 2015. pp. 149-274.

Noninvasive Ventilation

Ashwath Ram RN, Manu Sundaram

LEARNING OBJECTIVES

- Basic principles and mechanism of noninvasive ventilation (NIV)
- Indications and contraindications
- Noninvasive ventilation modes
- Types of NIV machines
- Components of NIV machine
- Types of interface
- Steps for initiating NIV
- Monitoring
- Troubleshooting
- Home mechanical ventilation
- High-flow nasal cannula oxygen therapy.

BASIC PRINCIPLES AND MECHANISM OF NONINVASIVE VENTILATION

Introduction

Until the early 1960s, negative-pressure ventilation in the form of tank ventilator was the most common type of mechanical ventilation outside the anesthesia suite.

With the introduction of nasal continuous positive airway pressure (CPAP) to treat obstructive sleep apnea (OSA) in the early 1980s, noninvasive positive-pressure ventilation (NIPPV) has rapidly displaced negative-pressure ventilation as the treatment of choice for chronic respiratory failure in patients with neuromuscular and chest wall deformities (Figs. 1A and B).

Over the past two decades, the use of NIPPV and noninvasive CPAP by mask has increased substantially for acutely ill patients. There are various studies in the adult practice that have supported the benefit of noninvasive ventilation (NIV) in select patients. NIV has been used in the setting of acute respiratory failure to avoid endotracheal intubation in different patient populations and settings, with variable success. In addition, NIPPV has been used to facilitate early liberation from conventional mechanical ventilation and to prevent reintubation.

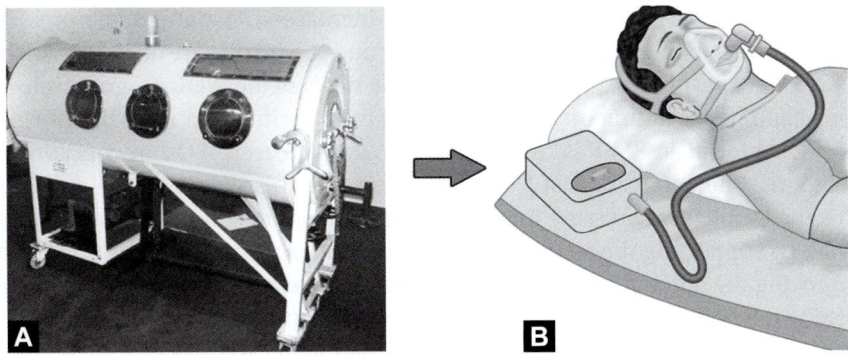

Figs. 1A and B: Negative-pressure ventilation and positive-pressure ventilation.

Definition of Noninvasive Ventilation

Mechanical ventilation is a lifesaving/supportive intervention both in adults and children. This is commonly provided invasively via an artificial airway in the form of an endotracheal tube (ETT) or tracheotomy tube in an intensive care unit (ICU) setting. NIV is providing mechanical ventilation support without any invasive artificial airway.

Noninvasive ventilation can be provided in the form of negative-pressure ventilators or positive-pressure ventilators. Today based on convenience and efficacy PPV are the common form of NIV support via the interfaces of nasal cannula, nasal masks, oronasal masks, etc.

Applied Physiology of Noninvasive Ventilation

There are certain peculiarities with regards to the physiology and anatomy in pediatric patients. In the very young children their muscle strength is determined by some structural and functional characteristics.
- The ability of the intercoastal muscle to contract is reduced as the rib cage is more circular than ellipsoidal compared to the adults. This results in a reduced bucket-handle movement of the ribs.
- As the amount of type 1 muscle fiber is less in infants, they are more prone to diaphragmatic fatigue compared to adults.
- The angle of insertion of the diaphragm on the ribs and flexibility of the ribs limit the stabilizing role of the rib cage in the opposing elastic forces of the lung.

Acute respiratory failure can be divided into type 1 or type 2 respiratory failure. It is easier to understand the physiological basis for using NIV as type 1 or type 2 respiratory failure. The NIV has a higher success rate in type 2 respiratory failure compared to type 1 respiratory failure as in type 2 respiratory failure a failed pump is replaced by the NIV machine as a pump. In type 1 respiratory, there is ventilation perfusion mismatch. In many conditions such as bronchiolitis, the respiratory failure is a combination of type 1 and type 2 respiratory failure.

The application of positive end-expiratory pressure (PEEP) during acute respiratory failure (ARF) in children has effects on:
- *Decreasing the patient's work of breathing (WOB)*: In ARF, the resistance is increased and compliance is decreased. Hence, the WOB needed to compensate for the inspiratory

load is significant. At the beginning of ARF, the increased transpulmonary pressure (PTP) value reflects the higher use of muscle capacity and the infants are at higher risk of fatigue from prolonged respiratory distress. At the same time, as the WOB progressively increases the end-expiratory volume increases resulting in hyperinflation from the intrinsic PEEP (PEEPi). This intrinsic PEEP is responsible for the increased WOB in conditions such as bronchiolitis. The application of CPAP can overcome this PEEPi. But to generate a tidal volume the esophageal pressure must be less than the atmospheric pressure. This reduces the WOB by supporting the respiratory muscles to work again below the critical threshold by improving the efficiency of muscular contractions to generate the tidal volume and by abolishing the harmful effects of PEEPi; resulting in significant decrease in WOB.
- *Improving the breathing pattern*: Tachypnea is the initial response to ARF to maintain the minute ventilation. This increase in respiratory rate (RR) is associated with shortening of the Ti and Te. The reduction in Te is associated with physiological changes during the ARF leading to PEEPi as seen in acute bronchiolitis. The improvement in tidal volume with the application of CPAP results in significant reduction in RR and reduction of dynamic airway obstruction from PEEPi. In addition, the application of the PEEP maintains the patency throughout the respiratory tract, from the upper airways to the smaller lower airways. This also helps in facilitating the expiratory flow in obstructive conditions of the airway.
- *Improving the functional residual capacity (FRC)*: In type 1 respiratory failure there is V-Q mismatch from either intra-alveolar factors such as secretions, fluid, and edema. In addition, there could be extra-alveolar factors such as pleural effusions or increased intra-abdominal pressure. The decreased in the FRC results in in hypoxemia from the shunting. If the alveolar collapse can be reversed then the shunting can be reduced. Various studies have shown the beneficial effects of PEEP on keeping the alveoli open during expiration and reducing shunting. The early use of PEEP can help in preventing alveolar collapse, which mainly occurs in expiration and the subsequent increase in the shunting over several respiratory cycles.
- *Effect on cardiac output*: The effect of NIV on cardiovascular system can be divided into the impact on right and left ventricular failure. The NIV may worsen the right ventricular dysfunction as the NIV can decrease the venous return due to the increased intrathoracic pressures. The NIV has an opposite effect on the left ventricular failure. The PEEP reduces the LV afterload and supports a failing left ventricle. The PEEP pressure splints the alveoli open and pushes out the fluid from the alveoli if there is pulmonary edema. The PEEP also keeps the alveoli open and in a stable state. This reduces the shunting and reduces the V/Q mismatch and improves the oxygenation. To summarize, the PEEP also reduces the WOB and left ventricular dysfunction and reduces the oxygen requirement.

Mechanics of Action of Noninvasive Ventilation

In summary, the two basic supports provided by NIV is inspiratory positive airway pressure (IPAP) and end-expiratory positive pressure or CPAP.

The inspiratory positive pressures help by:
- Providing inspiratory pressure support
- Reducing WOB
- Offloads the respiratory muscles.

The end-expiratory positive pressure helps by:
- Improving the FRC which in turn improves the oxygenation and lung compliance.
- Reduces the preload and afterload for the heart and improves the cardiac output, which enables better oxygen delivery to the tissues.
- Reduces auto PEEP and thereby improves the WOB.

Goals of Noninvasive Ventilation

Noninvasive ventilation is used for both acute and chronic settings and the goals vary depending on the indication of use.

In acute settings:
- Relieve hypoxemia and hypercapnia-related symptoms.
- Reduce WOB.
- Minimize complications related to invasive ventilation.
- Avoid intubation.
- Optimize patient comfort.

In chronic settings:
- Improve gas exchange
- Improve sleep duration and quality
- Maximize the quality of life
- Improve functional status
- Prolong survival.

Advantages of Noninvasive Ventilation

- May avert the need for invasive ventilation and related complications—airway trauma (ulceration, edema, subglottic stenosis), infections [ventilator-associated pneumonia (VAP), tracheitis, and related sepsis) and excessive sedation-related complications.
- Allows patients to eat orally, vocalize normally, and expectorate secretions.
- Need for less sedation.
- More comfortable.
- Can maintain this as intermittent support unlike invasive ventilation.
- May lower mortality and morbidity—especially in immunocompromised.
- Shortens length of ICU stay.
- Less expensive.

Disadvantages of Noninvasive Ventilation

- May cause delay in instituting invasive ventilation in deserving patients
- No airway protection—risk of aspiration
- Inability to do deep tracheal suctioning and clear secretions
- Claustrophobic
- Labor intensive
- Need unit to be familiar with the machine/usage/monitoring
- Pressure effects over the nose and face.

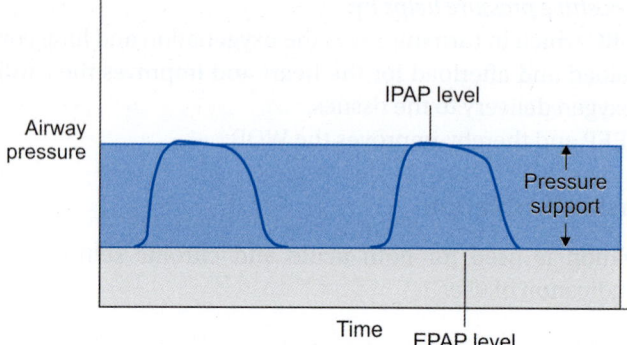

Fig. 2: Airway pressure curve showing inspiratory positive airway pressure (IPAP) and expiratory positive airway pressure (EPAP).

TERMINOLOGIES USED IN NONINVASIVE VENTILATION

- *Inspiratory positive airway pressure*: Application and maintenance of pressure throughout the phase of inspiration to achieve the desired tidal volume. This will ensure sufficient removal of carbon dioxide. This inspiratory support also helps to alleviate the sensation of breathlessness.
- *Expiratory positive airway pressure (EPAP)*: Application and maintenance of pressure at the airway throughout the phase of expiration. Splints airways open during expiration to overcome obstruction/airway collapse. Maintaining a positive pressure in the airways at the end of expiration will improve help recruit collapsed lung, improve V/Q mismatch, and improve the compliance of the lungs, making expansion during inspiration easier (Fig. 2).
- *Pressure support*: The pressure difference between the IPAP and EPAP. It is the amount of "help" which the ventilator will give for inspiration effort and is defined by the set IPAP for the controlled breath and the set pressure support for the spontaneous breath.
- *RR*: Is the desired minimal set rate for the patient.
- *I-time*: The time taken to deliver the required pressures.
- *Ramp time*: The interval during which time the ventilator linearly increases pressure, helping reduce patient anxiety.
- *Inspiratory trigger*: The trigger for initiating a breath.
- *Expiratory trigger*: The trigger to cycle to expiration.
- *FiO_2*: The fractional oxygen concentration to be delivered.
- *Leak*: Amount of leak the circuit or from around the interface-usually depicted in % or in L/m.
- *Rise time*: Speed with which the inspiratory pressure rises to the set target pressure.

INDICATIONS AND CONTRAINDICATIONS

Indications for Noninvasive Ventilation

Noninvasive ventilation can be used for acute conditions. Studies have shown that NIV is more successful in type 2 respiratory failure compared to type 1 respiratory failure as essentially in type 2 respiratory failure a failing pump is replaced by another pump, i.e. the NIV machine.

- *Hypoxemic respiratory failure (Type I)*: It is characterized by an arterial oxygen tension (PaO_2) lower than 60 mm Hg with a normal or low arterial carbon dioxide tension ($PaCO_2$). This is the most common form of respiratory failure, and it can be associated with virtually all acute diseases of the lung (bronchiolitis, asthma, pneumonia, acute respiratory distress syndrome (ARDS), atelectasis, pulmonary edema) which generally involve fluid-filling or collapse of alveolar units. Success rate for NIV in type 1 respiratory failure is around 60–70%. This is because some of the type 1 respiratory failure presents as an ARDS. In the presence of ARDS, an early intubation would be beneficial, if there is no response to NIV after a brief trial.
- *Hypercapnic respiratory failure (Type II)*: It is characterized by a $PaCO_2$ higher than 50 mm Hg. Hypoxemia is common in patients with hypercapnic respiratory failure who are breathing room air. The pH depends on the level of bicarbonate, which, in turn, is dependent on the duration of hypercapnia. This hypercapnic failure can be acute or chronic in presentation. Common etiologies causing acute hypercapnic respiratory failure include drug overdose, severe forms of acute asthma, bronchiolitis, acute onset neuromuscular disease, and other neurological causes affecting respiratory drive. Some of the situations causing chronic respiratory failure include congenital chest wall abnormalities, and severe congenital obstructive airway disorders, chronic neuromuscular disorders (myopathy, muscular dystrophies, etc.). Type 2 respiratory failure has an 80% success rate.
- *Acute respiratory failure in immunocompromised children*: Studies have shown that NIV can reduce intubation rate in the oncology patient. This reduces the probability of these children getting nosocomial infections. This would facilitate the early discharge of these children from the hospitals and reducing the rates of serious complications. Many of the immunocompromised children are fluid overloaded around the time of chemotherapy and hyperhydration regimes. Early used of NIV in these children have prevented deterioration and prolonged ICU stays associated with intubation. Cardiovascular dysfunction, severe illness scores, and solid tumors were predictive factors for NIV failure in these patients.
- *Weaning from invasive ventilation/handling extubation failure*: NIV has a role in weaning acute on chronic respiratory failure kids who have been intubated. Studies have supported the use of NIV in post-extubation respiratory failure to prevent reintubation. This has been very useful in children with neuromuscular conditions and children with chronic lung disease. However, NIV use should not delay the need for intubation in children with postextubation respiratory failure.
- *Airway obstruction*: NIV has been well-established as a modality for treatment of OSA in children. A recent observational study has shown improvement in the WOB in conditions causing obstruction of the larger airway like vocal cord palsy and tracheobronchomalacia.
- Palliative care in patients with "*do not intubate*" plan.

Contraindications for Noninvasive Ventilation

Historically, NIV has been used for support of breathing in long-term neuromuscular and respiratory conditions. Over the last few decades, with the availability of better interfaces and machines, NIV has been used for providing support for acute conditions. With the improvement in technologies the standard boundaries for the use of technologies are being challenged. Hence, the most import factor is the contraindications for the use of acute NIV.

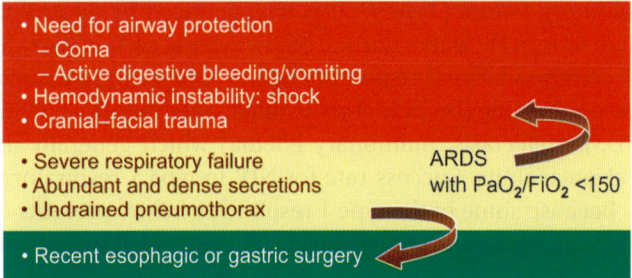

Fig. 3: Contraindications to noninvasive ventilation. (ARDS: acute respiratory distress syndrome)

This can be best explained by a traffic light signal gradation. But based on the experience and competencies of the teams with regards to the uses of acute NIV; some of relative contraindications could be an indication for the trail of NIV for another. But the most important thing is that this should not compromise on the safety of the patient. Hence, acute NIV is not a replacement for conditions where intubation is mandatory (Fig. 3).

Contraindications to NIV can be broadly considered as follows:
- *Inability to protect airway*: NIV is contraindicated in conditions where the airway cannot be protected; from either a low Glasgow Coma Scale or weak cough and gag reflex.
- *Vomiting and gastric bleeding*: In acute NIV, a full facemask or an oronasal interface is preferred. As there is a high risk of aspiration in the presence of vomiting and acute gastric bleeding, NIV is contraindicated.
- *Craniofacial trauma*: Fixation of interfaces becomes difficult in the presence of craniofacial trauma and burns of the neck and face; hence NIV is not suitable.
- *Hemodynamics instability*: In the presence of shock, the airway needs to be secured to conserve the energy that is used for the respiratory effort. Hence, it is better for these children to be intubated and the shock be managed appropriately. In early septic shock, the CPAP can be used early to support the cardiorespiratory system, especially in immunocompromised children.
- *Severe respiratory failure*: Various studies have shown that NIV has a higher mortality in moderate-to-severe ARDS. NIV is a relative contraindication in ARDS. NIV can be used for mild ARDS, where a short trial of NIV can be given as long as it does not delay intubation.
- *Abundant secretions*: The presence of oronasal interfaces reduces the ability for regular airway clearance when there are abundant secretions. The risk of NIV failure is higher when the abundant secretions cannot be cleared. Depending on the expertise of the team, various interventions such as regular physiotherapy, cough assist devices, and physiotherapy vests can be used to help clear secretions.

MODES IN NONINVASIVE VENTILATION

There are several modes of NIV depending upon the machine that is used. We will learn about the different machines in the next chapter. We describe the common modes of NIV here.

Commonly used modes in NIV:
- *HFNC*: High-flow nasal cannula oxygen therapy (discussed separately in later chapter)
- *CPAP*: Continuous positive airway pressure
- *S mode*: Spontaneous mode
- *ST mode*: Spontaneous-timed mode
- *PCV*: Pressure control ventilation mode
- *AVAPS/IVAPS*: Average volume-assured pressure support
- *NAVA mode*: Neurally adjusted ventilatory assist NIV

What define the modes are three main variables, very similar as in conventional ventilation:
1. *Trigger*: What initiates the breath
2. *Limit*: That which terminates inspiration
3. *Cycle*: That which switches from inspiration to expiration.

Continuous Positive Airway Pressure Mode

- In this mode, continuous positive pressure is maintained throughout both inspiration and expiration, by maintaining continuous flow as in NIV ventilators and/or a pressure valve as seen in conventional ventilators.
- All breaths are patient-triggered, patient-limited, and patient-cycled. In simple terms, it is basically provision of PEEP in a spontaneously breathing patient.
- Some ventilators (like the V60) provide a C-flex option, where the ventilator reduces the pressure at the beginning of expiration (to enable patient comfort) and sets to return the pressure to the set CPAP level at the end of exhalation (Fig. 4).

Spontaneous Mode

- Breaths are patient-triggered, pressure-limited, and patient-cycled.
- All breaths are patient-triggered. Trigger sensitivity can be set in some ventilators.
- The set IPAP pressure is delivered to the patient once the patient triggers a breath. And at the end of exhalation the EPAP pressure is reached.

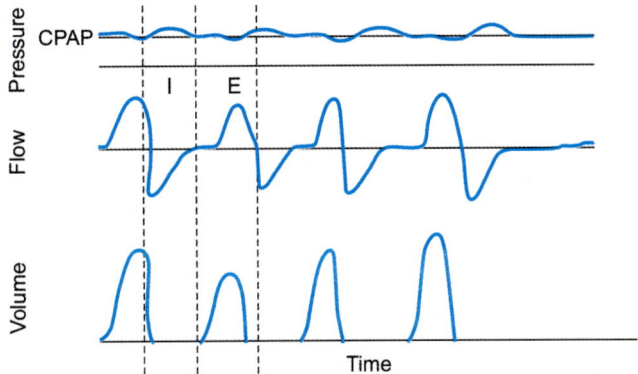

Fig. 4: Graphics displaying continuous positive airway pressure (CPAP) mode of noninvasive ventilation. Note the uniform flow in the flow–time scalars and the CPAP pressure in the pressure–time scales.

- The tidal volume obtained is the function of the difference in the pressure between the IPAP and the EPAP and the patient effort.
- Rise time can be set, which decides the time over which the desired IPAP pressure is delivered. This is mainly to satisfy the flow hunger for individual patients.
- The breath is limited by the generated pressure (IPAP).
- Cycling to expiration is controlled by the patients.
- Not ideal for patients who are unable to trigger all their breaths.

Spontaneous Timed Mode

- Two types of breath are delivered in this mode.
- *One*: Patient-triggered, pressure-limited (by the set IPAP), and patient-cycled breath.
- *Second*: Machine-triggered, pressure-limited (IPAP), time-cycled mandatory breaths. The mandatory breaths are delivered only if the patient fails to trigger a breath within the interval determined by the rate setting.
- Trigger sensitivity can be set in some ventilators.
- Rise time also can be set.
- Backup RR and inspiratory time is set—for mandatory breaths (Fig. 5).
- If the trigger is not sensitive enough, the patient may find they receive more mandatory breaths and can feel they are not synchronizing with the machine. In patients with poor triggering the backup rate should be sufficient to allow patient to achieve adequate ventilation.
- If the backup rate is too high, then the ventilator will interfere with patient's respiratory pattern.
- If inspiratory time is too long, then the patient will experience expiratory asynchrony small.

Pressure Control Ventilation Mode

- Breaths are patient/machine-triggered, pressure-limited, and time-cycled.
- Similar to (ST) mode as allows both patient-triggered assisted breaths and ventilator-triggered mandatory breaths.

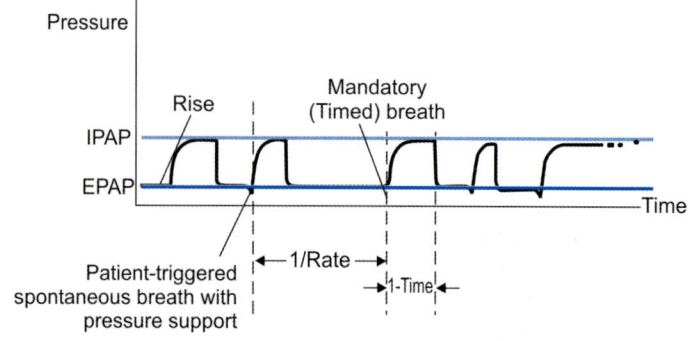

Fig. 5: Graphics displaying spontaneous timed (ST) mode. Note the trigger in the spontaneous breaths. Note the difference in the I-time between the spontaneous and mandatory breaths.
(EPAP: expiratory positive airway pressure; IPAP: inspiratory positive airway pressure).

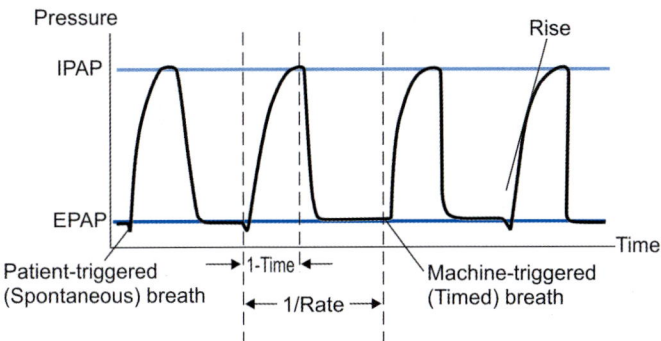

Fig. 6: Graphics displaying pressure control ventilation (PCV) mode. Note the trigger in the spontaneous/assisted breaths and the uniform I-time in both the breath types.
(EPAP: expiratory positive airway pressure; IPAP: inspiratory positive airway pressure).

- The difference from the ST mode is that the set inspiratory time apples to both patient-triggered and mandatory breaths.
- Allowing the ventilator to control the length of a spontaneous breath/assisted breath can help ensure that set pressures are reached and allow adequate lung expansion.
- This mode can be uncomfortable and difficult to synchronize with, particularly if the inspiratory time is not as per patient comfort/requirement (Fig. 6).

Average Volume Assures Pressure Support Mode

- The breaths are time-cycled mandatory breaths and pressure-supported spontaneous breaths similar to the ST mode.
- This mode delivers a set tidal volume by continually regulating the pressure applied through the circuit, by looking at the expired tidal volume, to reach the desired tidal volume.
- We need to set the minimum and maximum pressure that needs to be applied. The IPAP adjusts itself to meet the desired tidal volume within this pressure range.
- *Caution*:
  - The desired tidal volume may not be met, if the minimum and maximum pressures are outside the range of the targeted pressure required.
  - The expired tidal volume is not accurate in patients with huge leak (Fig. 7).

Table 1 summarizes the common pathologies causing respiratory failure along with the preferred mode.

TYPES OF NONINVASIVE VENTILATION MACHINES

Over the last two decades, there has been increase in the number of home NIV ventilators in the adults for conditions such as sleep disordered breathing, etc. Hence, there are more and better pediatrics home ventilators.

The NIV machines can be divided into three groups:
1. Home NIV ventilators
2. NIV-specific pediatric ICU (PICU) ventilators
3. Conventional ventilators with NIV option.

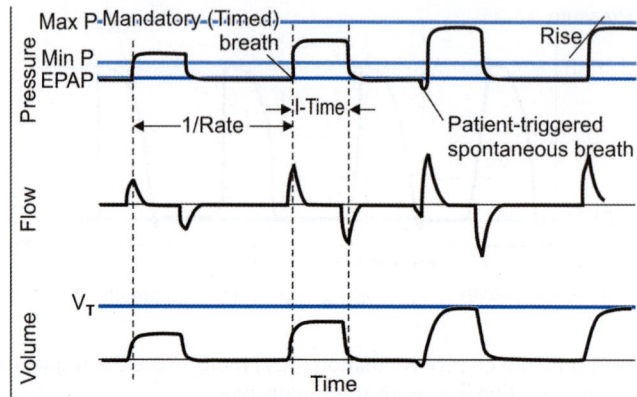

Fig. 7: Graphics displaying AVAPS mode. Note the Min and Max P set and the regulation of pressure to achieve the tidal volume.
(AVAPS: average volume-assured pressure support; EPAP: expiratory positive airway pressure)

Table 1: Choice of NIV modes depending upon the type of pathology.

Pathology causing respiratory failure	Preferred mode/suitable mode
Acute respiratory failure	CPAP/S/ST/PCV
Cardiogenic pulmonary edema	CPAP/ST
Obstructive sleep apnea	CPAP/ST
Restrictive lung	ST/AVAPS
Obstructive lung disease	ST/AVAPS

(AVAPS: average volume-assured pressure support; CPAP: continuous positive airway pressure; OSA: obstructive sleep apnea; PCV: pressure control ventilation; S: spontaneous; ST: spontaneous timed)

Home Noninvasive Ventilation Ventilator (Fig. 8)

The main differences in these ventilators compared to ICU ventilators are:
- Home NIV machines offer a more portable technology due to the reduced size of the air compressor. These compressors or turbines can generate very high flow rate of up to 150–180 liters per minute, hence can compensate well with leaks.
- Do not support pressures above 30 cm H_2O.
- Majority have single-limb tubing circuit.
- As it is a single limb circuit, exhalation ports or vented interfaces are required.
- Antiasphyxia valves are mandatory at home where power cut-off can occur.
- Lack of oxygen blender, hence, the maximum amount of oxygen that can be given is limited.
- No sophisticated alarm or battery backup systems.
- They do not need piped oxygen and air.

Examples of home NIV machines: ResMed Stellar 100, Stellar 150, Philips Trilogy, Breas VIVO 40, and Air-Liquide Monnal T-50.

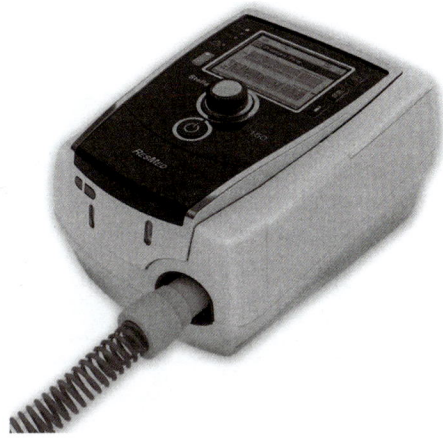

Fig. 8: Home noninvasive ventilation machine.

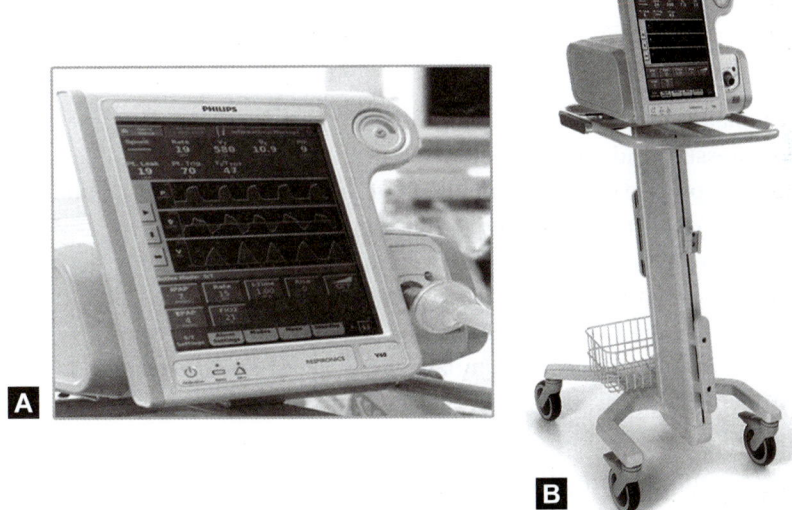

Figs. 9A and B: Noninvasive ventilation-specific hospital-based ventilator.

NIV-specific Hospital-based Ventilator (Figs. 9A and B)

Most of these ventilators are also turbine-driven ventilators. The main differences with a portable NIV machine are:
- Their ability to give up to 100% oxygen as they can be plugged into an oxygen port.
- Support pressures above 30 cm H_2O.
- Majority still have a have single-limb tubing circuit.
- As it is a single-limb circuit, exhalation ports or vented interfaces are required.
- Softwares to improve synchrony and better success in acute situations.

Examples of NIV-specific PICU ventilator: Philips V60 and Carina Dräger.

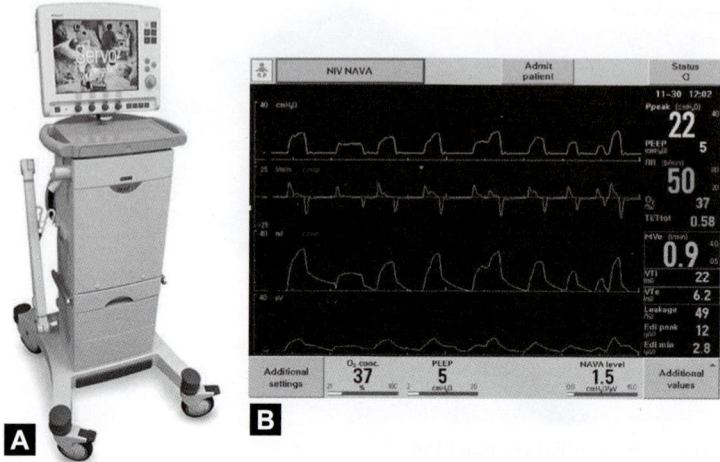

Figs. 10A and B: Conventional ventilators with NIV option.
(NAVA: neurally adjusted ventilatory assist; NIV: noninvasive ventilation).

Conventional Ventilators with NIV Option

Pediatric ICU ventilators are electronically controlled by a small embedded system to allow exact adaptation of pressure and flow characteristics to an individual patient's needs. This makes ventilation extremely precise including small infants and preterms (Figs. 10A and B).

The difference compared to the NIV ventilators are:
- Their ability to give up to 100% oxygen as they can be plugged into an oxygen port.
- They have double-limb tubing circuit for inspiration and exhalation.
- As it is a double limb circuit they do not need exhalation ports.
- Vented interfaces and interfaces with antiasphyxia valves should be avoided.
- As these are not turbine-driven ventilators, they do not cope as well as NIV specific ventilators with the leaks.

Examples of PICU ventilator with NIV option: MAQUET (Servo I), Dräger (VN500), Hamilton (G5), Purittan–Bennet, etc.

COMPONENTS OF NONINVASIVE VENTILATION MACHINES

Various components of NIV machines are:
- Humidification
- Expiratory port
- Antiasphyxia valve
- Battery support
- Oxygen
- Alarm

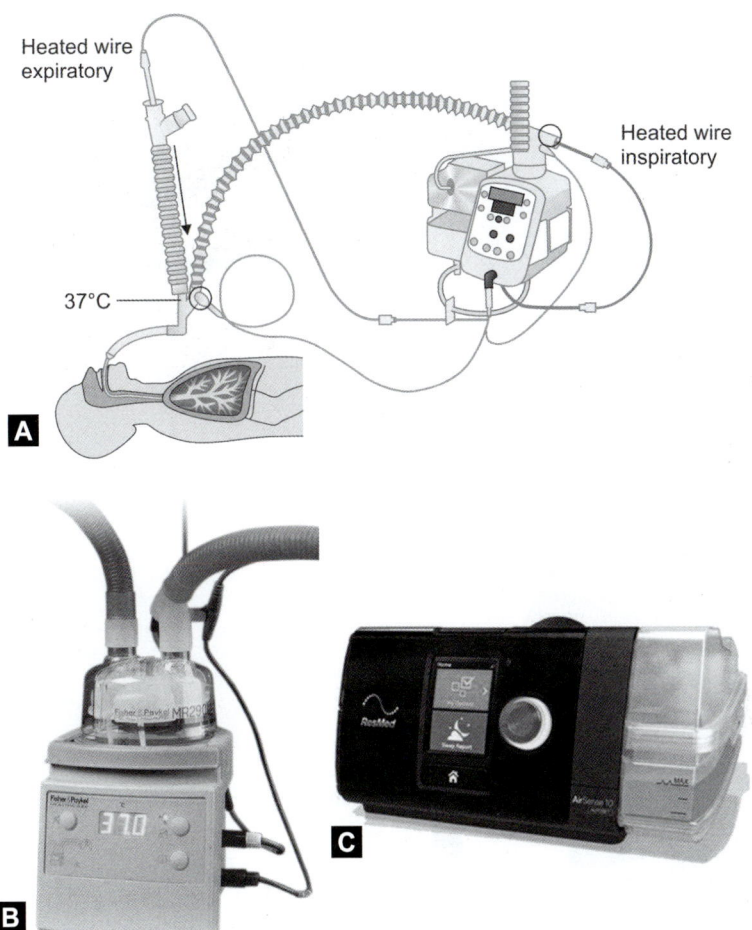

Figs. 11A to C: Various humidification devices.

Humidification (Figs. 11A to C)

- Air from the ventilator can be drying, particularly if wearing the machine for prolonged periods. This can be uncomfortable for the person using NIV. Heated humidification can help alleviate this.
- Should be considered in patients who struggle with retained secretions that may be dried out by the ventilator.
- Essential for tracheostomy patients as they bypass their own humidification system in their nose and mouth.
- Depending on the ventilator, the humidifier may attach directly to the machine or be a standalone unit.

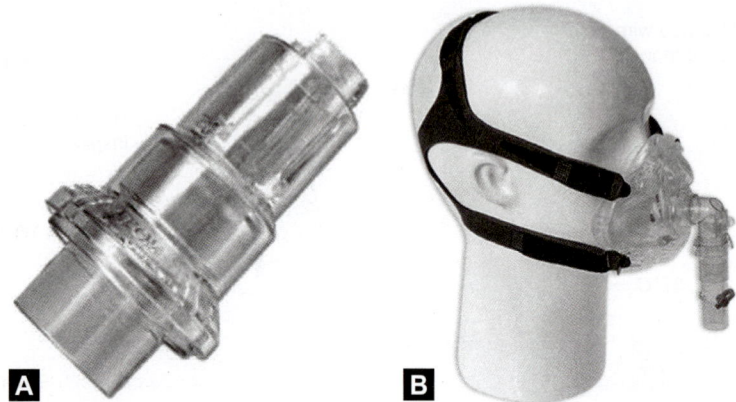

Figs. 12A and B: Expiratory port.

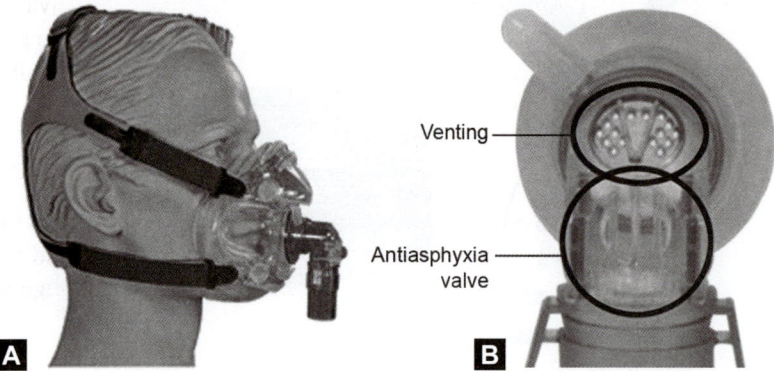

Figs. 13A and B: Difference between antiasphyxia valve and vent in the interface.

Expiratory Port (Figs. 12A and B)

- *An expiratory port*:
  - Is essential in any single limb circuit when non-vented interfaces are used.
  - To allow for carbon dioxide to be removed on expiration.
- Port can either be in the mask or circuit.
- Know where the port is and ensure it is not covered.

Antiasphyxia Valve (Figs. 13A and B)

- An antiasphyxia valve is not an expiratory port.
- It prevents the patient from asphyxia leading to hypoxia and hypercapnia if there is a mechanical failure. At the loss of pressure, the pressure valve opens to ambient air so that the patient can breathe in and out environmental air.

Battery Support

The ventilator should have an internal and if necessary external battery (which would prolong battery life of the vent) if:
- Person uses ventilator for prolonged periods.
- Person lives in an area with a high risk of power cuts.
- Person relies heavily on mandatory breaths from the machine.
- Person needs to be away for a power source while on the machine (e.g. when travelling/out and about).

Oxygen

Connector can either attach to machine directly, onto the circuit or entrained through connector on some masks.

Alarms

All tracheostomized patients should have their circuit disconnect alarm activated for safety. The alarms which can be set will depend on the needs of your patient and the policies of the NIV service who provide the machine. Available alarms will depend on the ventilator, but can include circuit disconnect, high and low RR, and high and low tidal volumes.

INTERFACES

Choosing the right interface is very essential for the success of NIV. A good mask fit is essential to ensure patient comfort, effective ventilation, and reduce pressure sores and eye irritation. For this, we need to consider ease of putting on the mask, if they breathe through their nose or mouth (Figs. 14 and 15).

Nasal Interfaces

- They are thin, flexible, and bridge material
- Dual density foam bridge forehead support
- Dual flap cushion.

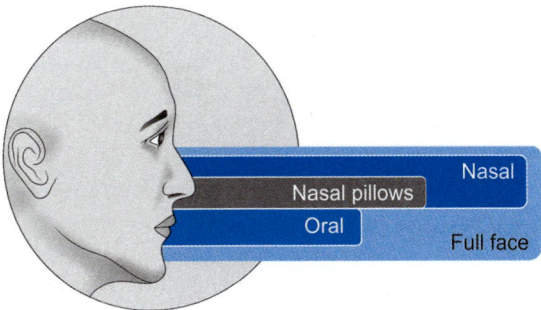

Fig. 14: Various types of interfaces.

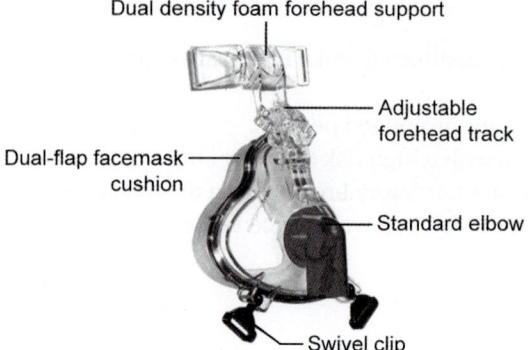

Fig. 15: Various components of interfaces.

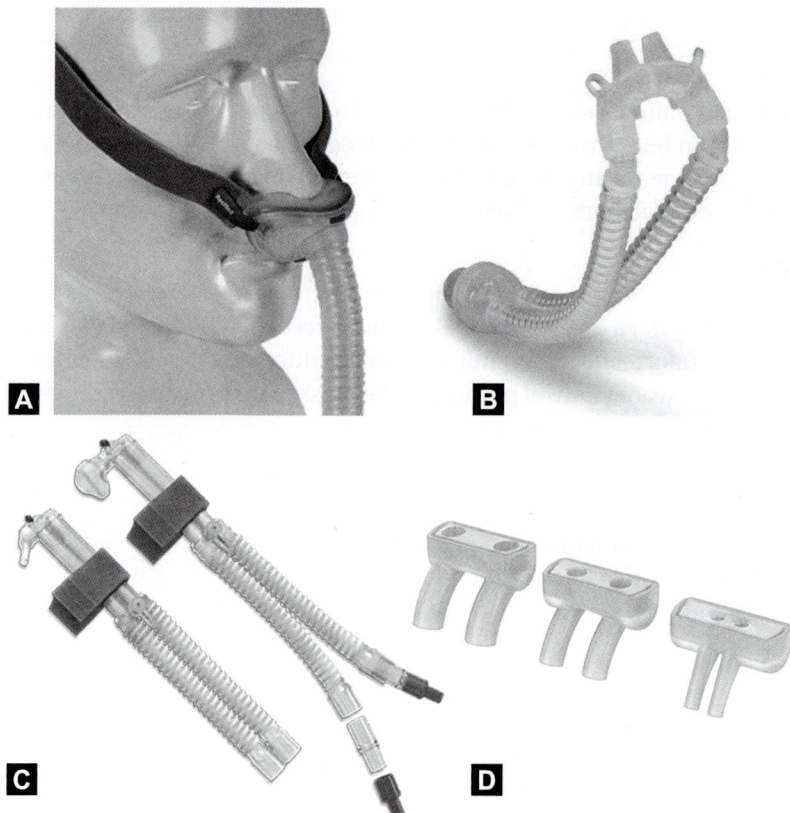

Figs. 16A to D: Nasal pillows and nasal prongs.

Nasal Pillows and Nasal Prongs (Figs. 16A to D)

Pros

- Small and unobtrusive
- Ideal to wear during the day

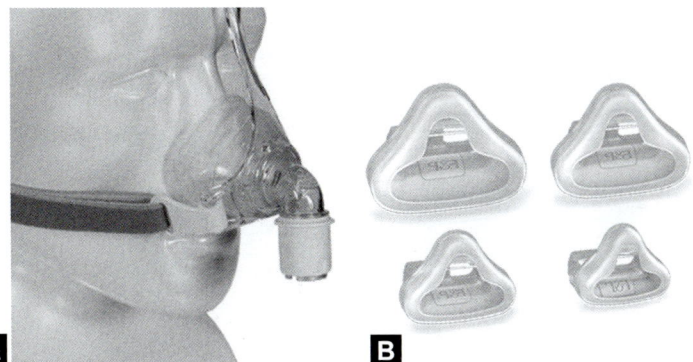

Figs. 17A and B: Nasal masks.

- Still able to talk, eat, etc.
- Preferable for claustrophobics.

Cons

- Can be uncomfortable as all air is directed into the nostrils
- Can cause irritation/dryness inside the nose
- Not effective for mouth breathers.

Nasal Masks (Figs. 17A and B)

Pros

- Relatively small and unobtrusive
- Ideal to wear during the day
- Can be less uncomfortable than nasal pillows
- Preferable for claustrophobics.

Cons

- Larger than nasal pillows
- Can cause irritation/dryness inside the nose
- Not effective for mouth breathers.

Full Facemask (Figs. 18A and B)

Pros

- Ideal for acute NIV. Hence, preferred option when children are unwell.
- Ideal for people who breathe through their mouth or are hypoxemic.

Cons

- Larger interfaces

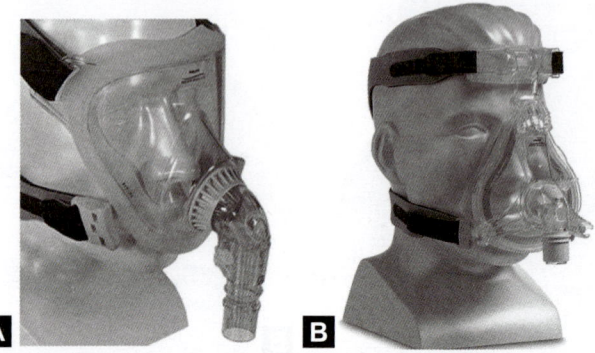

Figs. 18A and B: Full facemask.

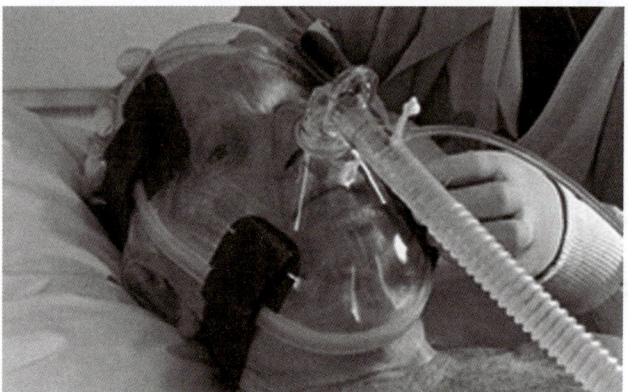

Fig. 19: Total facemask.

- Communication is much harder
- You are unable to eat and drink
- Can be difficult to wear, if you are claustrophobic.

Total Facemask (Fig. 19)

Pros

- Ideal for acute NIV. Hence, preferred option when children are unwell.
- Ideal for people who breathe through their mouth.
- Avoid skin sores of the nasal bridge.

Cons

- Much larger interfaces
- Communication is much harder
- You are unable to eat and drink
- Can be difficult to wear, if you are claustrophobic.

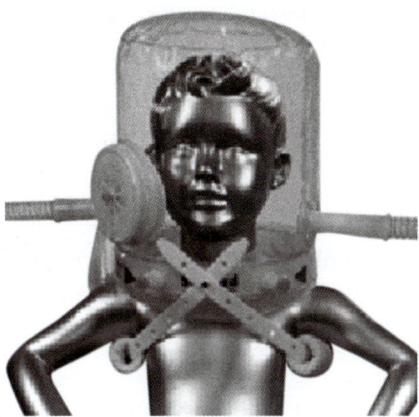

Fig. 20: Helmet mask.

Helmet (Fig. 20)

Pros

- Ideal for acute NIV. Hence, preferred option when infants are unwell.
- Well tolerated, ideal for people who breathe through their mouth.
- Avoids facial problems and skin sores.
- Less drying/irritation of the nose.

Cons

- Much larger interfaces.
- Communication is much harder.
- You are unable to eat and drink.
- Can be difficult to wear if you are claustrophobic.
- Less effective than standard interfaces in situations of resistive load.
- Not suitable for bilevel pressure. Asynchrony and worse CO_2 clearance.

STEPS OF INITIATING NONINVASIVE VENTILATION

- Choose ventilation mode, define your goals, and beware of possible complications.
- Using a sizing gauge, make sure a mask is chosen that is the proper size and fit.
- Attach the interface and circuit to the ventilator. Turn on the ventilator and adjust it initially to low pressure setting.
- Hold or allow the patient to hold the mask gently to the face until the patient becomes comfortable with it. Encourage the patient to use proper breathing technique.
- Monitor oxygen (O_2) saturation; adjust the fractional inspired oxygen (FiO_2) to maintain O_2 saturation above 90%.
- Secure the mask to the patient. Do not make the straps too tight.
- Titrate the inspiratory and end-expiratory positive airway pressures (IPAP 8 cm and EPAP 4 cm) to achieve patient comfort, adequate exhaled tidal volume, and synchrony with the ventilator.

- Check for leaks and adjust the straps if necessary. Ideally some leak is essential to prevent pressure sores and skin breakdown.
- Monitor the RR, heart rate (HR), level of dyspnea, O_2 saturation, minute ventilation, and exhaled tidal volume.
- Obtain blood gas values within 1 hour or monitor noninvasively using S/F ratio.

MONITORING

Once NIV is initiated, patients should be closely monitored in a critical care unit or a step-down unit until they are sufficiently stable to be moved to a regular ward.

Aim of Monitoring

The main aim of monitoring is to ensure relief of symptoms, reduced WOB, improved or stable gas exchange, good patient-ventilator synchrony, and patient comfort. A drop in the RR with improved oxygen saturation or improving pH with a lower $PaCO_2$, reduced HR, within the first 1 to 2 hours portends a successful outcome. The absence of these propitious signs indicates a poor response to NIV.

Potential Indicator of Success in Acute Noninvasive Ventilation

- Age older than 6 months
- Lower acuity of illness (APACHE score)
- Able to cooperate, better neurologic score
- Less air leaking
- Moderate hypercarbia ($PaCO_2$ > 45 mm Hg, < 92 mm Hg)
- Moderate academia (pH < 7.35, > 7.10)
- Improvements in gas exchange (S/F ratio > 200) and heart RRs within first 2 hours.

Possible Failure

- Worsening pH and $PaCO_2$
- Tachypnea persisting after couple of hours of NIV
- Hemodynamic instability
- Oxygen saturation by pulse oximeter (SpO_2) less than 90%
- Decreased level of consciousness
- Inability to clear secretions
- Inability to tolerate interface.

Noninvasive Ventilation Data Monitoring

- Data that can be collected includes mask leak, tidal volume, patient triggered breathing, and length of time the machine is used.
- The amount of data available is dependent on the company that produces the ventilators, although several companies are now trying to increase the amount of information that can be gained from their machines.

- There is a move toward monitoring and managing this data remotely using modems which attach to the ventilator. This could allow clinicians to monitor patients between reviews and can lead to more proactive management.

TROUBLESHOOTING

While on NIV the following are the common trouble that we might face:
- Equipment alarming
- Ventilator settings
- Interfaces
- Humidification devices
- Asynchrony.

Equipment Alarming

- Often the ventilator will come up with a message to say why it has been alarming which can help you troubleshoot.
- The alarms which have been set will vary depending on the patient and the policies of the NIV service providing the equipment.
- If there are any machine-related issues contact the services who have provided the equipment for support.

Ventilator Setting

- Persons who report they are not getting enough support from the machine or are more short of breath—usually need an increase in IPAP or rise time
- Persons who report they are getting morning headaches, pins and needles or excessive daytime sleepiness—need an increase in IPAP as these are signs of carbon dioxide elevation.
- Persons who report pressure is too much—reduce IPAP/EPAP and while person acclimatizes to ventilator. If person is struggling to wear the machine at night, advise trying during the daytime initially.

Interfaces

- Pressure sore should be prevented. Relief of pressure every 2–4 hours is strongly recommended at least for 1–2 minutes. Gentle massage in the area permits vascular flow and enhances tissue recovery.
- Rotation of interfaces ideally could work, but is not easy to have two different interfaces which fit the patient.
- Hydrocolloid dressings/gel pad should be placed in pressure points especially in hypoxemic patients who are not going to tolerate disconnections.
- Mask is noisy/air blowing outside of mask/dry sore eyes—check mask is cleaned properly/not old or damaged. If this is not a problem change interface.

Humidification

- Trial of adding active humidification if—person is complaining of a dry nose/mouth.
- *Secretions have become thicker and harder to clear since starting on NIV*: It is considered mandatory in neonates and infants, neuromuscular patients, cystic fibrosis patients, those patients requiring more than 50% of oxygen in a turbine-based ventilator and all patients on a PICU ventilator with NIV option (air and oxygen come from the flowmeter without humidity).
- *Water in hose/mask*: Turn down humidifier temperature, use less water in the humidification chamber, ensure that separate humidification unit is lower than machine.

Asynchrony

The asynchrony can be divided into two main types:
1. Inspiratory asynchrony
2. Expiratory asynchrony.

In invasive ventilation, asynchrony is a feature associated with negative outcomes like lengthening of mechanical ventilation or even worse outcomes, such as increased mortality in adult patients.

It is also a common reason for failing in NIV, so it is crucial to understand the major reasons of asynchrony in NIV and the best way to sort it out.

Hence, we need to teach our teams the correct selection of the interfaces and optimum fitting, because leaks are the major factor involved in asynchrony.

There are very few suitable oronasal interfaces for children younger than 3 years. Few years back only few interfaces were available for these children. Nasal interfaces have been commonly used in small infants and neonates. But with mouth open, leaks are common. Chin strap and pacifiers help to reduce oral leaks.

Inspiratory Asynchrony

This can be due to leaks, inadequate pressurization, ineffective triggering or autotriggering.

Leaks: In presence of leak, the machine does not reach the targeted IPAP. Hence, the machine prolongs the inspiration to compensate for the leaks and results in prolonged inspiration. If this leak cannot be reduced, then this can be managed by adjusting the inspiratory cycling. Cycling is the decrease to the predetermined fraction of the peak inspiratory flow. This usually set to percentage of the total inspiratory time. Hence when a percentage value of the pressure has been reached, the machine automatically cycles into the expiratory mode. The persisting leaks can also result in inadequate pressurization. The inadequate pressurization can be managed by changing the rise time, minimizing the leaks and changing to a ventilator with better pressurization.

Ineffective inspiratory trigger: The inspiratory muscle does not trigger the ventilator. This can happen in the presence of high leaks, high level of support, in presence of dynamic hyperinflation, and in presence of increased dead space from a filter.

This problem is commonly seen in NIV-specific ventilators when using in patients younger than 3 months (offlabel use). Many modern PICU ventilators with NIV option have inspiratory triggers more sensitive that can be used.

This can be solved by briefly (3–6 hours) removing the active humidification until patient improves and then is capable to generate a stronger inspiratory effort or change to T or P control mode. Appropriate inspiratory time and backup RR should be set in order to facilitate these small patients to adapt to NIV. Alternatively, you can change to ventilator with a more sensitive trigger (V60 with autotrack/NAVA).

Auto-trigger: Expiratory leaks can generate a pressure drop below the external PEEP level, in-turn simulating the patient's effort and triggering a ventilator breath. This results in shorter cycles and flow distortion. Hence the patient might not generate effort or fight the ventilator.

Autotriggering can be solved by decreasing trigger sensitivity by careful adjustment of settings and avoiding ineffective triggering.

Double triggering can happen because of insufficient level of pressure support or increased inspiratory demand or if the ventilator's pressurization time is too short.

Inspiratory cycling: Cycling is the decrease to the predetermined fraction of the peak inspiratory flow. This is usually set to percentage of the total inspiratory time.

Expiratory Asynchrony

Delayed cycling can result in expiratory asynchrony. This happens in the presence of leaks. This prolongs mechanical inspirations. The inspiration does not reach the cycling-off criterion and hence delaying cycling-off.

This can be solved by:
- Reducing the leaks with better selection of the interfaces and their position.
- Reducing the inspiratory time to 0.8–1.2 seconds.
- Reducing the IPAP and the pressure support level.
- Increasing the expiratory trigger to 50% of more.
- Higher value of the expiratory trigger reduces the expiratory cycling time.

HOME MECHANICAL VENTILATION

Advanced intensive care interventions have resulted in better survival with increased morbidity. At the same time, the increasing cost of healthcare, fear of hospital-acquired infections, and the recognized need for the child to be in a family environment that best suits its development is driving us to undertake early discharges to home wherever feasible. All this with improving rehabilitation technology has made home ventilation in a safe manner feasible and an expected service today.

The respiratory work is a balance between the neural mechanism including the neuromuscular system and the respiratory load toward airway, lung parenchymal and thoracic cage mechanics, the imbalance in which leads to respiratory failure and a sustained imbalance leads to chronicity in the respiratory failure (Fig. 21).

There can be broadly two categories of patients who need home ventilation:
1. Children who are dependent on ventilation for life support.
2. Children needing ventilation support for health maintenance, prevention of illness, reducing morbidity, reducing frequency and duration admission rates into hospital and improve quality of life.

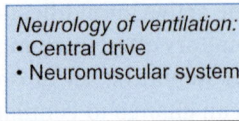 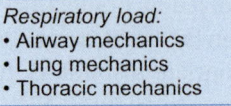

Fig. 21: The balance between the neural mechanism and respiratory load.

Patients can be ventilated at home by two methods:
1. Invasive ventilation (via tracheostomy/diaphragmatic pacemaker)
2. Noninvasive positive-pressure ventilation or noninvasive negative-pressure ventilation (NINPV).

The choice of methods depends upon:
- The age at which treatment begins
- Availability of appropriate noninvasive interface
- Pathology—airway/lung parenchymal/neuromuscular/central
- Degree of respiratory autonomy—ability to tolerate short breaks
- Family situation—caregiver's efficiency/financial status, etc.

Home Ventilation via Tracheostomy

Suitable for children being discharged from the hospital with otherwise stable medical condition and stable ventilator support over few weeks with following conditions:
- Children needing prolonged hours of ventilation support in a day—more than 16 hrs/day.
- Small infants and children dependent on ventilation for life sustenance, i.e. they do not tolerate even brief periods of discontinuation of ventilation support; Children with cord injury, moderate-to-severe parenchymal lung pathologies, severe neuromuscular disease, severe airway problems—severe tracheobronchomalacia and central hypoventilation.

Home Ventilation via Noninvasive Mask Interface

This may be suitable for children discharged from the hospital facility with stable medical condition and stable ventilator supports on NIV mask interface for few weeks, who have:
- Children who need support only during sleep
- Those who tolerate short periods off ventilator support with no life threats
- Could be an alternative to the tracheostomy group in selected situations with no major airway compromise.

For example; neuromuscular disease, restrictive lung diseases as in chest wall deformities, chronic lung disease, obesity hypoventilation, and some upper airway obstructions not surgically correctable.

Disease Specific Selection Guidelines for Long-term NIPPV

Restrictive Thoracic Disorders and Obesity Hypoventilation
- *Clinical*: Fatigue, morning headaches, hypersomnolence, enuresis, dyspnea, and nightmares.

- *Gas exchange criteria*: Daytime PCO_2 more than 45 mm Hg. Nocturnal desaturations (<88% for > 5 minutes or >10% of total monitoring time)
- Recovering from acute respiratory failure with PCO_2 retention.
- Needing repeated hospitalization for acute respiratory failure.

Obstructive Sleep Apnea/Central Sleep Apnea

- Polysomnogram showing OSA/central sleep apnea (CSA)/mixed patterns.
- Obstructive sleep apnea patient failing to improve or tolerate CPAP.
- Sustained desaturation nocturnally (<88% for >5 minutes or >10% of total monitoring time).
- Significant improvement in gas exchange on NIPPV based on oximetry or polysomnography.

Obstructive Lung Disease

- *Clinical*: Fatigue, hypersomnolence, and dyspnea.
- Failure to respond to maximal bronchodilator therapy/steroids/oxygen.
- *Gas exchange abnormalities*: $PaCO_2$ more than 52 mm Hg. Desaturations (<88% for >5 consecutive minutes despite oxygen supplementation).
- *On reassessment after 4 months*: Good compliance in usage (>4 hrs/day) or improvement in clinical situation.

Discharge Planning

These children will need the following preparation toward home transition.

Equipment Setup at Home

- Portable ventilator with good humidification, battery backup/alternative power provision, appropriate built-in alarms (low tidal volume, disconnection alarm, high pressure alarm, and power failure alarms).
- *For noninvasive interface patients*: Appropriate sized, shape mask to minimize dead space, leak, and pressure effect on the face or nose are mandatory. Suction facility at home—electrical/mechanical, with appropriate size suction catheters.
- Hand ventilation equipment (Ambu bag)
- Oxygen source—portable oxygen cylinder/oxygen concentrator
- Oxygen saturation monitor
- Nebulization kit, if needed with appropriate training in its usage.

Caregiver Preparation

- Staged discharge process ensuring caregivers understand the care process and are confident of caring for the child.
- 24/7 vigilante caregiver—at least 2 in number who understand the child's needs.
- Caregivers trained in basic cardiopulmonary resuscitation (CPR) and tracheostomy care including suction, changing tracheostomy tube, troubleshooting malfunction like obstruction.

- Educated in feeding process either orally, via NG tube, via gastrostomy and physiotherapy (chest/limbs).
- Clearly written comprehensive care plan at home discussed with the caregivers and ensure they understand the same.
- Clear follow-up plan with multidisciplinary home ventilation team comprising of pulmonologist, intensivist, and ear, nose, and throat (ENT) services.
- Emergency contacts numbers/tie up with nearest capable caring facility.

Follow-up Plan

- Multidisciplinary team comprising of general pediatrics, pulmonologist, ENT, and intensivist to be following up with.
- *Regular follow-up*: Weekly to begin with and later spaced out to 2–3 monthly in tracheostomy patients and 3–6 monthly in mask interface patients.
- Regular review for change in ventilator settings individualized to each patient based on clinical WOB, sleep studies, blood gases, and growth/development parameters.
- As needed counseling and psychological support for the child, parents, and caregivers.
- Appropriate transfer to adult caregivers based on their age and local health policies.

Situations where Long-term Home Ventilation is not Suitable Option

- Copious secretions difficult to manage for the family at home.
- Poorly motivated family/patient.
- Poor mask interface due to nonavailability or anatomic factors in the patient—consider tracheostomy.
- *Poor airway reflexes*: Mask interface not a good option, consider tracheostomy.
- Inability to comprehend and follow treatment plan and ventilator usage.
- Poor family resources and lack of accessible medical support in case of emergencies.

HIGH-FLOW NASAL CANNULA OXYGEN THERAPY

Noninvasive ventilation, provided by mask interface, in small children can be a challenging, but highly effective respiratory support modality. The challenges in the small children could be due to:
- Inability to get appropriate size masks.
- Children may not cooperate for the mask can be very threatening or claustrophobic.
- Injuries to the eye due to inappropriately sized masks.
- Pressure effects of the mask over the nose and cheeks.
- Speaking and eating needs removal of the masks interface in full facemasks.

High-flow nasal cannula oxygen therapy offers a great alternative in these situations. It is now the preferred mode of NIV in children, in select situations, especially small infants, neonates although it is not limited to this age group (Fig. 22).

High-flow nasal cannula system basically provides a mixture of humidified air and oxygen at flow rates greater than the peak inspiratory flow rates for the child.

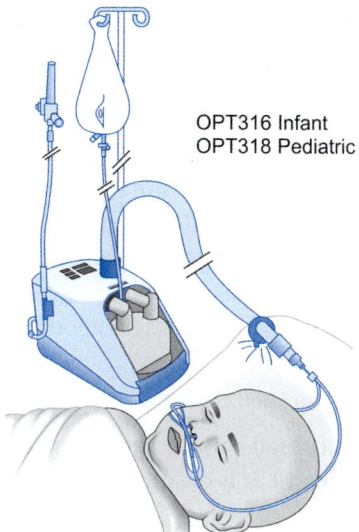

Fig. 22: High-flow nasal cannula (HFNC) machine with nasal cannula.

Machines

Three types of gas generators are currently available:
1. The first type uses an air/oxygen blender and is connected to a system to humidify and heat the gas, e.g. Optiflow System—Fisher and Paekel, Auckland, New Zealand, Precision Flow (Vapotherm, Exeter, UK, Comfort-Flo Teleflex Medical, Durham, NC, USA).
2. The second type uses a turbine + humidifier. This system has the advantage of not requiring an external source of gas, except oxygen. This device cannot be used with neonates, e.g. Airvo 2—Fisher and Paekel, Auckland, New Zealand.
3. The third type is based on a CPAP or conventional ventilator with an HFNC breathing circuit connected to the humidifier.

The system mainly comprises of:
- An air/oxygen blender
- An active humidifier
- A single heated circuit
- A nasal cannula.

Rationale and Physiological Effects

- *Reduction in anatomical dead space*: The high flow of oxygen "washes out" the end-expiratory oxygen-depleted gas from the anatomical dead space, oropharynx, and so in the next breath, the patient inhales pure oxygen. The extrathoracic dead space is proportionally two to three times greater in children than in adults. It may measure up to 3 mL/kg in newborns and becomes similar to the adult volume only after 6 years of age (0.8 mL/kg). This may contribute significantly for the WOB in small children. Consequently, the younger a child is, the greater the effect of a high flow on oxygenation and CO_2 clearance.

- *PEEP effect*: Although delivered through an open system, high flow overcomes resistance against expiratory flow and creates positive nasopharyngeal pressure. There is prevention of pharyngeal collapse. While the pressure is relatively low compared with closed systems, it is considered adequate to stent open the small airways and even increases lung volume or recruit collapsed alveoli.
- *Constant function of FiO_2 and WOB effects*: The difference between the inspiratory flow of patients and delivered flow is small and FiO_2 remains relatively constant.
- *Good humidification*: The gas in HFNC is humidified (95–100% relative humidity) and warmed to near body temperature. Because gas is generally warmed to 37°C and completely humidified, mucociliary functions remain good and little discomfort is reported.

Interfaces

Nasal cannula of different sizes (based on the age group/nostril size). The prong diameter should be about half that of the nostril. It is desirable to allow for leakage and avoid over pressure phenomenon.

Indications

- *Mild-to-moderate hypoxemic respiratory failure*: Saturations less than 90% despite standard oxygen flow and respiratory distress (bronchiolitis, pneumonia, pulmonary edema, asthma, atelectasis, etc.).
- Chronic hypercapnic respiratory failure (as in some CLD) and OSA.
- Respiratory support in chronic neuromuscular diseases.
- Weaning from invasive ventilation especially in small infants.
- Some use it preintubation for better tolerance of the apneic state during intubation.

Contraindications

- Severe hypoxemia respiratory failure
- Poor sensorium
- Poor airway reflexes with risk of aspiration
- Maxillofacial trauma
- Associated hemodynamic instability
- Presence of air leaks.

Advantages of High-flow Nasal Cannula

- Simple to use with need for minimal technical skills to set it up.
- Not claustrophobic, children can speak, eat, and drink freely.
- Humidified air—oxygen mix can be given.
- FiO_2 can be ascertained and set. High FiO_2 can be given.
- Pressure effects of mask NIV negated.
- Risk of aspiration minimized.

Steps Involved in Initiating and Monitoring of High-flow Nasal Cannula

Step 1:
- Select appropriate patient.
- Ensure no contraindications.
- Select appropriate size cannula (prong size ½ of the nostril).
- Explain procedure to family/patient where appropriate.
- Machine setup.

Step 2:
- Select desired flow and FiO_2
- *Keep flows in infants*: 1.5–2 L/kg/min and in children 1–1.5 L/kg/min
- FiO_2 to get saturations in 92–97% ranges (can start with high FiO_2 of about 50–60% and wean down depending on tolerance and saturations).

Step 3:
- *Monitor*: Consciousness, airway patency, RR, WOB, HR, blood pressure (BP), SaO_2, and blood gases.
- If improvement in parameters above in the next 2–4 hours—continue support.
- Expect FIO_2 to decrease to less than 40% or HR and RR to reduce by 20%, WOB to reduce.
- If no improvement or worsening, consider alternative supports—mask NIV.

Step 4:
- Wean FiO_2 gradually to attain saturations of 92–97% to as low as 21% if possible.
- Wean flows once the WOB is improving and the child is on more than 40% oxygen.
- Can wean off to nasal cannula oxygen or continue on low flow HFNC to wean off oxygen completely.

ACKNOWLEDGMENTS

We are extremely indebted to our advisor's Dr Marti Pons Odena, Pediatric Intensivist, University Hospital, Sant Joan de Déu, Barcelona, Spain, Chair of NIV in children for ESPINIC (Europe) and Dr Alberto Medina, Paediatric Intensivist, University Hospital, Central de Asturias, Spain for their extended support.

All Tables and Figures are adapted from NIV in Children Manual developed by Dr Ashwath Ram RN over the past 4 years.

SUGGESTED READING

1. Calderini E, Chidini G, Pelosi P. What are the current indications for noninvasive ventilation in children? Curr Opin Anaesthesiol. 2010;23:368.
2. Chisti MJ, Salam MA, Smith JH, et al. Bubble continuous positive airway pressure for children with severe pneumonia and hypoxaemia in Bangladesh: an open, randomised controlled trial. Lancet. 2015;386:1057.
3. Collins SP, Mielnicznik LP, Whittingham HA, et al. The use of noninvasive ventilation in emergency department patients with acute cardiogenic pulmonary edema: a systematic review. Ann Emerg Med. 2006;48:260-9.
4. de Miguel-DíezJ, Jiménez-García R, Hernández-Barrera V. National trends in hospital admissions for asthma exacerbations among pediatric and young adult population in Spain (2002-2010). Respir Med. 2014;108(7):983-91.

5. Dohna-Schwake C, Stehling F, Tschiedel E, et al. Non-invasive ventilation on a pediatric intensive care unit: feasibility, efficacy, and predictors of success. Pediatric Pulmonol. 2011;46:1114-20.
6. Essouri S, Chevret L, Durand P, et. al. Noninvasive positive pressure ventilation: five years of experience in a pediatric intensive care unit. Pediatr Crit Care Med. 2006;7(4):329-34.
7. Fartoukh M, Lefort Y, Habibi A, et al. Early intermittent non-invasive ventilation for acute chest syndrome in adults with sickle cell disease: a pilot study. Intensive Care Med. 2010;36:1355-62.
8. Fuchs H, Schoss J, Mendler MR, et al. The cause of acute respiratory failure predicts the outcome of noninvasive ventilation in immunocompromised children. Klin Padiatr. 2015;227:322-8.
9. Gupta P, Kuperstock JE, Hashmi S, et al. Efficacy and predictors of success of noninvasive ventilation for prevention of extubation failure in critically ill children with heart disease. Pediatr Cardiol. 2013;34:964-77.
10. Kneyber MCJ, Rimensberger PC. Recommendations for mechanical ventilation of critically ill children from the Paediatric Mechanical Ventilation Consensus Conference (PEMVEC). Intensive Care Med.2017;43:1764-80.
11. Kovacikova K, Skrak P, Dobos D, et al. Noninvasive positive pressure ventilation in critically ill children with cardiac disease. Pediatr Cardiol. 2014;35:676-83.
12. Lazner MR, Basu AP, Klonin M. Non-invasive ventilation for severe bronchiolitis: analysis and evidence. Pediatric Pulmonol. 2012;47:909-16.
13. Luo F, Annane D, Orlikowski D, et. al. Invasive versus non-invasive ventilation for acute respiratory failure in neuromuscular disease and chest wall disorders, 2017.
14. Mayordomo-Colunga J, Medina A, Rey C, et al. Noninvasive ventilation after extubation in paediatric patients: a preliminary study. BMC Pediatr. 2010;10:29.
15. Mayordomo-Colunga J, Medina A, Rey C, et al. Noninvasive ventilation in pediatric status asthmaticus: a prospective observational study. Pediatr Pulmonol. 2011;46:949-55.
16. Mayordomo-Colunga J, Medina A, Rey C, et al. Predictive factors of non-invasive ventilation failure in critically ill children: a prospective epidemiological study. Intensive Care Med. 2009;35(3):527-36.
17. Mayordomo-Colunga J, Pons-Òdena M, Medina A, et al. Non-invasive ventilation practices in children across Europe. Pediatr Pulmonol. 2018;53(8):1107-14.
18. Morley SL. Non-invasive ventilation in paediatric critical care. Paediatr Respir Rev. 2016;20:24-31.
19. Pancera CF, Hayashi M, Fregnani JH, et al. Noninvasive ventilation in immunocompromised pediatric patients: eight years of experience in a pediatric oncology intensive care unit. J Pediatr Hematol Oncol. 2008;30:533-8.
20. Piastra M, Luca De Le, Pietrini D, et al. Noninvasive pressure-support ventilation in immunocompromised children with ARDS: a feasibility study. Intensive Care Med. 2009;35:1420-7.
21. Silva CR, Andrade LB, Duarte MC, et al. Effectiveness of prophylactic non-invasive ventilation on respiratory function in the postoperative phase of pediatric cardiac surgery: a randomized controlled trial. Braz J Phys Ther. 2016;20(6):494-501.
22. Silva Pde S, Barreto SS. Non-invasive ventilation in status asthmaticus in children: levels of evidence. Rev Bras Ter Intensiva. 2015;27(4):390-6.
23. Walk J, Dinga P, Lang HJ, et al. Non-invasive ventilation with bubble CPAP is feasible and improves respiratory physiology in hospitalised Malawian children with acute respiratory failure. Paediatr Int Child Health. 2016;36(1):28-33.

Respiratory Monitoring in the Pediatric Intensive Care Unit

9

Vishram Buche, Anand Bhutada

LEARNING OBJECTIVES

- To learn clinical monitoring of the child in respiratory distress
- To understand the different modalities used in monitoring
- To understand capnography
- To understand acid-base balance and interpret blood gas analysis

INTRODUCTION

Respiratory monitoring in pediatric intensive care unit (PICU) is an essence of critical care. Be it clinical, invasive, or noninvasive, monitoring remains crucial in overall assessment of a critically ill child with cardiorespiratory problems. A functioning knowledge of the various tools of monitoring is essential in applying their use to patient care. This chapter discusses traditional methods of evaluation of respiratory system and newly established gold standard techniques as well. Attention is also given to newer modalities, including those that are investigational or currently limited to bench application that give promise for future application in PICU clinical practice. Pulse oximetry and capnography are the most commonly employed monitoring modalities, which have transformed the practice of critical care in the last 10 years. Arterial blood gases (ABGs) and calculated oxygen indices have been most commonly used and form essential part of monitoring in PICU. However, may be the excellent information is provided by respiratory monitors, it cannot replace careful bedside clinical examination.

Essentially, respiratory monitoring consists of:
- Physical examination
- Noninvasive monitoring
- Invasive monitoring.

PHYSICAL EXAMINATION

Measuring the respiratory rate (Table 1) is easy and has got a good accuracy in prediction of lower respiratory tract infection. Presence of increased work of breathing is suggested by flaring

Table 1: Normal respiratory rates.

Age	Respiratory rate
Infant (birth–1 year)	30–60
Toddler (1–3 years)	24–40
Preschooler (3–6 years)	22–34
School-age (6–12 years)	18–30
Adolescent (12–18 years)	12–16

Table 2: Silverman–Anderson Index.

Features	Score 0	Score 1	Score 2
Chest movement	Equal	Respiratory lag	See-saw respiration
Intercostal retractions	None	Minimal	Marked
Xiphoid retraction	None	Minimal	Marked
Nasal flaring	None	Minimal	Marked
Expiratory grunt	None	Audible wheeze by stethoscope	Audible

of alae nasi, suprasternal, intercostal, and subcostal retractions, use of accessory muscles of respiration, and paradoxical breathing.

Cyanosis of tongue and oral mucosa indicates oxygen saturation [oxygen saturation of arterial blood (SaO_2)] of less than 80%. However, there is significant interobserver variability and difficulty in SaO_2 interpretation.

When a neonate is a premature, or has underlying pathology, then expiratory grunting, retraction of the chest wall muscles, and other signs of respiratory distress may be readily seen. The Silverman–Anderson Index, commonly referred to as the Silverman retraction score, was developed as a systematic means of assessing newborn respiratory status, particularly when respiratory distress is suspected.

The parameters are assessed by inspection and auscultation of the upper and lower chest and nares on a scale of 0, 1, or 2. As it is observed in Table 2, the higher the score, the more severe is the respiratory distress.

NONINVASIVE RESPIRATORY MONITORING

Pulse oximetry is now an integral part of PICU monitoring, which helps in the assessment of the patient's cardiorespiratory (oxygenation) status. It is a simple, noninvasive, and continuous method of monitoring the SaO_2 and now widely accepted as the fifth vital sign. The pulse oximeter is a convenient, cost-effective way to monitor the patient's oxygenation status (and thereby O_2 content) and determine the changes before they are clinically apparent. It is important to know how oximeters work in order to maximize their performance and avoid errors in the interpretation of results.

Pulse oximetry is based on principles of spectrophotometry governed by Beer-Lambert law. The mandatory condition for interpretation of SaO_2 is the presence of a pulsatile arteriolar blood flow.

How does a Pulse Oximeter Work?

Interpretation of SaO_2 is based on the fact that oxygenated hemoglobin (HbO_2) and deoxygenated hemoglobin (Hb) have different absorption spectra. Currently available pulse oximeters use two light-emitting diodes (LEDs) that emit light at the 660 nm (red) and the 940 nm [infrared (IR)] wavelengths. These two wavelengths are used because HbO_2 and Hb have different absorption spectra at these particular wavelengths. In the red region, HbO_2 absorbs less light than Hb, while the reverse occurs in the IR region. The ratio of absorbencies at these two wavelengths is calibrated empirically against direct measurements of SaO_2 in volunteers, and the resulting calibration algorithm is stored in a digital microprocessor within the pulse oximeter. During subsequent use, the calibration curve is used to generate the pulse oximeter's estimate of arterial saturation (SpO_2). In addition to the digital readout of O_2 saturation and pulse rate, most pulse oximeters display a plethysmographic waveform which can help clinicians to distinguish an artifactual signal from the true signal.

There are two techniques of measuring SaO_2: transmission and reflectance. In the transmission method, the emitter and photodetector are opposite of each other with the measuring site in-between. The light can then pass through the site. In the reflectance method, the emitter and photodetector is next to each other, and on top the measuring site. The light bounces from the emitter to the detector across the site. The transmission method is the most common type of method of choice in use.

The normal SpO_2 value for adolescents and elders is greater than 95%, and for children, a level greater than 90–92% is normal. SpO_2 can be misleading as other factors must be considered when determining whether this SpO2 is normal for the particular patient.

Critical Discussion on Pulse Oximetry ($SpO_2 = SaO_2$)

- SaO2 gives fairly good idea of not only saturation but also of oxygen content (CaO_2) provided carboxyhemoglobin (COHb) and methemoglobin (MetHb) are expected in normal amounts. Since 98% of CaO_2 is contributed by saturated hemoglobin, hence it is a good idea that one should always calculate CaO_2, every time, after observing SpO_2 since CaO_2 is the better indicator of oxygenation.

  $CaO_2 = SaO_2 (98\%) + PaO2 (2\%)$

  $[CaO2 = 1.34 \times Hb \times SaO_2 + PaO_2 \times 0.003]$

  Interpretation of SpO_2 should always be done in context of the oxygen dissociation curve (ODC) (Figs. 1 and 2), since conditions causing a left shift can have a normal saturation but the patient may be hypoxic [low partial pressure of arterial oxygen (PaO_2)]. Similarly, conditions causing right shift may have low SaO_2 but the patient may not be hypoxic.

Limitations of Pulse Oximetry

Oximeters have a number of limitations which may lead to inaccurate readings. Shape of ODC, COHb, MetHb anemia, dyes, nail polish, ambient light, motion artifact, skin pigmentation, and low perfusion states are other causes as well.

Pulse oximeters measure SpO_2 that is physiologically related to arterial oxygen tension (PaO_2) according to the oxyhemoglobin dissociation curve (ODC). Because the ODC has a

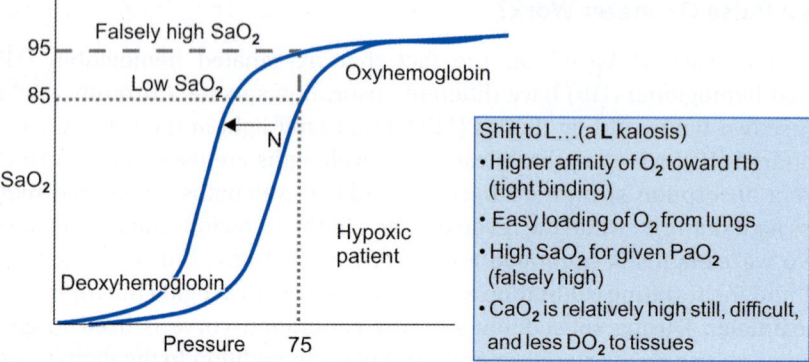

Fig. 1: Oxygen dissociation curve (ODC) with left shift.
(CaO_2: oxygen content; DO_2: oxygen delivery; Hb: hemoglobin; O_2: oxygen; SaO_2: oxygen saturation of arterial blood).

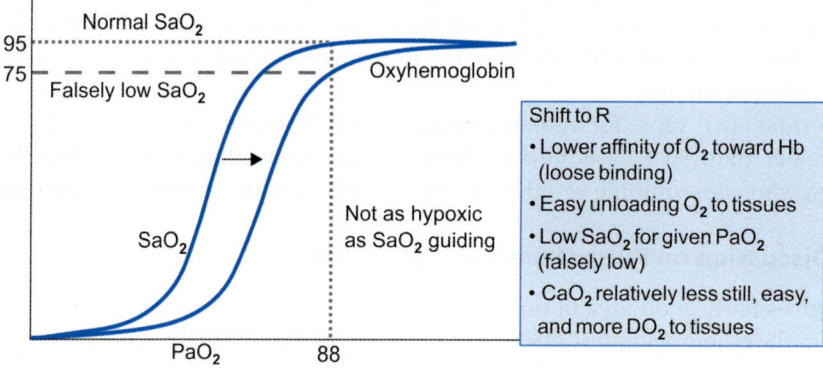

Fig. 2: Oxygen dissociation curve (ODC) with right shift.
(CaO_2: oxygen content; DO_2: oxygen delivery; Hb: hemoglobin; O_2: oxygen; PaO_2: partial pressure of arterial oxygen; SaO_2: oxygen saturation of arterial blood).

sigmoid shape, oximetry is relatively insensitive in detecting the development of hypoxemia in patients with high baseline levels of PaO_2 (upper flat portion of ODC curve).

Since pulse oximeters use only two wavelengths of light, it can distinguish only two substances, Hb and HbO_2. When COHb and MetHb are also present, four wavelengths are required to determine the "fractional SaO_2", i.e. $(HbO_2 \times 100)/(Hb + HbO_2 + COHb + MetHb)$ and this can be measured by co-oximetry. In the presence of elevated COHb levels, oximetry consistently overestimates the true SaO_2 by the amount of COHb present since it has got same absorption spectrum as of HbO_2. Elevated MetHb levels also may cause inaccurate oximetry readings. Anemia does not appear to affect the accuracy of pulse oximetry even in nonhypoxemic patients with acute anemia; pulse oximetry was accurate in measuring O_2 saturation. Severe hyperbilirubinemia (mean bilirubin, 30.6 mg/dL) does not affect the accuracy of pulse oximetry.

Intravenous dyes such as methylene blue, indocyanine green and indigo carmine can cause falsely low SpO_2 readings. Nail polish, if blue, green, or black, causes inaccurate SpO_2 readings, whereas acrylic nails do not interfere with pulse oximetry readings. Falsely low and high SpO_2 readings occur with fluorescent and xenon arc surgical lamps.

Motion artifact continues to be a significant source of error and false alarms. In a recent, prospective study in an intensive care unit setting, SpO_2 signals accounted for almost half of a total of 2,525 false alarms.

Inaccurate oximetry readings have been observed in pigmented patients, but not by all investigators. Low perfusion states, such as low cardiac output, vasoconstriction, and hypothermia may impair peripheral perfusion and may make it difficult for a sensor to distinguish a true signal from background layers.

An under-recognized and worrisome problem with pulse oximetry is that many users have a limited understanding of how it functions and the implications of its measurements. In a recent survey, 30% of physicians and 93% of nurses thought that the oximeter measured PaO_2. Some clinicians also have a limited knowledge of the ODC, and they do not recognize that SpO_2 values in the high 80s represent seriously low values of PaO_2. In the above survey, some doctors and nurses were not especially worried about patients with SpO_2 values as low as 80% (equivalent to $PaO_2 \leq 45$ mm of Hg).

Conventional pulse oximetry has problems during ambient light, abnormal hemoglobin, pulse rate, and rhythm, vasoconstriction and cardiac function, physical motion, and low perfusion and that has great impact on when making critical decisions. ABG tests have been used to supplement or validate pulse oximeter readings. The advent of "Next-generation" pulse oximetry technology has demonstrated significant improvement in the ability to read through motion and low perfusion, thus making pulse oximetry more dependable to take decisions during critical period.

It is important to remember that pulse oximeters assess oxygen saturation only and thereby oxygenation status and gives no indication of the level of CO_2 and thereby ventilation status. For this reason, they have a limited benefit in patients developing respiratory failure due to CO_2 retention.

The pulse oximeter may be used in a variety of situations that require monitoring of oxygen status and may be used either continuously or intermittently. It is not a substitute for an ABG, but can give clinicians an early warning of decreasing arterial oxyhemoglobin saturation prior to the patient exhibiting clinical signs of hypoxia. The pulse oximeter is a useful tool but the patient must be treated, not the numbers. As with all monitoring equipment, the reading should be interpreted in association with the patient's clinical condition. If a patient is short of breath and bluish with a saturation reading of 100%, check for possible causes due to artifact. Never withhold therapeutic oxygen from a patient in distress while waiting to get a reading. If the patient appears to be in perfect health and the saturation is reading 70%, this should alert you to the possibility of interference. Never ignore a reading which suggests the patient is becoming hypoxic. The main disadvantage of pulse oximeter is its inability to use in cases of hyperoxia at saturations between 90% and 100%.

Masimo Pulse Oximetry: A New Promising Way of Measuring Arterial Saturation

What Makes Masimo Pulse Oximetry Different from Conventional Pulse Oximetry?

Conventional pulse oximetry assumes that arterial blood is the only blood moving (pulsating) in the measurement site. During patient motion, the venous blood also moves, which causes conventional pulse oximetry to under-read because it cannot distinguish between the arterial and venous blood. Masimo signal technology identifies the venous blood signal, isolates it, and cancels the noise and extracts the arterial signal, and then reports the true arterial oxygen saturation and pulse rate.

Following setbacks of conventional pulse oximetry for inaccurate monitoring or signal dropout during the reading are rectified by Masimo technology:

- Patient motion or movement
- Low perfusion (low signal amplitude)
- Intense ambient light (lighting or sunlight)
- Electrosurgical instrument interference.

CAPNOGRAPHY

End-tidal CO_2 (EtCO_2) monitoring is an exciting noninvasive technology that is more commonly used in the emergency department, intensive care units, and in the prehospital settings. Its main use has been in verifying endotracheal tube (ETT) position during mechanical ventilation and cardiopulmonary resuscitation (CPR), but it is being studied and used for other purposes as well. The American Heart Association new guidelines state that the secondary confirmation of proper ETT placement in all patients by exhaled CO_2 immediately after intubation and during transport is essential.

End-tidal CO_2 monitoring is an exciting new technology that measures CO_2 in the exhaled breath continuously and noninvasively. CO_2 is produced during cellular metabolism, transported to the heart, and exhaled via the lung and so EtCO_2 reflects ventilation, metabolism, and circulation. If any two systems are kept constant, then changes in the third system reflect changes in EtCO_2. This was first studied clinically by Smallhout and Kalenda in the 1970s, and in the late 1980s to 1990s this methodology has been studied extensively in various clinical settings. The most common use of EtCO_2 is to verify ETT position. It is being increasingly studied and used during CPR and other clinical settings.

What is Capnography?

It is a graphical representation of noninvasive, continuous measurement of exhaled carbon dioxide (EtCO_2) concentration over time accompanied by digital display that provides EtCO_2 value and distinct waveform (tracing) for each respiratory cycle.

Some Definitions: Capnometry

- *Capnometer*: Provides only a numerical measurement of carbon dioxide.
- *Capnogram*: It is a waveform display of carbon dioxide over time.
- *Capnography*: A numerical value of the EtCO_2 and a waveform of the concentration of CO_2 present in the airway, and respiratory rate detected from the actual airflow. The normal capnogram is shown in Figure 3.

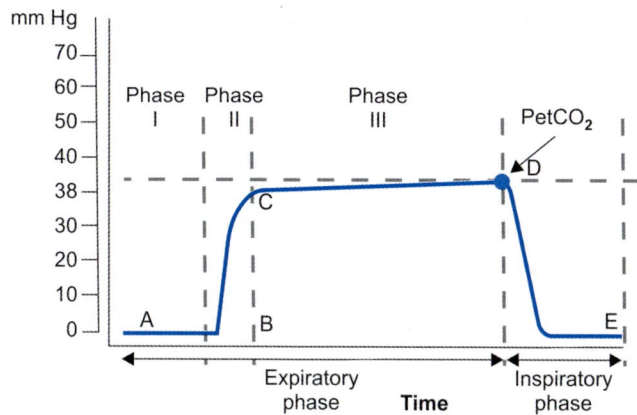

Fig. 3: Normal capnogram.
($PetCO_2$: end-tidal carbon dioxide)

The capnogram is divided into four distinct phases:
1. Phase I (A–B) is the beginning of exhalation. It represents most of the anatomical dead space. CO_2 is almost zero.
2. Phase II (B–C) is where the alveolar gas begins to mix with the dead space gas and the CO_2 begins to rapidly rise.
3. Phase III (C–D) represents the alveolar gas, usually has a slight increase in the slope as "slow" alveoli empty. The "slow" alveoli have a lower V/Q ratio and therefore have higher CO_2 concentrations. In addition, diffusion of CO_2 into the alveoli is greater during expiration. This is more pronounced in infants. $EtCO_2$ is measured at the maximal point of phase III (D).
4. Phase IV (D–E) is the inspirational phase.

Note that the presence of the alveolar plateau confirms that the measurement is end-tidal. Without a capnography, you cannot be sure that a measured CO_2 value is really end-tidal.

A normal value for $ETCO_2$ is approximately 38–40 mm Hg.

Types of Carbon Dioxide Monitors

There are two types of CO_2 monitors:
1. Mainstream
2. Side stream

Mainstream

Salient features are:
- The IR sensor is located in the airway adapter, between the ET tube and the breathing circuit tubing.
- Response time is faster and may be as little as 40 msec.
- Water cannot be drawn-in to disrupt sensor function, and since no mixing of gases in the sample tube, it is nearly a very accurate one.
- Difficult to calibrate without disconnecting (makes it hard to detect rebreathing)

- More prone to the reading being affected by moisture
- Sensor device is larger in size hence can kink the tube.
- Adds dead space to the airway.
- Bigger chance of being damaged by mishandling.

Side Stream

Salient features are:
- Can be used in intubated or nonintubated patients thus have wider applications
- The airway adapter is positioned at the airway (whether or not the patient is intubated) to allow aspiration of gas from the patient's airway back to the sensor, which lies either within or close to the monitor, thus gas is sampled through a small tube.
- Analysis is performed in a separate chamber.
- Very reliable
- Time delay of 1–60 seconds
- Less accurate at higher respiratory rates
- Prone to plugging by water and secretions
- Ambient air leaks are common.

Clinical Applications of Carbon Dioxide Monitoring

The $EtCO_2$ level read on the display of the monitor depends upon the proper functioning of the following:
- Lungs and airways
- Patient ventilation system
- Respiratory mechanism
- Patient's metabolism and circulation.

Malfunctions of the lungs and airway or the patient's ventilation system can be depicted as follows (Table 3):
- Upper airway obstruction—reflected by an increased $EtCO_2$
- Apnea—reflected by a sudden cessation of $EtCO_2$ readings
- Improper ventilator operation—reflected by either high or low $EtCO_2$ readings
- Hyperventilation—reflected by a decreased $EtCO_2$
- Hypoventilation—reflected by an increase in $EtCO_2$
- A faulty one-way valve—reflected by an increased inspired CO_2 and increased $EtCO_2$
- Esophageal intubation—reflected by no $EtCO_2$ reading
- Respiratory depression (from anesthesia)—reflected by a decreased $EtCO_2$
- Increased level of muscle relaxation—reflected by a decreased $EtCO_2$
- Reversal of muscle relaxant and resulting improvement in muscle tone—reflected by an increased $EtCO_2$
- Malignant hyperthermia—reflected by an increased $EtCO_2$

Differential Diagnosis of Abnormal Capnogram

It is shown in Table 3.

Table 3: Differential diagnosis of abnormal capnogram.

Symptom	Possible cause	
Sudden drop of $EtCO_2$ to zero	• Esophageal intubation • Ventilator disconnection or malfunction • Defect in CO_2 analyzer • Dislodged or obstructed endotracheal tube	
Sudden fall of $EtCO_2$ (not to 0)	• Leak in ventilator system, obstruction • Partial disconnect in ventilator circuit • Partial airway obstruction (secretions)	
Exponential fall of $EtCO_2$	• Cardiac arrest • Hypotension (sudden) • Severe hyperventilation • Cardiopulmonary bypass • Pulmonary embolism	
Change in CO_2 baseline	• CO_2 absorber saturation (anesthesia) • Calibration error • Water droplet in analyzer • Mechanical failure (ventilator)	
Sudden increase of $EtCO_2$	• Accessing an area of lung previously obstructed • Release of tourniquet • Sudden increase in blood pressure	
Gradual lowering of $EtCO_2$	• Hypovolemia • Decreasing cardiac output • Decreasing body temperature, hypothermia, drop in metabolism	
Gradual increase in $EtCO_2$	• Rising body temperature • Hypoventilation • CO_2 absorption • Partial airway obstruction (foreign body), reactive airway disease	
Constantly high $EtCO_2$	• Respiratory depression due to drugs • Metabolic alkalosis (respiratory compensation) • Insufficient minute ventilation	

($EtCO_2$: end-tidal carbon dioxide)

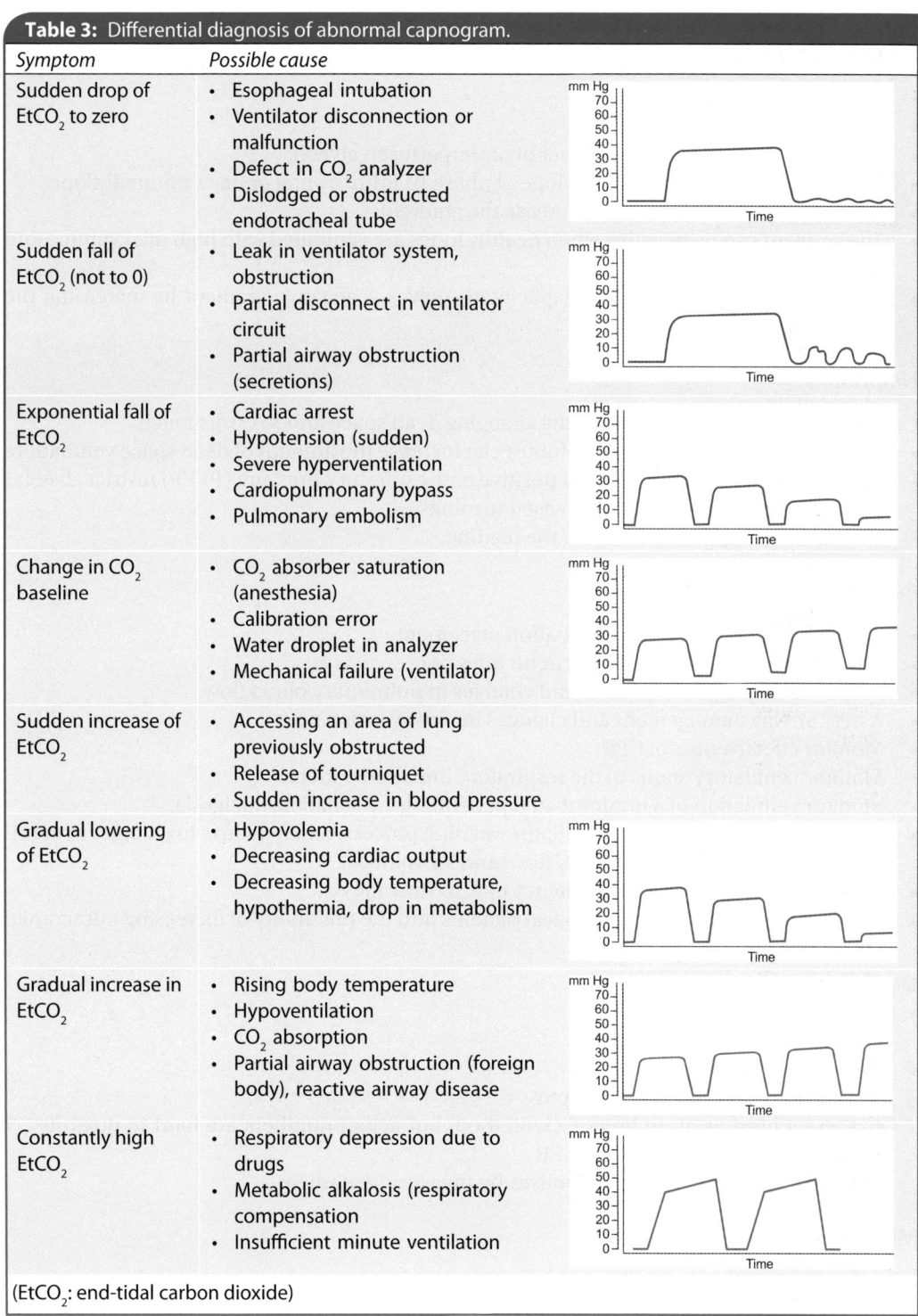

Partial Pressure of Carbon Dioxide-end-Tidal CO_2 ($PaCO_2$-$EtCO_2$) Gradient

- It is usually less than 6 mm Hg.
- $EtCO_2$ is usually less.
- Difference depends on the number of underperfused alveoli.
- Tend to mirror each other if the slope of phase III is horizontal or has a minimal slope.
- Decreased cardiac output will increase the gradient.
- The gradient can be negative when healthy lungs are ventilated with high tidal volume and low rate.
- Decreased functional residual capacity also gives a negative gradient by increasing the number of slow alveoli.

Limitations

Critically ill patients often have rapidly changing dead space and V/Q mismatch.
- Higher rates and smaller tidal volumes can increase the amount of dead space ventilation.
- High mean airway pressures and positive end-expiratory pressure (PEEP) restrict alveolar perfusion, leading to falsely decreased readings.
- Low cardiac output will decrease the reading.

Indications for Capnography

- Confirm and verify tracheal intubation placement.
- Evaluate ventilator settings and circuit integrity.
- Assess cardiopulmonary status and changes in pulmonary blood flow.
- Assess airway management and changes in airway resistance.
- Monitor effectiveness of CPR.
- Monitor ventilatory status of the respiratory impaired patient.
- Monitor ventilation of a nonintubated patient during sedation/analgesia.
- Monitor the effectiveness of ventilator weaning process, and response to changes in ventilator settings (i.e. respiratory rate, flow, and/or volume).
- Reduce the number and/or frequency of ABG drawings.
- Aids in the treatment of neurological patients and the possibility of increasing intracranial pressures.

Other uses:
- Metabolic
  - Assess energy expenditure
- Cardiovascular
  - Monitor trend in cardiac output
  - Can be used as an indirect Fick method, but actual numbers are hard to quantify
  - Measure of effectiveness in CPR
  - Diagnosis of pulmonary embolism by measuring gradient

Microstream Technology

It is a third-generation technology which can be used with intubated or nonintubated patients and requires low sample flow rate—50 mL/min. It allows its use in neonate and pediatric patients. In this technology, sampling lines are not flooded with moisture.

Microstream improves upon conventional side stream sampling based upon the principle that CO_2 molecules absorb infrared (IR) radiation at specific wavelengths.

Advantages

- No sensor at airway
- Intubated and nonintubated patients (neonatal through adult)
- No routine calibration
- Automatic zeroing
- Accurate at small tidal volumes and high respiratory rates
- Superior moisture handling.

PULMONARY FUNCTION TESTS

Few of the numerous pulmonary function tests currently available have an impact upon clinical management of the a critically ill child, particularly if the patient has to be moved to a laboratory. A number of other tests require highly specialized equipment and fulfill a predominant research role.

Clinically Relevant Tests

Tests which are relevant clinically are given in Table 4.

Research Tests (Examples)

Research tests are given in Table 5.

Table 4: Clinically relevant tests.

Measurement	Tests	Common clinical use
PaO_2, SaO_2, $PaCO_2$	Arterial blood gases	Oxygenation, ventilation status
SpO_2	Pulse oximetry	Oxygen saturation, content status
End-tidal PCO_2	Capnography	Ventilation status
Vital capacity, tidal volume	Spirometry, electronic flow-metry	Serial measurement of borderline function (VC < 10–15 mL/kg), e.g. Guillain–Barré syndrome
Peak expiratory flow rate	Wright peak flow meter	(Spontaneous ventilation) asthma
FEV_1, FVC	Spirometry, electronic flow-metry	(Spontaneous ventilation) asthma, obstructive/restrictive disease
Lung/chest wall compliance	Pressure–volume curve	Ventilator adjustments, monitoring disease progression
Flow volume loop, pressure volume loop	Pneumotachograph* manometry	Ventilator adjustment

*Pneumotachograph: An apparatus for recording the rate of airflow to and from lungs.

(FEV1: forced expiratory volume in one second; FVC: forced vital capacity; $PaCO_2$: partial pressure of arterial carbon dioxide; PaO_2: partial pressure of arterial oxygen; PCO_2: partial pressure of carbon dioxide; SaO_2: oxygen saturation of arterial blood; SpO_2: arterial saturation; VC: vital capacity)

Table 5: Research tests.

Measurement	Tests	Research use
Diaphragmatic strength (trans-diaphragmatic pressure)	Gastric and esophageal manometry	Respiratory muscle functions, weaning
Pleural (intrathoracic) pressure	Esophageal manometry	Ventilator trauma, work of breathing, weaning
Functional residual capacity	Closed circuit helium dilution (bag-in-box) open circuit N_2 washout	Lung volumes, compliance
Ventilation–perfusion relationship	Multiple inert gas elimination techniques, isotope technique	Regional lung ventilation–perfusion, pulmonary gas exchange
Pulmonary diffusing capacity	Carbon monoxide uptake	Pulmonary gas exchange

Notes:
- Compliance equals the change in pressure during a linear increase in volume above functional residual capacity (FRC).
- The Bohr equation calculates physiological dead space (VD); normally it is less than 30%.
- The shunt equations estimate the proportion of blood shunted past poorly ventilated alveoli (Qs) compared with total lung blood flow (QT).

These useful equations are supplement to assess pulmonary function and ventilation/perfusion mismatch.
- V/Q = 1, Ventilation and perfusion are well matched.
- V/Q > 1, increased dead space (where alveoli are poorly perfused but well ventilated)
- V/Q < 1, increased venous admixture or shunt (where alveoli are well perfused but poorly ventilated)

1. *Alveolar gas equation*:
   $PAO_2 = FiO_2 (PB - PH_2O) - (PaCO_2/RQ)$ [RQ = 0.8]
2. *Calculating the alveolar*: Arterial oxygen gradient: (A-a) DO_2, normal is 10–15 mm of Hg
3. *Bohr equation*: $VD/VT = (PaCO_2 - $ expired $PCO_2)/PaCO_2$
4. *Shunt equation*: $Qs/QT = (CCO_2 - CaCO_2)/(CCO_2 - CvO_2)$ where CCO_2 = end capillary O_2 content; a = arterial; v = mixed venous
5. Expected $PaO_2 = FiO_2 \times 5$. A very useful equation with limitations.

Pressure–Volume Curve Relationship

It is shown in Figure 4.

X-ray

A very commonly ordered investigation in PICU, which has diagnostic, therapeutic, and prognostic value is X-ray chest (this has been discussed in detail in other chapter in this book).

INVASIVE MONITORING

ARTERIAL BLOOD GAS ANALYSIS

The term *arterial blood* refers to a specific set of tests performed on arterial blood sample. It provides four key points information: pH, PO_2, $[HCO_3]$, and PCO_2. The name *blood gas* is

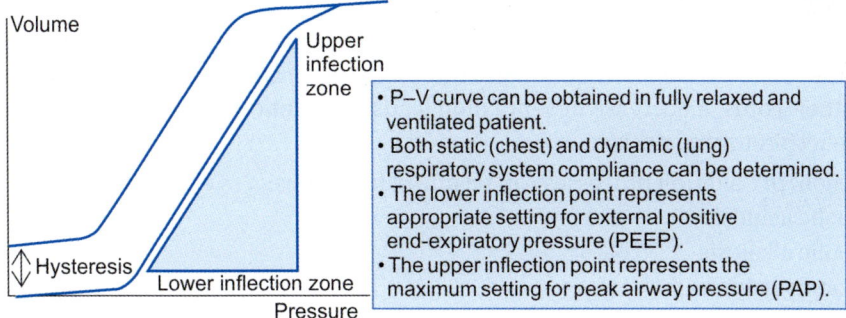

Fig. 4: Pressure–volume (P–V) curve relationship.

really a partial misnomer since H⁺ and HCO_3 are not gases. It is a gold standard investigation to assess pulmonary and cardiac functions as well.

Basic Concepts

- Arterial blood gas
- Gas exchange
- Acid–base disturbances.

Systematic Analysis of Arterial Blood Gases

- Oxygenation
- Stepwise approach to acid-base disorders.

Basic Introduction of Arterial Blood Gases

The term hypoxia refers to reduced O_2 delivery to tissues. The term hypoxemia refers to reduced O_2 content in arterial blood. A normal arterial pressure of O_2 is dependent on the atmospheric pressure, temperature, inspired O_2 content, and the patient's age.

Hypoxemia can be for two basic reasons: Oxygen may not be delivered to the alveolar air sacs (hypoventilation) or oxygen in the alveoli may not enter into the blood stream. A patient can be hypercarbic (high levels of CO_2) or hypocarbic (low level of CO_2), which is due to an inability to normally exchange gases in the lungs.

The terms acidemia and alkalemia refer to alterations in blood pH, and are the result of underlying disturbance (s) (metabolic and/or respiratory). The terms acidosis and alkalosis refer to the processes that alter the acid–base status. There can be (and often are) more than one of these processes simultaneously in a patient.

Diseases that alter the acid–base status of a patient can be divided into:
- Metabolic
- Respiratory.

Metabolic processes are those that primarily alter the HCO_3 concentration in the blood. A decrease in serum HCO_3 (an alkali or base) leads to a metabolic acidosis, while an increase in serum HCO_3 leads to a metabolic alkalosis.

Respiratory processes alter the pH by changing the CO_2 levels. CO_2 accumulation causes an acid state in the blood (through carbonic acid), and as respirations (respiratory rate and/or tidal volume) increase, the body eliminates more CO_2 (acid) and is left with a respiratory alkalosis. In other words, a decrease in ventilation leads to retention and increased levels of CO_2, and thus a respiratory acidosis.

In conclusion, pH-altering processes can be one of four types:
1. Metabolic acidosis
2. Metabolic alkalosis
3. Respiratory acidosis
4. Respiratory alkalosis.

Again, one or more of these processes may be present in a patient with an abnormal acid–base status.

Systematic Analysis of Arterial Blood Gases

Arterial blood gases are obtained for two basic purposes:
1. To determine oxygenation
2. To determine acid–base status

Let us elaborate now, how to determine oxygenation, and then evaluate the acid-base status systematically.

Determining oxygenation i.e. alveolar: arterial oxygen gradient: (A-a) DO_2: [Age and fraction of inspired oxygen (FiO_2)-dependent derivative]

An important part of interpreting blood gases is to assess oxygenation. An arterial oxygen concentration (PaO_2) of less than 60 mm Hg, associated with an oxygenation (SaO_2) of less than 90%, is poorly tolerated in humans; therefore a PaO_2 of less than 60 is termed hypoxemic. However, "normal" oxygenation decreases with age as the lungs become less efficient at diffusing oxygen from the alveolus to the blood. Again, normal oxygenation for age can be estimated as $PaO_2 = 104.2-(0.27 \times age)$ or more crudely, normal oxygenation for age is roughly one-third of the patient's age subtracted from 100. Using this estimation, for example, a 60-year-old patient should have a PaO_2 of 80 and a 15-year-old patient should have a PaO_2 of 95. Values less than this would be considered hypoxemic for age.

Calculating the alveolar: arterial oxygen gradient (Figs. 5A and B): (A-a) DO_2 can determine if hypoxia is a reflection of hypoventilation (in other words, decreased because of a rise in $PaCO_2$) or due to deficiency in oxygenation. Unlike oxygen (for which alveolar concentrations are higher than arterial concentrations), CO_2 freely diffuses across the lung such that the arterial and alveolar concentrations are identical. As a patient hypoventilates, CO_2 will accumulate in the body (more CO_2 is produced through metabolism than can be eliminated) and thus in the blood (where we measure it as $PaCO_2$). The carbon dioxide displaces the oxygen in the alveolus. This reciprocal relationship between oxygen and carbon dioxide in the alveolus is described by the alveolar gas equation:
- PAO_2 (partial pressure of oxygen in the alveolus) = $150-1.25 (PACO_2)$
  PA = partial pressure of a gas in the alveolus;
  Pa = partial pressure of a gas in the arterial blood

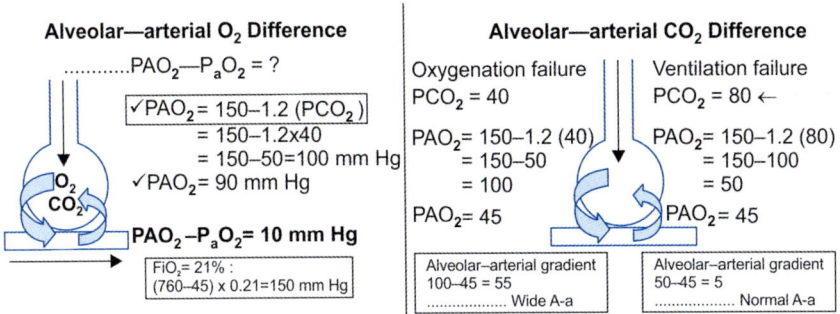

Figs 5A and B
(PaO_2: partial pressure of arterial oxygen; PAO_2: partial pressure of oxygen in the alveolus; PCO_2: partial pressure of carbon dioxide)

This equation assumes that the patient is breathing room air (21% O_2) at atmospheric pressure (Figs. 5A and B).

Where does 150 come from?
- (Atmospheric P − water vapor P) × FiO_2. At room temperature, at sea level, atmospheric pressure = 760 mm Hg;
- In the lung, the air is fully saturated with water, giving a water vapor pressure of about 47; room air is about 21%, thus at room air, the PAO_2 = 0.21 (760−47) = 149.7, or about 150;

And where does 1.25 come from?
This is a fudge factor which is derived from the respiratory quotient (RQ). The formula actually requires that the $PACO_2$ be divided by the RQ, which is defined as the ratio of CO_2 produced to O_2 consumed (and which depends on diet and metabolism). We estimate the RQ to be 0.8, and the reciprocal of 0.8 is 1.25.

This value is the partial pressure of O_2 within the alveolus. Because the CO_2 freely diffuse from arterial blood to alveolar airspaces, the $PACO_2$ is equal to the $PaCO_2$, which is measured in the ABG. The above equation can then be rewritten as:

PAO_2 = 150 − 1.25 ($PaCO_2$)
Thus, A−a DO_2 = PAO_2 − PaO_2 or
A−a DO_2 = [150 − 1.25 ($PaCO_2$)] − PaO_2

A normal A−a gradient is 10–20 mm Hg, with the normal gradient increasing within this range as the patient ages. An increased A−a gradient identifies decreased O_2 in the arterial blood compared with the O_2 in the alveolus. This suggests a process that interferes with gas transfer, or in general terms, suggests ventilation-perfusion mismatch. A normal A−a gradient in the face of hypoxemia suggests that the hypoxemia is due to hypoventilation and not due to underlying lung disorders.

When the patient is not breathing room air, then:
A−a gradient = [(FiO_2) (760−47) − (1.25) ($PaCO_2$)] − PaO_2.

Stepwise Approach to Diagnosing Acid–Base Disorders

In order to understand the various processes that can co-exist in a patient, one must systematically evaluate blood gases and serum electrolytes. The simple method of six steps to analyze the acid–base status of the patient is presented here.
1. pH and HCO_3 ...Moves in same direction
2. pH and PCO_2 ....Moves in opposite direction
3. HCO_3 and PCO_2 ...Moves in same direction
4. Simple disorder
5. HCO_3 and PCO_2 ... Moves in opposite directions
6. Mixed disorder

Normal values of ABG:
- pH: 7.35–7.45
- PCO_2: 35–45
- HCO_3: 22–26
- PaO_2: 90–99

Steps in Acid–Base Analysis

- *Step 1*: Consider the clinical settings! Anticipate the disorder!
- *Step 2*: Look at pH.
- *Step 3*: Who is the culprit for changing pH? Metabolic/respiratory process
- *Step 4*: If respiratory, acute and/or chronic and is metabolic compensation appropriate?
- *Step 5*: If metabolic acidosis, is respiratory compensation appropriate?
  - Anion gap increased and/or normal or both?
- *Step 6*: Is more than one disorder present? Mixed one?

Step 1

Clinical assessment based on clinical settings is an essential first step. From the history, examination, and initial investigations, make a clinical decision as to what is the most likely acid–base disorder (s).

This is very important but be aware that in some situations, the history may be inadequate, misleading, or the range of possible diagnoses large. Mixed disorders are often difficult; the history and examination alone are usually insufficient in sorting these out.
- *Vomiting*: Metabolic alkalosis
- *Diarrhea*: Metabolic acidosis
- *Septicemia*: Lactic acidosis
- *Hypotension, hypoxemia, shock*: Lactic acidosis
- *Diabetes mellitus*: Ketoacidosis
- *Pneumonia*: Respiratory alkalosis/acidosis
- *Bronchial asthma*: Respiratory alkalosis/acidosis
- *Hepatic failure*: Respiratory alkalosis, metabolic alkalosis
- *CNS disorders*: Respiratory alkalosis
- *Renal disorders:* Metabolic acidosis

Key point: Metabolic alkalosis and acidosis can exist together with any respiratory either acidosis or alkalosis. Both two respiratory disorders cannot occur simultaneously.

Step 2

Look at the pH.

The pH of the ABG measurement identifies the disorder as alkalemic or acidemic.
- pH > 7.4, alkalosis; pH < 7.4, acidosis
- pH = 7.4 normal or mixed disorder

(Only chronic respiratory alkalosis can have normal value of pH)

Step 3

Who is responsible for this change in pH? Who is the culprit?
- HCO_3...... Metabolic PCO_2 ...... Respiratory
    - \> 26 ..... Met. alkalosis   > 45 ...... Resp. acidosis
    - < 22 ......Met. acidosis   < 35 ...... Resp. alkalosis

It is essential to determine whether the disturbance affects primarily the arterial $PaCO_2$ or the serum HCO_3.
- Respiratory disturbances alter the arterial $PaCO_2$ (normal value 35–45).
- Metabolic disturbances alter the serum HCO_3 (normal value 22–26).

If the pH is low (i.e. the primary and controlling disturbance is acidosis causing acidemia), either the $PaCO_2$ is high or the HCO_3 is low (these are the only ways in which the pH can be low). A high $PaCO_2$ defines a primary respiratory acidosis and a low HCO_3 defines a primary metabolic acidosis.

Conversely, if the pH is high (i.e. the primary and controlling disturbance is alkalosis causing alkalemia), either the $PaCO_2$ is low or the HCO_3 is high (these are the only ways in which the pH can be high). A low $PaCO_2$ defines a primary respiratory alkalosis and a high HCO_3 defines a primary metabolic alkalosis.

Step 4

If it is a primary respiratory disturbance, is it acute and/or chronic?

For 10 mm change in pCO_2:

pH changes as:
- Acidosis (↑CO_2).....pH ↓ ... acute......by 0.08, chronic...by 0.03
- Alkalosis (↓CO_2).... pH ↑... acute...... by 0.08, chronic...by 0.03

HCO3 compensates as:
- Acidosis (↑CO_2).....HCO_3↑......... acute......by 1, chronic...by 3
- Alkalosis (↓CO_2) ... HCO_3↓......acute......by 2, chronic...by 5

For example,
- In an acute respiratory acidosis, if the PCO_2 rises from 40 to 50, you would expect the pH to decline from 7.40 to 7.32.
- In an acute respiratory alkalosis, if the PCO_2 falls from 40 to 30, you would expect the pH to rise from 7.40 to 7.48.
- In chronic respiratory disturbances, there are renal mediated shifts of bicarbonate that alter and partially compensate for the pH shift for a change in the $PaCO_2$.

- In a chronic respiratory acidosis, if the PCO_2 rises from 40 to 50, you would expect the pH to decline from 7.40 to 7.37.
- In a chronic respiratory alkalosis, if the PCO_2 falls from 40 to 30, you would expect the pH to rise from 7.40 to 7.43.

Remember to suspect if:
- Compensated HCO_3 is more than expected: Additional metabolic alkalosis is there.
- Compensated HCO_3 is less than expected: Additional metabolic acidosis is there.

Step 5

If it is a primary metabolic disturbance, whether respiratory compensation appropriate?
For metabolic acidosis: Expected $PCO_2 = [1.5 \times (HCO_3)] + 8 \pm 2$ Winter's formula
OR Expected CO_2 is equal to last two digits of pH (important and easy to remember)
For metabolic alkalosis: Expected $PCO_2 = 6$ mm for 10 mEq rise in bicarbonate.

Uncertain compensation:

Remember to suspect if:
- Compensated PCO_2 is more than expected: Additional respiratory acidosis is there.
- Compensated PCO_2 is less than expected: Additional respiratory alkalosis is there.

Processes that lead to a metabolic acidosis can be divided into:
- Increased anion gap
- Normal anion gap.

The anion gap is the difference between the measured serum cations (positive) and the measured serum anions (negative). (Of course, there is no real gap; in the body the numbers of positive and negative charges are balanced. The gap refers to the difference in positive and negative charges among cations and anions which are commonly measured.) The commonly measured cation is sodium. (Some people also use potassium to calculate the gap, which results in a different range of normal values.) The measured anions include chloride and bicarbonate. Thus, the anion gap can be summarized as: $AG = [Na^+] - ([Cl^-] + [HCO_3^-])$.

The normal anion gap is 12. An anion gap of more than 12 is increased. Anion gap more than 25 has got distinct value having significant acidosis. This is important, because it helps to significantly limit the differential diagnosis of a metabolic acidosis. The most common etiologies of a metabolic acidosis with an increased anion gap include:
- Commonest pediatric causes are lactic acidosis, diabetic ketoacidosis, and renal failure.
- Aspirin, ketones (starvation, alcoholic and diabetic ketoacidosis)
- Uremia (renal failure), lactic acidosis, ethanol, paraldehyde, and other drugs
- Methanol, other alcohols, and ethylene glycol intoxication.

Key point: The true anion gap is underestimated in hypoalbuminemia (fall in unmeasured anions); AG must be adjusted. Remember to adjust AG—for every 1.0 fall in albumin, increase the AG by 2.5.

Step 6

- Is more than one disorder present?
    - Proper clinical history

- pH normal, and PCO_2 and HCO_3 out of range
- PCO_2 and HCO_3 moving in opposite directions
- Degree of compensation for primary disorder is inappropriate.

KEY MESSAGES

- Respiratory monitoring helps in the early diagnosis of change in a physiological parameter of oxygenation and ventilation, and provides guidelines toward institution of appropriate therapy.
- Basic knowledge of the principles of monitoring tools and correct interpretation of data is important since failure to do so can result in misdirected therapy.
- Pulse oximetry and capnography are the essential monitors in PICU which need clinical correlation.
- Arterial blood gas analysis is an integral part of respiratory monitoring in PICU.
- No amount of monitoring, though excellent information provided by monitors, however, can replace careful bedside clinical signs.

SUGGESTED READING

1. Abelow B. Understanding Acid–Base. Baltimore, MD: Williams and Wilkins; 1998. pp. 52-4.
2. Barker SJ, Tremper KK, Hyatt J. Effects of methemoglobinemia on pulse oximetry and mixed venous oximetry. Anesthesiology. 1989;70:112-7.
3. Barker SJ, Tremper KK. The effect of carbon monoxide inhalation on pulse oximeter signal detection. Anesthesiology. 1987;67:599-603.
4. Bhende MS. Capnography in the paediatric emergency department. Peds Emerg Care 1999;15:64-9.
5. Buche VB. Systematic analysis of blood gases. Intensivist. 2006.
6. Hayden WR. Respiratory monitoring. In: Rogers Textbook of Pediatric Intensive Care. 2007. pp. 205-13.
7. Jay GD, Hughes L, Renzi FP. Pulse oximetry is accurate in acute anemia from hemorrhage. Ann Emerg Med. 1994;24:32-5.
8. Jubran A. Pulse oximetry. In: Tobin MJ (Ed). Principles and Practice of Intensive Care Monitoring. New York: McGraw Hill, Inc.; 1998. pp. 261-87.
9. Martin L. All you really need to know to interpret arterial blood gases. 1992.
10. Singer M, Webb AR. Oxford Hand Book of Critical Care. 2005. pp. 94-7.
11. Swedlow DB. Noninvasive respiratory monitoring. In: Zimmerman JJ. Pediatric Critical Care. 2011. pp. 99-109.

Acute Respiratory Distress Syndrome

10

Vinay Joshi, Gaurang Upadhyay

LEARNING OBJECTIVES

- To be able to define acute respiratory distress syndrome (ARDS) and understand the evolution of the definition
- To understand the etiopathogenesis
- To apply the principles of safe ventilation
- To apply appropriate adjunctive therapy

INTRODUCTION

Acute respiratory distress syndrome (ARDS), first described in pathology in 1967 by Ashbaugh, manifests as pulmonary inflammation, alveolar edema, and hypoxemic respiratory failure. The pathophysiology is characterized by inflammatory, proliferative, and fibrotic phases.

Over fifty years, there have been multiple revisions of the definition. Although these diagnostic criteria were developed primarily for use in the adult population, until recently, they have been used in children (Table 1).

DEFINITIONS

A major development in the history of acute lung injury (ALI) and its more severe form, ARDS, came in 1994 with the establishment of consensus diagnostic criteria.

The 1994 American European Consensus Conference (AECC) definition was proposed and used as standard in clinical and experimental studies (Box 1). This standardization has also created opportunities to evaluate the impact of novel therapies early in the course of disease.

Over this same time, however, a number of issues with the AECC definition have become apparent. Some investigators have reported problems with its use and implementation. In one study enrolling adult patients, Esteban et al., compared clinical criteria for ARDS with autopsy findings and found that accuracy of the AECC definition was only moderate (i.e. sensitivity

Table 1: Differences in pediatric and adult physiology.

Feature	Child	Adult
Airway cartilage formation	Incomplete	Complete
Airway resistance	Greater increase in airway resistance with reduction in airway radius	Smaller increase in airway resistance with reduction in airway radius
Chest-wall compliance	Greater compliance in view of incomplete ribcage ossification	Less compliant in view of ribcage ossification
Alveolar maturation and impact on FRC	20–300 million alveoli (age-dependent); lower FRC	300 million mature alveoli; higher FRC
Respiratory muscle reserve	More reliant on diaphragm	Less reliant on diaphragm
Risk of pulmonary vascular remodeling	Greater due to higher pulmonary vascular resistance during perinatal transition	Lower
Metabolic requirements	Higher	Lower

(FRC: functional residual capacity)

75%, specificity 84%. There is evidence to suggest that risk factors for ARDS in the pediatric population differ from those in the adult population (Box 2).

A number of other problems have been encountered with this definition. ALI, as defined using the AECC criteria, has been seen to be under-recognized by clinicians. The AECC definition requires that onset of respiratory failure to be acute, but does not explicitly define the specific timeframe (e.g., hours, days, or weeks). The hypoxemia criterion has generated concerns because ratio of partial pressure of arterial oxygen and fraction of inspired oxygen (PaO_2/FiO_2) may vary with FiO_2, and also in response to other ventilator settings, particularly positive end-expiratory pressure (PEEP). The chest X-ray criterion has only moderate inter-observer reliability even when applied by experts, although this can be improved through use of a training set of radiographs. Finally, although the AECC definition includes a pulmonary artery wedge pressure (PAWP) less than 18 mm Hg (when measured), patients with hallmark findings of ARDS often have an elevated PAWP because of elevated pleural pressures and/or vigorous fluid resuscitation. The use of

Box 1: American European consensus conference definition of acute respiratory distress syndrome.

In the presence of risk factors and in the absence of chronic lung disease
- Acute onset disease
- Bilateral infiltrates on chest radiograph
- No evidence of elevated left atrial pressure (PAWP < 18 mm Hg) (Noncardiac origin)
- Two categories:
  - ALI: PaO_2/FiO_2 ratio ≤ 300
  - ARDS: PaO_2/FiO_2 ratio ≤ 200

(ALI: acute lung injury; ARDS: acute respiratory distress syndrome; FiO_2: fraction of inspired oxygen; PaO_2: partial pressure of arterial oxygen; PAWP: pulmonary arterial wedge pressure)

pulmonary artery catheters has also been decreasing in recent years, thus precluding its use to diagnose ARDS.

These problems have led to another proposed definition to diagnose ARDS in an attempt to overcome these limitations. This has been proposed as the "Berlin Definition" and essentially attempts to refine the AECC definition further (Table 2).

The proposal to change the definition is based on the following observations:

Observational data suggest that the majority of patients with ARDS are identified within 72 hours of the recognition of the underlying risk factors, with nearly all patients identified within 7 days.

There is poor interobserver consensus in interpreting chest radiographs. To help address this issue, an attempt has been made to make the chest radiograph criterion more explicit specifying that it should include bilateral opacities consistent with pulmonary edema that are not fully explained by effusions, lobar/lung collapse, or nodules/masses on chest radiograph as a defining criterion for ARDS.

Given the declining use of pulmonary artery catheters worldwide and the recognition that hydrostatic edema and ARDS may coexist, the PAWP criterion was removed. It has been proposed that patients whose respiratory failure is not fully explained by cardiac failure or fluid overload as judged by the treating physician using all available data may qualify as having ARDS. Nevertheless, if no known etiologic risk factor for ARDS is apparent (Table 2), objective evaluation of cardiac function (e.g., echocardiography or cardiac output measurement) is required to help rule out hydrostatic edema secondary to heart failure.

Box 2: Risk factors for acute respiratory distress syndrome.

- Pneumonia
- Nonpulmonary sepsis
- Aspiration of gastric contents
- Major trauma
- Pulmonary contusion
- Pancreatitis
- Inhalational injury
- Severe burns
- Non-cardiogenic shock
- Drug overdose
- Transfusion-related acute lung injury (TRALI)
- Pulmonary vasculitis
- Drowning

Table 2: Berlin definition of acute respiratory distress syndrome.

Timing	Within 1 week of a known clinical insult or new or worsening respiratory symptoms
Chest imaging	Bilateral opacities—not fully explained by effusions, lobar/lung collapse, or nodules
Origin of edema	Respiratory failure not fully explained by cardiac failure or fluid overload; need objective assessment (e.g. echocardiography) to exclude hydrostatic edema, if no risk factors
Oxygenation	
Mild	200 mm Hg < PaO_2/FiO_2 ≤ 300 mm Hg with PEEP or CPAP ≥ 5 cm H_2O
Moderate	100 mm Hg < PaO_2/FiO_2 ≤ 200 mm Hg with PEEP ≥ 5 cm H_2O
Severe	PaO_2/FiO_2 ≤ 100 mm Hg with PEEP ≥5 cm H_2O
(CPAP: continuous positive airway pressure; FiO_2: fraction of inspired oxygen; PaO_2: partial pressure of arterial oxygen; PEEP: positive end expiratory pressure)	

Since, PEEP can affect the reliability and specificity of PaO_2/FiO_2, to classify the severity of ARDS, a minimum level of 5 cm H_2O PEEP (or noninvasive CPAP for mild ARDS) has been included in the updated definition.

The term acute lung injury was removed from the ARDS definition, due to the perception that many clinicians and researchers viewed ALI as a category. The creation of the mild ARDS categorises with a less severe form of the syndrome but by applying the term ARDS, it recognizes the severity of their illness (mortality 27% and response to lung protective ventilation).

Previous application to pediatrics of the adult-based ARDS definitions, with the requirement to measure arterial oxygenation, may have led to an underestimation of the prevalence of ARDS in pediatrics, given the less common use of arterial lines in infants and children.

Due to the important limitations of the previous adult-based definitions, the pediatric acute lung injury consensus conference (PALICC) published in 2015 a pediatric-specific definition for ARDS. However, acute hypoxemia unique to the perinatal period or related to congenital abnormalities are excluded. The PALICC definition eliminates the requirement for bilateral pulmonary infiltrates on chest imaging due to a lack of evidence that etiology, management, and outcomes differ between patients with unilateral versus bilateral disease (Table 3).

To overcome the limitation of using PaO_2/FiO_2, the PALICC definition relies on the oxygenation index (OI) [(FiO_2 × mean airway pressure × 100)/PaO_2] or the oxygen saturation index (OSI) [(FiO_2 × mean airway pressure × 100)/SpO_2] when an arterial blood gas is not available) to assess the degree of hypoxemia in PARDS. It is important to note that the recommendation be titrated to achieve peripheral capillary oxygen saturation (SpO_2) the 88–97% range. Mild PARDS is defined as an OI of 4–8 (OSI = 5–7.5), moderate as an OI of 8–16 (OSI = 7.5–12.3), and severe as an OI more than 16 (OSI > 12.3).

Given the increasingly common use of noninvasive ventilation in pediatrics, PALICC included this approach in the PARDS definition as long as the patient is receiving a minimum CPAP (expiratory positive airway pressure) of 5 cm H_2O. This helps to promote earlier diagnosis, and intervention, for those with significant lung injury. Other elements of the PALICC definition, similar to the Berlin definition, include onset within 7 days of a known clinical insult and the presence of respiratory failure not fully explained by cardiac failure or fluid overload.

PALICC included recommendations for defining PARDS in infants and children with chronic lung disease, cyanotic congenital heart disease, and left ventricular dysfunction. Given variable baselines, values of OI (or OSI) should not be used to risk stratification of PARDS in these specialized, higher-risk subpopulations.

Pediatric-specific criteria may provide the ability to promptly recognize and diagnose PARDS in clinical practice. Improvements in prognostication and stratification of disease severity may help guide therapeutic interventions.

INCIDENCE AND EPIDEMIOLOGY

Population-based studies in the United States, Europe, Australia, and New Zealand using the AECC definition suggest that the incidence of ARDS in adults ranges from 17.9 per 100,000

Table 3: PALICC definition of pediatric acute respiratory syndrome.

Age	Exclude patients with perinatal-related lung disease			
Timing	Within 7 days of known clinical insult			
Origin of edema	Respiratory failure not fully explained by cardiac failure or fluid overload			
Chest imaging	Chest imaging findings of new infiltrates consistent with acute pulmonary parenchymal disease			
Oxygenation	**Noninvasive ventilation**	**Invasive mechanical ventilation**		
	No severity stratification	Mild	Moderate	Severe
	Total facemask bilevel ventilation or CPAP ≥5 cm H_2O PaO_2/FiO_2 ratio ≤ 300 SpO_2/FiO_2 ratio ≤ 264	$4 ≤ OI < 8$ $5 ≤ OSI < 7.5$	$8 ≤ OI < 16$ $7.5 ≤ OSI < 12.3$	$OI ≥ 16$ $OSI ≥ 12.3$

Special populations
Cyanotic heart disease: Standard criteria above for age, timing, origin of edema, and chest imaging with an acute deterioration in oxygenation not explained by underlying cardiac disease.
Chronic lung disease: Standard criteria above for age, timing, and origin of edema with chest imaging consistent with new infiltrate and acute deterioration in oxygenation from baseline that meet oxygenation criteria above.
Left ventricular dysfunction: Standard criteria for age, timing, and origin of edema with chest imaging changes consistent with new infiltrate and acute deterioration in oxygenation that meet criteria above not explained by left ventricular dysfunction.

(OI: oxygenation index; OSI: oxygen saturation index; PARDS: pediatric acute respiratory distress syndrome)

person-years to 81.0 per 100,000 person-years. In contrast to adults, the incidence of ARDS in the United States, European, Australian, and New Zealand children is 2.0–12.8 per 100,000 person-years. Although mortality from ARDS is lower in clinical trials, population-based studies suggest that the overall mortality of ARDS in adults is 27–45%. ARDS attributable mortality in children is lower than in adults (18–27%), although data from Australia suggest that pediatric and adult mortality from ARDS may be similar (35%).

Immunodeficiency is a common preexisting condition in both pediatric and adult patients that develop ARDS and most studies show increased mortality among immunodeficient patients who develop ARDS. Pneumonia, sepsis, aspiration, and trauma account for 63–92% of ARDS in both adults and children.

PATHOPHYSIOLOGY

Host Genetic Factors

Over the past decade, much effort has been extended to apply techniques from molecular genetics to understanding the role of host factors by linking the presence of specific genetic polymorphisms to the development and/or severity of ARDS. In particular, specific polymorphisms in genes that govern endothelial barrier function, proinflammatory, and anti-inflammatory cytokine production, the transcription regulator nuclear factor- kB (NF-kB) and its inhibitor NF-kB1A, pattern recognition receptors (PRRs) of the innate immune system, oxidant-mediated injury, surfactant protein B production, angiotensin-converting enzyme, and the coagulation cascade have all been associated with either susceptibility to ARDS or the severity of its presentation.

Initiating Factors

ARDS develops following either direct or indirect lung injury. Pneumonia and pulmonary aspiration are among the most common conditions with the potential to inflict direct lung injury and ARDS, but submersion injury and inhalational injury are other relative common causes of direct lung injury. The most common forms of indirect lung injury include systemic conditions, such as sepsis, shock, cardiopulmonary bypass, and transfusion-related lung injury. Each of these pathways is associated with distinct pathologic changes in respiratory system mechanics that may be associated with distinctly different clinical outcomes. For example, direct injury is suspected of causing regional consolidation from destruction of the alveolar architecture; while indirect injury is believed to be associated with pulmonary vascular congestion, interstitial edema, and less severe alveolar involvement.

PHASES OF THE DISEASE

Regardless of the inciting factors, ARDS commonly progresses through stages defined by their associated clinical, radiographic, and histopathological features.
- *Exudative phase*: This is characterized by the acute development of decreased pulmonary compliance and arterial hypoxemia, tachypnea, and hypocarbia. The chest X-ray usually reveals diffuse alveolar infiltrates from pulmonary edema. This usually lasts 1–3 days.
- *Fibro-proliferative phase*: In this stage, increased alveolar dead space and refractory pulmonary hypertension may develop as a result of chronic inflammation and scarring of the alveolar capillary unit. This may last up to 2 weeks.
- *Recovery phase*: There is restoration of the alveolar epithelial barrier, gradual improvement in pulmonary compliance and resolution of arterial hypoxemia, and eventual return to premorbid pulmonary function in many patients.

Alveolar Capillary Barrier Dysfunction and Edema Formation

The edema in ARDS results from disruption of the structural components that regulate alveolar fluid balance under normal conditions. The key pathophysiologic event in ALI and ARDS is injury to the alveolar epithelium and/or pulmonary capillary endothelium, directly as the result of parenchymal injury or following a distant or systemic disease process that provokes the host immune response, causing neutrophil activation and elaboration of proinflammatory cytokines. This results in opening of tight junctions and unregulated leakage of fluid, protein, and other solutes into the interstitium and, subsequently, into the alveolar space, which creates multiple mechanisms for impairment of gas exchange. The permeability edema that is the defining feature of early ARDS sets the stage for reduced compliance and an end-expiratory lung volume (EELV) that decreases below functional residual capacity (FRC) to a point approaching closing capacity, creating conditions that favor the development of regional atelectasis, intrapulmonary shunt, and alveolar hypoxia.

Surfactant Dysfunction and Alteration of Pulmonary Mechanics

Injury to the pulmonary surfactant system is one of the more serious manifestations of damage to the alveolar epithelium and subsequent alveolar flooding. Following lung injury, surfactant production declines because of damage to alveolar epithelial cells, and the surface activity of any surfactant remaining in the alveolar space is impaired because of alterations in its phospholipid constituents, as well as from inactivation by alveolar exudates. Loss of surfactant results in collapse of alveolar units with higher pressures required to achieve and maintain lung recruitment and an overall decrease in lung compliance that is evident throughout the respiratory cycle.

Impaired Alveolar Fluid Clearance

The alveolar epithelial damage that occurs in ALI creates conditions that compromise the capacity of membrane proteins to regulate alveolar fluid balance. Exposure of alveolar epithelium to hypoxia inhibits transepithelial sodium transport and decreases overall alveolar fluid clearance.

Alterations in Gas Exchange

Edema in the interstitial compartment or in the alveolar space inhibits gas exchange and pulmonary blood flowing past compromised or collapsed lung units remains poorly oxygenated. The phenomenon of intrapulmonary shunt is ameliorated to some degree by pulmonary vasoconstriction, which redirects blood toward better ventilated lung units. In ALI and ARDS, consolidation and collapse of lung units are widespread and fluid-filled alveoli act as low V/Q lung units. Consolidation of diseased alveoli creates radial traction on neighboring lung units that result in alveolar overdistension and pulmonary capillary narrowing, creating high V/Q areas and adding to alveolar dead space.

Effects on Cardiovascular Function

The development of permeability edema, leading to alveolar hypoxia, thrombotic obstruction of the pulmonary microvasculature, and eventual interstitial fibrosis leads to increase in pulmonary vascular resistance (PVR), adding to right ventricular afterload and potentially compromising cardiac output. Overdistension of alveolar units with ventilation can also compress pulmonary vessels and increase PVR. Increases in PVR and right ventricular afterload at the extremes of lung volume can ultimately reduce systemic cardiac output, by shifting the interventricular septum toward the left, resulting in decreased left ventricular (LV) compliance and poor LV filling. These cardiopulmonary interactions suggest that strategies that emphasize the maintenance of alveolar volume while avoiding alveolar overdistension are not only necessary to improve gas exchange, but they are also likely to have a favorable effect on cardiovascular performance in ALI and ARDS.

CLINICAL FEATURES AND INVESTIGATIONS

Tachypnea and hypoxemia are the cardinal clinical features of ARDS primarily due to decrease in lung compliance. The eventual leakage of proteinaceous fluid into the alveolar spaces interferes with native surfactant function, creating conditions that favor regional atelectasis and small-airways closure, as well as a decrease in EELV to a point near or below closing capacity. At this point, hypoxia rapidly worsens and breathing becomes more labored in an effort to generate transpulmonary pressures sufficient to maintain alveolar patency. At this stage, the hypoxemia is refractory to oxygen, and positive pressure ventilation (PPV) is required to open a sufficient number of atelectasis lung units for adequate gas exchange.

Arterial blood gas analysis and chest radiograph are two important investigations required initially for the diagnosis and management of patients of ARDS. Repeated investigations are needed to assess the improvement or worsening of the disease and to monitor the beneficial or ill effects of ventilation and other interventions.

MANAGEMENT

The mainstay of therapy remains supportive care, of which a critically important component is the application of PPV.

Positive Pressure Ventilation

The decrease in pulmonary compliance, EELV, and V/Q mismatch in ARDS explain why the hypoxia is refractory to supplemental O_2. This explains why application of PPV is needed. It is also important to recognize the potential for PEEP to augment anatomical dead space by distending large airways, and potentially adding to alveolar dead space. In heterogeneous conditions, such as ALI and ARDS, it is difficult to know what level of PEEP will open enough alveoli to produce adequate oxygenation without creating conditions for ongoing stress-induced lung injury. The minimum PEEP that allows for a PaO_2 in the range of 55–80 mm Hg, with SpO_2 of 88–95%, using FiO_2 of 0.5–0.6. The tidal volume (VT) to be selected also merits careful consideration because studies have proven that phasic stretch during ventilation and alveolar overdistension at end-expiration actually potentiates and propagates the proinflammatory cytokine cascade in ARDS.

Tidal Volume

A landmark study in the history of ARDS by the ARDS network published in 2000 established that patients randomized to receive a VT of 6 mL/kg (predicted body weight) with plateau pressure limitation to 30 cm H_2O had a mortality reduction of 22% relative to those receiving a VT of 12 mL/kg (predicted body weight) with allowable plateau pressures of 50 cm H_2O. The investigators were also able to demonstrate a significant reduction in plasma levels of the proinflammatory cytokine IL-6 among patients in the low VT group. Other studies have also proven a greater reduction in plasma levels of proinflammatory cytokines among those patients who were randomized to receive lower VTs. This low VT ventilator strategy is now standard practice in management of ARDS.

Pediatricians extrapolate the adult-based recommendation of 6 mL/kg VT for ARDS to infants and children or rely on observational pediatric data. The studies by Erickson et al., and Khemani et al., demonstrated an inverse relationship between VT and mortality in children. The same finding was seen by Zhu et al., in infants.

PALICC recommended that for any invasively mechanically ventilated pediatric patient, the delivered VT should be "in or below the range of physiologic VT for age or body weight (i.e., 5–8 mL/kg predicted body weight) according to lung pathology and respiratory system compliance", when evaluating the full component of ARDS data on VT and outcome (pediatric and adult data), PALICC recommended using "patient-specific VTs" according to disease severity. Tidal volumes should be 3–6 mL/kg ideal (predicted) body weight for patients with poor respiratory system compliance and closer to the physiologic range (5–8 mL/kg ideal body weight) for patients with better preserved respiratory system compliance."

Optimum Positive End-expiratory Pressure

Positive end-expiratory pressure should be titrated to avoid alveolar collapse at end expiration (atelectrauma). Three randomized controlled trials (RCTs) in adults with ARDS studied higher versus lower PEEP levels according to PEEP or FiO_2 tables but did not analyze PEEP in relation to collapse during end expiration. There was no difference in outcome. However, two subsequent meta-analyses suggest that higher levels of PEEP as part of a lung-protective strategy may be associated with lower hospital mortality in adults with ARDS as defined by PaO_2/FiO_2 ratio less than or equal to 200 mm Hg. However, this positive data, effect of PEEP was not seen in those with more mild forms of acute lung injury. Unfortunately, data are lacking with regard to PEEP management for PARDS.

In the absence of definitive pediatric data, moderately elevated levels of PEEP (10–15 cm H_2O) should be titrated in patients with severe PARDS to the observed oxygenation and hemodynamic response. PEEP levels more than 15 cm H_2O may be needed for severe PARDS with attention paid to limiting the peak airway pressure less than 28. With higher PEEP, it is important to closely monitor markers of oxygen delivery, respiratory system compliance, and hemodynamics.

Peak Inspiratory Pressure and Plateau Pressure

There is a linear association between mortality and peak inspiratory pressure (PIP). The plateau pressure, in the absence of transpulmonary pressure measurements, should be limited "to 28 cm H_2O, allowing for slightly higher plateau pressures (29–32 cm H_2O) for patients with increased chest wall elastance (i.e., reduced chest wall compliance)".

Driving Pressure

Driving pressure has been suggested by Amato and colleagues to be the key variable for optimization when performing mechanical ventilation in patients with ARDS. Driving pressure (ΔP) is the ratio of VT to (static) respiratory system compliance (Crs); i.e.,

ΔP = VT/Crs. Driving pressure (ΔP) can be calculated at the bedside as plateau pressure minus positive end-expiratory pressure (Pplat – PEEP).

Recent data in the adult ARDS population have shown that the driving pressure is more closely related to mortality than PIP or PEEP alone. A single standard deviation (SD) increment in driving pressure (approximately 7 cm H_2O) was shown to be associated with higher mortality with a relative risk of 1.41. No corresponding data exist for PARDS, and thus difficult to use relatively new concept in clinical care in pediatrics at present.

Recruitment

Recruitment refers to the concept of increasing transpulmonary pressure from lower levels to higher levels (through increments in PEEP) to achieve optimal distension of alveoli in ARDS.

The ability to recruit diseased lung depends on several factors, including the type of lung disease (e.g., diffuse alveolar disease vs. focal alveolar consolidation), time course of the lung disease process, and respiratory system compliance.

Thus the optimal PEEP will keep the lung open (open lung concept) and lesser distending pressures (plateau pressures) will be needed during ventilation thereby potentially reducing shear stress on alveoli and damage due to repeated opening and closing of alveolar units. It is, however, important to avoid overdistension during this procedure as well. Two large, multicenter, randomized, controlled trials were published in 2008 that examined the question of whether using higher levels of PEEP to stabilize alveolar volume at end expiration could enhance the established mortality benefits of tidal volume reduction and plateau pressure limitation. While one study allowed higher PEEP and recruitment with plateau pressures up to 40 cm H_2O while maintaining VTs of 6 mL/kg, the other adjusted the PEEP to achieve plateau pressures less than 30 and similar low VTs. Neither trial was able to demonstrate a mortality benefit. However, the trial in which PEEP was titrated according to plateau pressure and in which plateau pressure was more conservatively managed did manage to show a significant increase in the median number of ventilator free days.

With the lack of convincing adult-based data and no definitive pediatric data, significant controversy continues to exist on how best to apply recruitment maneuvers, if at all, in clinical pediatric practice. PALICC recommended that careful recruitment maneuvers by slow incremental and decremental PEEP steps be formed in an attempt to improve severe oxygenation failure. However, sustained inflation was not recommended due to a lack of available data.

High Frequency Ventilation

Ongoing interest in the lung-protective merits of low VT ventilation has led to the expectation that high-frequency oscillatory ventilation (HFOV) would have an important role in the management of patients with ALI and ARDS because it uses VTs below dead space volume in the setting of continuous alveolar recruitment. Theoretically, high-frequency ventilation should provide the ultimate open-lung strategy of ventilation, with preservation of EELV, minimization of cyclic stretch, and avoidance of parenchymal overdistension at end-inspiration, amounting to ventilation on the most compliant portion of the volume-pressure curve while avoiding extremes of lung volume.

The first and largest multicenter, randomized trial to evaluate the effect of HFOV versus conventional ventilation in children was a crossover design that enrolled children with diffuse alveolar disease and/or air leak. The investigators randomized 70 patients to receive (a) conventional ventilation with limitation of peak inspiratory pressure, or (b) HFOV using a strategy that targeted a lung volume at which optimal oxygenation occurred (SaO_2 90% and $FiO_2 < 0.6$). The study found no difference in survival or duration of mechanical ventilation between the 2 groups, but significantly fewer children randomized to receive HFOV remained dependent on supplemental O_2 at 30 days.

A recent retrospective pediatric study on HFOV of 20 pediatric ARDS patients ventilated with HFOV after conventional ventilation failed showed that after initiation of HFOV, there was immediate and sustained increase in PaO_2/FiO_2 ratio. The ratio remained elevated and OI decreased significantly after 10–20 minutes and maintained for at least 48 hours. 13 of the 20 patients were successfully weaned. No significant change in the mean arterial pressure and heart rate was noted after HFOV and the overall survival rate was 65%.

Bateman et al., recently published a secondary propensity score analysis of the 353 subjects enrolled in the randomized evaluation of sedation titration for respiratory failure (RESTORE) study that were managed with HFOV. Early application of HFOV was associated with a significantly longer duration of mechanical ventilation and greater use of sedation and pharmacologic paralysis. However, no mortality association was noted. The authors speculated that the increased length of ventilation with early HFOV use could be related to variations in the management of HFOV (specifically HFOV weaning) across the multiple centers or due to HFOV itself. The lack of randomization of HFOV and the lack of standardization of ventilator management limit the conclusions that can be drawn.

Since the publication of OSCAR and OSCILLATE in 2013, adult practitioners have trended away from HFOV use for ARDS. In pediatrics, the use of HFOV for PARDS remains controversial, with practice generally based on institutional experience. Until additional PARDS studies are performed, HFOV use in pediatrics will probably remain center-dependent and even clinician-dependent.

HFOV should be considered as an alternative ventilator mode for those patients with moderate-to-severe PARDS "in whom plateau airway pressures exceed 28 cm H_2O in the absence of clinical evidence of reduced chest-wall compliance". It seems prudent to adopt the routine use of lung-protective conventional ventilation for PARDS and transition to HFOV in selected patients, followed by aggressive weaning as the disease process (es) resolves and pulmonary compliance improves.

Prone Positioning

Alveolar consolidation occurs along the gravitational axis in ALI and ARDS, and pulmonary blood flow is distributed preferentially to dorsal lung regions. The dorsal lungs are perfused but not contributing to ventilation. Placing a patient prone might reduce chest wall compliance, thus transmitting airway pressure to the alveoli more efficiently and stabilizing alveolar volume over a larger portion of previously nonaerated dorsal lung units. Studies have shown that prone positioning actually reduces stress strain and actually attenuates ventilator-associated lung injury.

A number of studies have been conducted on the benefits of prone positioning in ARDS. Most of these studies have found improvements in oxygenation. None, however, have shown any significant survival benefit.

Although the process of proning appears safe, no differences in the primary outcome variable of ventilator-free days or any of the secondary outcome parameters were seen in most studies. Thus, the role of prone position for PARDS remains uncertain.

Noninvasive Respiratory Support

Much attention has been paid to noninvasive ventilation in the pediatric population over the past couple of years. An RCT comparing nasal intermittent positive pressure ventilation (NIPPV) with control group demonstrated that heart rate and respiratory rate improved with NIPPV. The frequency of endotracheal intubation was also significantly lowered from 60% to 28% (p = 0.045) in mild form of ARDS. Similar to noninvasive ventilation, the use of high-flow nasal cannula continues to increase in the pediatric critical care environment without definitive data. A systematic investigation of the use of high-flow nasal cannula support for PARDS is needed.

OTHER ADJUNCTS TO THERAPY

Fluid Management

A multicenter randomized control trial to evaluate the effects of various fluid-management protocols on outcomes in ALI and ARDS using a contemporary open lung, low VT strategy in 1,000 adults with ALI/ARDS showed that mortality is the same whether conservative or liberal fluid strategy is used, but the conservative strategy was associated with an improvement in OI and a significant increase in ventilator-free days during the first 28 days of therapy. Thus, after the initial resuscitative phase of ARDS, a conservative fluid administration policy may be beneficial.

Surfactant Therapy

Dysfunction of surfactant has been found to be one of the pathophysiological alterations in ARDS. Surfactant replacement has hence been postulated to be of benefit in these patients.

Evidence on the use of surfactant in children comes in large part from a recent multicentered double-blinded placebo controlled trial that compared administration of modified bovine surfactant (Calfactant) with air placebo in 152 infants and children with ALI and ARDS. The authors reported a significant reduction in mortality in the surfactant patients, compared with the placebo patients (19% vs. 36%), as well as significant improvements in OI. The study, however, was underpowered, making it difficult to identify which patients with pediatric ALI/ARDS might benefit best from Calfactant.

The ideal surfactant dose and composition, the timing of its administration, and the number of doses to be administered are currently not standardized and need further clarification.

Inhaled Nitric Oxide

Nitric oxide (NO) has been known for some time as the endogenous endothelium-derived relaxing factor that couples with cyclic guanosine monophosphate (c-GMP) system to mediate vasodilation by local smooth muscle relaxation and to modify immune function and platelet aggregation. Inhaled NO (INO) is, theoretically, a selective pulmonary vasodilator due to its local activity and very short half-life. Because vasodilation predominantly occurs in adequately ventilated regions of the lung, blood is shunted away from more poorly ventilated regions. INO has been postulated as a therapeutic approach to ARDS by reducing ventilation/perfusion mismatch via a reduction in dead space ventilation and a resultant improvement in oxygenation via relieving microvascular obstruction by reducing platelet aggregation, and potentially reducing neutrophil adhesion and local inflammation.

However, 3 RCTs have been performed in children with ARDS, and each has shown that INO does not improve outcome for PARDS.

Corticosteroids

Numerous clinical trials have attempted to establish a role for corticosteroids in modulating the role of the immune response to improve clinical outcomes in patients with ALI and ARDS. Corticosteroids are understood to limit transudation of plasma across the capillary endothelium and exert anti-inflammatory effects by downregulating expression of steroid-responsive genes coding for proinflammatory cytokines while upregulating those encoding for anti-inflammatory agents, such as IL-10.

A study by the ARDS network in 2006 which enrolled 180 adults with persistent ARDS and administered steroids after 7 days found that use of steroids was associated with increased number of ventilator-free and shock-free days during the first 28 days, with improvement in oxygenation, respiratory-system compliance, and blood pressure with fewer days of vasopressor therapy. However, increased 60- and 180-day mortality rates among patients enrolled 14 days after onset of ARDS were noticed. The rate of infectious complications did not increase but patients who received steroids showed a higher rate of neuromuscular weakness. Use of steroids in ARDS was not recommended by the authors in view of the increased mortality.

Meduri et al., conducted a prospective, double-blinded, randomized, placebo-controlled group sequential clinical trial in which steroids were started early within 72 hours of diagnosis in the form of low-dose prolonged methylprednisolone. A loading dose of 1 mg/kg, infusion of 1 mg/kg/day from days 1–14; 0.5 mg/kg/day days 15–21; 0.25 mg/kg/day from days 22–25; 0.125 mg/kg/day from days 26–28 was used. Protocol was advanced to day 15 if patient was extubated before day 14 and enteral dosing started when patient started tolerating enteral feeds. Almost 50% more patients in the treatment group had improved lung function and more than double the treated patients were extubated at 7 days.

A critical appraisal of the study by Meduri et al., concluded that steroids in early ARDS cannot be recommended as standard therapy at this time because of limitations in the study design.

A prospective, observational, single-center PARDS study by Yehya et al., investigated corticosteroid administration for a variety of indications in a cohort of 283 children. This study demonstrated that corticosteroid exposure for more than 24 hours was associated with increased mortality, fewer ventilator-free days (at 28 days), and a longer length of ventilation in survivors as compared with those without corticosteroid exposure or corticosteroid exposure for less than 24 hours.

Given the available pediatric literature, it is determined that corticosteroids cannot be recommended as routine therapy for PARDS.

Neuromuscular Blockade

In the adult population, neuromuscular blockade during the initial 48 hours of ARDS demonstrated improved survival and time off the ventilator in those with severe lung disease. For infants and children, the topic of neuromuscular blockade for PARDS has not been adequately studied.

Nutritional Support

Over the past several years, a number of reports support the concept that enteral, rather than parenteral, nutrition can preserve functional integrity of the gastrointestinal mucosal barrier and decrease the potential for intestinal bacterial translocation and systemic infection. A recent multicenter randomized trial examined whether mechanically ventilated patients with ALI would benefit more from receiving low volume enteral feedings as compared with full volume enteral feedings for the first 6 days of supportive care. This trial was unable to demonstrate a benefit of trophic enteral feedings relative to full enteral feedings, with respect to the primary outcome measure (ventilator-free days: 14.9 days vs. 15.0 days; 95% CI, -1.4 to 1.2 days; $p = 0.89$).

Blood Transfusion

Packed red blood cells transfusion should not be done in clinically stable children with evidence of adequate oxygen delivery except congenital cyanotic heart disease, bleeding, and severe hypoxemia, if hemoglobin is more than 7 g/dL.

Role of ECMO

The use of veno-venous extracorporeal membrane oxygenation (ECMO) for refractory ARDS continues to increase, especially in the adult population. Despite decades of use, the optimal timing for cannulation remains uncertain and continues to be controversial. Khemani et al., reported a mortality rate for PARDS of 40% when the OI exceeds 16. Survival rates more than 70% have been reported with veno-venous ECMO for viral-induced ARDS. The key to optimal outcomes for severe PARDS is balancing risk versus benefit to the right patient at the right time. Data from the extracorporeal life support organization (ELSO) registry indicate an average overall survival to discharge of 75% in this cohort. Unfortunately, data to assist with this complex clinical decision-making process are lacking.

OUTCOMES IN PEDIATRIC ARDS

Recent data indicates that mortality in pediatric ALI and ARDS seems to be decreasing. While retrospective case series published 15–20 years ago documented mortality rates of 50-75%, at least one recent and carefully controlled clinical trial has documented a mortality rate of less than 10% for pediatric ALI or ARDS. Outcome improvements over the past 15 years extend even to immunocompromised children with ALI or ARDS, a subgroup that has historically demonstrated particularly high mortality rates. The general trend has been one of decreasing mortality for PARDS, especially for those without preexisting comorbidities. The presence of one or more nonpulmonary organ failures correlates with a six- to eightfold increase in the likelihood of mortality.

Patient-level meta-analysis of 4,188 patients with ARDS from 4 multicenter clinical datasets and 269 patients with ARDS from 3 single-center datasets (adults and children) containing physiologic information showed that the stages of mild, moderate, and severe ARDS were associated with mortality of 27%, 32%, and 45%, respectively.

KEY MESSAGES

- The PALICC has provided the critical care community with the first pediatric-focused definition for ARDS.
- OSI should be used when an OI is not available for stratification of risk for patients receiving invasive mechanical ventilation. Oxygen saturation SF ratio can be used when PF ratio is not available to diagnose PARDS in patients receiving noninvasive full facemask ventilation (CPAP or BiPAP) with a minimum CPAP of 5 cm H_2O.
- Oxygen therapy should be titrated to achieve an SpO_2 between 88% and 97%.
- Consider early NIV for alveolar recruitment in alert, cooperative patient with mild and in early moderate forms of ARDS.
- Ventilation in patients with ARDS should be with low VT (4–6 mL/kg), adequate PEEP and should ensure plateau pressures less than 28 cm H_2O while allowing hypercapnia, so as to prevent progression of lung injury.
- Use of high frequency ventilation, inhaled nitric oxide, surfactant and prone positioning offers improvement in oxygenation in selected patients but does not improve outcomes.
- Short-term administration of neuromuscular blockers (NMBs) to facilitate mechanical ventilation may benefit patients with severe disease and it is important to give daily NMBs infusion interruption and discontinue as soon as feasible.
- The routine use of corticosteroids is not recommended at present.
- Adequate attention to hemodynamics and other organ dysfunction is crucial to outcomes.
- Although outcomes for PARDS have improved over the past decade, mortality, and morbidity remain significant.

SUGGESTED READING

1. Abraham E, Matthay MA, Dinarello CA, et al. Consensus conference definitions for sepsis, septic shock, acute lung injury, and acute respiratory distress syndrome: Time for a reevaluation. Crit Care Med. 2000;28:232-5.
2. Amato MB, Meade MO, Slutsky AS, et al. Driving pressure and survival in the acute respiratory distress syndrome. N Engl J Med. 2015;372(8):747-55.
3. ARDS Definition Task Force. Ranieri VM, Rubenfeld GD, Thompson BT, et al. Acute respiratory distress syndrome: the Berlin definition. JAMA. 2012;307(23):2526-33.

4. Arnold JH, Hanson JH, Toro-Figuero LO, et al. Prospective, randomized comparison of high-frequency oscillatory ventilation and conventional mechanical ventilation in pediatric respiratory failure. Crit Care Med. 1994;22:1530-9.
5. Bateman ST, Borasino S, Asaro LA, et al. Early high frequency oscillatory ventilation in pediatric acute respiratory failure: a propensity score analysis. Am J Respir Crit Care Med. 2016;193(5): 495-503.
6. Bernard GR, Artigas A, Brigham KL, et al. The American-European Consensus Conference on ARDS: definitions, mechanisms, relevant outcomes, and clinical trial coordination. Am J Respir Crit Care Med. 1994;149(3 Pt 1):818-24.
7. Broccard A, Shapiro RS, Schmitz LL, et al. Prone positioning attenuates and redistributes ventilator-induced lung injury in dogs. Crit Care Med. 2000;28:295-303.
8. Broccard AF, Shapiro RS, Schmitz LL, et al. Influence of prone position on the extent and distribution of lung injury in a high tidal volume oleic acid model of acute respiratory distress syndrome. Crit Care Med. 1997;25:16-27.
9. Chu EK, Whitehead T, Slutsky AS. Effects of cyclic opening and closing at low- and high-volume ventilation on bronchoalveolar lavage cytokines. Crit Care Med. 2004;32:168-74.
10. Curley MA, Hibberd PL, Fineman LD, et al. Effect of prone positioning on clinical outcomes in children with acute lung injury: a randomized controlled trial. JAMA. 2005;294(2):229-37.
11. Curley MA, Wypij D, Watson RS, et al. Protocolized sedation vs. usual care in pediatric patients mechanically ventilated for acute respiratory failure: a randomized clinical trial. JAMA. 2015;313(4):379-89.
12. Drago BB, Kimura D, Rovnaghi CR, et al. Double-blind, placebo-controlled pilot randomized trial of methylprednisolone infusion in pediatric acute respiratory distress syndrome. Pediatr Crit Care Med. 2015;16(3):e74-81.
13. Ferguson ND, Fan E, Camporota L, et al. The Berlin definition of ARDS: an expanded rationale, justification, and supplementary material. Intens Care Med. 2012;38:1573-82.
14. Ferguson ND, Meade MO, Hallett DC, et al. High values of the pulmonary artery wedge pressure in patients with acute lung injury and acute respiratory distress syndrome. Intens Care Med. 2002;28:1073-7.
15. Fineman LD, La Brecque MA, Shih MC, et al. Prone positioning can be safely performed in critically ill infants and children. Pediatr Crit Care Med. 2006;7(5):413-22.
16. Gao L, Barnes KC. Recent advances in genetic predisposition to clinical acute lung injury. Am J Physiol Lung Cell Mol Physiol. 2009;296:L713-25.
17. Gattinoni L, Caironi P, Pelosi P, et al. What has computed tomography taught us about the acute respiratory distress syndrome? Am J Respir Crit Care Med. 2001;164:1701-11.
18. Gattinoni L, Pelosi P, Suter PM, et al. Acute respiratory distress syndrome caused by pulmonary and extrapulmonary disease. Different syndromes? Am J Respir Crit Care Med. 1998;158:3-11.
19. Gattinoni L, Tognoni G, Pesenti A, et al. Effect of prone positioning on the survival of patients with acute respiratory failure. N Engl J Med. 2001;345:568-73.
20. Henderson WR, Chen L, Amato MB, et al. Fifty years of research in ARDS: respiratory mechanics in acute respiratory distress syndrome. Am J Respir Crit Care Med. 2017.
21. Hu X, Qian S, Xu F, et al. Chinese Collaborative Study Group for Pediatric Respiratory Failure: Incidence, management and mortality of acute hypoxemic respiratory failure and acute respiratory distress syndrome from a prospective study of Chinese paediatric intensive care network. Acta Pediatr. 2010;99:715-21.
22. Khemani RG, Conti D, Alonzo TA, et al. Effect of tidal volume in children with acute hypoxemic respiratory failure. Intens Care Med. 2009;35(8):1428-37.
23. Khemani RG, Smith LS, Zimmerman JJ, et al. Pediatric Acute Lung Injury Consensus Conference Group. Pediatric acute respiratory distress syndrome: definition, incidence, and epidemiology: proceedings from the Pediatric Acute Lung Injury Consensus Conference. Pediatr Crit Care Med. 2015;16(5 Suppl 1):S23-40.

24. Khemani RG, Thomas NJ, Venkatachalam V, et al. Comparison of SpO2 to PaO2-based markers of lung disease severity for children with acute lung injury. Crit Care Med. 2012;40(4):1309-16.
25. Lamm WJ, Graham MM, Albert RK. Mechanism by which the prone position improves oxygenation in acute lung injury. Am J Respir Crit Care Med. 1994;150:184-93.
26. Meade MO, Cook DJ, Guyatt GH, et al. Ventilation strategy using low tidal volumes, recruitment maneuvers, and high positive end-expiratory pressure for acute lung injury and acute respiratory distress syndrome: A randomized controlled trial. JAMA. 2008;299:637-45.
27. Meduri GU, Golden E, Freire AX, et al. Methylprednisolone infusion in early severe ARDS: results of a randomized controlled trial. Chest. 2007;131:954-63.
28. Mercat A, Richard JC, Vielle B, et al. Positive end-expiratory pressure setting in adults with acute lung injury and acute respiratory distress syndrome: A randomized controlled trial. JAMA. 2008;299: 646-55.
29. National Heart Lung and Blood Institute Acute Respiratory Distress Syndrome ARDS Clinical Trials Network. Wheeler AP, Bernard GR, Thompson BT, et al. Pulmonary-artery versus central venous catheter to guide treatment of acute lung injury. N Engl J Med. 2006;354:2213-24.
30. Papazian L, Forel JM, Gacouin A, et al. Neuromuscular blockers in early acute respiratory Distress syndrome. N Engl J Med. 2010;363(12):1107-16.
31. Pediatric Acute Lung Injury Consensus Conference Group. Pediatric acute respiratory distress syndrome: consensus recommendations from the Pediatric Acute Lung Injury Consensus Conference. Pediatr Crit Care Med. 2015;16(5):428-39.
32. Randolph AG, Meert KL, O'Neil ME, et al. The feasibility of conducting clinical trials in infants and children with acute respiratory failure. Am J Respir Crit Care Med. 2003;167:1334-40.
33. Rimensberger PC, Cheifetz IM. Pediatric Acute Lung Injury Consensus Conference Group. Ventilatory support in children with pediatric acute respiratory distress syndrome: proceedings from the pediatric acute lung injury consensus conference. Pediatr Crit Care Med. 2015;16(5 Suppl 1): S51-60.
34. Steinberg KP, Hudson LD, Goodman RB, et al. National Heart, Lung, and Blood Institute Acute Respiratory Distress Syndrome (ARDS) Clinical Trials Network. Efficacy and safety of corticosteroids for persistent acute respiratory distress syndrome. N Engl J Med. 2006;354:1671-84.
35. The Acute Respiratory Distress Syndrome Network. Ventilation with lower tidal volumes as compared with traditional tidal volumes for acute lung injury and the acute respiratory distress syndrome. N Engl J Med. 2000;342:1301-8.
36. Thomas NJ, Shaffer ML, Willson DF, et al. Defining acute lung disease in children with the oxygenation saturation index. Pediatr Crit Care Med. 2010;11(1):12-7.
37. Timmons OD, Dean JM, Vernon DD. Mortality rates and prognostic variables in children with adult respiratory distress syndrome. J Pediatr. 1991;119:896-9.
38. Valentine SL, Nadkarni VM, Curley MA. Pediatric Acute Lung Injury Consensus Conference Group. Non-pulmonary treatments for pediatric acute respiratory distress syndrome: proceedings from the Pediatric Acute Lung Injury Consensus Conference. Pediatr Crit Care Med. 2015;16(5 Suppl 1): S73-85.
39. Ventre KM, Arnold JH. Acute lung injury and acute respiratory distress syndrome. In: Nichols DG, Shaffner DH (Eds). Rogers' Textbook of Pediatric Intensive Care, 4th edition. Philadelphia: Lippincott Williams and Wilkins; 2008: pp. 731-52.
40. Yehya N, Servaes S, Thomas NJ, et al. Corticosteroid exposure in pediatric acute respiratory distress syndrome. Intens Care Med. 2015;41(9):1658-66.

Hemodynamic Monitoring

11

Vasanth Kumar, Suchitra Ranjit

LEARNING OBJECTIVES

- Understanding the concepts in invasive and noninvasive hemodynamic monitoring (HD) monitoring
- Applying these at the bedside
- Correctly interpret the results in order to apply therapeutic interventions.

INTRODUCTION

Hemodynamic monitoring refers to measurements of the functional characteristics of the heart and the circulating system that affect the oxygenation and perfusion of tissues. Successful use of hemodynamic measurements necessitates that the clinician possess the requisite skills, be aware of the multiple potential risks and be able to successfully interpret the information provided by the measurement. Hence, these devices should serve as adjuncts and not replacements for clinical skills.

The objectives of monitoring in a critically ill child are:
- Diagnostic—to assess the severity of the underlying condition.
- Therapeutic—to indicate the need and timing for intervention.
- Surveillance—assess response to therapy.
- Prognostic—trends during monitoring help in the prediction of outcome.
- Warning—audiovisual alarms in various monitors alert the clinician to untoward events.

CLINICAL EXAMINATION

Forward flow to vital organs, necessary for oxygen delivery, depends on the presence of a pressure gradient or perfusion pressure. Mean arterial pressure (MAP) is more appropriate than isolated systolic or diastolic blood pressure (BP) for goal directed therapy in shock.

Systemic perfusion: Since pressure does not equal flow, evaluation of indirect signs of blood flow and systemic vascular resistance (SVR) is required. This can be done by monitoring the perfusion, i.e., the presence and volume of central and peripheral pulses and assessing the end organ perfusion and function. A discrepancy in the volume of peripheral and central pulses may be caused by vasoconstriction or decreased cardiac output. Broadly, a narrow pulse pressure suggests increased SVR compared to a wide pulse pressure which suggests decreased SVR.

End-organ Perfusion

- Mottling, pallor, delayed capillary refill and peripheral cyanosis are indicative of poor skin perfusion.
- Urine output is directly proportional to renal blood flow and glomerular filtration rate thereby making it a very good indicator of renal perfusion.
- Altered consciousness of any degree may be an indicator of impaired brain perfusion.

Blood Pressure

Blood pressure measurement is integral in the support of the critically ill patient and is determined by both cardiac output and systemic vascular resistance. It is very important to remember that pressure does not equal flow. When cardiac output falls, normal blood pressure is maintained by compensatory vasoconstriction causing high systemic vascular resistance, even though blood flow to various organs is reduced. Hypotension is, therefore, a late sign of cardiovascular decompensation, and one must not feel reassured by the presence of a normal blood pressure.

Noninvasive Blood Pressure Monitoring (NIBP)

The oscillometric technique is the most commonly used one to measure arterial pressure. MAP is the most accurate by this method and diastolic pressure is the least accurate.

The major limitations of NIBP are:
- Readings can be fallacious in the presence of hypoperfusion or peripheral vasoconstriction
- It gives intermittent readings
- Accuracy of readings are dependent on appropriate cuff size and placement.

Invasive Hemodynamic Monitoring

Invasive BP monitoring is considered the gold standard for arterial pressure monitoring in an ICU. It is indicated in situations where there is need for continuous, reliable BP recording along with the need for frequent arterial blood sampling. The BP measured by this method is unaffected by poor flow or perfusion in the limb. IBP is a relatively safe procedure. Some of the complications include hemorrhage, hematoma, arterial thrombosis, vasospasm, ischemia and infection.

The equipment required for invasive BP monitoring includes an arterial cannula with a heparinized saline column and flushing device, a transducer, an amplifier and a monitor. A continuous column of fluid from the blood vessel lumen to the transducer diaphragm transmits variations in intraluminal pressure, causing changes in resistance and current that is converted into an electrical signal, which is amplified to display a waveform and digital pressure on the bedside monitor.

Pressure is usually measured with a transducer, which is a device that coverts pressure in a fluid-filled system to electric waveform. Three factors have to be considered when using a transducer:
- Calibration
- Zero setting
- Leveling

Calibration: The precision and accuracy of arterial pressure system depends on meticulous calibration that must be carried out regularly.

Zero setting: Why is zeroing important? The process of eliminating the atmospheric pressure is called "zeroing," and what is essentially being done is opening the fluid column on the measuring device to atmosphere, so that atmospheric pressure is the starting value or zero.

Leveling: Leveling eliminates the influence of hydrostatic pressure on the transducer. A transducer that is positioned below the patient's heart will produce falsely elevated pressure and a transducer positioned above the patient's heart will produce falsely low pressure. Pressure measurements in a fluid-filled system are relative to a reference point. A widely used reference point is the phlebostatic axis which corresponds to the midpoint of the right atrium, because this is where blood comes back to the heart and this is also the pressure that provides the preload for the heart as a whole. The phlebostatic axis is determined by the junction of the two lines, a transverse line along the fourth intercostal space and a vertical line midway between the anterior and posterior chest wall.

The system should be arranged such that the reference stopcock of the transducer (that is opened for zeroing the transducer) must be leveled to the phlebostatic axis.

Pressure versus Flow

Clinicians caring for sick children must remember that BP and heart rate often do not reflect blood flow. The distinction between pressure and flow is very important. For instance, when evaluating a "shocky" patient on vasopressors, an increase in blood pressure is often assumed to indicate an increase in systemic blood flow, but the opposite effect (a decrease in flow) is also possible.

Note that as the pressure wave moves toward the periphery, the systolic pressure gradually increases, and the systolic portion of the waveform narrows. The systolic pressure can increase as much as 20 mm Hg from the proximal aorta to the radial or femoral arteries (distal pulse amplification). This increase in peak systolic pressure is offset by the narrowing of the systolic pressure wave, so that the mean arterial pressure remains unchanged. Therefore, the mean arterial pressure is a more accurate measure of central aortic pressure.

Mean Arterial Pressure (MAP)

The MAP has two features that make it superior to the systolic pressure for arterial pressure monitoring. First, the MAP is the true driving pressure for peripheral blood flow. Second, the MAP does not change as the pressure waveform moves distally, nor is it altered by distortions generated by recording systems.

Preload Assessment

Preload is one of the three major determinates of stroke volume and the other two include contractility and afterload. Ensuring optimum preload is the primary cornerstone of therapy in pediatric septic shock. Preload measurements may be static or dynamic.

Static Preload Measurements

These are central venous pressure (CVP) (right atrium), the pulmonary artery occlusion pressure (P_{pao}) (left atrial filling pressure), assessments of right ventricular end-diastolic volume (RVEDV) or global end-diastolic volume (GEDV).

Central Venous Pressure (CVP) Monitoring

Central venous pressure is the most commonly used measure of preload; however, this modality has many fallacies and reliance on CVP has been deemphasized. The trends of CVP recordings are more important than a single value. It is important to recognize the optimal value that supports adequate cardiac output for an individual patient rather than aiming for a standard value. Observation of the response to volume helps in deciding adequacy of fluids and need for vasoactive drugs. An initial high value of CVP however should prompt more careful evaluation before attributing it to fluid overload. Pericardial effusion, tamponade, constrictive pericarditis, high ventilatory pressure/PEEP, pulmonary thromboembolism, pulmonary hypertension are some of the conditions where the CVP may be misleadingly high in spite of poor ventricular filling. An echocardiography may assist in better evaluation at this juncture.

Dynamic Indices of Preload

In contrast to static measures, dynamic indices rely on the changing physiology of heart lung interactions to determine whether a patient will benefit from increased preload. An understanding of the Frank-Starling curve (Fig. 1) is fundamental to understanding the concept of preload responsiveness. The slope of the relationship between ventricular preload and stroke volume (SV) depends on ventricular contractility. As contractility increases, the Starling curve shifts upward and to the left and increases its slope. Increasing preload serves to augment ventricular output predominantly on the steep portion of the curve. As seen in Figure 1, augmenting preload on the flat portion of the curve produces minimal increases in SV. A preload that would indicate volume responsiveness in the normal heart may not apply to a failing heart.

Dynamic indices apply a controlled and reversible preload variation and measure the hemodynamic response to positive pressure ventilation, or to reversible preload-increasing maneuvers, such as passive leg raising (PLR).

During positive pressure inspiration, preload to the right heart is decreased, because of increased intrathoracic pressure, both from compression of the vena cava (decreased venous return) and increased right atrial pressure. This decrease in right ventricular (RV) preload leads to a decrease in RV output, which subsequently leads to a decrease in pulmonary artery blood flow, LV filling, and LV output. The end result of these pressure changes is that LV stroke volume (SV) increases, while RV SV decreases during positive pressure inspiration. The delay of pulmonary blood transit time results in decreased RV SV translating to a decreased LV SV a few heartbeats later (i.e., usually during expiration).

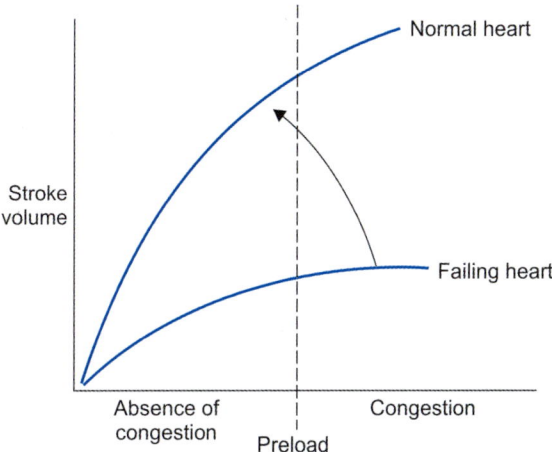

Fig. 1: Frank–Starling curves demonstrating relationship between changes in preload to change in stroke volume (SV) in a normal and failing ventricles. A given change in preload may cause variable changes in SV, depending on the slope of the curve.

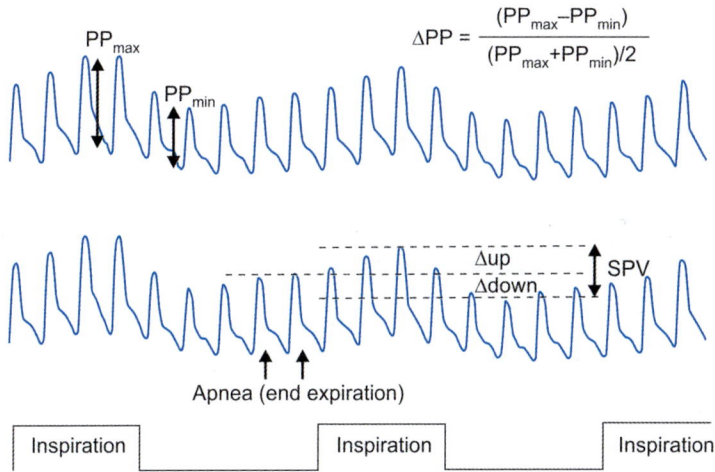

Fig. 2: Measures of arterial blood pressure variability during mechanical ventilation. (PPMAX = maximal pulse pressure, PPMIN = minimal pulse pressure, SPV = systolic pressure variation).

These phasic differences are exaggerated in the setting of hypovolemia as the underfilled vena cava is more collapsible, and the underfilled right atrium is more susceptible to increased intrathoracic pressure. This increased variation in pressures between the inspiratory phase and the expiratory phase can be used to identify hypovolemia and volume responsiveness.

The various dynamic indices of preload or fluid responsiveness are stroke volume variation (SVV), systolic pressure variation (SPV) and pulse pressure variation (PPV) (Fig. 2).

Large variability of the arterial pressure suggests that measures to increase preload, (e.g., fluid volume administration) will increase stroke volume. The top panel demonstrates the

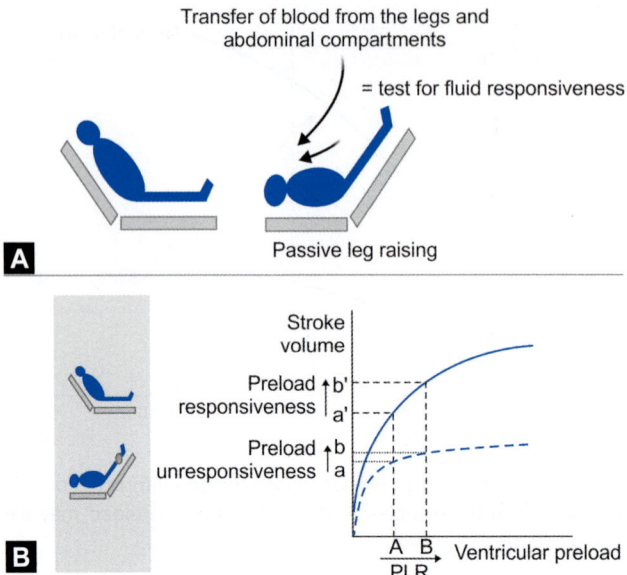

Figs. 3A and B: Passive leg raise. The passive leg raising test consists in measuring the hemodynamic effects of a leg elevation up to 45°.

calculations for PPV. At commencement of inspiration with PPV, an initial rise in systolic blood pressure (delta-up) occurs, possibly due to the emptying of pulmonary capacitance vessels and secondary to the effect of decreasing afterload. However, the positive-pressure breath also decreases systemic venous return and; thus, right-heart preload, which is transferred to the left heart by the end of the inspiratory breath and continues into early expiration. The net effect is a drop in systolic blood pressure (delta-down), which will return to baseline by end of expiration.

Passive Leg Raising (Figs 3A and B)

Passive leg raising (PLR) is a form of reversible volume challenge that can be used to evaluate which patients will benefit from intravenous fluid and increased preload. Elevating a patient's legs allows a passive transfer of blood from the lower part of the body toward the central circulation. If the right ventricle cannot increase cardiac output with increased preload, the left ventricle will not see the increased preload, and cardiac output will not improve. Importantly, PLR can be used in spontaneously breathing patients and in patients without a sinus rhythm. The increase in preload from the maneuver is reversed completely when the legs are returned to horizontal. International consensus guidelines now recommend PLR to evaluate fluid responsiveness in patients with shock with a sensitivity of 97% and specificity of 94%. Studies have found that the PLR-induced changes in aortic blood flow and arterial pulse pressure variation (PPV) were predictive of volume responsiveness, but change in aortic blood flow was more accurate than the change in PPV. Increase of cardiac output or SV of greater than 12% with PLR predicted volume responsiveness.

Further studies are needed to clarify the use of PLR in young infants (in whom the lower extremity blood volumes may be low) and patients on vasoconstrictors. PLR must be avoided in patients with raised intra-abdominal pressures and raised ICP.

Dynamic indices repeatedly have been shown to be superior to static measures for determining preload responsiveness in critically ill patients. However, except PLR, the conditions under which most dynamic indices may be performed are stringent (controlled ventilation with tidal volume at least 8 mL/kg, no spontaneous efforts, etc., sinus rhythm) which only a few real-world ICU patients will satisfy. Further, the requisite increase in stroke volume or cardiac output must be measured, rather than easily available measures, such as BP or HR. Moreover, it is important to remember that preload responsiveness does not equate to needing more preload. Healthy individuals are preload-responsive and will increase their cardiac output in response to a fluid challenge, but they do not require increased blood volume. Therefore, even with accurate measures of preload responsiveness, clinical judgment remains essential. Similarly, some patients maybe preload responsive, but their lungs maybe congested and it may not be safe to fill. So, prior to volume administration, it is mandatory to answer the following two questions:
- Is the given child with shock preload responsive?
- If so, is it safe to fill? If the answer to both questions is yes, one proceeds with volume administration.

Cardiac Output Assessment

Assessment of cardiac output (CO) in the PICU setting is challenging and prone to potential errors. Moreover, in children CO varies with body surface area (BSA), therefore, it is essential to use cardiac index (CI) L/(min/m^2), which is CO/BSA (Appendix 1). In normal children, CI of 2 L/(min/m^2) is adequate. But in septic shock, the American College of Critical Care Medicine (2017) recommends a target CI of 3.3–6 L/(min/m^2) to maintain tissue perfusion.

There are various methods to measure CO, a few are outlined below.

Thermodilution

Thermodilution, through a pulmonary artery catheter (PAC), is the gold standard method for measurement of CO, using bolus injections of iced or room temperature saline. However, it is invasive, technically difficult, time-consuming and prone to complications.

Thoracic Electrical Bioimpedance

The measurement is based on the observation that blood flow in the thoracic aorta can be quantified by continuously assessing the impedance to an AC current applied to thorax with the help of electrodes applied in neck and chest. Bioimpedance is defined as the ratio of voltage detected to the current applied. The concept is that during systole RBCs move in a parallel fashion permitting the electric current to flow easily with maximum electrical velocity and limited impedance. Whereas the exact opposite happens in diastole when RBCs are arranged randomly, increasing the impedance to the electric current and thereby decreasing the

Appendix 1: Common hemodynamic variables.

Parameter	Formula	Normal range	Unit
Cardiac index	CI = CO/BSA	3.5–5.5	L/min/m²
Stroke index	SI = CI/heart rate	30–60	mL/m²
Systemic vascular resistance index	SVRI = 80 × (MAP–CVP)/CI	800–1,600	Dyne-sec/cm²/m²
Pulmonary vascular resistance index	PVRI = 80 × (MAP–LAP)/CI	80–240	Dyne-sec/cm²/m²
Left ventricular stroke work index	LVSWI = SI × MAP × 0.0136	50–62 (adult)	g-m/m²
Right ventricular stroke work index	RVSWI = SI × MAP × 0.0136	5.1–6.9 (adult)	g-m/m²
Arterial oxygen content	CaO_2 = (1.34 × Hb × SaO_2) + (PaO_2 × 0.003)		mL/m²
Oxygen delivery	DO_2 = CI × CaO_2	570–670	mL/min/m²
Fick principle	CI = VO_2/CaO_2–CvO_2	160–180 (infant VO_2) 100–130 (child VO_2)	mL/min/m²
Mixed venous oxygen saturation		65–75%	
Oxygen extraction ratio	OER = (SaO_2–SvO_2)/SaO_2	0.24–0.28	

electrical velocity. The changes of impedance overtime are integrated in a complex algorithm that allows to measure CO, preload (thoracic fluid index; TFI), afterload (SVR) and many other hemodynamic parameters. Electrical cardiometry is FDA approved and validated for use in neonates, children and adults.

Esophageal Doppler

A Doppler probe placed in the esophagus calculates stroke volume from the velocity of blood flow in the aorta. It also provides indirect measures of preload and afterload.

Two-dimensional Transthoracic Echocardiography

Echo can reliably measure the SV, thereby the CI and SVRI. The blood pumped out of the heart assumes the shape of a virtual cylinder in the LV outflow tract (LVOT). By measuring the LVOT diameter (base of a cylinder), the LVOT area is calculated (πr^2). Similarly, the height is measured using pulsed wave Doppler to obtain the velocity time integral (VTI). Finally, the stroke volume can be calculated as the product of VTI and the LVOT area. While the advantage is the noninvasive nature and the availability of the echo machine, a major downside is the potential for large errors with very small changes in angle of the probe, further it is a time-consuming process, needing expertise and manual calculations. Hence, 2D echocardiography may be logistically difficult for frequent, serial hemodynamic assessment in critically ill children.

Arterial Pulse Contour Methods

A variety of methods exist for continuous arterial pulse-contour analysis of CO on a beat to beat basis, all of which utilize a combination of calculations for aortic impedance, aortic compliance, systemic vascular resistance, pressure wave reflection. All methods require an indwelling CVP and arterial catheter to measure changes in stroke volume, and an alternative method for cardiac output measurement, (i.e., transpulmonary thermodilution, lithium dilution) for (re) calibration.

Assessment of Afterload

Afterload is assessed by measuring the SVR. The resistance (R) in any circuit is the pressure gradient (ΔP) divided by the flow (R = ΔP/Flow). SVR is the pressure gradient between MAP at the exit of the left ventricle and at entrance of the right atrium (CVP) divided by the flow (CO); [SVR = (MAP–CVP)/CO]. SVRI [(MAP–CVP)/CI], becomes independent of body size. The SVRI measured in Wood units is multiplied by 80 to convert to dynes/cm^2. SVRI is usually measured by echocardiography and Doppler based methods as described earlier. Although there is still no clear evidence that monitoring CI and SVRI improves the outcome of children in septic shock, it makes physiological sense and provides objective parameter to intensivist to titrate vasoactive therapy.

Assessment of Tissue Oxygenation

Because of the technical difficulties of measuring cardiac output in clinical practice, several measures of adequacy of organ flow and oxygen delivery DO_2 are employed. The balance between DO_2 (delivery) and VO_2 (consumption) is of vital importance in critically ill patients. The main goal of any hemodynamic intervention is to improve DO_2 while maintaining an adequate perfusion pressure. Monitoring tissue oxygenation is important as standard measures of hemodynamics (such as BP and by near infrared spectroscopy (NIRS), orthogonal polarization spectral (OPS), tissue capnometry).

Venous O_2 Saturation

Mixed (SVO_2)/Central venous Oxygen Saturation ($ScvO_2$)

- Mixed venous blood is defined when all sources of systemic venous return (superior vena cava, inferior vena cava, and coronary sinus) have mixed, which occurs in the normal heart in the RV and pulmonary artery.
- Mixed venous saturation will decrease when oxygen delivery falls or oxygen consumption increases.

The normal mixed venous oxygen saturation is ~73% (range 65–75%), but it is obviously less in cyanosed patients. The typical range for the arteriovenous oxygen saturation difference is 20–33%. Because of the difficulty in accessing mixed venous blood, central venous saturation has been suggested as an alternative in both pediatric and adult practice.

Both global oxygenation and regional oxygenation indices may be measured. Since there are no direct measures of tissue oxygenation, indirect measures of tissue oxygenations are often used which are described in Appendix 2.

Appendix 2: Common oxygenation indices.

Index/parameter	Value
Oxygen delivery DO_2	Normal 900–1,000 mL/min DO_2 360–600 mL/min /m²
Oxygen consumption (VO_2)	Normal 220–290 mL/min VO_2 110–160 mL/min/m²
Oxygen extraction ratio (OER)	Normal 0.20–0.30
Cardiac index–OER ratio	Normal 12 Ratio <10 = inadequate cardiovascular response necessitating increased OE *Note:* In septic shock, ratio <10 –myocardial depression or inadequate fluid resuscitation
Mixed venous oxygen saturation (SvO_2)	Normal 65–75% <50% = Severe oxygen deficit
Central venous oxygen saturation ($ScvO_2$)	Normal 70%
Lactate	Normal <2 mmol/L Monitor trends, failure to decrease with treatment has poor prognostic implications Rule out other causes of increased lactate levels (adrenal, washout effect).

- Some global oxygenation indices include lactate levels, central venous oxygen saturation ($ScvO_2$), and mixed venous oxygen saturation (MvO_2 or SvO_2).

Regional oxygenation may be measured be sampled from the superior vena cava just before it enters the right atrium because samples taken from a right atrial catheter may selectively draw blood from the coronary sinus, which is relatively desaturated (typical values 30–37%).

The superior vena cava is preferred over the inferior vena cava because oxygen saturation in the inferior vena cava (IVC) depends can vary widely, this is due to tissue beds with widely varying saturations draining into the inferior vena cava, ranging from muscle (60–71%), to gut or liver (66%), to renal (92%). Thus, if the inferior vena cava is used for central venous sampling, the catheter tip should lie above the hepatic veins.

Interpreting Central venous Oxygen Saturation ($ScvO_2$)

A decrease in SvO_2 below 70% indicates that systemic O_2 delivery (DO_2) is impaired. A decrease in DO_2 can be the result of a low cardiac output (Q), anemia (low Hb), or hypoxemia. A decrease in SvO_2 to 50% indicates a global state of actual or impending tissue hypoxia.

Near-infrared Spectroscopy

It is a noninvasive method which allows continuous monitoring of the regional tissue saturation and oxygen extraction. Electrodes are placed depending on the target organ to be assessed, e.g., forehead, kidneys, abdomen or muscles. Near-infrared spectroscopy (NIRS) principle is similar to pulse oximetry where the electrode emits infrared light from one end, and based on the amount of light absorbed by the hemoglobin, the receptor measures the regional O_2 saturation at the other end. NIRS emits an infrared light continuously, thus providing a measurement of O_2 saturation mainly at the venous side (70%). Therefore, NIRS should be considered as a noninvasive alternative to $ScvO_2$.

SUGGESTED READING

1. Beaulieu Y, et al. Specific skill set and goals of focused echocardiography for critical care clinicians. Crit Care Med. 2007;35(5)Suppl:S144-9.
2. Brown JM. Use of echocardiography for hemodynamic monitoring. Crit Care Med. 2002;30: 1361-64.
3. Bur A, Herkner H, Vleck M, et al. Factors influencing the accuracy of oscillometric blood pressure measurements in critically ill patients. Crit Care Med. 2003;31(3):793-9.
4. Damen J, Weaver J: The use of balloon-tipped pulmonary artery catheters in children undergoing cardiac surgery. Intensive Care Med 1987;13:266-72.
5. Davis AL, Carcillo JA, Aneja RK, et al, American College of Critical Care Medicine Clinical Practice Parameters for Hemodynamic Support of Pediatric and Neonatal Septic Shock. Crit Care Med. 2017;45(6):1061-93.
6. Fathi EM, Narchi H, Chedid F. Noninvasive hemodynamic monitoring of septic shock in children. World J Methodol. 2018;8(1):1-8.
7. Lemson J, Nusmeier A, van der Hoeven JG. Advanced hemodynamic monitoring in critically ill children. Pediatrics. 2011;128(3):560-71.
8. Pershad J, Myers S, Plouman C, et al. Bedside limited echocardiography by the emergency physician is accurate during evaluation of the critically Ill Patient. Pediatrics. 2004;114:e667-71.
9. Pickering TG, Hall JE, Appel LJ, et al. Recommendations for blood pressure measurement in humans and experimental animals, part 1: Blood pressure measurement in humans: a statement for professionals from the Subcommittee of Professional and Public Education of the AHA Council on HBP. Circulation. 2005;111:697-716.
10. Pinsky MR. Hemodynamic evaluation and monitoring in the ICU. Chest. 2007;132(6):2020-9.
11. Pulmonary Artery Catheter Consensus conference: Consensus statement. Crit Care Med 25(6): 910-25.
12. Shoemaker WC, Kram HB, Appel PL. Therapy of shock based on pathophysiology, monitoring, and outcome prediction. Crit Care Med. 1990;18(1 Pt 2):S19-25.
13. Vignon P, Chastagner C, Francois B, et al. Diagnostic ability of hand-held echocardiography in ventilated critically ill patients. Crit Care. 2003;7(5):R84-91.
14. Vincent JL, Rhodes A, Perel A, et al. Clinical review: Update on hemodynamic monitoring–a consensus of 16. Crit Care. 2011;15(4):229.

Acute Heart Failure 12

Vikas Taneja, Manvinder Singh Sachdev

LEARNING OBJECTIVES

- *Core concepts*:
  - Definition
  - Factors affecting cardiac output
  - Pathophysiology of symptoms in acute heart failure
- *Clinical recognition*:
  - Etiology of acute heart failure
  - Classification of acute heart failure
  - Clinical presentation
- *Management skills*:
  - Investigations
  - Clinical management
  - Recent advances
  - Drug doses
- *Key messages*

CORE CONCEPTS

Acute heart failure (AHF) in children is different from adults. Several definitions have been proposed, but despite years of research, AHF still is not completely understood. Though there are established protocols for management of heart failure in adults, there are no established national or international guidelines on the management of cardiac failure in children. Consequently, the approach to treatment of AHF in children is based on a combination of clinical experience and data extrapolated from adult studies.

Definition

According to the American Heart Association (AHA) practice guidelines 2005, the term "heart failure" is used instead of "congestive heart failure." AHF is a clinicopathophysiological state or syndrome, in which there is an abnormality of cardiac function either from volume or pressure overload or both, which results in its inability to meet the metabolic requirements of the body. In case of children, this requirement includes growth and development.

Factors Affecting Cardiac Output

The cardiac output (CO) is dependent on stroke volume (SV) and heart rate (HR). The SV further depends on the preload, myocardial contractility, and afterload.
- *Preload*, defined as the degree of end-diastolic fiber stretch, determines the end-diastolic volume. This is influenced by the intravascular volume status of the patient and ventricular wall thickness. For clinical purposes, central venous pressure (CVP) although with limitations, is an indicator of the preload status.
- *Myocardial contractility* is characterized by the force and velocity of myocardial contraction, but, clinically the contractile state is often expressed as the ejection fraction (EF).
- *Afterload*, the force resisting myocardial fiber shortening after stimulation from the relaxed state, is a reflection of the work the myocardium has to do. Clinically, the afterload is referred to as the resistance against which the heart has to function.
- *The HR and rhythm* are also important contributors to AHF. It may be worth noting that arrhythmia may be the cause or may precipitate AHF.

Frank–Starling Principle

Under most circumstances, the CO is directly proportional to the amount of blood coming into it. This is a direct effect of the muscle stretch which results in muscle to contract with a greater force. This is the Frank–Starling principle. This mechanism operates in AHF, but as ventricular function is abnormal, the response is inadequate. If the Frank–Starling curve is depressed, fluid retention, vasoconstriction, and a cascade of neurohumoral responses lead to the syndrome of AHF. Over time, left ventricle (LV) remodeling with dilatation and hypertrophy further compromises cardiac performance, especially during physical stress.

Pathophysiology of Symptoms in Acute Heart Failure

Left Ventricle Failure

In LV failure, as the CO declines, the left atrial pressure increases resulting in an increase in pulmonary venous pressure. Dyspnea or increased work of breathing correlates with elevated pulmonary venous pressure. When fluid extravasates into the interstitial space and alveoli, it significantly alters pulmonary mechanics and results in ventilation/perfusion mismatch. This results in intrapulmonary shunting of unoxygenated blood. A combination of alveolar hyperventilation due to increased lung stiffness and reduced PaO_2 is a characteristic of LV failure. Arterial blood gas analysis reveals an increased pH and a reduced $PaCO_2$ (respiratory alkalosis) with low SO_2 reflecting increased intrapulmonary shunting. A raised $PaCO_2$ signifies alveolar hypoventilation possibly due to respiratory muscle failure and requires ventilatory support.

Right Ventricle Failure

In right ventricle (RV) failure, systemic venous congestive symptoms develop. Pleural effusions usually accumulate in the right hemithorax and later bilaterally. Hepatic dysfunction commonly occurs secondary to RV failure, with increase in hepatic enzymes [aspartate transaminase (AST), alanine transaminase (ALT)]. Reduced aldosterone breakdown by the impaired liver further contributes to fluid retention. It is worth noting that ventricular cross-talk, a significant phenomenon seen in infants, results in RV failure in LV failure. This explains the finding of hepatomegaly in isolated L to R shunts resulting in AHF.

CLINICAL RECOGNITION

Etiology of Acute Heart Failure

The causes of AHF can be grouped in many ways. These can be:
- *LV failure/RV failure*: Left ventricle failure characteristically develops in congenital defects [e.g., large left to right shunts like ventricular septal defect (VSD), patent ductus arteriosus (PDA), common atrioventricular (AV) canal, anomalous left coronary artery from pulmonary artery (ALCAPA), left-sided obstructive lesions (aortic stenosis, CoA, and other forms of interrupted aortic arch)], most forms of cardiomyopathy, tachyarrhythmias, and myocarditis. Post-cardiopulmonary bypass is also an important cause of LV dysfunction.

    Right ventricle failure is most commonly caused by prior LV failure and tricuspid regurgitation. Mitral stenosis, pulmonary hypertension, pulmonary artery (PA) or valve stenosis are also the causes.
- *Systolic dysfunction/diastolic dysfunction*: Acute heart failure commonly manifests as systolic dysfunction. Systolic dysfunction has numerous causes; the most common being myocarditis. More than 20 viruses have been identified as causal. Toxic substances damaging the heart include a variety of organic solvents, certain chemotherapeutic drugs (e.g., doxorubicin), β-blockers, calcium (Ca) blockers, and antiarrhythmics.

    Diastolic dysfunction accounts for 20–40% of cases of AHF. It is generally associated with prolonged ventricular relaxation time, as measured during isovolumic relaxation (the time between aortic valve closure and mitral valve opening when ventricular pressure falls rapidly). Diastolic failure per se as a cause of AHF is rare except in setting of postoperative RV failure, e.g., Tetralogy of Fallot (TOF).
- *High output failure/low output failure*: High output failure is associated with a persistent high CO that eventually results in ventricular dysfunction. Conditions associated with high CO include anemia, beriberi, thyrotoxicosis, pregnancy, advanced Paget's disease, and arteriovenous fistula. AHF in such states is often reversible by treating the underlying cause.

    Low output failure includes all causes discussed above as well as in postoperative congenital heart disease (CHD).

Etiology of Acute Heart Failure Based on Pathophysiology

On the basis of pathophysiology, the etiology of AHF may be classified into:
- Increased preload (volume overload) may stretch the muscle fiber beyond physiologic states resulting in an effective decrease in cardiac function. This is seen in volume loading

conditions like left to right shunts, mitral regurgitation, aortic regurgitation, and complete heart block (unusually increased end-diastolic volume due to a highly prolonged diastole).
- Impaired myocardial contractility results in a decreased myocardial function as in myocarditis (viral or metabolic), cardiomyopathy, and ALCAPA.
- Increased afterload (pressure overload), when ventricles work against abnormally high systemic vascular resistance that result in myocardial failure, e.g., coarctation of aorta (CoA), aortic stenosis, and interrupted aortic arch.
- Inadequate diastolic filling would result in a low CO due to decreased filling. This would typically be seen in tachyarrhythmias, constrictive pericarditis, and ventricular hypertrophy. Under these conditions, initially, various compensatory mechanisms come into play, which have got salutary effects. But the same compensatory mechanisms if pressed into play indefinitely cause nonsalutary effects and potentiate heart failure (Table 1).

Table 1: Salutary and nonsalutary effects of compensatory mechanisms in acute heart failure.

Compensatory mechanism	Salutary effects	Nonsalutary effects
Increase in end-diastolic volume and pressure	This increases myocardial contractory force through Frank–Starling mechanism	When end-diastolic pressure reaches high levels, pulmonary, and peripheral congestion and edema develop
Increase in sympathetic tone	This augments heart rate and myocardial contractility, which helps to maintain tissue perfusion pressure	When sympathetic action is intense, tachycardia and peripheral vasoconstriction (increased afterload) lead to substantial increase in myocardial oxygen consumption, increased cardiac work, and reduced coronary perfusion
Stimulation of renin–angiotensin-aldosterone system	This causes renal retention of salt and water, which increases diastolic filling pressure. It causes vasoconstriction to maintain tissue perfusion pressure	When these effects are excessive, it causes systemic and pulmonary venous congestion on one hand and increases afterload on the other. As cardiac function deteriorates, renal blood flow decreases in proportion to the reduced CO, the GFR falls, and blood flow within the kidney is redistributed. The filtration fraction and filtered Na decrease, but tubular reabsorption increases
Atrial natriuretic peptide (ANP) released in response to increase in atrial volume and pressure B-type natriuretic peptide (BNP) is produced in response to increase in ventricular pressure and volume	These peptides enhance renal excretion of Na, but in patients with acute heart failure (AHF), the effect is blunted by decreased renal perfusion, receptor down-regulation, and enhanced enzymatic degradation	When these effects are excessive, marked sodium and water retention occurs leading to fluid overload.

Contd...

Contd...

Compensatory mechanism	Salutary effects	Nonsalutary effects
Release of arginine vasopressin peptide (AVP) in response to a fall in extracellular fluid (ECF) volume and by various neurohormonal stimuli.	It diminishes excretion of free water by the kidney and contributes to the hyponatremia of AHF	When these effects are excessive, marked sodium and water retention occurs leading to fluid overload
Ventricular hypertrophy	This provides more contractile elements increasing myocardial contraction	Progressive hypertrophy leads to abnormal diastolic relaxation leading to pulmonary and systemic congestion

Etiology Based on Age of Onset of Acute Heart Failure

In pediatrics, the age of onset of AHF is a useful guide to the underlying etiology. For the purpose of classification, the pediatric age range can be divided into three stages: fetal development, infancy, and childhood and adolescence. In infancy, the etiologies vary from birth to 1 year of age (Table 2).

Acute Heart Failure in Postoperative Congenital Heart Disease

- *Systemic ventricular failure*: The pathophysiology of postoperative AHF is based on the pathophysiology of the congenital heart defect as well as on the cardiopulmonary bypass.

    Left ventricle failure occurs postoperatively if the LV is subjected to volume overload, e.g., systemic to PA shunts if the shunt is large, pulmonary atresia with remaining large aortopulmonary collaterals. Aortic regurgitation causes LV volume overload following aortic valvotomy for aortic stenosis, or following VSD repair that results in distortion of aortic cusp. Postoperative mitral regurgitation can also cause LV volume overload after repair of endocardial cushion defects.

    Left ventricle failure also occurs due to myocardial ischemia following cardiopulmonary bypass. The risk of this depends on the duration of the aortic cross-clamp time and myocardial preservation techniques. Myocardial dysfunction also occurs in d-transposition of the great arteries (d-TGA), where the LV functions as the pulmonary ventricle and if surgery is delayed beyond the first month, the LV is unable to take the systemic afterload and fails. In patients with d-TGA undergoing atrial switch operation (Senning operation), the anatomic RV functions as the systemic ventricle and deterioration of the ventricle function has been reported postoperatively.
- *RV failure*: Postoperative RV failure most commonly occurs as a result of RV hypertension, e.g., in residual PA stenosis after repair of TOF, obstruction of the RV to PA conduit, and acute pulmonary hypertension. Patients who have undergone Fontan procedure (cavo-pulmonary anastomosis for single ventricle complexes) often have significant RV failure in the early postoperative period. Pulmonary insufficiency especially after a pericardial patch is placed across the pulmonary valve annulus or a nonvalved RV to PA conduit is placed, usually well tolerated but RV dysfunction if associated with pulmonary hypertension.

Table 2: Causes of acute heart failure (AHF) according to age at presentation.

Age at presentation	Causes (by descending order of occurrence)
Fetus	Tachyarrhythmia Third-degree atrioventricular (AV) block Anemia Valvular insufficiency Arteriovenous malformation Premature closure of foramen ovale Fetomaternal transfusion
Neonatal	Birth asphyxia Tachyarrhythmia Large PDA Hypoplastic left heart syndrome, coarctation of aorta Obstructive TAPVC Critical aortic stenosis, critical pulmonary stenosis Tricuspid regurgitation Truncus arteriosus Persistent pulmonary hypertension Myocarditis (Coxsackie, adenovirus) Sepsis Cardiomyopathy Heart block Infant of diabetic mother Postcardiopulmonary bypass
Infancy	Coarctation of aorta Large left to right shunts (PDA, VSD, atrioventricular septal defects) Common mixing lesions Tachyarrhythmias Postcardiopulmonary bypass Anomalous left coronary artery from pulmonary artery Unobstructed TAPVC Myocarditis (Coxsackie, adenovirus) Familial cardiomyopathy Pompe's disease Carnitine deficiency Mitochondrial cardiomyopathy
More than 1 year old	Cardiomyopathy Rheumatic heart disease Congenital valve disease—MR, TR, AR subaortic stenosis Pulmonary atresia with large collaterals Postoperative – Tetralogy repair, Fontan, Senning Myocarditis, endocarditis Collagen vascular disease Kawasaki's disease Tachyarrhythmias Anemia

(AR: aortic regurgitation; MR: mitral regurgitation; PDA: patent ductus arteriosus; TAPVC: total anomalous pulmonary venous connection; TR: tricuspid regurgitation; VSD: ventricular septal defect)

Table 3: Ross classification for staging the severity of acute heart failure (AHF) in infants.

Class	Symptoms
Class I	No limitations or symptoms
Class II	Mild tachypnea or diaphoresis with feeding in infants Dyspnea on exertion in older children No growth failure
Class III	Marked tachypnea or diaphoresis with feeds or exertion Prolonged feeding times Growth failure from chronic heart failure (CHF)
Class IV	Symptoms at rest with tachypnea, retractions, grunting, or diaphoresis

Classification of Acute Heart Failure by Severity

Part of classifying AHF is also defining the spectrum of severity. The well-established New York Heart Association (NYHA) Heart Failure Classification is not applicable to most of the pediatric population. The Ross Heart Failure Classification was developed to provide a global assessment of heart failure severity in infants, and has subsequently been modified to apply to all pediatric ages. The modified Ross Classification incorporates feeding difficulties, growth problems, and symptoms of exercise intolerance into a numeric score comparable with the NYHA classification for adults (Table 3).

Clinical Presentation

Irrespective of the etiology, the first manifestation of AHF is sinus tachycardia. A sustained HR of more than 160 beats per minute (bpm) in infants and more than 100 bpm in older children is typically seen with AHF. This represents the adaptive mechanism to increase the CO by increasing the HR when stroke volume is diminished. However, HR of more than 220–240 bpm in infants and 150–170 bpm in older children should raise the possibility of supraventricular tachycardia which would prove to be the underlying cause of AHF. An obvious exception to this finding occurs in AHF due to a primary bradyarrhythmia or complete heart block. Various clinical features are mentioned in Table 4.

Important Points

- The clinical features of AHF in a newborn may be nonspecific; sometimes resembling septicemia. A high index of suspicion is required.
- Initial presentation in an interrupted aortic arch or CoA in neonates can be AHF (in presence of PDA). When the ductus closes, these babies present with acute shock.
- CoA does not cause AHF after 1 year of life, when sufficient collaterals have developed.
- Central cyanosis associated with AHF and soft or no murmurs in a newborn, should raise the suspicion of transposition of great arteries with intact septum, obstructed total anomalous pulmonary venous connection, etc.
- Acyanotic heart lesions like ASD or VSD does not cause AHF in first 2 weeks of life because of increased pulmonary pressures. Their presence with AHF should prompt evaluation for associated TAPVC or CoA respectively.

Table 4: Pathophysiology of clinical features in acute heart failure.

Symptom/sign	Pathophysiology
Tachypnea	Increase in left ventricular volume and pressure leads to increase in pulmonary venous pressure. This leads to increase in capillary permeability and accumulation of fluid in the interstitium and alveoli. Mediated by vagus nerve or J receptors in pulmonary interstitium.
Dyspnea	Due to pulmonary venous congestion Due to pulmonary edema.
Wheezing	Due to compression of bronchi by dilated pulmonary artery (PA) or atria. Usually seen in older children
Feeding difficulty	Lack of energy to suck and tire quickly
Failure to thrive	Deficiency in calories due to poor intake and extra work of breathing causes increased metabolic demand
Irritability	Reduced O_2 transport
Sweating	Increased sympathetic activity that occurs when they are challenged with eating in respiratory distress
Reduced urine output	Reduced renal perfusion
Tachycardia	Increased sympathetic activity as an adaptive mechanism to provide more O_2 to tissues
Cool extremities, reduced capillary filling	Reduced tissue perfusion
Pulsus paradoxus	Due to fluctuations in cardiac output (CO) with respiration
Increased precordial activity	Chamber dilatation or hypertrophy
Gallop sounds	Increased afterload, reduced compliance
Crepitations	Alveolar edema
Hepatomegaly and edema	Systemic venous congestion

- A premature newborn with significant respiratory distress and a systolic murmur should be evaluated for PDA causing AHF.
- Several children with CHD or cardiomyopathies have associated chromosomal anomalies or extracardiac manifestations which provide clues for diagnosis.
- Older children with TOF physiology can have AHF due to complicated course (anemia, infective endocarditis, bicuspid aortic valve with aortic regurgitation) or over shunting from aorto-pulmonary shunts.

MANAGEMENT SKILLS

Investigations

Diagnosis of AHF is based primarily on clinical grounds and supported by laboratory tests to define the nature of specific disease, functional status of myocardium, and comorbid features.

Radiography

Chest radiograph should be done in all patients with suspected AHF; an echocardiogram is not a substitute for radiograph. It helps to assess the cardiac size, quantification of pulmonary blood flow, presence of associated chest infection, pleural effusion etc., as well as being pathognomonic in certain disease states. A cardiothoracic ratio of more than 0.6 in neonates and more than 0.55 in infants and older children on an inspiratory film suggests cardiomegaly. Left lower lobe collapse due to compression of the left lower lobe bronchus by the enlarged left atrium can be seen. Pleural effusions are seen in systemic venous congestion. Pericardial effusion is suggested by globular appearance of the cardiac shadow. Parenchymal diseases can be ruled out especially coexistent pneumonia.

Typical radiographs strongly suggestive of certain diagnosis include those with transposition of great arteries (egg-on-side), obstructed total anomalous pulmonary venous connection (TAPVC; snowstorm appearance), unobstructed TAPVC (Figure of 8 appearance), truncus arteriosus (waterfall appearance of hila), Ebstein's anomaly (globular cardiomegaly with decreased pulmonary flow), etc.

Electrocardiography

The electrocardiogram (ECG) provides supportive data like ventricular hypertrophy, atrial enlargement or changes in the ST segment or T wave. ECG may also give a clue to diagnosis in certain conditions like arrhythmias, heart block, myocarditis, and ALCAPA. ALCAPA presents with pathologic q waves in anterolateral leads. A prolonged QTc interval with terminal T-wave inversion is suggestive of hypocalcemia as the cause of left ventricular dysfunction.

Echocardiography

The echocardiogram has expanded the ability of the cardiologist to establish anatomic diagnosis, functional status, and follow-up assessment of response to therapy. Two-dimensional echo provides details of the cardiac anatomy in CHD. Assessment of regional wall motion abnormality by two-dimensional imaging helps in determining the etiology as well as response to therapy in AHF. Continuous wave and color flow Doppler detects any intracardiac shunting, valvular regurgitation, and stenosis. They also help in calculating gradients across the stenotic lesions as well as the CO. Antenatal echo can diagnose fetal AHF, which can manifest as fetal hydrops.

Pulse Oximetry

Pulse oximetery, and a hyperoxia test in newborns, is useful tests in detecting any cardiac lesion. SpO_2 in room air is a reliable measure of oxygenation. The partial pressure of arterial oxygen (PaO_2) when the patient is receiving 100% oxygen (hyperoxia test) helps in distinguishing intracardiac malformations from pulmonary disease in the setting of hypoxia.

Blood Gas and Electrolytes

In early AHF, respiratory alkalosis is seen due to alveolar hyperventilation. As CO falls metabolic acidosis is usually seen. PaO_2 is low due to pulmonary congestion and ventilation perfusion mismatch. Rising $PaCO_2$ is an indicator of respiratory muscle fatigue or severe AHF whereby CO is so low that it affects cerebral perfusion leading to central hypoventilation. At this point, arterial blood gas (ABG) usually shows a combination of respiratory and metabolic

Table 5: Algorithm for inotropic management in acute heart failure.

Clinical condition	Interpretation	Treatment strategy
Tachycardia, poor pulses, cool extremities, delayed CFT, decreased urine output, low BP, lactate high	Low CO	Dopamine 10 µg/kg/min, dobutamine 10 µg/kg/min, may increase up to 15 µg/kg/min, try Fluid bolus cautiously (5 mL/kg that too in aliquots, 5 ml for infants and 10 mL for children); elective ventilation
Tachycardia, poor pulses, cool extremities, CFT delayed, urine output low, BP maintained, lactate high	Low CO	Add lasix infusion 0.05–0.1 mg/kg/hr Add inodilators
Tachycardia settling, good central pulses, cold extremities, urine output better, BP normal to high, lactate high	High afterload	Add milrinone
HR increases, good pulses, warm extremities, urine output decreases, BP normal to low, lactate high	Relative hypovolemia (vasodilatation due to milrinone)	Give fluid challenge
HR increases, good pulses, cold extremities, urine output decreases, BP normal to high, Lactate increases	High afterload	Increase milrinone
HR increases, low pulses, cold extremities, urine output high, BP low, lactate increases	Hypovolemia	Give fluid bolus
HR settled, good pulses, warm extremities, good urine output, normal BP, normal lactate	CO optimized	Maintain same inotropic support, plan weaning and extubation
HR increases, good pulses, warm extremities, urine output decreases, normal BP, lactate increases	Fall in CO	Increase inotropic support, preferably milrinone
HR settled, good pulses, warm extremities, good urine output, normal BP, normal lactate	CO optimized	Add digoxin, taper IV inotropes

Tapering of inotropes:
- *Add digoxin*: Slow digitalization preferred
- Once digitalization is done, taper dopamine @ 0.1 µg/kg/min every 1–2 hours till 5 µg/kg/min. Follow the clinical signs and lactates. Tapering may have to be done slower than expected.
- Then taper dobutamine similar to dopamine.
- Once dopamine and dobutamine have reached 5 µg/kg/min, oral vasodilator is added in the form of enalapril. First dose hypotension is to be looked for.
- Milrinone is decreased to half after first dose enalapril, and stopped after the second dose.
- After this if hemodynamics maintained, dopamine is tapered as above and stopped followed by dobutamine.

(BP: blood pressure; CFT: capillary filling time; CO: cardiac output; HR: heart rate)

acidosis. Plasma lactate is an important marker and can be followed up serially to determine the physiological condition as well as response to treatment. An algorithm following clinical signs and blood gas lactates serially to determine treatment strategies is shown in Table 5.

Hyponatremia may be seen in AHF and reflects hemodilution due to water retention. Hyperkalemia may be associated with metabolic acidosis as well as due to reduced glomerular filtration rate (GFR). Hypochloremia, metabolic alkalosis, and hypokalemia are usually caused by diuretic therapy and need regular electrolyte monitoring.

Miscellaneous Tests

Hypoglycemia has been associated with AHF in infants and hypocalcemia noted with LV failure in neonates. CPK MB and troponin I levels are supportive in detecting coronary insufficiency, myocarditis, and asphyxia-related AHF. Severe anemia can itself precipitate and accentuate AHF associated with any primary cardiac defect. Autoimmune disorders can be ruled out by rheumatoid factor (RF), anti-dsDNA, and antinuclear antibody (ANA) assays. Blood levels of carnitine, lactate, and glucose help to detect mitochondrial cardiomyopathies.

Cardiac Catheterization

The need for cardiac catheterization in the evaluation of AHF has declined with the development of echocardiography. However, interventional catheterization is still required to perform procedures like balloon atrial septostomy in TGA, valvotomies in stenotic lesions which help in the management of AHF. Myocardial biopsy for histological and PCR testing may be helpful in diagnosing underlying cause like myocarditis.

Clinical Management

The goal in management of AHF is to optimize the CO so as to meet the metabolic demands adequately. The goals are defined based on the pathophysiology of AHF and include:
- *Optimizing preload*: Relief of pulmonary and systemic congestion
- Increasing myocardial performance
- Optimizing the afterload
- Optimizing the HR
- Improving the oxygen carrying capacity of the blood
- Removing the underlying cause.

Optimize Preload

This requires restriction of fluids (2/3rd of maintenance rate) as well as pharmacological therapy in the form of diuretics. Diuretics are used mainly to relieve the systemic and pulmonary congestion. Major diuretics used are loop diuretics, thiazides, and aldosterone antagonists. These act directly on kidneys to inhibit solute and water reabsorption thereby promoting excretion of excess salt and water.

Furosemide is the drug of choice in acute AHF. It has a rapid onset (2–5 minutes) and duration of action (3 hours). It can also be used as a continuous infusion which causes less hemodynamic instability and electrolyte disturbances. Side effects include hypokalemia, metabolic alkalosis, hyponatremia, and hyperuricemia. Ototoxicity has been reported rarely in children and is usually reversible.

Thiazides have a slower onset of action, are available in oral form so their use in AHF is limited.

Spironolactone (aldosterone antagonist) is a weak diuretic and is rarely used alone. It is added to thiazides or loop diuretics to counter their kaliuretic action. It is given orally and the onset of action takes 2–3 days.

Increase Myocardial Performance

Inotropes are the mainstay of treatment to optimize the CO. For precise control of blood pressures inotropes like dopamine and dobutamine are initially given as continuous infusions and later oral inotropes in the form of digoxin can be added.

Dopamine: Dopamine is a catecholamine with inotropic and chronotropic effects. Its action is dependent on norepinephrine stores to produce the desired effects. It has β1-adrenergic and dopaminergic effects in lower doses and α-adrenergic at higher doses. It is given as continuous infusion. Dose of 5–15 μg/kg has inotropic effect and increases myocardial contractility. However, doses above 15 μg/kg/min lead to severe vasoconstriction, compromising renal flow, increasing systemic vascular resistance, and LV afterload. Doses of 5 μg/kg/min or less, initially thought to improve renal flow and natriuresis, are not used now because of lack of evidence.

Dobutamine: Dobutamine is a synthetically altered catecholamine with powerful inotropic effects, moderate chronotropy, and vasodilatation. It differs from dopamine by its dominant action on aα1-receptors and by not dependent on norepinephrine stores to produce the desired effects. It causes inotropy with vasodilatation and thus increases the CO. The benefit over dopamine is that it does not increase the myocardial oxygen demand, is less arrhythmogenic and reduces the systemic vascular resistance with minimal alteration of blood pressure and HR. Dobutamine does not stimulate the dopaminergic receptors and so does not alter renal blood flow.

Epinephrine: Epinephrine has mixed β and α effects. It may improve CO in AHF and in postoperative situations with inotropic effect. Its use in AHF has gone down as it causes intense vasoconstriction and markedly increases the afterload. It can be arrhythmogenic by its excessive chronotropic action and causes downregulation of β receptors on long-term use. It should be given as short-term treatment for patients unresponsive to other inotropes.

Isoproterenol: Isoproterenol is a sympathomimetic amine and a pure β-adrenergic agonist. By its $β_1$ and $β_2$ effects, isoproterenol augments myocardial contractility and HR along with vasodilatation. Despite reducing afterload, it increases ventricular oxygen demand by its positive inotropic and chronotropic effects. It is useful in AHF complicated by increased reactive pulmonary vascular resistance or complete heart block. Its use is often limited by tachycardia.

Digoxin: Digoxin is the most widely used and studied oral inotrope for management of AHF. Mechanism of action is by inhibition of sarcolemmal Na^+K^+-ATPase activity leading to increased intracellular calcium and hence increases ventricular contractility. It slows HR and conduction by blocking the AV node. Major indication in AHF is to improve myocardial contractility. It is also useful in treating fetal AHF induced by tachycardia.

Despite the lack of data regarding its use in children, digoxin is frequently used in the treatment of heart failure in children as evidenced in a survey by Jain S et al.

The results of survey were as follows:
- Use of digoxin is indicated in children with primary myocardial disease with ventricular dysfunction.
- It is also indicated in symptomatic children with left to right shunts and with valvular regurgitations.
- Digoxin has also been used in patients with heart failure due to myocarditis, but caution needs to be exercised and lower dosages are used in these patients.
- In patients with heart failure due to tachyarrhythmias and those symptomatic patients in heart failure due to other causes rapid digitalization may be done if they have not received digoxin earlier.
- No improvement in long-term survival in pediatric heart failure patients was noticed with use of digoxin but it nevertheless helps in managing acute exacerbations of heart failure in these patients.
Anorexia, nausea, vomiting, visual disturbances, AV block, and dysrhythmias are the common side effects. Dose should be adjusted in the presence of hypokalemia, renal dysfunction and when combined with quinidine, verapamil, and amiodarone.

Optimize Afterload

- *Inodilators*: Phosphodiesterase III inhibitors amrinone and milrinone are bipyridine derivatives. They increase cyclic adenosine monophosphate (cAMP) by inhibiting phosphodiesterase III, an enzyme that reduces adenyl cyclase activity. These are potent vasodilators and inotropes. These are commonly used in low CO states as they optimize CO by altering afterload. Onset of action is slower than adrenergic agents so they require a loading dose to achieve full effect. In view of its vasodilating effects, blood pressure is to be monitored frequently and intravascular volume to be adequate. Milrinone is free of harmful side effects than amrinone. Side effects of amrinone include hypotension, ventricular ectopy, and thrombocytopenia. Amrinone is used less frequently due to its long half-life. Milrinone is used in dosage of 0.3–0.75 µg/kg/min.
- *Vasodilators*: Vasodilators (sodium nitroprusside and nitroglycerine) are not an important modality for treatment of AHF in children. They play a vital role in management of postoperative low CO, severe atrioventricular valve regurgitation, and dilated cardiomyopathy. They cause vasodilatation and reduce afterload by their direct action on the vascular smooth muscle and have no direct cardiac or renal effects.
- *Angiotensin converting enzyme (ACE) inhibitors*: These are competitive inhibitors of ACE and reduce the production of vasoconstricting hormone angiotensin II. They also inhibit the breakdown of bradykinin, a potent vasodilator. Thus, they cause vasodilatation, reduce afterload, increase renal blood, and cause diuresis. ACE inhibitors are used to wean off intravenous inodilators. Captopril, the first known ACE inhibitor, is well tolerated. Side effects include rashes, taste impairment, mild gastrointestinal (GI) disturbances, and neutropenia. Potassium supplementation should be avoided to prevent hyperkalemia. Enalapril is a newer agent with the advantage of less frequent dosing. Blood pressure, renal function, and neutrophil count should be monitored.

Adjunctive Therapy

- *Position*: Semi-Fowler position either by cardiac chair or elevating head and shoulders to an angle of 45° improves pulmonary function by easing respiration and reducing pulmonary pooling.
- *Oxygen*: Oxygen through mask or nasal prongs with adequate humidification helps to loosen secretions and improve oxygenation. Caution must be applied for duct-dependent lesions in neonatal period.
- *Positive pressure ventilation*: Patients in AHF usually are in severe respiratory distress, which add to the metabolic demands of the myocardium. Hence artificial ventilation, sedation and paralysis help to reduce the workload of the myocardium. Ventilation helps the myocardium by improving the oxygenation as well as in the cardiac physiology. Ventilatory rate and tidal volume are adjusted as per the age and according to the PCO_2 levels. Positive end-expiratory pressure (PEEP) has both beneficial and detrimental effects on the heart depending on whether the AHF is primarily right sided or left sided. In RV failure, PEEP increases the afterload on the RV by increasing the intra-alveolar pressures and compressing the pulmonary vascular bed thereby increasing the pulmonary vascular resistance. In LV failure, PEEP helps by optimizing the preload to the LV and thereby improving the LV end diastolic volume. PEEP also helps by opening up the alveoli collapsed due to edema and thus improving the ventilation perfusion mismatch.

    Weaning for AHF patients should be planned once the CO has been optimized and the end-organ damage has been reversed: warm peripheries, good urine output, good bowel sounds, and normal lactates. The patient should be monitored during weaning for any increase in respiratory distress, decrease in peripheral temperatures and increase in lactates or fall in urine output. Accordingly, the weaning process and extubation should be done. The inotropic support should not be changed prior to weaning.
- *Blood transfusion*: This helps to improve the oxygen-carrying capacity of the blood in case of low hemoglobin, which potentiates AHF. Packed cell transfusion should be given slowly under strict cardiac monitoring to maintain the hemoglobin above 10 g%. Overuse of the blood products should be avoided as they can have deleterious effects by increasing the preload and worsening of AHF.
- *Prostaglandin E1*: PGE_1 is useful to maintain the ductal patency in conditions with duct-dependent systemic circulation, like tight coarctation of the aorta, interruption of aortic arch, critical aortic stenosis (AS), hypoplastic left heart syndrome (HLHS), and TGA with intact septum and restrictive inter-atrial communication. These disorders require prostaglandin infusion till the time more definitive treatment can be employed. This consists of percutaneous procedures for critical AS (valvuloplasty), TGA (balloon atrial septostomy) as well as surgical procedures for neonatal CoA, HLHS, etc. In cases where surgery for CoA is not possible due to severe comorbid conditions, a balloon dilatation is performed initially and once the baby has been stabilized, corrective surgery is performed later.
- *Diet*: Adequate calories and protein are required to meet the increased metabolic needs. Caloric requirement may be up to 130–170 kcal/kg/day in infants. Nasogastric tube feeds help by saving the energy used in feeding in severely symptomatic children.

Treatment of Underlying Condition

Transcatheter interventions may have to be carried out in patients with Frank AHF to treat underlying defects like critical AS, interrupted aortic arch or CoA. Early surgical correction of large left to right shunts has to be planned after initial stabilization. Control of infection, anemia, arrhythmias, hypertension and metabolic deficiencies can help to control AHF early. Intravenous immunoglobulin has been proved to be useful in myocarditis. Role of steroids in rheumatic heart disease with AHF may be lifesaving but controversial. Treating the mother antenatally with digoxin helps to control supraventricular tachycardia causing failure in the fetus. The final option for end-stage failure would be cardiac transplant.

Recent Advances

Drugs

- *Beta-blockers*: The use of beta-blockers in heart failure has seen a sea change over the last few years. Beta-blockers like metoprolol and carvedilol have shown to improve myocardial contractility, help in remodeling of dilated ventricles, reduce symptoms and improve survival in patients with heart failure. Most studies regarding the use of beta-blockers have been conducted in adults and the same are being extrapolated to children now. Beta-blockers help in heart failure by their ability to counteract the neurohormonal effects of norepinephrine in heart failure patients.

    They are initiated in heart failure due to decreased myocardial contractility as in patients with myocarditis and dilated cardiomyopathy. They do not seem to have a role in pediatric patients with structural heart disease (left to right shunts). They are usually not initiated in the acute stage in view of their propensity to cause hypotension and bradycardia but only after the hemodynamic stability has been achieved. Carvedilol remains the most widely used beta blocker in heart failure. Dose ranges from 0.05 mg/kg/day to 1 mg/kg/day. It is started at the lower dose which is gradually stepped up on a weekly basis till an optimal dosage has reached.

- *Levosimendan*: Calcium sensitizers are a new class of inotropes that share the properties of calcium sensitization and phosphodiesterase inhibition. Levosimendan is a calcium sensitizer, which stabilizes the interaction between calcium and troponin C by binding to troponin C in a calcium-dependent manner. It improves myocardial contractility (inotropy) without adversely affecting myocardial relaxation (lusitropy). It also causes vasodilatation, through activation of several potassium channels. Levosimendan does not lead to increase in myocardial oxygen consumption, proarrhythmia, or neurohumoral activation, unlike the conventional inotropes. In large, well-controlled trials in patients with decompensated heart failure, intravenous levosimendan was significantly more effective than placebo or dobutamine for overall hemodynamic response rate (primary endpoint).

- *Nesiritide*: B-type natriuretic peptide (BNP) is an endogenous cardiac neurohormone, which is produced by the ventricles when intraventricular volume or pressure increases. Nesiritide is similar to BNP and acts by causing preload and afterload reductions, natriuresis, diuresis, suppression of the renin-angiotensin-aldosterone system, and lowering of norepinephrine. This helps in improving the myocardial performance.

Nesiritide results in balanced vasodilatation of arteries and veins, and may be suitable for patients presenting with decompensated heart failure due to volume overload. Nesiritide also lowers pulmonary capillary wedge pressure, pulmonary artery pressure, right atrial pressure, and systemic vascular resistance, as well as increases cardiac index and stroke volume index. Experience with nesiritide in children is limited but has shown promising results.

Mechanical Afterload Reduction

- *Intra-aortic balloon pump (IABP)*: Intra-aortic balloon counterpulsation provides circulatory support by decreasing left ventricular afterload during systole and augmenting aortic perfusion pressure during diastole. This is achieved by repetitive cycle synchronized pneumatic inflation and deflation of a catheter mounted balloon placed in the thoracic aorta. Before the onset of systole, the balloon is deflated thus reducing left ventricular afterload. Inflation of the balloon occurs immediately after the closure of the aortic valve thereby increasing aortic perfusion. This results in better myocardial perfusion during diastole. CO increases which results in increase in perfusion pressure in cerebral and renal vascular beds.

  Intra-aortic balloon pump has not been used widely as analogous clinical settings are few in children unlike adults and due to technical problems related to catheter size. They might be useful in coronary artery disease as in Kawasaki or ALCAPA and in postoperative setting with reduced cardiac output that is refractory to medical management. Technical obstacles in children include rapid heart rates, more compliant aortas, small femoral arteries and aortic collaterals that tend to make IABP less effective and more problematic.
- *Extracorporeal membrane oxygenation (ECMO)*: It has been more widely used for children requiring cardiopulmonary support in either perioperative period or in end-stage heart failure as a bridge to cardiac transplant. However, studies have shown poor transplant survival with ECMO particularly in children less than 1 year of age and those with complex CHD. For children requiring a long-term mechanical support as a bridge to cardiac transplantation, ventricular assist devices are being used with increasing frequency.
- *Ventricular assist device (VAD)*: It can be used as a bridge to transplant or in difficulty in weaning from bypass. These devices can offer univentricular or biventricular circuit support. The newly developed pulsatile, paracorporeal ventricular assist devices designed for long-term assist in children have demonstrated their ability to provide excellent results beyond the abilities of extracorporeal membrane oxygenation and centrifugal pumps.

Stem-cell Therapy

Stem-cell therapy has generated more interest in children with end-stage heart failure. This form of therapy is being investigated worldwide under experimental settings, for children with refractory heart failure who are not candidates for transplantation.

Potential indications for stem cell use in pediatric heart failure include repair of ventricular myocardium and creation of biological heart valves, tissue-engineered vessels, and biological pacemakers. Increasing knowledge about genetic and genomic aspects of pediatric heart disease is also expected to help in treatment and risk stratification.

Heart Transplantation

Heart transplantation remains the therapy of choice for end-stage heart failure in children refractory to surgical and medical therapy. Heart transplantation has been used for treatment of end-stage heart disease in children for nearly four decades with first infant transplant done in late 1960s. Current 1-year survival after heart transplantation in children is 85% and overall survival of 20 years after transplantation is 40%. The Pediatric Heart Transplant Study, a prospective event-driven registry, has collected extensive information on children listed for heart transplant since 1993 in the United States, the Canada, and the United Kingdom. Analyses performed by the Pediatric Heart Transplant Study have identified risk factors for poor outcome after listing and transplantation in both cardiomyopathy and CHD patients, some of which are amenable to intervention.

Drug Doses (Table 6)

Table 6 describes the drug dosages.

Table 6: Drug doses.

Drug/Class	Dose	
Diuretics		
Furosemide	0.5–1 mg/kg/dose, max 2 mg/kg/dose, qid, 0.05–0.1 mg/kg/hr infusion	
Chlorthiazide	1–4 mg/kg/dose IV bd, 20–40 mg/kg/day PO bd	
Metolazone	0.2–0.4 mg/kg/day PO qd	
Spironolactone	1–3.5 mg/kg/day PO qd/bd	
Inotropes		
Dopamine	5–20 µg/kg/min as infusion	
Dobutamine	5–20 µg/kg/min as infusion	
Adrenergic agent		
Epinephrine	0.05–1 µg/kg/min	
Norepinephrine	0.05–1 µg/kg/min	
Isoproterenol	0.05–1 µg/kg/min inotropic, 0.01–0.05 µg/kg/min for bradycardia	
Digoxin	**Total digitalization dose**	**Maintenance dose**
Term infant	30 µg/kg	8–10 µg/kg
Infants < 2 years	30–40 µg/kg	10 µg/kg
Child > 2 years	40 µg/kg	10 µg/kg
For rapid digitalization ½ of loading dose is given initially, ¼ 6–12 hours later and remaining ¼ 24 hours after the first dose. Half-life of digoxin is 20 hours in infants and 40 hours in older children.		
PDEIII inhibitors		
Amrinone	0.75 mg/kg loading dose × 3 times, over 15 minutes each, then 5–10 µg/kg/min infusion	
Milrinone	50 µg/kg loading dose IV over 15–30 minutes, followed by 0.25–0.75 µg/kg/min infusion	

Contd...

Contd...

Drug/Class	Dose
Vasodilators	
Sodium nitroprusside	0.5–8 µg/kg/min IV infusion (needs titration)
Nitroglycerine	0.5–5 µg/kg/min IV infusion (needs titration)
Prazosin	0.01–0.05 mg/kg/dose PO q tid, max dose 0.1 mg/kg
ACE inhibitors	
Captopril	0.1–0.5 mg/kg/dose PO tid, up to 4 mg/kg/day
Enalapril	0.1–0.4 mg/kg/day PO qd/bd
Beta-blockers	
Atenolol	1–2 mg/kg/day PO qd
Carvedilol	0.05 mg/kg/dose PO bd/tid, up to 0.5 mg/kg/dose
Metoprolol	1–2 mg/kg/dose PO bd
Esmolol	100–500 µg/kg IV loading dose in 1–2 minutes, 50–500 µg/kg/min infusion
Miscellaneous drugs	
PGE_1	0.05–0.1 µg/kg/min infusion
Carnitine	20–35 mg/kg/dose PO tid
Morphine	40 µg/kg loading followed by 40–80 µg/kg/hr as infusion
Fentanyl	2 µg/kg loading followed by 1–5 µg/kg/hr as infusion
Vecuronium	0.1 mg/kg prn, duration of action 45 min, no cardiovascular effects

(ACE: angiotensin converting enzyme; PDE: phosphodiesterase; PGE: prostaglandin)

OUTCOME

Outcomes of heart failure in children depend on the underlying cause. Because of advances in surgical and other interventional strategies, morbidity, and mortality associated with structural heart disease have declined significantly. However, little progress has been made in improving the significant mortality and morbidity associated with symptomatic heart failure in children with cardiomyopathies.

CONCLUSION

Acute heart failure in children is a complex syndrome with varied etiology and presentation. Unlike adults, AHF in children is commonly due to structural heart disease and reversible conditions, thus making it amenable to definitive therapy. The overall outcome with AHF is better in children than that in adults. Clinical presentation of AHF in younger children can be nonspecific requiring high degree of suspicion. In particular, some conditions that can present with acute shock are important to recognize, as they can be effectively treated or palliated on an urgent basis. While the general principles of management are similar to those in adults, there is a dearth of evidence base in pediatric AHF. It would require a judicious balance of extrapolation from adult medicine and development of children-specific treatments to optimize the outcomes in this challenging field.

KEY MESSAGES

- The diagnosis of AHF in infants and children need high index of suspicion, especially during the neonatal period and in cases of arrhythmias and myocarditis.
- The AHF in pediatric age group can be classified in many ways, based on pathophysiology, age at presentation or type of dysfunction.
- The echocardiogram has expanded the ability of the cardiologist to establish anatomic diagnosis, functional status and follow-up assessment of response to therapy in AHF, but it's not a substitute for chest radiograph or ECG.
- Medical management is of utmost importance both for medical causes of AHF and for pre- and postoperative stabilization in congenital heart defects.
- Advances in the surgical and interventional strategies in the management of structural heart defects have improved survival but not much progress has been made in our understanding and management of myocarditis and cardiomyopathies.

SUGGESTED READING

1. Balaguru D, Artman M, Auslender M. Management of heart failure in children. Curr Probl Pediatr. 2000;30:5-30.
2. Colluci WS, Wright RF, Braunwald E. New inotropic agents in the treatment of congestive heart failure. New Engl J Med. 1986;314:349-55.
3. Das BB. Current state of pediatric heart failure: Review. Children. 2018;5:88-103.
4. Deiwick M, Hoffmeier A, Tjan TD, et al. Heart failure in children—mechanical assistance. Thorac Cardiovasc Surg. 2005;53(Suppl 2):S135-40.
5. Freed MD. Congestive heart failure. In: Nadas' Pediatric Cardiology. US: Elsevier Health; 1994. pp. 63-72.
6. Hsu DT, Pearson GD. Heart failure in children – Part I: History, etiology, and pathophysiology. Circ Heart Fail. 2009;2:63-70.
7. Hsu DT, Pearson GD. Heart failure in children – Part II: Diagnosis, treatment, and future directions. Circ Heart Fail. 2009;2:490-8.
8. Jain S, Vaidyanathan B. Digoxin in management of heart failure in children: Should it be continued or relegated to the history books? Ann Pediatr Card. 2009;2:149-52.
9. Kantor PF, Mertens LL. Heart failure in children. Part I: Clinical evaluation, diagnostic testing, and initial medical management. Eur J Pediatr. 2010;169:269-79.
10. Kantor PF, Mertens LL. Heart failure in children. Part II: Current maintenance therapy and new therapeutic approaches. Eur J Pediatr. 2010;169:403-10.
11. Metra M, Giubbini R, Nodari S. Differential effects of beta blockers in patients with congestive heart failure: prospective, randomized, double-blinded comparison of long-term effects of metoprolol vs carvedilol. Circulation. 2000;102:546-51.
12. O'Laughlin MP. Congestive heart failure in children. Pediatr Clin North Am. 1999;46(2):263-73.
13. Scholz H. Inotropic drugs & their mechanism of action. J Am Coll Cardiol. 1984;4:389-98.
14. Shaddy RE, Curtin EL, Sower B, et al. The pediatric randomized carvedilol trial in children with heart failure: Rationale and design. Am Heart J. 2002;144(3):383-9.
15. Talner NS. Heart failure. In: Emmanouilides GC, Riemenschneider TA, Allen HD, et al., eds. Moss and Adams' Heart Disease in Infants, Children and Adolescents, including the Fetus and Young Adult, 5th edn. Baltimore: Williams and Wilkins; 1995.
16. Turanlahti M, Boldt T, Palkama T, et al. Pharmacokinetics of levosimendan in pediatric patients evaluated for cardiac surgery. Pediatr Crit Care Med. 2004;5(5):457-62.

Cardiac Arrhythmias 13

Sanah Merchant-Soomar, Vishal Baldua

LEARNING OBJECTIVES

- To understand and interpret cardiac arrhythmias
- To treat these arrhythmias.

INTRODUCTION

Arrhythmias are being increasingly recognized and more effectively treated today as compared to a decade ago. The overall incidence of arrhythmias is about 55 per 100,000 pediatric emergency visits in the United States. The most common dysrhythmias are sinus tachycardia (50%), supraventricular tachycardia (13%), bradycardia (6%), and atrial fibrillation (4.6%). Though more common in postoperative cardiac patients, it is important to recognize and treat common arrhythmias as timely management can be lifesaving.

The self-explanatory diagram (Fig. 1) shows the correlation between the different phases of the cardiac cycle with that of the pattern generated on the electrocardiogram. A basic understanding of this helps interpret arrhythmias better.

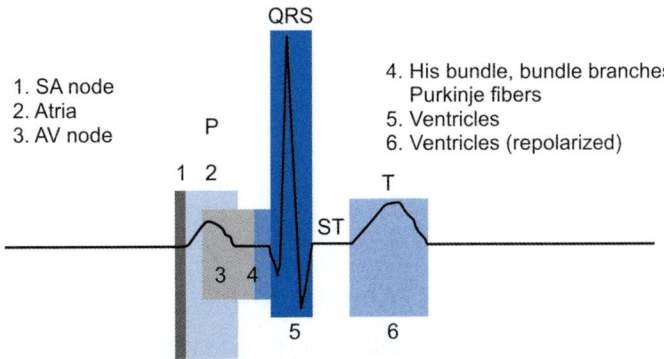

Fig. 1: Components of a normal ECG.
(AV: atrioventricular; ECG: electrocardiogram; SA: sinoatrial)

Table 1: Normal range of heart rate as per age.

	Sleeping HR	Resting awake HR	Maximum with exercise/fever
Newborn	80–160	100–180	220
1–12 weeks	80–160	100–180	220
3–24 months	70–120	80–180	200
2–10 years	60–90	70–110	180
>10 years	50–90	55–90	180
(HR: heart rate)			

It is important to know the upper and lower limits of heart rate (Table 1) for children across all ages to label dysrhythmias.

TACHYARRHYTHMIAS

Tachycardias can be classified broadly into those that originate from foci at and above the atrioventricular (AV) node (i.e., supraventricular) and those originating within the ventricle. The majority of tachycardias are supraventricular (SVT) in origin. Those that are ventricular in origin are associated typically with hemodynamic compromise. Tachyarrhythmias are more common than bradyarrhythmias in the pediatric population.

SUPRAVENTRICULAR TACHYARRHYTHMIAS

Arrhythmias can be classified on the basis of their underlying mechanism which may be reentry or triggered, i.e. ectopic or automatic. Reentrant tachycardia is defined as a continuous repetitive propagation of an excitatory wave traveling in a circular path, returning to its site of origin to reactivate that site. Reentry tachycardias include AV tachycardias in which the circular path involves the atrium, the AV node, and the ventricle. In atrial flutter and fibrillation the reentry circuit is intra-atrial and does not involve the AV node. Reentrant tachycardias are amenable to pacing and cardioversion while "automatic" tachycardias are not.
- *"Reentrant" atrioventricular tachycardias*:
  - Atrioventricular reciprocating tachycardia (AVRT): Accessory pathway-mediated
  - Atrioventricular nodal reentry tachycardia (AVNRT)
- *"Reentrant" atrial tachycardias*:
  - Atrial flutter and fibrillation
- *"Automatic" tachycardias*:
  - Sinus tachycardia
  - Ectopic atrial tachycardia (EAT)
  - Multifocal atrial tachycardia.

REENTRANT ATRIOVENTRICULAR TACHYCARDIAS

This includes the typical tachycardias for which the term "SVT" is commonly used. SVT is the most common symptomatic dysrhythmia in infants and children. The heart rate is greater

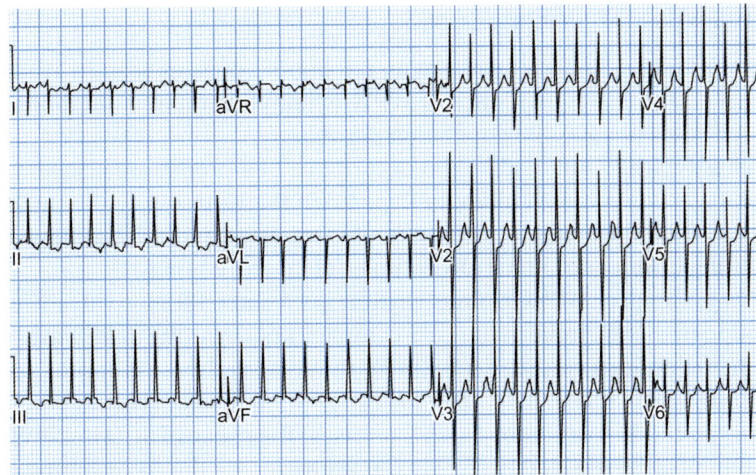

Fig. 2: ECG trace showing narrow complex tachycardia (rate >240/min) with no discernible P-wave – s/o SVT. (ECG: electrocardiogram; SVT: supraventricular)

than 220 BPM in newborns and young infants and more than 180 BPM in older children. The electrocardiogram (ECG) (Fig. 2) shows a narrow complex tachycardia, either without discernible P waves or with retrograde P waves with an abnormal axis. The QRS duration is usually normal with little or no variation in the heart rate. Rarely, wide complex SVTs may be seen with aberrancy, bundle blocks or antidromic SVTs. For practical purposes, broad QRS tachyarrhythmias are treated as ventricular tachycardia unless proven otherwise.

Atrioventricular Reciprocating Tachycardia

Reentry occurs when an impulse initiates the following sequence: An ectopic atrial focus is blocked in the accessory pathway due to longer refractory period and is transmitted down to the ventricles via the AV node. This impulse then travels retrograde from the ventricular end of the accessory pathway, which is no longer refractory to impulse transmission. This orthodromically conducted impulse may reach the AV node again. If it finds the AV node to be in a refractory state, further impulse propagations would stop. However, if the AV node has recovered, the impulse will be transmitted though it and up the accessory pathway again, setting up a "circus" reentrant arrhythmia. This is the most common variety, especially in young infants and children. The reverse mechanism wherein the impulse travels down the accessory pathway in an antegrade manner and then up the AV node to reach the atria and set-up reentrant arrhythmias is referred to as antidromic conduction .Incidence of orthodromic SVTs is much more than antidromic ones. The QRS complex is narrow in orthodromic conduction and broad in antidromic conduction as the accessory pathway depolarizes the ventricle before the "AV node-His bundle" axis does.

Wolff–Parkinson–White Syndrome

A common example of a "bypass" pathway is the bundle of Kent seen in Wolff–Parkinson–White (WPW) syndrome. The incidence of WPW is fairly common with approximately four newly diagnosed cases per 100,000 population per year.

Tachycardia is typically initiated by the occurrence of a premature atrial beat (PAB). The PAB impulse travels down the AV node to depolarize the ventricle as the bundle of Kent is initially refractory from the previous sinus beat. The impulse then travels retrograde the accessory bundle setting up a reentrant narrow complex tachyarrhythmia.

Typical ECG findings of WPW in sinus rhythm are a short PR interval, a wide QRS and a positive inflection in the upstroke of the QRS complex, known as the delta wave.

The incidence of sudden cardiac death (SCD) in WPW syndrome is approximately 1 in 100 symptomatic cases when followed for up to 15 years. Although relatively uncommon, SCD may be the initial presentation in as many as 4.5% of cases. The cause of SCD in WPW syndrome is rapid conduction of atrial fibrillation (AF) to the ventricles via the AP, resulting in ventricular fibrillation (VF).

Atrioventricular Nodal Reentrant Tachycardia (Fig. 3)

This is a cyclical reentrant pattern involving dual (slow and fast) pathways within the AV node. These pathways have different conduction velocities and refractoriness and are depolarized simultaneously. During tachycardia, the impulse typically conducts in an antegrade manner through the slow pathway and in a retrograde manner through the fast pathway, resulting in a reentry circuit. The PR interval is longer than the RP interval during tachycardia. It is more common in adolescents.

AVRT—via accessory pathway	AVRT—dual pathways within the AV node
ST-T Changes >50% cases R-P interval >70 seconds	Lesser frequency of ST-T changes R-P interval <70 seconds
Inverted P waves: Never an AV block	P waves often hidden in QRS: Occasionally, AV block
Termination with adenosine is abrupt without P wave	Adenosine terminates abruptly with a P wave

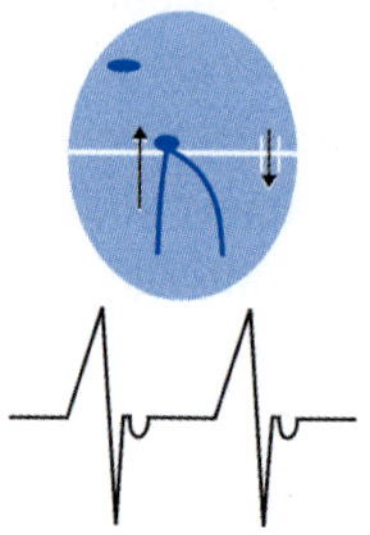

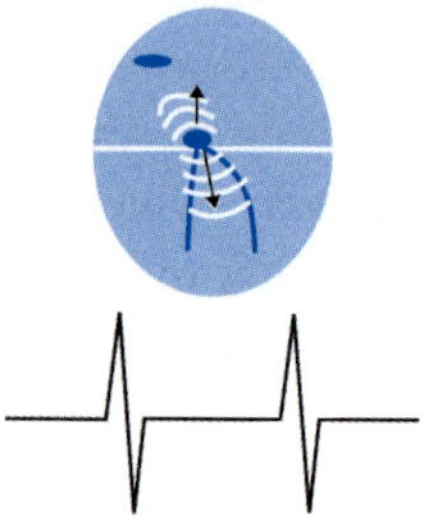

Fig. 3: AV nodal (AVNRT) reentrant tachycardia.
(AV: atrioventricular; AVNRT: atrioventricular nodal reentry tachycardia; AVRT: atrioventricular reciprocating tachycardia)

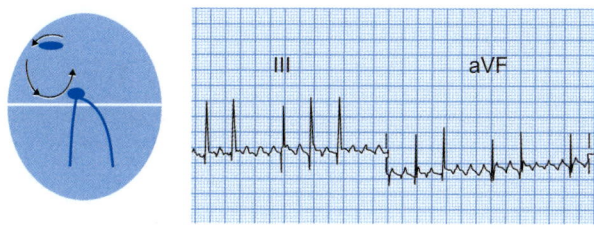
Saw-tooth appearance of P waves

Fig. 4: Atrial flutter.

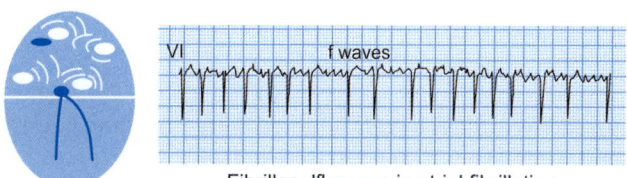
Fibrillary 'f' waves in atrial fibrillation

Fig. 5: Atrial fibrillation.

Atrial Flutter (Fig. 4)

Atrial flutter is common in the fetus and newborn and becomes very rare again until adult life. Causes of atrial flutter in children are attributed largely to structural heart disease with dilated atria, myocarditis, acute infection, or postoperative cardiac patients. On an ECG, the hallmark pattern is "saw-toothed" flutter waves, which is best, viewed in leads II, III, and V1. The atrial rate is typically over 300/minutes. Atrial flutter can be well-tolerated and may even be asymptomatic, if there is a high degree of AV node block and the ventricular rate is near normal. If there is 2:1 AV conduction the ventricular rate may be too fast. Incomplete ventricular relaxation may decrease the diastolic filling time and thereby decrease the stroke volume and cardiac output. However, if AV nodal conduction is brisk, 1:1 AV conduction can occur, that inevitably leads to circulatory compromise or death. It is an important cause of fetal hydrops.

Atrial Fibrillation (Fig. 5)

Atrial rates range from 350 BPM to 600 BPM and the rhythm is described as being "irregularly irregular", with beat-to-beat variability of the atrial size and shape. This is best recognized in lead V1. The QRS complexes appear normal. Atrial fibrillation is also associated with decreased cardiac output due to loss of atrial "kick".

Sinus Tachycardia

Sinus tachycardia is identified by QRS axis and a P wave that precedes every QRS complex. Sinus tachycardia can be associated with underlying conditions as fever, hypoxia, anemia, hypovolemia, shock, myocardial ischemia, and medications (most commonly catecholamines).

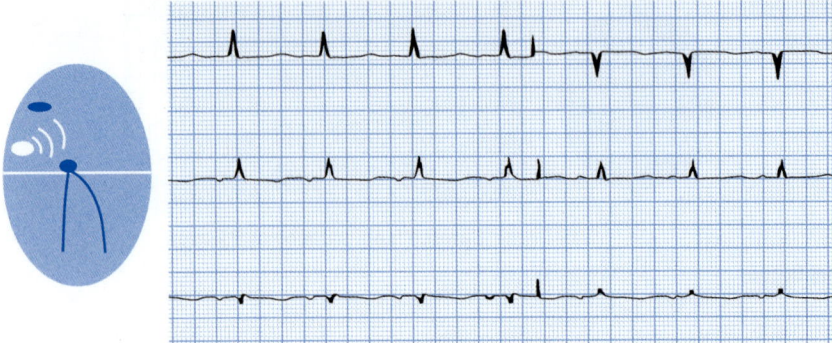

Fig. 6: Ectopic atrial tachycardias with electrocardiogram showing P wave of altered morphology.

The treatment of sinus tachycardia is largely targeted at treating the underlying disorder, rather than treating the tachycardia itself. It may be confused with SVT.

Ectopic Atrial Tachycardia

This is also a supraventricular tachyarrhythmia which occurs due increased automaticity of a focus in the atrium or close to the AV node (Fig. 6). The hallmark is the presence of abnormal P wave morphologies. Each P wave is conducted to the ventricle and the ectopic atrial focus takes over the rate determination. It has a gradual onset and the occasional AV block (especially, if 2:1) may be diagnostic. It has a warm up phenomenon and differing P axis and morphology. The P waves are distinct and identical and the P-R interval is normal or minimally prolonged. In case of multiple such foci, P waves would have different morphologies in the same strip. This is referred to as multifocal atrial tachycardia (MFAT).

Junctional Ectopic Tachycardia

Junctional ectopic tachycardia is a supraventricular tachycardia due to increased automaticity in the region of the AV node. It is more commonly seen in postoperative cardiac patients (especially those involving VSD closure) as compared to the congenital form. Poor postoperative myocardial function coupled with loss of AV synchrony can lead to significant reduction in cardiac output.

A standard approach to SVTs is given in Flowchart 1.

PRESENTATION AND CLINICAL FEATURES OF SVTs

The majority of infants with SVT present at less than 4 months of age—50% have an idiopathic cause, 24% are associated with fever and drug exposure, 23% are caused by congenital heart disease (most commonly Ebstein's anomaly and L-transposition), and 10–20% are the result of WPW syndrome. Among older children, causes are more likely to be WPW, concealed bypass tracts, or congenital heart disease. The AV reentrant type of tachycardia is more common in children less than 12 years of age, whereas the AVNRT becomes more evident in adolescents.

Flowchart 1: Algorithmic approach to supraventricular tachycardias.

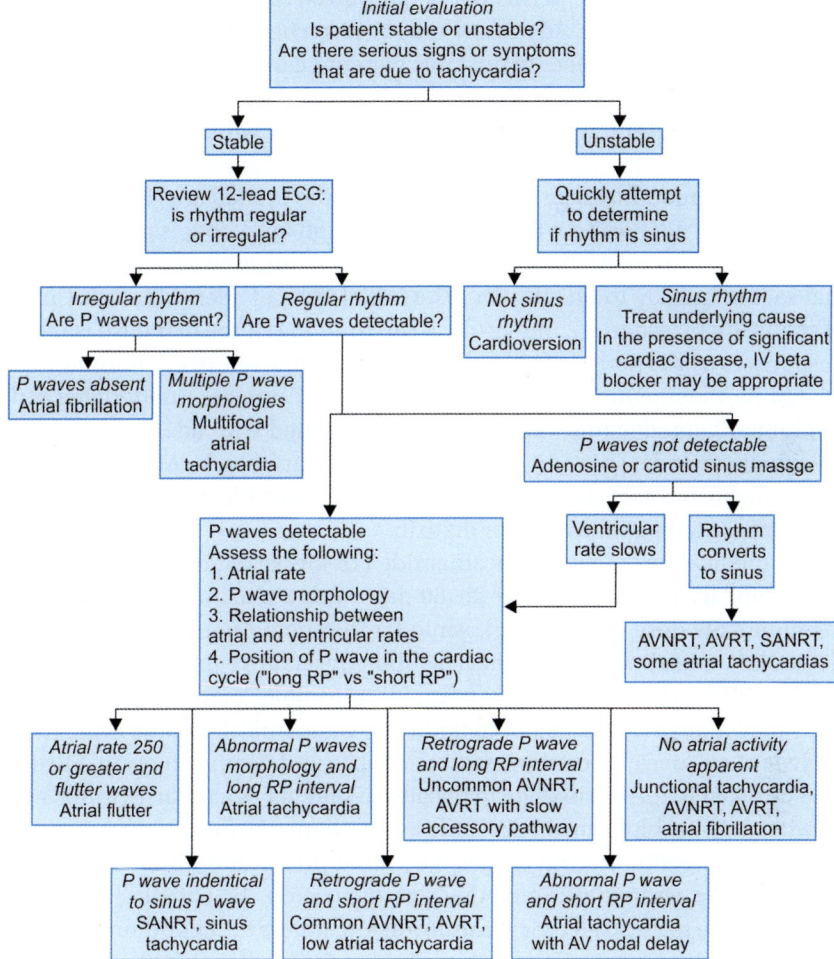

(*Note*: RP interval – Onset of QRS to the next visible P wave - best noted in leads II and V1)
(AV: atrioventricular; AVNRT: atrioventricular nodal reentry tachycardia; AVRT: atrioventricular reciprocating tachycardia; ECG: electrocardiogram)

Infants often present with nonspecific complaints such as "fussiness", lethargy and simply "not acting right" or with florid signs of congestive failure. They may present as dilated cardiomyopathy or as SIDS. Palpitations and syncope may be noted in older children. A family history of sudden death or cardiac disease should be sought.

MANAGEMENT OF SUPRAVENTRICULAR TACHYCARDIAS

The management of SVT always begins with ensuring that the patient is maintaining airway, breathing and cardiovascular status. It is important to promptly administer oxygen and differentiate between stable and unstable patients. In a child presenting with unstable SVT with severe heart failure and poor perfusion, synchronized cardioversion is initiated at 0.5 J/kg and can be increased up to 1 J/kg. Adenosine may be given before cardioversion, if intravenous access has already been established. In unstable patients, cardioversion should not be delayed for attempts at IV access or sedation.

In children who present with asymptomatic SVT or with mild heart failure, vagal maneuvers, such as ice to the face in an infant or blowing through a straw in an older child may be attempted (carotid massage and pressure over the eyeball are NOT to be performed). If that is unsuccessful, adenosine is administered through an IV that is preferably close to the heart. Because of its extremely short half-life, adenosine must be pushed and flushed (with 5 cc normal saline) quickly to be effective. The initial dose of adenosine is 0.1 mg/kg (up to 6 mg) and can be increased to 0.2 mg/kg/dose (up to 12 mg) if the first dose is ineffective. An effective response is a brief period of asystole on ECG, with the return of a normal sinus rhythm. Adenosine can be therapeutic as well as diagnostic as it unmasks underlying atrial flutter. There are minimal hemodynamic consequences associated with adenosine administration. Contraindications include second- or third-degree heart block. Additionally, adenosine can worsen bronchospasm in asthmatics and increase heart block or precipitate ventricular arrhythmias in those taking verapamil, or digoxin.

Alternative medications include procainamide (15 mg/kg, IV, over 30–60 min or at 20–80 µg/kg/min), amiodarone (5 mg/kg over 20–60 min, with a maximum single dose of 150 mg and a maximum daily dose of 15 mg/kg). Amiodarone should not be used in newborns during the first month of life because of benzyl alcohol preservative that may cause fatal gasping syndrome. Beta (β) blockers, such as propranolol or esmolol may be used but with caution because they may induce hypotension. In addition, verapamil should be avoided in children less than 1 year of age because cardiovascular collapse and death can occur. Further precautions should be taken in the use of digoxin because it may act as a proarrhythmic agent in SVT associated with WPW by blocking the AV node as mentioned before.

Patients in atrial reentrant arrhythmias, i.e., atrial flutter and fibrillation may be hemodynamically unstable warranting immediate cardioversion. In patients who are receiving digoxin, it is advisable to avoid electrical cardioversion, unless the condition is life threatening, because the combination is associated with malignant ventricular arrhythmias due to digoxin-induced AV block. Heparin may be added to prevent embolization. Alternatives include rapid atrial pacing with catheterization or lower current settings. If patient is hemodynamically stable, digoxin is administered to increase AV blockade, thereby slowing the ventricular rate. Propranolol, 1.0–4.0 mg/kg/day, orally in divided doses, three to four times a day may be added. Esmolol and procainamide are alternatives to propranolol. Recurrences are then prevented in consultation with an expert cardiologist.

Ectopic atrial tachycardia may be difficult to treat and often polytherapy is needed using drugs as propafenone, sotalol, flecainide, and amiodarone under supervision of an expert cardiologist. Junctional ectopic tachycardia may also be difficult to manage and treatment involves cooling, avoiding sympathomimetic drugs as may be possible, the use of amiodarone and in some cases overdrive pacing.

The long-term management of SVT may include β-blockers, procainamide, sotalol, amiodarone, or flecainide. Radiofrequency catheter ablation has an 85–95% success rate of preventing recurrence of SVT. The evaluation of SVT includes electrolytes (especially potassium, calcium, magnesium, and glucose), complete blood count, toxicology screen, blood gas, and thyroid function tests. Once stabilized, the majority of patients who present with SVTs will need to be investigated for the underlying cause of SVT and long-term control. Death seen rarely is due to long-standing SVT leading to dilated cardiomyopathy, rapid antidromic conduction predisposing to VF or incorrect use of drugs as verapamil that may lead to cardiogenic shock in infants.

VENTRICULAR TACHYARRHYTHMIAS

Premature Ventricular Contractions

A premature ventricular contraction (PVC) is a premature, wide QRS complex that has a distinct configuration and is not preceded by a P wave (Fig. 7). They may appear in a pattern of two consecutive PVCs (couplet), alternating PVC with a normal QRS complex (bigeminy), or in which every third beat is a PVC (trigeminy). The occurrence of three or more consecutive PVCs is considered ventricular tachycardia. The sinoatrial (SA) node maintains a normal conduction pace and the PVC replaces a normal QRS wave while maintaining a rhythm.

Most children who have PVCs are otherwise healthy. PVCs can also be associated with congenital heart disease, long QT syndrome, cardiomyopathies, electrolyte imbalances, drug toxicities (e.g. digoxin, catecholamines, sympathomimetics), cardiac injury, cardiac tumors, myocarditis, or hypoxia. PVCs are considered malignant, if they are associated with underlying heart disease; there is a history of syncope or family history of sudden death; precipitated by or increased with activity; exhibit multiform morphology; they are symptomatic of runs of PVCs; or there are frequent episodes of paroxysmal ventricular tachycardia. Children presenting with PVCs require evaluation whenever there are two or more PVCs in a row, they are multifocal in origin, there is an "R-on-T" phenomenon, or if there is underlying heart disease. The R-on-T phenomenon is an instance in which a PVC occurs on the T wave, which is considered a vulnerable period of stimulating abnormal rhythms. This can be seen with hypoxia or hypokalemia and may result in life-threatening arrhythmias. For those patients who have an

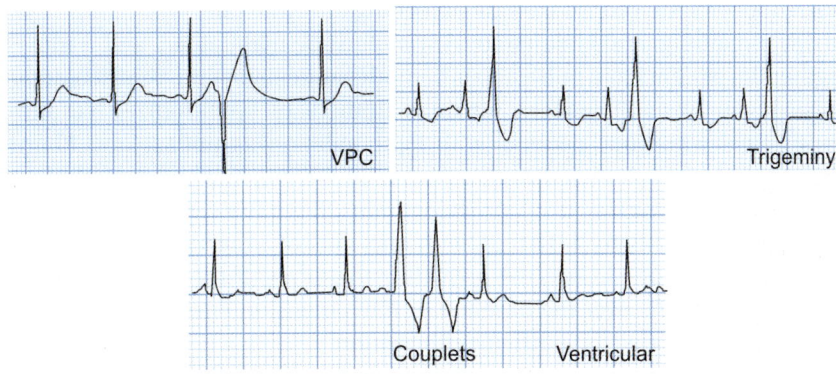

Fig. 7: Premature ventricular contractions (PVC).

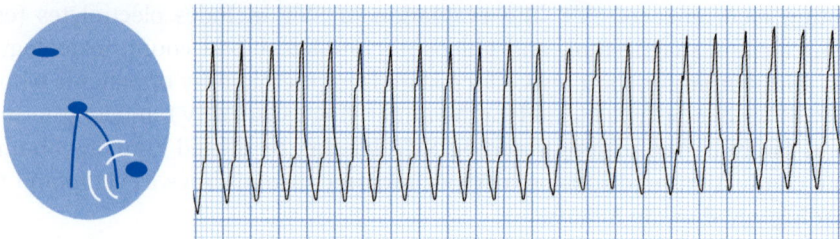

Fig. 8: Wide complex ventricular tachycardia.

underlying cause (e.g. electrolyte abnormality, hypoxia, or severe acidosis), the treatment consists of managing the underlying cause. The treatment consists largely of IV lidocaine (1 mg/kg/dose), followed by a lidocaine drip (20–50 µg/kg/min). Amiodarone, procainamide, and β blockers are reserved for conditions that are refractory to lidocaine. In asymptomatic patients who present with isolated PVCs and normal cardiac structure and function, no treatment is necessary.

Ventricular Tachycardia

Three or more consecutive contractions of ventricular origin define this life-threatening rhythm (Fig. 8). These contractions are hemodynamically inefficient and can decompensate into ventricular fibrillation, which is a nonperfusing, terminal arrhythmia. Ventricular tachycardia may result from electrolyte disturbances (hyperkalemia, hypokalemia, and hypocalcaemia), metabolic abnormalities, congenital heart disorders, myocarditis, or drug toxicity. Other causes include cardiomyopathies, cardiac tumors, acquired heart disease, prolonged QT syndrome, and idiopathic causes.

ECG—The QRS duration is prolonged, ranging from 0.06 seconds to 0.14 seconds. Complexes may appear monomorphic with a uniform contour and absent or retrograde P waves. Alternatively, the QRS complexes may appear polymorphic or vary randomly as is seen in torsades de pointes. EKG findings that further support the presence of VT include the presence of AV dissociation with the ventricular rate exceeding the atrial rate.

The airway, breathing, and circulation (ABCs) must be maintained, and it must be determined whether the patient has a pulse and is hemodynamically stable. Ventricular tachycardia with a pulse in an unstable patient warrants immediate synchronized cardioversion at 0.5–1 J/kg. Pretreat conscious patients with light sedation as midazolam. Pharmacologic interventions include amiodarone (5 mg/kg IV over 20–60 min; maximum single dose, 150 mg; maximum daily dose, 15 mg/kg/days), procainamide (15 mg IV over 30–60 min), or lidocaine (1 mg/kg IV bolus, repeat every 5–10 min, with max total of 3 mg/kg). When using procainamide, the infusion is stopped once the arrhythmia resolves, if the QRS complex widens to more than or equal to 50% over the baseline or if hypotension ensues. Pulseless ventricular tachycardia should be treated as ventricular fibrillation.

After cardioversion, the return to normal sinus rhythm is usually transient. The medication used to achieve sinus rhythm must be given as a continuous infusion using lidocaine (20–50 µg/kg/min), amiodarone (7–15 mg/kg/day), or procainamide [20–80 µg/kg/min (maximum

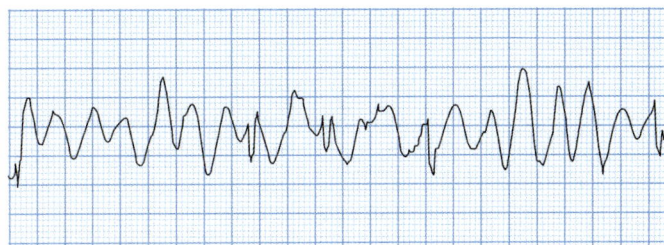

Fig. 9: Ventricular fibrillation.

dose of 2 g/24 hours)]. In polymorphic ventricular tachycardia, temporary atrial or ventricular pacing may be required.

Ventricular Fibrillation (Fig. 9).

On the ECG, the rhythm is one of bizarre QRS complexes with varying sizes and configurations and a rapid, irregular rate. Causes of VF include postoperative complications from congenital heart disease repair, severe hypoxemia, hyperkalemia, medications (digitalis, quinidine, catecholamines, and anesthesia), myocarditis, and myocardial infarction.

Automated external defibrillators (AEDs) may be used in 1–8-year-old children who have no signs of circulation, ideally with the pediatric dose. For documented VF or pulseless VT, defibrillation is recommended .Because ventricular fibrillation is a nonperfusing rhythm, cardiopulmonary resuscitation (CPR) must be initiated immediately. Defibrillation is initiated at 2 J/kg, increased from 2 to 4 J/kg, and then followed by a third shock at 4 J/kg. If defibrillation is unsuccessful, epinephrine (0.01 mg/kg, 1:10,000 solutions) should be given and repeated every 3–5 minutes as necessary.

If pulseless ventricular tachycardia is refractory to defibrillation, antiarrhythmic drugs are indicated, such as amiodarone (5 mg/kg, IV bolus) or lidocaine (1 mg/kg, IV bolus, and repeated to a maximum of 3 mg/kg). Although the pediatric dosing of amiodarone has not been clearly established, the recommended loading dose of 5 mg/kg IV may be given over 20–60 min and the dose may be repeated in increments of 5 mg/kg IV, to a maximum of 15 mg/kg/day IV. For polymorphic VT (torsades des pointes), the treatment is magnesium (20–50 mg/kg, IV).

Long QT Syndrome

Long QT syndrome (LQTS) is a disorder of delayed ventricular repolarization and is characterized by prolongation of the QT interval. It may be either hereditary (channelopathy) or acquired. The delayed repolarization properties may be patchy within the myocardium thus creating a substrate for transmural reentry. Patients may be triggered into polymorphic torsades with sympathetic stimulation, such as sudden anxiety and loud noise. The most common acquired causes are medications and electrolyte abnormalities, such as hypokalemia, hypocalcemia, and hypomagnesemia.

Patients with LQTS commonly present with recurrent episodes of near or frank syncope that are often precipitated by intense emotion, vigorous physical activity, or loud noises and may be mistaken for seizures because they can result in the loss of consciousness and tonic–clonic movements. Approximately, 10% of children with LQTS present with sudden death or with milder symptoms, such as diaphoresis, palpitations, or lightheadedness.

A markedly prolonged QT interval is calculated with the Bazett formula. $QTc=QT/\sqrt{}$ preceding RR interval; e.g., $QTc=0.452/\sqrt{0.612}$, then $QTc=578$ msec.

To account for the normal physiologic shortening of the QT interval that occurs with increasing heart rate, the corrected QT interval (QTc) is calculated using the Bazett formula $QTc=QT/\sqrt{RR}$. The current practice identifies a QTc interval of more than or equal to 460 ms as prolonged. Most deaths are seen when the QTc exceeds 500 ms.

The hallmark dysrhythmia of LQTS is torsades de pointes ("twisting of the points) wherein the cardiac output is markedly impaired, often resulting in syncope or seizures. Although often self-limiting with spontaneous return of consciousness, the dysrhythmia has the potential to degenerate into ventricular fibrillation and sudden death.

LQTS should be considered and an ECG be obtained on any patient presenting with a suggestive history, including first-degree relatives of known LQTS carrier, a family history of syncope, seizures, sudden death, SIDS, a seizure of unknown cause or an unexplained near-drowning.

Patients presenting with an episode of polymorphic VT or torsades de pointes of unknown origin should receive magnesium (25–50 mg/kg, IV, maximum 2 g). Serum electrolytes and a toxicology screen should be obtained. Beta blockers may be useful in suppressing catecholamine surges and any further dysrhythmic activity. Patients with recurrent ventricular tachycardia may require temporary transcutaneous ventricular pacing. Once a patient is diagnosed with LQTS, an ECG should be performed on all other family members.

Beta blockers are generally recommended as the initial therapy for long-term management and have been shown to effectively eradicate dysrhythmias in 60% of patients and to decrease mortality significantly. The most commonly used β-blocker is propranolol (2–4 mg/kg/day, maximum 60 mg/day). Patients with severe asthma, in whom β blockers are contraindicated, may be candidates for implantable cardioverter-defibrillator (ICD) under the guidance of an electrophysiologist.

Of note, more than 12 types of LQTS have been identified, though the first 3 account for more than 90% cases.

LQTS 1	Most common: Precipitated Precipitated by exertion	K channelopathy	Beta-blockers/ICD indicated
LQTS 2	Precipitated by sudden noises/startling situations	Na channelopathy	?ICD
LQTS 3	More commonly during sleep	Na channelopathy	Beta-blockers

BRADYARRHYTHMIAS

Mechanisms of bradycardia include depression of the pacemaker in the sinus node or conduction system blocks. Bradyarrhythmias may manifest as repeated syncopal attacks, dizziness and rarely as sudden death.

Sinus Bradycardia

P waves precede each QRS complex on the ECG. Usually, the heart rate is less than 80 BPM in infants and less than 60 BPM in older children. The adequacy of the patient's oxygenation and ventilation should be assessed rapidly. It can also be associated with hyperkalemia, hypercalcemia, hypoxia, hypothermia, hypothyroidism, and medications (e.g., digitalis and β blockers). As with sinus tachycardia, the treatment of sinus bradycardia is targeted at the treatment of the underlying cause.

Distinction must be made from junctional (nodal) bradycardia which has either no P waves or inverted P waves after QRS complexes and may occur in an otherwise normal heart or postoperatively, with digitalis toxicity or with increased vagal tone. If the patient is asymptomatic, no treatment is indicated or else atropine or pacing may be indicated.

Conduction Abnormalities

First-degree Atrioventricular Block

First-degree AV block is an abnormal delay in conduction through the AV node that manifests as a prolonged PR interval on electrocardiography with a normal QRS configuration. There are no dropped beats. Common causes include otherwise healthy children with an infectious disease. It may further be associated with myocarditis (e.g., rheumatic fever and Lyme disease), cardiomyopathies, and congenital heart disease (ASD and Ebstein's anomaly) (Fig. 10).

Second-degree Atrioventricular Block: Mobitz Type I (Wenckebach) and Type II

In the Mobitz type I block, otherwise known as the Wenckebach phenomena, the PR interval lengthens progressively until a QRS complex is dropped. The block is caused by an increased refractory period at the level of the AV node. Although this can be seen in otherwise healthy individuals, it can also be seen in patients who have myocarditis, myocardial infarctions, cardiomyopathies, congenital heart disease, digoxin toxicity, and postoperative cardiac repairs. The Mobitz type II second-degree heart block, there is either normal AV conduction with a normal PR or RR interval before a dropped QRS or a completely blocked conduction (Fig. 11).

Third-degree Heart Block

Third-degree heart block, otherwise known as complete heart block, occurs when none of the atrial impulses is conducted to the ventricles. There is a complete loss of rhythm conduction

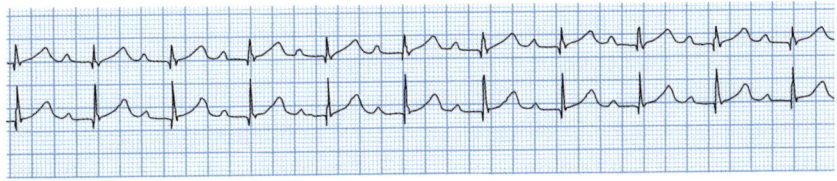

Fig. 10: First degree atrioventricular block.

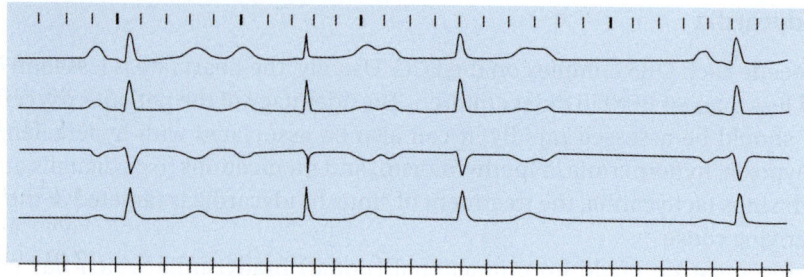

Fig. 11: Second degree atrioventricular block.

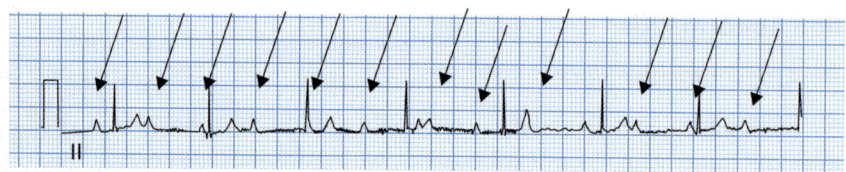

Fig. 12: Third degree atrioventricular block.

from a working atrial pacemaker, thereby allowing the ventricular pacemaker to take over. On electrocardiography, the P waves are completely dissociated from the QRS waves. Even though they are dissociated, both the atrial and ventricular rhythms are regular, maintaining regular PP and RR intervals, respectively. The QRS duration is usually normal if the block is usually proximal to the bundle of His, whereas a wide QRS complex indicates that the block is most likely in the bundle branches (e.g., surgically-induced complete heart block). Oftentimes, the ventricular rhythm is slower than normal (Fig. 12).

Complete heart block (CHB) may be congenitally associated with structural lesions, such as in L-transposition of the great arteries and maternal lupus. Acquired heart block may result from cardiac surgery, especially when there is suturing in the atrium. This effect can be either transient, resolving within a week postoperatively or permanent. Other causes include infectious causes, such as myocarditis, Lyme disease, rheumatic fever, diphtheria, and inflammatory disorders, such as Kawasaki disease and SLE. CHB is also associated with myocardial ischemia, cardiac tumors, muscular dystrophies, hypocalcemia and drug overdoses.

Children presenting with first-degree heart block are largely asymptomatic but have the potential to progress to further heart block, including second- and third-degree heart blocks. Second degree, type II, block frequently progresses to complete heart block. Those children, who present with complete heart block, most notably in infancy, may present with signs of congestive heart failure. Older children may present with syncopal attacks, otherwise known as Stokes–Adams attacks, with heart rates less than 40–45 BPM or even sudden death.

Treatment of Bradyarrhythmias

Bradycardia in children may be attributable to vagal stimulation, hypoxemia, acidosis, or an acute elevation of intracranial pressure. The management of bradycardia includes the identification and treatment of the cause and appropriate cardiopulmonary resuscitation, with assisted ventilation, oxygenation, and chest compressions as indicated.

If symptomatic bradycardia persists despite initial resuscitative measures, pharmacologic intervention is initiated with epinephrine (0.01 mg/kg IV; 0.1 mL/kg of 1:10,000 solution) or atropine (0.02 mg/kg, IV, minimum 0.1 mg; maximum single dose is 0.5 mg in children and 1 mg in adolescents). Epinephrine is the initial drug of choice in children with symptomatic bradycardia. Chest compressions are indicated for neonates or children with heart rates less than 60 BPM with hemodynamic compromise. Emergency transcutaneous pacing may be lifesaving if the bradycardia is due to complete heart block or sinus nodal dysfunction unresponsive to ventilation, oxygenation, chest compressions, and medications, especially if it is associated with congenital or acquired heart disease. Pacing is not useful for asystole or bradycardia due to postarrest insult. No treatment is indicated for a first-degree degree heart block. For second-degree heart blocks, treatment is directed at the underlying cause. In patients who have Mobitz type II second-degree heart block, a prophylactic pacemaker may be warranted because there is a risk of progressing to complete heart block. For those who present with a complete heart block, the mainstay of therapy is a pacemaker. While awaiting pacemaker insertion, it may be necessary to administer atropine or isoproterenol, which temporarily increases the heart rate.

Asystole/Pulseless Electrical Activity

These rhythms are the common ECG manifestations of most pediatric cardiorespiratory arrests. Rarely, as in adults, the collapse rhythm may be ventricular tachycardia or fibrillation especially in children with underlying structural heart disease or familial history of sudden death. As with bradyarrhythmias or tachyarrhythmias, the 4 Hs and 4 Ts (Table 2) may be the initiating or perpetuating causes for asystole and PEAs.

TESTS USED IN DIAGNOSIS AND MANAGEMENT OF ARRHYTHMIAS

Electrophysiological Testing

12-lead ECG is a must except where the rhythm is life threatening and needs immediate treatment. Detailed 24–48 hours Holter monitoring may also be very useful as often some arrhythmias may be paroxysmal in nature. Exercise testing when indicated should be done under expert supervision. Detailed intracardiac studies involve detailed mapping of the

Table 2: Treatable causes for bradyarrhythmias.

Four Hs	Four Ts
Hypoxemia	Tamponade
Hypovolemia	Tension pneumothorax
Hypothermia	Toxins/drugs
Hyper/hypokalemia	Thromboembolism

conduction pathways allowing better understanding of etiopathogenesis of ectopic foci, accessory conduction bundles and heart blocks with simultaneous treatment possibility in the same setting.

Echocardiogram

This is needed to rule out structural heart disease as a cause of arrhythmias (e.g., WPW syndrome with Ebstein's anomaly) and any dysfunction as cause (DCM) or effect (tachycardia-induced cardiomyopathy).

TREATMENT OF PEDIATRIC ARRHYTHMIAS (TABLE 3 AND FLOWCHARTS 2 TO 4)

It involves pharmacotherapy and often electrical cardioversion, defibrillation, and pacing. Commonly used drugs in the management of arrhythmias are discussed below and a few in more detail.

Table 3: Drugs used in the management of tachyarrhythmias (Ref. American Pharmacists Association).

Antiarrhythmics (Class and mechanism of action)	Commonly used drug and their dosages	
Class I Sodium channel blockers (depress automaticity and conduction velocity) Procainamide, lidocaine, flecainide	Procainamide	15 mg/kg IV/IO over 30–60 min, *Adult dose*: 20 mg/min IV infusion up to total max dose 17 mg/kg
	Lidocaine	Bolus: 1 mg/kg IV/IO, Max dose: 100 mg ET*: 2–3 mg, Infusion: 20–50 µg/kg/min
Class II Beta adrenergic blockers—(depress automaticity and conduction velocity: Especially useful in long QTS which is a catecholaminergic driven tachycardia Propranolol, esmolol	Propranolol	1 mg/kg/dose 3–4 times a day
	Esmolol	0.6 mg/kg f/b infusion of 0.2 mg/kg/min
Class III Potassium channel blockers—Prolong refractory period of conducting tissues Amiodarone, Sotalol (shorter acting)	Amiodarone	5 mg/kg IV/IO; repeat up to 15 mg/kg, maximum 300 mg
Class IV Calcium channel blockers—slows SA and AV node Verapamil, diltiazem	Verapamil	0.1 mg/kg/dose (Maximum 5 mg/dose)
Others (Unclassified) *Adenosine*: 0.1 mg/kg (maximum 6 mg): Repeat: 0.2 mg/kg (maximum 12 mg) *Digoxin*: 5–25 µg/kg (half of digitalization dose) *Atropine*: 0.02 mg/kg IV/IO, 0.03 mg/kg ET*Minimum dose: 0.1 mg: Maximum single dose: Child 0.5 mg, Older: 1 mg *Magnesium sulfate*: 25–50 mg/kg IV/IO in 10–20 min; faster in torsades. Maximum dose: 2 g : May cause hypotension *Adrenaline*: 0.01 mg/kg i.e. 0.1 mL/kg of 1:10,000 (for asystole, bradycardia, ventricular tachycardia/fibrillation)		
(AV: atrioventricular; IO: intraosseous; IV: intravenous; SV: sinoventricular)		

Flowchart 2: Algorithm for tachyarrhythmias (PALS).

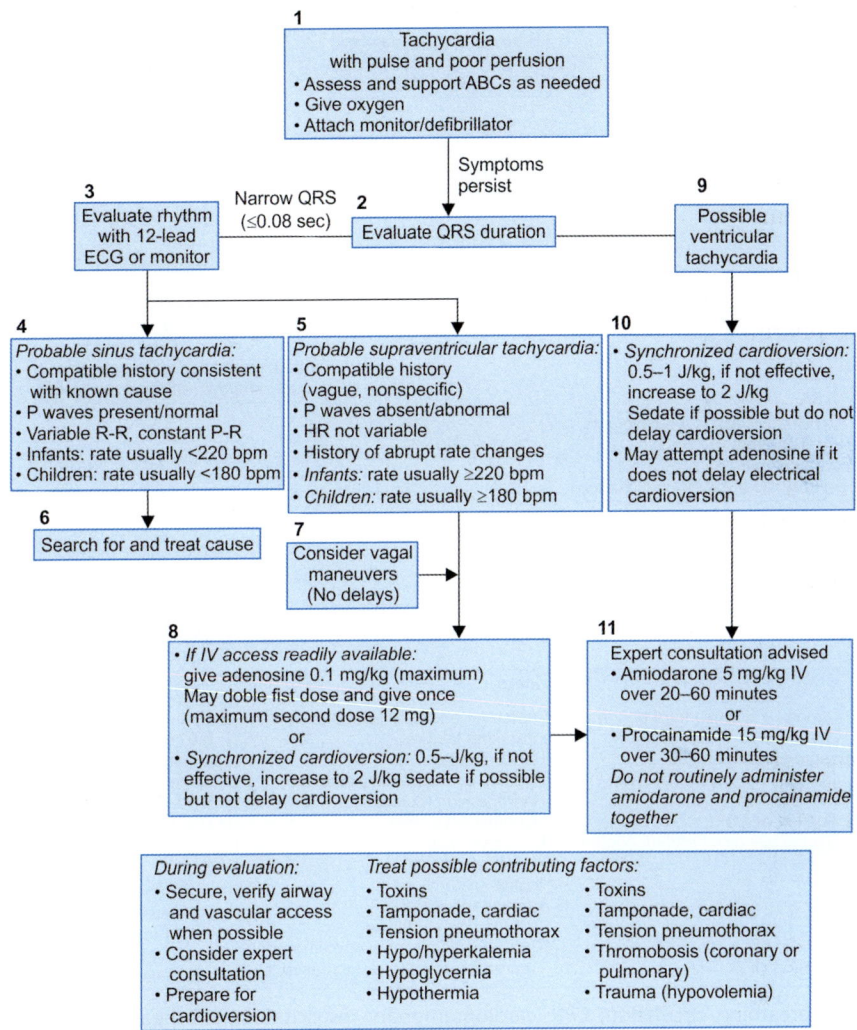

(ECG: electrocardiogram; IV: intravenous).

Commonly Used Drugs

Adenosine

It is metabolized rapidly by RBCs and has a half-life of less than 10 seconds. It needs to be given by two syringe "rapid push" technique using. Dose is 0.1 mg/kg and may be doubled if no response. It is helpful in differentiating reentrant tachycardias (where the rate decreases immediately due to the blocking of impulses at the AV node) from those due to increased automaticity. Bronchospasm, apneas, and prolonged asystole may occur. It causes a sense of impending doom and older patients may need to be warned of the same. Aminophylline causes reversible antagonism of adenosine.

Flowchart 3: Pediatric bradycardia algorithm (with a pulse and poor perfusion): PALS.

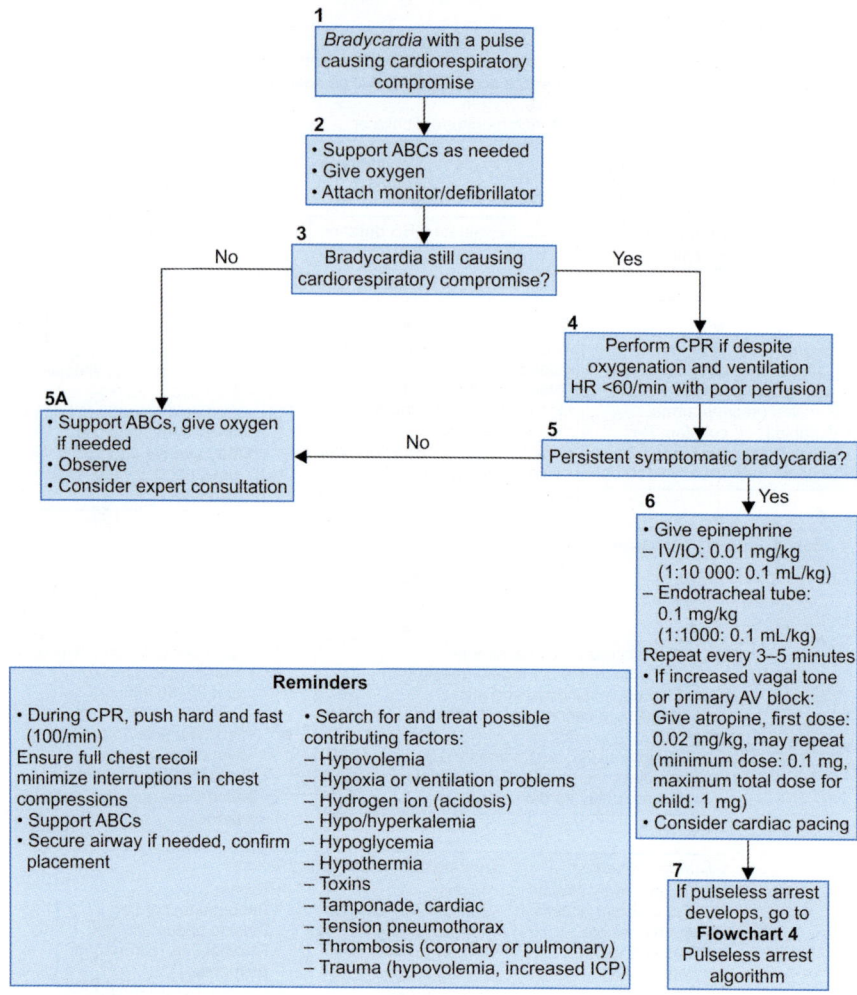

(ABC: airway breathing circulation; CPR: cardiopulmonary resuscitation; HR: heart rate; VF: ventricular fibrillation; VT: ventricular tachycardia)

Amiodarone

It is a potent versatile drug. Contraindicated in those sensitive to Iodine. It may cause hypotension, especially if loading dose is used. Vasodilatory and negative inotropic effects may be seen. Bradycardias may be resistant to atropine and contradict usage, if coexisting heart blocks known. Range is 5–15 µg/kg/min (7–21 mg/kg/day). It may be considered in the treatment of both supraventricular and ventricular tachycardias and even shock-refractory or recurrent VT/VF. The latter recommendation is extrapolated from adult studies showing increased survival.

Cardiac Arrhythmias

Flowchart 4: Pulseless arrest algorithm: PALS.

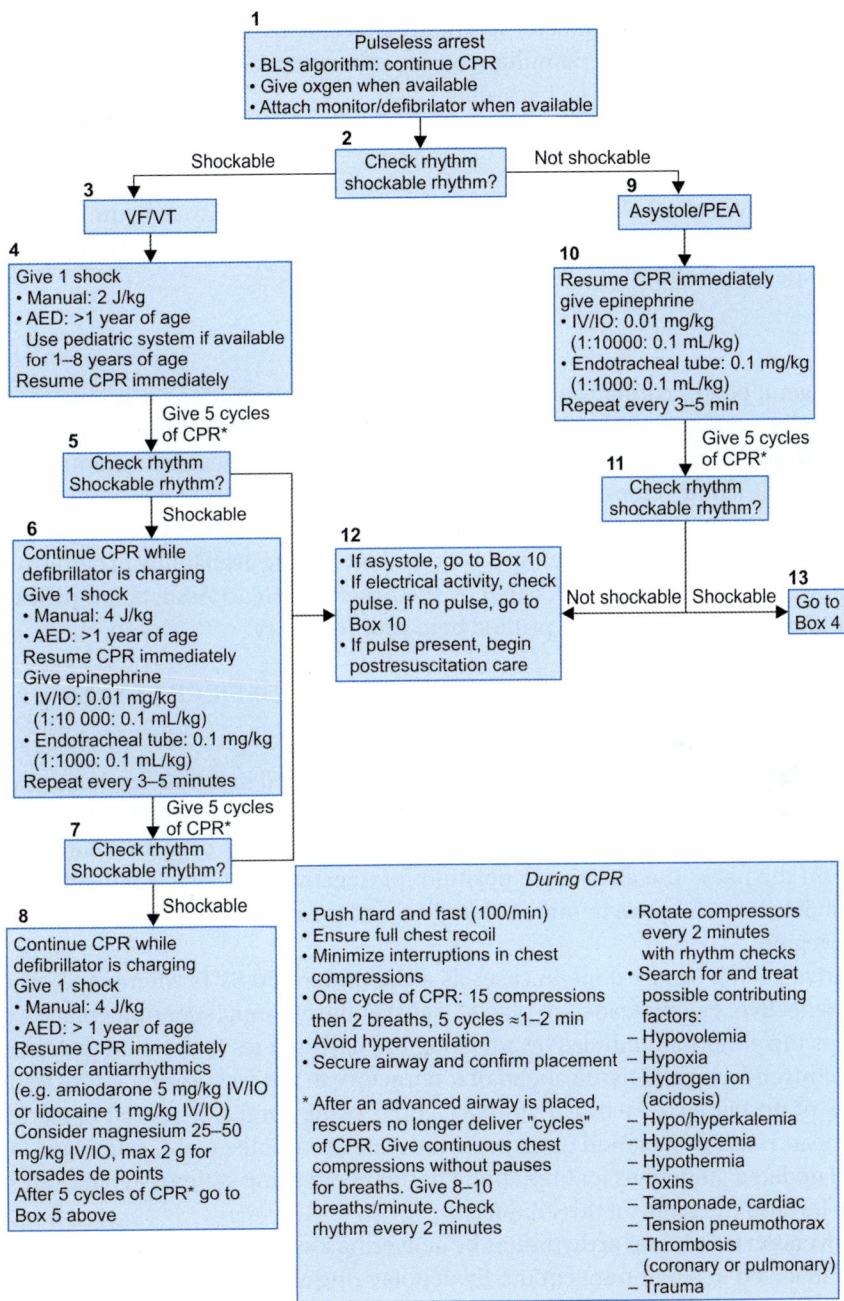

(AED: automated external defibrillator; BLS: basic life support; CPR: cardiopulmonary resuscitation; VF: ventricular fibrillation; VT: ventricular tachycardia)

Digoxin

This is proarrhythmic drug with safer alternatives available. Blocks AV node and thus may worsen atrial tachycardias by simultaneously enhancing conduction through accessory pathways leading to ventricular tachycardias.

Flecainide

It may cause bradycardia, heart blocks, and worsening of ventricular arrhythmias. Dose varies from 1 mg/kg/day to 4 mg/kg/day in 3 divided doses and may be increased under the supervision of an expert cardiologist.

Lidocaine

A class IB agent, blocks cardiac sodium ion channels, which shortens action potential duration, decreasing cardiac muscle refractoriness and shortening QRS duration and QT interval. Its effects are most pronounced in diseased cardiac tissue, decreasing automaticity and suppressing ventricular ectopy.

The outcome of pediatric dysrhythmias has improved over the last decade due to availability of better drugs with improved safety profile and increasing availability of cardioverters and defibrillators. The PALS guidelines issued by the American Heart Association provide a stepwise algorithmic approach and are printed below for reference.

TRANSCUTANEOUS PACING, OVERDRIVE PACING, DEFIBRILLATION AND CARDIOVERSION

Transcutaneous pacing is not well-studied and recommended in the pediatric age group. They may be used for heart blocks and sinus bradycardias that cause profound hemodynamic compromise. The usual position for placing the negative electrode is over the heart and positive electrode on the back. The alternative position for negative electrode is left side of the chest over fourth intercostals space in mid axillary line and positive electrode over right side infraclavicular region.

Overdrive pacing can be done in cases as atrial flutter and SVTs where medical management is ineffective. Pacing leads are placed transvenously though centrally placed catheters and it stops the abnormal impulse by adjusting the pacing rates faster than the spontaneous rates thereby rendering the tissue ahead of it refractory to the tachycardia. More frequent use is in cases of postsurgical tachyarrhythmias as JET using surgically placed epicardial leads. The American Heart Association (AHA) and the American College of Cardiology (ACC) have published updated guidelines for implanting permanent pacing systems in children, details of which are beyond the scope of this chapter.

Cardioversion terminates arrhythmias by delivering a synchronized shock that depolarizes the tissue involved in a reentrant circuit. By depolarizing all excitable tissue of the circuit and making the tissue refractory, the circuit is no longer able to propagate or sustain reentry. As a result, cardioversion terminates those arrhythmias resulting from a single reentrant circuit, such as atrial flutter, AVNRT, AVRT, or monomorphic ventricular tachycardia. In contrast, in nonorganized rhythms, such as polymorphic ventricular tachycardia and ventricular fibrillation, the wave fronts are multiple and involve more myocardial mass, thereby requiring more energy for termination.

Use of a larger pad or paddle surface is associated with a decrease in resistance and increases in current and may cause less myocardial necrosis. For children more than 10 kg weight, adult paddles may be used. Apply firm pressure on the paddles (manual) placed over the right side of the upper chest and the apex of the heart (to the left of the nipple over the left lower ribs). Alternatively, place one electrode on the front of the chest just to the left of the sternum and the other over the upper back below the scapula. Ensure good sedation, good surface to paddle contact, and sufficient jelly at the interface (to avoid skin burns). Also, the longer the arrhythmia has been presented, more difficult it is to revert. Newer biphasic waveform-based machines are more efficient than the older machines that deliver monophasic energy.

Defibrillation may be lifesaving in cases of ventricular fibrillation or unresponsive ventricular tachycardias where earlier use has been shown to have higher success rates for conversion to sinus rhythm. The initial dose may be 2 J/kg that can be increased to 4 J/kg. It is important to minimize interruptions in chest compressions while intermittently using the defibrillator. Ensure oxygen delivery and use of epinephrine alongside defibrillation to ensure best possible outcomes in these otherwise fatal arrhythmias.

KEY MESSAGES

- Pediatric dysrhythmias may be too slow (bradycardia), too fast (tachycardia), or collapse (arrest) rhythm.
- Identify whether the child is hemodynamically stable or unstable.
- Basic cardiopulmonary resuscitation should be initiated when needed and should take precedence over specific antiarrhythmia measures.
- Identify and treat the reversible causes of arrhythmias like hypoxemia, hypovolemia, hypothermia, hyper/hypokalemia (4 Hs) and tamponade, tension pneumothorax, toxins/drugs and thromboembolism (4 Ts).
- The specific therapy of symptomatic bradycardia is oxygenation, epinephrine and consider atropine or pacing according to the underlying cause.
- The management options for SVT include vagal maneuvers, IV/IO adenosine and synchronized cardioversion.
  - For wide complexes tachycardia treatment should be based with pulses one can consider cardioversion or alternative medication like amiodarone, procainamide or lidocaine.
- VF and pulseless VT should be immediately reverted by defibrillation and the use of epinephrine.

SUGGESTED READING

1. American Heart Association guidelines - Part 12: Pediatric Advanced Life Support. Circulation. 2010;112.
2. Chang PM, Silka MJ, Moromisato DY, et al. Amiodarone versus procainamide for the acute treatment of recurrent supraventricular tachycardia in pediatric patients. Circ Arrhythm Electrophysiol. 2010;3(2):134-40.

3. Davis AM, Gow RM, McCrindle BW, et al. Clinical spectrum, therapeutic management, and follow-up of ventricular tachycardia in infants and young children. Am Heart J. 1996;131(1):186-91.
4. Gewitz MH, Woolf PK. Cardiac emergencies. Textbook of Pediatric Emergency Medicine. 5th edition. 2006:717-58.
5. Kaltman J, Shah M. Evaluation of the child with an arrhythmia. Pediatr Clin North Am. 2004; 51(6):1537-51.
6. Samson RA, Atkins DL. Tachyarrhythmias and defibrillation. Pediatr Clin North Am. 2008;55(4): 887-907.
7. Samson RA, Nadkarni V, Bingham R, et al. Use of automated external defibrillators for children: an update. Circulation. 2003;107:3250-5.
8. Song MK, Baek JS, Kwon BS, et al. Clinical spectrum and prognostic factors of pediatric ventricular tachycardia. Circ J. 2010;74(9):1951-8.
9. Wiley JF. Tachycardia/palpitations. In: Fleisher GR, Ludwig S (Eds). Textbook of Pediatric Emergency Medicine. 5th edition. 2006:657-68.
10. Zipes DP, Ackerman MJ, Estes NA, et al. Task force 7: arrhythmias. J Am Coll Cardiol. 2005;45(8): 1354-63.

14. Vasoactive Agents

Rekha Solomon, Isha Bhagat

LEARNING OBJECTIVES

- Understand the effects of each agent on the cardiovascular system
- Choose the appropriate agent in a given clinical scenario
- Optimal dosing and safe administration of vasoactive agents
- Nursing care during administration.

INTRODUCTION

Vasoactive agents are primarily drugs which modify the cardiovascular system to maintain adequate organ perfusion. It is important to use clinical judgment as well as available invasive tools to guide the therapy. Shock can be categorized in terms of cardiac output (CO) and systemic vascular resistance (SVR), as low CO with decreased SVR (previously called warm shock), or low CO with increased SVR (cold shock).

Appropriate manipulation of cardiac contractility, heart rate (HR), diastolic function, and systemic and pulmonary vascular tone helps to improve organ perfusion, which is the ultimate goal in shock management (Box 1). The relationship between CO, perfusion pressure [mean arterial pressure–central venous pressure (MAP–CVP)] and SVR is as follows: CO = (MAP–CVP)/SVR. Fluid resuscitation is the first most crucial step of shock. Therapy with vasoactive agents is initiated in fluid refractory shock, low CO state, post-cardiac surgery as well as during hypertensive emergencies.

> **Box 1:** Steps in the management of shock.
>
> - Fluid resuscitation is the first step
> - Start vasoactive agent during or after fluid boluses if the patient remains hypotensive.
> - Clinically judge whether inotrope or vasopressor is needed.
> - Frequent bedside reassessment of heart rate, CRT, pulse volume, urine output, sensorium, respiratory rate, work of breathing is a must.
> - ECG monitoring, invasive BP monitoring, central venous access, urinary catheterization should be done when on vasoactive agents.
>
> (BP: blood pressure; CRT: cardiac resynchronization therapy; ECG: electrocardiography)

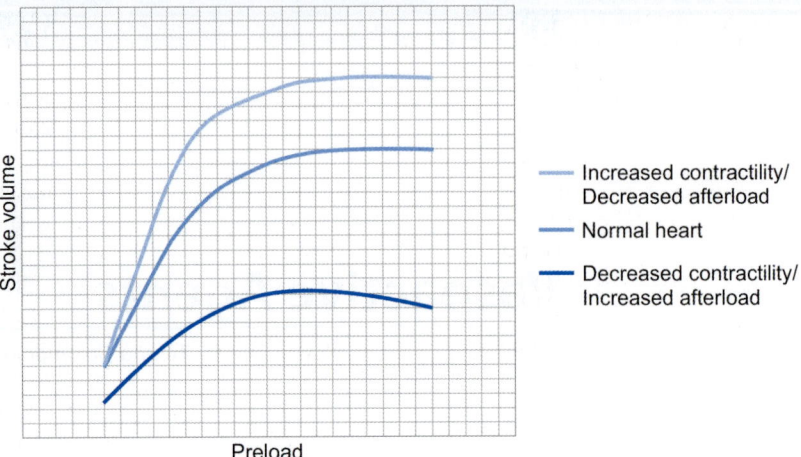

Fig. 1: Frank-Starling curve.

CLASSIFICATION OF VASOACTIVE AGENTS

- *Inotrope*: Increases force of cardiac muscle contraction and thereby stroke volume (isoprenaline).
- *Vasopressor*: Vasoconstriction (noradrenaline, phenylephrine). Several agents have a dose-dependent mix of inotropic and vasopressor activity.
- *Inopressor*: Increases cardiac contractility and causes vasoconstriction (highdose adrenaline, dopamine).
- *Inodilator*: Inotropic agents which cause vasodilation (milrinone, levosimendan, lowdose adrenaline, dobutamine).
- *Vasodilator*: Vasodilation (nitroglycerine, nitroprusside, phenoxybenzamine).

In Figure 1, the CO can be increased by increasing inotropy. In children with myocardial dysfunction, vasodilation helps in improving CO. Vasopressors increase the venous tone and improve venous return thus improving CO; however, they are to be avoided in myocardial dysfunction as they can increase afterload and worsen CO.

MECHANISM OF ACTION

The main categories of adrenergic receptors relevant to vasopressor activity are the alpha-1, beta-1, and beta-2 adrenergic receptors, as well as the dopamine receptors (Table 1 and Fig. 2). The final common pathway of adrenergic drugs is by alteration of calcium concentration in the cytosol.

- *Alpha adrenergic*: Activation of alpha-1 adrenergic receptors located in vascular walls induces significant vasoconstriction. Alpha-1 adrenergic receptors are also present in the heart and can increase the duration of contraction without increased chronotropy. However, the clinical significance of this phenomenon is unclear.
- *Beta adrenergic*: Beta-1 adrenergic receptors are most common in the heart and mediate increases in inotropy and chronotropy with minimal vasoconstriction. Stimulation of beta-2 adrenergic receptors in blood vessels induces vasodilation.

Table 1: Vasoactive agents: Site and mechanism of action, agonists.

Target	Important location	Main action	Agonist
α_1 receptor	Arterioles Heart	Vasoconstriction Inotropy	Adrenaline, noradrenaline, dopamine
α_2 receptor	Arterioles—mainly coronary and renal	Vasoconstriction	Epinephrine, noradrenaline
β_1 receptor	Conducting system of heart Atrial and ventricular muscle Arterioles in skeletal muscle and heart	Chronotropy Inotropy Vasodilation	Isoprenaline, adrenaline, dopamine, dobutamine
β_2 receptor	Vascular smooth muscles	Vasodilation	Isoprenaline, adrenaline, dopamine, dobutamine
D_1 receptor	Post-synaptic receptor in peripheral vasculature	Vasodilation	Dopamine
D_2 receptor	Pre-synaptic receptor in peripheral vasculature	Vasodilation	Dopamine
Vasopressin-1 receptor	Vascular smooth muscles	Vasoconstriction	Vasopressin
Phosphodiesterase III enzyme inhibition	Vascular smooth muscle Heart	Vasodilation Inotropy, lusitropy	Milrinone
Calcium sensitizer	Heart Vascular smooth muscle	Inotropy Lusitropy	Levosimendan
Nitric oxide release	Vascular smooth muscle	Arterial and venous dilatation	Sodium nitroprusside, Nitroglycerine

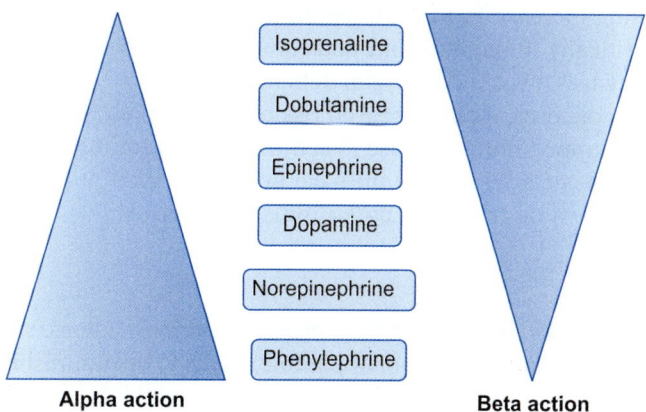

Fig. 2: α and β actions of catecholamines. Modified from Hollenberg.

Dopamine: Dopamine receptors are present in the renal, splanchnic (mesenteric), coronary, and cerebral vascular beds; stimulation of these receptors leads to vasodilation. A second subtype of dopamine receptors causes vasoconstriction by inhibiting noradrenaline reuptake at the synapse, improving inotropy and increasing peripheral vascular resistance.

Calcium sensitizers: Some agents increase the sensitivity of the myocardial contractile apparatus to calcium, causing an increase in myofilament tension development and myocardial contractility (e.g., pimobendan and levosimendan). These agents have additional pharmacologic properties, such as phosphodiesterase inhibition, which may increase inotropy and vasodilation and contribute significantly to their clinical profile, the details of which are discussed separately.

Angiotensin: Angiotensin receptors (AT_1 and AT_2) are G-coupled protein receptors with angiotensin II as their ligand. Angiotensin II is a vasoconstrictor that is part of the renin-aldosterone-angiotensin system (RAAS). When receptors are stimulated, cytosolic calcium concentration increases to mediate vasoconstrictive effects as well as aldosterone and vasopressin secretion.

Vasopressin receptors: V1, V2, V3. V1 receptors are present throughout the smooth muscle vasculature and activation leads to vasoconstriction.

INDIVIDUAL VASOACTIVE AGENTS

Dopamine

Dopamine is a precursor of norepinephrine and epinephrine. It acts on dopaminergic as well as adrenergic receptors. It has dose-dependent pharmacological action. At doses of 0.5–3 µg/kg/min, it stimulates dopaminergic D1 receptors and causes vasodilation in the renal and mesenteric bed. It also has direct natriuretic effects through its action on renal tubules. Though it increases urine output, it does not increase glomerular filtration rate (GFR) and renal protective effect has not been demonstrated. At dose 3–10 µg/kg/min, it acts on β_1 adrenergic receptors and increases cardiac contractility and HR. Above the dose 10 µg/kg/min, α_1 action predominates causing increase in SVR. However, there is significant overlap in these dose-related effects in critically ill patients and bedside titration is needed. It causes significant tachycardia and increases myocardial oxygen demand.

There have been concerns about increased risk of arrhythmias, decreased mucosal blood flow in gut, pituitary suppression, decrease in cell-mediated immunity, and impaired thyroid function. Though doses of 3–20 µg/kg/min have been described, it is prudent to add on a catecholamine early when more than 10 µg/kg/min is needed.

Clinical Usage

Fluid refractory septic shock. However, in view of accumulating evidence supporting early use of adrenaline or noradrenaline, the role of dopamine seems to be diminishing.

Dobutamine

Dobutamine is a synthetic catecholamine introduced in the late 1970s. Dobutamine is a racemic mixture of two isomers—D isomer which acts on β_1 and β_2 adrenergic receptors and L isomer with β_1 and α_1 adrenergic effects. It has a strong affinity for both β_1 and β_2 receptors which it binds in a 3:1 ratio. It is a potent inotrope with weaker chronotropic activity. It causes vasodilation particularly at low doses (<5 µg/kg/min). It reduces systemic and pulmonary vascular resistance. Unlike dopamine, it increases blood pressure (BP) by increasing cardiac contractility without causing vasoconstriction. Hence, it soon became the drug of choice in cardiogenic shock. However, further studies showed development of pharmacological tolerance when used beyond 72 h. At higher doses >15 µg/kg/min, it causes tachycardia, myocardial ischemia, and arrhythmias. Two studies reported that the left ventricular stroke work index increased by 23–58% at mean dobutamine doses of 5–12 µg/kg/min. Similar increases in right ventricular stroke work were also observed in these studies. It significantly increases myocardial oxygen consumption; hence, milrinone is preferred over dobutamine when inodilator is needed especially in post-cardiac surgery patient. Dobutamine and isoprenaline may cause hypokalemia due to β-agonist effect.

Clinical Usage

- It is the drug of choice in patients with cardiogenic shock with adequate filling pressures.
- In septic shock, it is used as an adjunct to norepinephrine to improve organ perfusion.

Epinephrine

Epinephrine or adrenaline is a hormone that is secreted principally by the adrenal medulla in response to physical or mental stress. It is an endogenous catecholamine with a high affinity for $β_1$, $β_2$, and α1 receptors. At lower doses (<0.3 µg/kg/min), β effects are more prominent and α effects at higher doses (>0.3 µg/kg/min). It also increases pulmonary vascular resistance and pulmonary blood flow. High-dose therapy for prolonged duration can cause direct myocardial contraction band necrosis, stimulate myocardial apoptosis. It increases metabolism and stimulates glycolysis, thus increasing lactate levels.

Clinical Usage

- During cardiopulmonary resuscitation (CPR), adrenaline increases diastolic pressure and helps maintain coronary perfusion. Adrenaline infusion is used to treat the hemodynamic instability post-cardiac arrest.
- Anaphylactic shock.
- Shock with increased SVR (cold shock). Traditionally used a second-line agent in fluid refractory, dopamine resistant shock, currently, it has replaced dopamine as first-line agent for cold shock in children. Though the usage up to 1 µg/kg/min has been described, in higher doses (>0.3 µg/kg/min), adverse effects predominate.
- Cardiogenic shock with low BP. Recent evidence suggests that adrenaline may worsen the outcome of cardiogenic shock. In high resource settings, early institution of mechanical support [e.g., extracorporeal membrane oxygenation (ECMO) and left ventricular assist device (LVAD)] may improve outcome.
- Low CO state post-cardiac surgery.

Norepinephrine

It is a major catecholamine liberated by postganglionic adrenergic nerves. It is a potent vasopressor acting on $α_1$ adrenergic receptors. It increases systolic, diastolic, and pulse pressure and has minimal inotropic action. It has minimal chronotropic action, hence is desirable when tachycardia is to be avoided. It increases coronary perfusion by increasing the diastolic pressures. It decreases pulmonary vascular resistance. It also causes venoconstriction and improves venous return and thus CO. Prolonged high-dose infusion can cause ischemic effects and limb discoloration. Extravasation may cause tissue necrosis; this may be treated with local infiltration by injecting phentolamine, an α blocker.

Clinical Usage

- It is the drug of choice in distributive shock. Typically first-line drug in adult septic shock, recent evidence has emerged that vasodilation is common in pediatric septic shock as well and noradrenaline helps reduce fluid requirement and increase MAP.
- It should be used with caution in cardiogenic shock as the increase in afterload will not be tolerated by a failing ventricle.
- It is also useful in spinal shock and patients with raised intracranial pressure to maintain cerebral perfusion pressure.

Vasopressin

Vasopressin is a peptide hormone synthesized in the hypothalamus and stored in the posterior pituitary gland. It is a stress hormone released in response to hypovolemia, hypotension, and increased osmolality. It acts on the V1 receptor in vascular smooth muscle and causes vasoconstriction, V2 receptors in renal collecting duct increasing water reabsorption. It also increases the responsiveness to catecholamines. In low doses, it causes vasodilatation in pulmonary, cerebral, and pulmonary vascular beds by stimulating oxytocin receptor and stimulating NO release. Unlike catecholamines, even in severe metabolic acidosis, vasopressin receptor sensitivity is well preserved. Increased levels have been observed in hemorrhagic shock and initial few hours of septic shock, but decrease thereafter causing relative vasopressin deficiency due to depletion of the stores. Vasopressin as well as other vasopressors may reduce splanchnic blood flow.

Clinical Usage

- Low-dose vasopressin has emerged as a rescue therapy in refractory septic shock to improve the BP in volume optimized patients especially with a low SVR. It is added to norepinephrine and has been found to reduce norepinephrine requirements as well. However, it is advisable to use it as a replacement therapy for relative deficiency rather than as a vasopressor titrated to effect as in higher doses ischemic effects over coronary, splanchnic, and peripheral circulation predominate.
- It is also used as a short-term rescue therapy for post-cardiopulmonary bypass vasoplegic shock.
- It may have a role in CPR; however, current evidence does not support its routine use.

Levosimendan

Levosimendan is a calcium sensitizing agent which does not increase cyclic adenosine monophosphate (c-AMP) or calcium, both of which have adverse effects. It enhances troponin C sensitivity to calcium, augmenting contractility. It causes peripheral vasodilation by opening smooth muscle ATP-dependent K channels. It also inhibits phosphodiesterase 3 (PDE3) enzyme. It facilitates diastolic relaxation as well by potentiating cross-bridge formation. Data from clinical trials indicate that levosimendan improves hemodynamics with no attendant significant increase in cardiac oxygen consumption and relieves symptoms of acute heart failure;[7] these effects are not impaired or attenuated by the concomitant use of beta-blockers. Levosimendan also has favorable effects on neurohormone levels in heart failure patients. It is used at doses of 0.1–0.4 µg/kg/min (usually 0.2 µg/kg/min). Hemodynamic effects are maintained up to 3–7 days after stopping levosimendan infusion, due to the formation of an active metabolite, designated OR-1896.

Clinical Usage

- Congestive heart failure and cardiogenic shock with normal BP
- Dilated cardiomyopathy
- Post-cardiac surgery.

Phosphodiesterase III Inhibitors

This category includes amrinone, milrinone, enoximone, and olprinone; of which milrinone is the strongest and shortest acting and most commonly used. Milrinone is an inodilator and also has lusitropic (diastolic relaxation) properties. In the cardiac myocytes, inhibition of PDE3 increases c-AMP and increases calcium entry in the myocytes which increases myocardial contractility. Whereas in vascular smooth muscle, PDE3 inhibition increases removal of calcium from the vascular smooth muscle leading to smooth muscle relaxation and vasodilation. It causes pulmonary vasodilation, reduces pulmonary pressures and is useful in pulmonary hypertension. However, it can cause hypotension and increase the requirement of vasopressors, especially in patients with low filling pressures. It is renally excreted and should be avoided in patients with impaired creatinine clearance. The main drawback for use in septic shock is its relatively long half-life (2–4 h) if hypotension or arrhythmias occur, these adverse effects persist for hours in contrast to dobutamine. Continuous infusion of 0.25–0.75 µg/kg/min is generally reasonable. Loading dose may cause hypotension.

Clinical Usage

- Because of its nonadrenergic mechanism of action, lusitropy, less chronotropy (as compared to dobutamine) it has evolved as an indispensable agent in post-cardiac surgery patients especially with right ventricle (RV) dysfunction and pulmonary hypertension [tetralogy of Fallot (TOF)].
- It is especially useful in chronic heart failure states where adrenergic receptor downregulation/desensitization occurs due to chronic beta agonist administration.

Isoprenaline

It is a potent, nonselective β agonist, with very low affinity for α receptors. It has potent inotropic and chronotropic action, causes significant systemic and pulmonary vasodilatation. Isoproterenol is also a potent bronchodilator. As it causes severe tachycardia and potent systemic vasodilatation, it is not commonly used in the pediatric intensive care unit (PICU).

Clinical Usage

- The positive chronotropic effects of isoproterenol may be useful in children with bradycardia and mild heart blocks.
- The drug is increasingly used in electrophysiology suites to facilitate the detection of abnormal conduction pathways in infants and children under general anesthesia.

Phenylephrine

It is a potent α agonist with virtually no β action. It causes systemic and splanchnic vasoconstriction and has no effect on the heart though it may reduce CO by raising the afterload. Evidence for use in septic shock is lacking.

Clinical Usage

- It is used mainly as a rapid bolus for sudden severe hypotension, usually during anesthesia to raise MAP. It can be used for vagally mediated hypotension in diagnostic and therapeutic procedures.
- It is used in treatment of cyanotic spell in children with tetralogy of Fallot to increase SVR and reduce right to left shunting.

Nitroprusside

It causes venous and arteriolar dilatation by release of nitric oxide. It reduces both pulmonary and SVR. Peak action is seen within 2 min and it is cleared within 3 min of stopping the drug. It is inactivated in alkaline conditions and in the presence of light; hence, tubing needs to be covered with paper or foil. The dose is 0.5–8 µg/kg/min and should be titrated to effect. Side effects are cyanide toxicity, methemoglobinemia, hypotension, rebound hypertension, increased cerebral blood flow, and tachyphylaxis. Nitroprusside should be avoided in patients with liver or renal failure and those with raised intracranial pressure. Cyanide toxicity may present with altered sensorium or metabolic acidosis. Methemoglobinemia due to nitroprusside toxicity should not be treated with methylene blue as it may lead to further increase in cyanide levels.

Clinical Usage

- It can be used in the management of ventricular dysfunction with normal BP as it decreased both preload and afterload.
- It is used in the management of hypertensive emergency.

Nitroglycerine

Nitroglycerine is converted to nitric oxide which increases cyclic guanosine monophosphate (c-GMP) levels in vascular smooth muscle. Nitroglycerine primarily causes venodilatation leading to decreased preload. At doses >3 µg/kg/min, it causes arteriolar dilatation as well. It is generally used in a dose of 0.5–10 µg/kg/min. In hypovolemic patients, use of nitroglycerine may further compromise endorgan perfusion.

Clinical Usage

- Heart failure or cardiogenic shock with normal BP
- In patients with coronary insufficiency, it is helpful by decreasing preload and improving pulmonary blood flow.

NEWER AGENTS

Angiotensin II: It has been tried recently in vasodilatory shock refractory to high doses of vasopressors and has been shown to have three times greater likelihood of achieving an acceptable BP. It targets the RAAS pathway and is a powerful mediator of arterial BP. Angiotensin II is 40 times more potent than noradrenaline. Its onset of action is 10–20 s with a half-life of a few minutes; it is degraded to angiotensin III. Mechanisms of action include direct vasoconstriction by activating angiotensin I receptors, enhancement of peripheral noradrenergic neurotransmission, increased sympathetic discharge [central nervous system (CNS)], and release of catecholamines from the adrenal medulla. In the treatment of pediatric septic shock not responding to the conventional drugs, angiotensin II may have a useful role pending for further studies.

Methylene blue: Methylene blue has been used as a treatment for refractory distributive shock due to sepsis or anaphylaxis. It is a selective inhibitor of nitric oxide–cyclic guanosine monophosphate (NO–cGMP) pathway. However, definitive evidence is lacking and no mortality benefit has been documented. The ideal dose is unknown, but based on existing literature and safety profile, a single bolus of 1–2 mg/kg may be tried when patients do not respond to standard therapy.

Istaroxime: It inhibits Na^+/K^+ ATPase activity, increases intracellular calcium during systole, and improves cardiac contractility.[4] It increases systolic BP and decreases HR and may have a role in heart failure states.

Omecamtiv Mecarbil: It is a novel agent which acts as a cardiac myosin activator. It increases the efficiency of cardiac contractions without increasing oxygen consumption. It is not available for clinical practice as yet (Table 2).

There are various factors which affect vasoactive agent action such as genetic polymorphisms in the signaling cascade, receptor downregulation, developmental variations, hypoxia, and acidosis. Hence, close monitoring and dose titration at the bedside is essential.

NURSING CARE/PRACTICAL TIPS

- Vasoactive agents should be given via syringe pumps to ensure accurate delivery. Even when using syringe pumps, rate <1 mL/h might not deliver accurately.
- It takes 15–20 min for the drug to reach the circulation especially when given via long central lines. It is not advisable to bolus inotropes, higher infusion rates can be set initially to ensure faster delivery.
- Always ensure the syringe pumps are connected to a continuous power source and infusions are not interrupted. Any alarm should be attended immediately.
- Nursing staff should be trained in preparing inotropes, using syringe pumps, managing central and arterial lines, monitoring hemodynamics.

Table 2: Dosing and administration.

Medication	Vial strength	Usual dose (μ/kg/min)	Dilution in 50 mL	Diluent	IV infusion rate
Dopamine (central line concentration)	1 mL/40 mg	5–15	30 mg/kg	NS/D5	1 mL/h = 10 μg/kg/min
Dopamine (peripheral line concentration)	1 mL/40 mg	5–15	3 mg/kg	NS/D5	1 mL/h = 1 μg/kg/min
Dobutamine (central line concentration)	1 mL/50 mg	5–15	30 mg/kg	NS	1 mL/h = 10 μg/kg/min
Dobutamine (peripheral line concentration)	1 mL/50 mg	5–15	3 mg/kg	NS	1 mL/h = 1 μg/kg/min
Epinephrine	1 mL/1 mg	0.01–1.0	0.3 mg/kg	NS/D5	1 mL/h = 0.1 μg/kg/min
Norepinephrine	1 mL/1 mg	0.05–0.5	0.3 mg/kg	D5	1 mL/h = 0.1 μg/kg/min
Vasopressin	1 mL/20 units	0.0001–0.0005 units/kg/min	0.3 units/kg	NS/D5	1 mL/h = 0.0001 unit/kg/min
Milrinone	1 mL/1 mg	0.3–0.9	1.5 mg/kg	NS	1 mL/h = 0.5 μg/kg/min
Sodium nitroprusside (SNP) (to be covered with foil)	1 mL/25 mg	0.5–8	3 mg/kg	D5	1 mL/h = 1 μg/kg/min
Nitroglycerine (NTG)	1 mL/5 mg	0.5–10	3 mg/kg	D5	1 mL/h = 1 μg/kg/min
Phenylephrine	1 mL/10 mg	0.1–0.5	0.3 mg/kg	D5/NS	1 mL/h = 0.1 μg/kg/min

(IV: intravenous; NS: normal saline)

- Ensure a dedicated port for inotrope infusion—appropriately labeled.
- The syringe must be labeled with the amount of drug and dilution.
- Continuous monitoring and documentation of HR, BP, complement fixation test (CFT), pulses, urine output, inotropic therapy is a must.
- The bedside nurse should be alert and commence piggy backing/double pumping when 1 h/5 mL of infusion is remaining (start a fresh infusion when the syringe is about to empty to ensure continuous delivery).
- When inotropes have been discontinued, block the line and do not give bolus through the line. The line should not be used for several hours. Alternatively, a normal saline infusion at a low rate may be started to flush the line.

Vasoactive Agents

- Vasoactive agents can be given by peripheral line, external jugular vein or intraosseous route until central line access is obtained.[1] Extravasation of vasoconstrictors may cause severe tissue necrosis. In the case of extravasation injury due to alpha adrenergic agonists, phentolamine can be injected locally. Vasoconstrictors can also worsen skin or limb ischemia in children with thrombosis.

GOALS OF VASOACTIVE THERAPY

The ultimate goal in shock management is to increase CO and maintain organ perfusion. BP is the most commonly chased parameter, but it is a pressure measure and does not reflect flow. Certain vasoactive agents increase BP at the cost of perfusion (Fig. 3). Clinical judgment with multimodal monitoring is needed to decide if an agent is needed that increases heart contractility or modifies vascular tone (Table 3 and Flowchart 1).

In spite of having normal BP, regional perfusion may remain poor. Hence, rather than a single parameter, one should rely on a comprehensive evaluation including bedside clinical evaluation along with blood markers of tissue perfusion, functional echocardiography, along with the latest gadgets for CO measurement (if available). Nothing can replace frequent bedside clinical assessment of mental status, skin temperature, color, pulse volume, cardiac resynchronization therapy (CRT), HR, urine output, BP, respiratory rate, and work of breathing. Clinical assessment is supplemented with blood lactates and mixed venous oxygen saturations. Lactate level is related to morbidity and mortality and is useful in detecting patients with subclinical shock who have deceptively reassuring clinical signs due to catecholamine storm. Mixed venous oxygen saturation reflects the balance between oxygen delivery and oxygen consumption. Low values indicate increased oxygen extraction due to CO not being high enough to meet the tissue needs. Functional echocardiography and invasive CO monitoring is now available and is useful in severe shock to guide therapy. Vasoactive

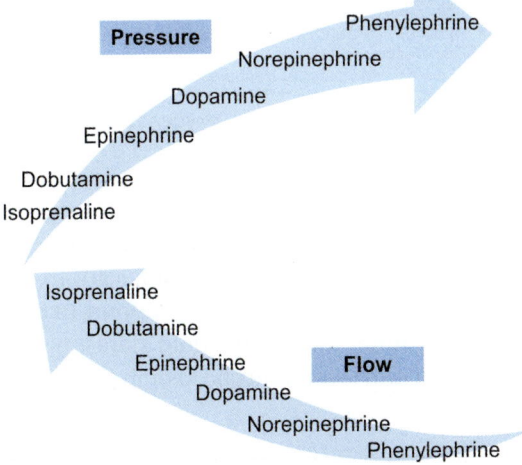

Fig. 3: Effects of vasoactive agents on blood pressure and blood flow. Modified from Hollenberg.

Table 3: Vasoactive agent indicated according to type of shock.

Hemodynamic parameter	Treatment
Low CI, high SVR, normal BP	Inodilators (e.g. milrinone, dobutamine, levosimendan)
Low CI, high SVR, low BP	Adrenaline, optimize fluid therapy If BP still low, noradrenaline If BP normalizes and perfusion still poor, add inodilator
Low CI, low SVR, low BP	Noradrenaline, optimize fluids Vasopressin

Normal cardiac index (CI): 3.3–6 L/min/m². Normal systemic vascular resistance index (SVRI): 700–1600 Dynes/s/cm⁵/m².
(BP: blood pressure)

Flowchart 1: Choice of vasoactive agents in different types of shock.

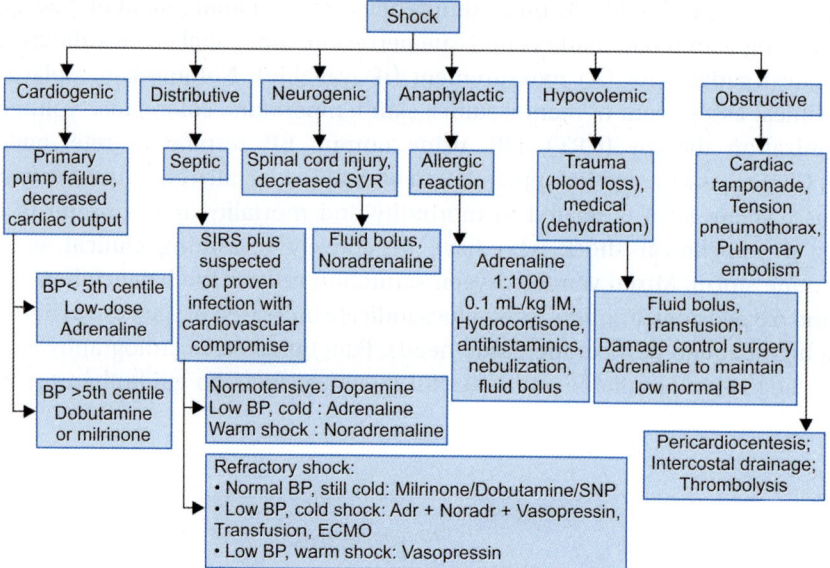

(BP: blood pressure; ECMO: extracorporeal membrane oxygenation; SNP: sodium nitroprusside; SIRS: systemic inflammatory response syndrome)

agents should be used with an intention to target normal pressure and perfusion. Declining lactates, with improving tissue perfusion are a reassuring sign. In face of persistent clinical signs of shock and low mixed venous levels, inotropic support may have to be increased. In addition to increasing inotropes, other factors like fluid status, need for transfusion, source control, and electrolytes (e.g., calcium level) must be kept in mind.

CONCLUSION

Timely and appropriate vasoactive agent therapy may save lives. However, evidence of their impact on clinical outcomes in randomized trials has been minimal, despite their widespread

use in cardiovascular illness. Hence, bedside evaluation of physiologic state, selection of vasoactive agent according to action desired (contractility or manipulation of vascular tone) and titration of dose to desired effect is essential.
- Norepinephrine is considered the first-line vasopressor in vasodilatory shock (warm shock).
- Dobutamine or milrinone is used in shock associated with decreased CO (cardiogenic shock).
- Epinephrine is the first-line catecholamine in CPR and is replacing dopamine as initial agent in cold shock.
- Vasopressin in replacement doses should be considered in refractory septic shock.

KEY MESSAGES

- Use vasoactive agents at the lowest dose required for the shortest possible time.
- Rather than using very high doses of a single inotrope, adding another vasoactive agent based on physiological state is preferable.
- Dobutamine/milrinone should be added when signs of hypoperfusion are ongoing despite adequate volume and mean arterial pressure (MAP).
- Add vasopressin for refractory septic shock in replacement doses.
- Noradrenaline should be considered when pulse pressure is high and cardiac function is good.
- In cardiogenic shock, inodilators and low-dose inotropes are preferable.

ACKNOWLEDGMENTS

We thank Dr Dinesh Chirla and Dr Rakshay Shetty, who wrote the chapter in the previous edition.

SUGGESTED READING

1. Backer D, Aldecoa C, Njimi H, et al. Dopamine versus norepinephrine in the treatment of septic shock: A meta analysis. Crit Care Med. 2012;40(3):725-30.
2. Belletti A, Benedetto U, Biondi-Zoccai G, et al. The effect of vasoactive drugs on mortality in patients with severe sepsis and septic shock, a network meta-analysis of randomized controlled trials. J Crit Care. 2017;91-8.
3. Bishop NB, Greenwald BM, Notterman BA. Pharmacology of the cardiovascular system. In: Fuhrman BP, Zimmerman JJ (Eds). Fuhrman and Zimmerman's Pediatric Critical Care, 5th edition. Philadelphia: Elsevier; 2016. pp. 352-79.
4. Christopher B, Overgaard, Vladimir D. Inotropes and vasopressors. Circulation. 2008;118:1047-56.
5. Davis A, Carcillo J, Aneja R, et al. American College of Critical Care Medicine Clinical Practice parameters for hemodynamic support of pediatric and neonatal septic shock. Crit Care Med. June 2017;45(6):1061-92.
6. Francis G, Bartos J, Adatya S. Inotropes. J Am Coll Cardiol. May 2014;63(20):2069-78.
7. Hollenberg SM. Inotrope and vasopressor therapy of septic shock. Am J Respir Crit Care Med. 2011;187:847-55.

8. Leopold V, Gayat E, Pirrachio R, et al. Epinephrine and short-term survival in cardiogenic shock: an individual data meta-analysis of 2583 patients. Intensive Care Med. June 2018;44(6):847-56.
9. Levy MM, Evans LE, Rhodes A. The surviving sepsis campaign bundle: 2018 update. Crit Care Med. 2018;46(6);997-1000.
10. Tume S, Schwartz S, Bronicki R. Pediatric Cardiac Intensive Care Society 2014 Consensus Statement: Pharmacotherapies in cardiac critical care treatment of acute heart failure. Pediatr Crit Care Med. March 2016;17(3):S16-19.

Hypertensive Crises 15

Indira Jayakumar, U Sridhurga

LEARNING OBJECTIVES

- To understand the terms associated with the condition
- To understand the physiological basis of the condition
- To be able to manage hypertension in the urgent setting

INTRODUCTION

Hypertension is prevalent in 2–5% of pediatric population and hypertensive emergencies account for 1% of emergency department visits. Children with severe hypertension or rapid increase in blood pressure (BP) can present with life-threatening condition.

ACUTE SEVERE HYPERTENSION

The term acute severe hypertension encompasses both hypertensive emergency and urgency. Acute severe hypertension is usually associated with rapid increase in BP and the absolute value is often 30 mm Hg above stage II hypertension (as defined later).

HYPERTENSIVE EMERGENCY

It is defined as severe symptomatic elevation of BP associated with potentially life-threatening symptoms or with acute target organ damage. The organs that can be affected are brain (hypertensive encephalopathy), heart (congestive heart failure), kidney [acute kidney injury (AKI)], and retina (papilledema, exudates, and hemorrhages).

HYPERTENSIVE URGENCY

It is defined as severe symptomatic elevation of BP with no life-threatening symptoms or target organ damage. They present with mild symptoms like headache and vomiting.

Table 1: Definitions of BP categories of and stages.	
For children aged 1–13 years	*For children aged ≥13 years*
• *Normal BP*: <90th percentile	• *Normal BP*: <120/<80 mm Hg
• *Elevated BP*: ≥90th percentile to <95th percentile or 120/80 mm Hg to <95th percentile (whichever is lower)	• *Elevated BP*: <120/<80 mm Hg to 129/<80 mm Hg
• *State 1 HTN*: ≥95th percentile to <95th percentile + 12 mm Hg or 130/80 to 139/89 mm Hg (whichever is lower)	• *Stage 1 HTN*: 130/80 mm Hg to 139/89 mm Hg
• *Stage 2 HTN*: ≥95th percentile + 12 mm Hg or ≥ 140/90 mm Hg (whichever is lower)	• *Stage 2 HTN*: ≥140/90 mm Hg

Source: American Academy of Pediatrics (AAP), 2017.
(BP: blood pressure; HTN: hypertension)

MALIGNANT HYPERTENSION

It is defined as acute elevation in BP with impairment of at least three different target organs or the presence of microangiopathic hemolytic anemia. Previously, the same was defined as acute increase in BP with or without previous hypertension, associated with stage III or IV retinopathy.

Blood pressure levels should be interpreted based on age, sex, height, based on which new normative table has been proposed in the fourth report (Task Force Report on the diagnosis, evaluation and treatment of high BP in children and adolescents from 1 year to 18 years of age). The normative curve in second report is still used to define hypertension in infants.

- *Normal blood pressure*: Systolic and diastolic BP less than 90th centile or 120/80 mm Hg. Definitions of BP categories of and stages (Table 1).
- *Elevated blood pressure*: Systolic and/or diastolic BP between 90th centile and 95th centile or 120/80 to 129/80, whichever is lower.
- *Stage I hypertension*: Systolic and/or diastolic BP between 95th centile and 95 + 12 mm of Hg or 130/80 to 139/89, whichever is lower.
- *Stage II hypertension*: Systolic and/or diastolic BP more than 95th centile + 12 mm of Hg or more than 140/90, whichever is lower.

APPLIED PHYSIOLOGY

Blood pressure = Cardiac output × Systemic vascular resistance.

Based on the above physiological equation, BP can be elevated due to either increased cardiac output or systemic vascular resistance. Irrespective of the primary cause, hypertension results in endothelial damage, activates local coagulation cascade, platelet clumping, and fibrinoid necrosis. This causes organ dysfunction as well as increase in systemic vascular resistance perpetuating the elevated BP. The other factors which increase BP are increased sympathetic activation and fluid overload. In addition, increased BP causes pressure natriuresis, volume depletion, and secondary activation of renin–angiotensin–aldosterone system (RAAS).

When BP is above the higher level of autoregulation, it affects cerebral blood vessels leading to vasogenic edema and resultant "reversible encephalopathy syndrome", which manifests as blurring of vision, altered sensorium, seizures, and stroke (Fig. 1).

In the hypertensive patient, the organ autoregulation curves (coronary, cerebral, and renal) are shifted to the right. Sudden, rapid drop in perfusion pressures could cause life-threatening organ ischemia.

ETIOLOGY

Table 2 summarizes the etiology of hypertension.

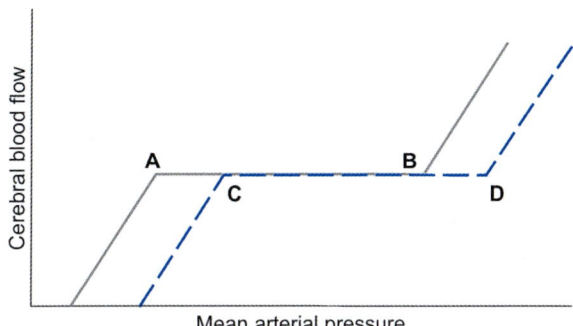

Fig. 1: Autoregulation of cerebral blood flow.
A–B normal range 60–150 mm Hg. C–D shifts to the right in chronic hypertension

Table 2: Etiology of hypertension.	
Renal	• Glomerulonephritis • Pyelonephritis • Hemolytic uremic syndrome • Obstructive uropathy • Reflux nephropathy • Renal anomalies • Renal tumors • Renal trauma
Renovascular	• Renal artery stenosis • Renal vein thrombosis • Renal artery thrombosis • Vasculitis
Endocrine causes	• Hyperthyroidism • Cushing syndrome • Congenital adrenal hyperplasia • Primary hyperaldosteronism • Catecholamine secreting tumors
Cardiovascular	• Coarctation of aorta • Middle aortic syndrome
Miscellaneous	• Liddle's syndrome • Glucocorticoid remediable aldosteronism • Apparent mineralocorticoid excess • Pseudohypoaldosteronism type II • Drug-induced steroids, cyclosporine, cyclophosphamide • Hyperkalemia • *Neurological causes*: GBS, familial dysautonomia
Primary hypertension	
(GBS: Guillain–Barré syndrome)	

Table 3: Clinical features.

System	Symptoms and signs
Neurology	Altered sensorium, headache, seizures, stroke, visual loss, posterior reversible encephalopathy syndrome (PRES)
Cardiovascular	Palpitation (pheochromocytoma), dyspnea, orthopnea, paroxysmal nocturnal dyspnea, raised jugular venous pressure (JVP), gallop, radiofemoral delay (coarctation of aorta)
Respiratory	Rales, dyspnea, hemoptysis (vasculitis)
Abdomen	Hepatomegaly, mass (neuroblastoma), renal artery bruit (renal artery stenosis)
Eye	Visual disturbance, fundus changes
Skin	Petechiae, purpura (vasculitis)
Renal	Hematuria, generalized edema

CLINICAL PRESENTATION

The clinical presentation depends on the target organ affected and the etiology (Table 3).

INVESTIGATIONS

The investigations can be divided into:
- To identify severity of end-organ damage: This includes fundoscopy, echo, renal functions, and computed tomography (CT) scan or magnetic resonance imaging (MRI).
- To ascertain etiology of hypertension:
  - Urine for proteinuria, hematuria, casts, spot protein/creatinine ratio (PCR), and 24 hours urinary protein
  - Blood urea, serum creatinine, and serum electrolytes
  - Ultrasound abdomen—to look for renal size, discrepancy in renal size, and mass
  - Renal vein Doppler—it is useful in children more than 8 years who are cooperative. If there is a strong suspicion of renal artery stenosis either CT or MR angiography can be done.

Based on clinical suspicion, further workup for etiology can be done as follows:
- Vasculitis workup
- *Central nervous imaging*: CT/MRI brain
- Renal biopsy
  - *Endocrine workup*: 24 hours urinary metanephrines and normetanephrines, cortisol level, thyroid profile, porphyrins plasma renin activity and aldosterone levels
- *Echocardiography*: To look for coarctation of aorta or left ventricular hypertrophy
- *Drug levels*: Tacrolimus and cyclosporine

MANAGEMENT

Initial Stabilization

As for any other emergency, the airway, breathing, and circulation must be assessed and stabilized. *Always remember to measure four-limb blood pressure.*

Measurement of Blood Pressure

Invasive BP monitoring is the gold standard. But if unavailable or not feasible either oscillometric techniques validated for children or auscultatory method can be used with appropriate size cuff. The bladder width should be 40% of mid-arm circumference measured between acromion process and olecranon. The length of the bladder should be 80% of the mid-arm circumference.

Target

In case of life-threatening symptoms, the rate of reduction of BP should be slow and gradual as given below:
- Reduction targets
- First 8–12 hours: 20–25% of the target
- Next 8–12 hours: Next 25%
- *Next 24 hours*: 50%.

Subsequently the BP is gradually reduced to 90th from the 95th centile over days. In case of comorbidities like chronic kidney disease (CKD), diabetes mellitus, the target is 50th to 90th centile.

Drugs Used (Table 4)

Vasodilators:
- *Direct vasodilators*:
  - Hydralazine
  - Sodium nitroprusside
  - Diazoxide
  - Minoxidil.

Calcium channel blockers:
- Nifedipine
- Nicardipine
- Amlodipine.

Vasodilators can cause reflex tachycardia and fluid retention. It is optimum to combine with sympatholytic drugs. Sodium nitroprusside causes cyanide toxicity when there is associated renal failure or prolonged/high-dose infusion. Nifedipine through sublingual route is not preferred due to the risk of rapid drop in BP and end-organ damage. Vasodilators cause increase in intracranial pressure (ICP) due to dilatation of cerebral blood vessels and increase in cerebral blood flow, so contraindicated in hypertension associated with raised ICP.

Table 4: Antihypertensive drugs.

Class	Drugs	Mechanism of action	Side effects
Direct vasodilators	Hydralazine Sodium nitroprusside Diazoxide Minoxidil	Decreases systemic vascular resistance	Reflex tachycardia Fluid retention Cyanide toxicity
Calcium channel blockers	Nifedipine Nicardipine Amlodipine	Decreases systemic vascular resistance	Reflex tachycardia Fluid retention
Sympatholytic	α- and β-blockers: Labetalol β-blocker: Esmolol α-blocker: Phenoxybenzamine Central $α_2$-agonist: Clonidine	β-blocker: Decreases RAAS α–blocker: Decreases SVR	• Hyperglycemia, bradycardia • Contraindicated in asthma, acute heart failure
ACE inhibitor	Enalaprilat	Blocks RAAS and causes vasodilatation	Precipitous drop in BP, hyperkalemia, dry cough
Diuretics	Furosemide Torsemide Spironolactone	Reduces preload and reduces cardiac output	Dyselectrolytemia

(ACE: angiotensin-converting enzyme; RAAS: renin–angiotensin–aldosterone system; SVR: systemic vascular resistance)

Sympatholytic agents:
- *Labetalol*: Alpha- and beta-blocker (1:7)
- *Esmolol*: Beta-blocker
- *Phenoxybenzamine*: Alpha-blocker
- *Clonidine*: Central alpha-agonist.

Beta-blockers are contraindicated in asthma and acute heart failure. They can cause hyperglycemia and bradycardia. Labetalol is the first-line of management in hypertensive emergencies. Phenoxybenzamine is used in pheochromocytoma where isolated beta-blocker can cause unopposed alpha-mediated hypertension. Clonidine can be used orally in hypertensive urgency.

Drugs blocking renin–angiotensin–aldosterone system:
Enalaprilat: It can cause precipitous fall in BP, hyperkalemia, and AKI.

Diuretics:
- Furosemide
- Spironolactone.

Furosemide is used in hypertension in renal causes associated with volume overload. Spironolactone is useful in certain types of monogenic hypertension.
- Fenoldopam, a newer drug, is a dopamine receptor agonist—limited experience in pediatrics.

Specific Conditions

In hypertensive emergencies intravenous drugs are preferred for controlled reduction of BP, whereas in hypertensive urgencies oral drugs can be used if able to take orally.
- *Aortic dissection*: Rapid reduction of systolic BP is needed. Beta-blockers are the preferred agents.
- *Coarctation of aorta*: Beta-blockers (esmolol) and RAAS blockade
- *Antiseizure medication*: If indicated.

Drug Dosage of Commonly Used Drugs

- *Labetalol*: Bolus 0.2–1 mg/kg/dose up to 40 mg/dose. Infusion 0.25–3 mg/kg/h
- *Esmolol*: 100–500 mg/kg/min
- *Sodium nitroprusside*: 0.5–10 mg/kg/min
- *Hydralazine*: 0.2–0.6 mg/kg, maximum single dose 20 mg
- *Nifedipine*: 0.25–0.5 mg/kg/dose, 6 hourly
- *Clonidine*: 2–5 mg/kg/dose to a maximum of 10 mg/kg PO and can be repeated hourly to a maximum of eight times till BP under control.

KEY POINTS

- Acute severe hypertension includes hypertensive emergency and urgency.
- Hypertensive emergency is associated with life-threatening symptoms or target organ damage.
- Hypertensive urgency is associated with severe hypertension, but no life-threatening symptoms and target organ damage.
- Controlled reduction of BP is important to avoid ischemia.

SUGGESTED READING

1. Ellis D, Miyashita Y. Management of the hypertensive child. In: Avner ED, Harmon WE, Niaudet P, Yoshikawa N, Emma F, Goldstein SL (Eds). Pediatric Nephrology, 7th edition. New York: Springer; 2016. pp. 2023-98.
2. Flynn JT. Acute severe hypertension. In: Fuhrmann BP (Ed). Pediatric Critical Care, 5th edition. Philadelphia, PA: Elsevier; 2017.
3. Flynn JT, Kaelber DC, Baker-Smith CM, et al. Clinical Practice Guideline for Screening and Management of High Blood Pressure in Children and Adolescents. Pediatrics. 2017;140(3):e20171904.
4. Lurbe E, Agabiti-Rosei E, Cruickshank J, et al. 2016 European Society of Hypertension guidelines for the management of high blood pressure in children and adolescents. J Hypertens. 2016:34(10): 1887-920.
5. Ofori-Amanfo G, Smerling A, Schleien CL. Hypertensive Crisis. In: Nichols DG, Shaffner DH (Eds). Roger's Textbook of Pediatric Intensive Care. 5th edition. Philadelphia: Wolters Kluwer; 2016.
6. Report of the second task force on blood pressure control in children–1987. Task force on blood pressure control in children. National Heart, Lung, and Blood Institute, Bethesda, Maryland. Pediatrics. 1987;79(1):1-25.

Sepsis and Septic Shock

16

Soonu Udani

LEARNING OBJECTIVES

- To learn new concepts in the definitions of sepsis
- To understand briefly, the pathophysiology
- To familiarize the reader with the latest guidelines of the Surviving Sepsis Campaign

INTRODUCTION

Septic shock remains a major cause of morbidity and mortality among children, mainly due to acute hemodynamic compromise and multiple organ failure. Guidelines undergo modification every few years and it is important to keep up with best practice standards. Emphasis remains on early recognition and aggressive therapy of septic shock and a bundled approach to the entire management.

PATHOPHYSIOLOGY

Shock refers to a dangerous, systemic, and pathological process under the effect of various drastic etiological factors, characterized by acute circulatory failure including decreased effective circulatory volume, inadequate tissue perfusion, cellular metabolism impediment, and multiple organ failure. Compensatory mechanisms and microcirculatory changes set in which are outlined in brief.

Microcirculatory Changes

- Small blood vessel constriction
- Precapillary resistance increases more than postcapillary resistance.
- Closed capillary increased resistance leads to further tissue hypoperfusion.
- Arteriovenous shunts at the tissue levels open up.
- This results in inflow to the tissues being less than outflow leading to oxygen by pass of tissues.

Compensatory Mechanisms

Decreased circulating volume→Activation of sympathetic-adrenal system → Vasoconstrictive substance increase (catecholamine, angiotension II, vasopressin, TAX2, endothelin) → a) Activation of α-receptors and constriction of blood capillaries; Plus (b) Activation of β-receptors →Opening of A-V shunts.

This results in acidosis, the local accumulation of metabolic products, an alteration of platelet function and procoagulant and anticoagulant balance disturbance, endotoxin production, and effects of humoral factors. There is effective microcirculatory stasis which reduces circulating blood volume, lowers vascular resistance and blood pressure, thereby blood supply for vital organs and causing dysfunction.

DEFINITIONS

While the early recognition of shock relies on simple clinical parameters, it is recognized that shock can exist with normal clinical parameters and may be recognized by additional biochemical markers of poor perfusion like acidosis, increasing lactates, and lowered mixed venous saturations (Box 1).

Hypotension is not necessary for the clinical diagnosis of septic shock; however, its presence in a child with clinical signs of an infection is confirmatory and sinister.

Box 1: Clinical parameters for shock.
- Decreased or altered mental status
- Prolonged capillary refill of more than 2 seconds (cold shock)
- Diminished and differential pulses (cold shock).
- Mottled cool extremities (cold shock), or flash capillary refill (warm shock)
- Bounding peripheral pulses and wide pulse pressure (warm shock)
- or decreased urine output of less than 1 mL/kg per hour.

The American College of Critical Care Medicine, in 2017, redefined the terms used in the general discussion and research on sepsis and septic shock to enable the dialog to be more specific, prevent overlapping terminology, and achieve greater clarity.

Old Definition

Systemic inflammatory response syndrome (SIRS): If two or more of the following criteria are not:
- Temperature >38°C or <36°C
- Heart rate >90/min
- Respiratory rate >20/min or $PaCO_2$ <32 mm Hg (4.3 kPa)
- White blood cell count >12,000/mm³ or <4,000/mm³
- or >10% immature bands
  There was an overemphasis on inflammation.

New Definition

What is sepsis: Sepsis is a multifaceted host response to an infecting pathogen. It is the host's deleterious, nonresolving inflammatory response to infection that leads to organ dysfunction and is not the same as sterile inflammation. It differs from sterile inflammation, by the presence of an underlying infectious process that may be significantly amplified by endogenous

Table 1: Sequential organ failure assessment.	
Variable	Points
• Respiratory rate >22/min	1
• Altered mentation	1
• Systolic blood pressure <100 mm Hg (adults)	1
qSOFA ≥2 identified patients more likely to have ICU stay ≥3 days or to die in the hospital	

factors. Sepsis is now recognized to involve early activation of both pro- and anti-inflammatory responses along with major modifications in nonimmunologic areas like cardiovascular, neuronal, autonomic, hormonal, bioenergetic, metabolic, and coagulation.

Redundant terms to be avoided include: "Sepsis syndrome" and "sepsis with SIRS".

Severe sepsis is replaced by *sepsis with organ dysfunction* denoting organ hypoperfusion but not requiring vasopressors to maintain perfusing pressure.

It is also important to realize that specific infection can cause a single organ dysfunction without a dysregulated immune response, e.g., pneumonia.

Adult scoring places emphasis on the qSOFA or sequential organ dysfunction score of more than 2 points from the baseline consequent to infection (Table 1).

This is a purely clinical score, requires no laboratory tests, is quick and repeatable but not often used in children as the values for respiratory rate and blood pressure need to be age adjusted.

Septic shock is a subset of sepsis in which underlying circulator and cellular/metabolic abnormalities are profound enough to substantially increase mortality. Criteria to define shock include:
- Persisting hypotension requiring vasopressors to maintain mean arterial pressure (MAP) for age.
- Serum lactate level more than 2 mmol/L (18 mg/dL) despite adequate volume resuscitation.

With these criteria, hospital mortality is in excess of 40%.

The guidelines and Surviving Sepsis Campaign recommend a "BUNDLED" approach whereby a standard fairly protocolized approach could be used by an institution to deliver timely and standardized care with an aim toward improving sepsis outcomes globally. Institutions should form their own workable bundles according to needs and compliance factors.

In an understandable way and to get across the urgency, Jean Louis Vincent explained the phases of sepsis in this simple way which would correspond to bundles and each unit could make their own corresponding sets within the principles of management.

These are expanded below to cover the major components of management (Table 2):
- *Salvage*

  Recognition and IV access in 15 minutes: To recognize sepsis using clinical and biochemical parameters within the first 15 minutes. If the patient meets criteria for severe sepsis, anticipate fluids, antibiotics, cultures, and laboratories being ordered if not done yet.

  Resuscitation: As soon as shock is recognized, the patient should be given 100% oxygen if the airway is maintainable. Crystalloid fluid normal saline (NS) boluses up to 30 mL/kg.

Table 2: Phases and components in the management of septic shock.

Salvage	Optimize	Stabilize	De-escalate
Provide minimum acceptable blood pressure	Provide adequate oxygenation	Organ support	Wean from vasoactive agents
Lifesaving measures	Optimize cardiac output, ScVO$_2$, Lactate	Minimize complications	Achieve negative fluid balance

Source: Adapted from Vincent JL, De Backer D. Circulatory shock. NEJM. 2013.

Here the 2017 guidelines make a distinction from the earlier use of liberal fluids with these caveats (Box 2):

Getting intravenous access may be difficult early in the course of shock especially in small children and rapid use of intraosseous access should be utilized which is useful for the administration of all fluids and medication. Time should not be wasted in attaining a central line. Each fluid bolus should be followed by quick assessment of clinical parameters like improvement in heart rate as per age, capillary refill time (CRT), equalizing of peripheral and central pulses, blood pressure, sensorium and urine output. Hypoglycemia and hypocalcemia should be corrected.

Box 2: 2017 guidelines basic tenets of fluid resuscitation.
- Some do and some do not
- Shock may be euvolemic or even hypervolemic
- Anemic patients require platelet RBCs
- Malnourished patients require slow fluids
- Cardiac failure patients require inotropes and less or no fluids
- First bolus 10–20 mL/kg
- No more than 40 mL/kg without full assessment for overload and myocardial dysfunction (USG, Echo)
- Suggest adding albumin in patients who require repeated boluses of crystalloids
- Slow boluses rather than rapid in certain situations
- Restore mean arterial pressure rather than systolic blood pressure

Monitoring should include pulse oximetry, continuous electrocardiography, blood pressure, and pulse pressure (noninvasive blood pressure is only reliable when pulses are palpable). Note pulse pressure and diastolic pressure to help distinguish between low systemic vascular resistance (SVR) [wide pulse pressure: pulse pressure >50% systolic blood pressure (SBP)] and high SVR (narrow pulse pressure <1/3rd of SBP). Temperature, urine output, glucose, and ionized calcium should also be checked (anion gap and lactate, if facilities available).

- *Fluids:* Crystalloids remain the mainstay of resuscitation. Start with boluses of 20 mL/kg, titrated to clinical parameters of cardiac output (CO) including heart rate, peripheral pulses, CRT <3, improved sensorium, and urine output. Initial volume resuscitation requirements may be 10 mL/kg if crepitations or hepatomegaly are present but 40–60 mL/kg is not uncommon in the first 1–3 hours. Patients who do not respond to fluid boluses, should be considered for invasive hemodynamic monitoring, preferably after 30 mL/kg. This can be helpful to optimize preload and CO. Observation of little change in the central venous pressure (CVP) (<2 cm H$_2$O) in response to a fluid bolus suggests that the venous system is not overfilled and that more fluid may be tolerated or needed. Observation that an increasing CVP more than 5 cm H$_2$O is met with reduced MAP–CVP suggests that too much fluid has been given. This remains a loose guide and has its own fallacies.

Large volumes of fluid for acute stabilization in children have not been shown to increase the incidence of the acute respiratory distress syndrome (ARDS) or cerebral edema and fluids should not be withheld at this acute stage (Box 3).

> **Box 3:** Principles of fluid administration.
> - Quantity more important—liberal use
> - Crystalloids initially 30 mL/kg
> - No hexaethyl starch
> - Albumin if "large" quantities of crystalloids needed or gelatin-based colloids
> - Restore BP to minimal acceptable for age
> - Achieve reversal of signs of shock
> - Heart rate, equal central per pulses and temperature, sensorium, urine output, capillary refill time <3

- *Antibiotics*: Broad-spectrum antibiotics should be administered early preferably within first hour of therapy after taking appropriate cultures but should not delay therapy, as each passing hour increase chances of mortality. Antibiotics should be chosen based on suspected community-acquired or hospital-acquired infection, local resistance pattern of organism, site of infection, and whether immune-compromised or immune-competent and past history of chronic illness. Any site of localized pus collection should be drained once child is stable enough for procedure. Antibiotics can be de-escalated later according to culture sensitivity reports. The dose should be maximised for bodyweight and volume of distribution of edema fluid and given to optimize drug levels. Subsequent doses could be adjusted for creatinine clearance.
- *Within 1–3 hours of severe sepsis*:
  - Measure lactate level
  - Obtain blood cultures prior to administration of antibiotics
  - Administer broad-spectrum antibiotics
  - Minimum 30 mL/kg crystalloid for hypotension or lactate more than or equal to 4 mmol.
- *Airway and breathing*: Airway and breathing should be rigorously monitored and maintained especially earlier than fluid resuscitation if it is unmaintainable. Lung compliance and work of breathing may change precipitously. In early sepsis, patients often have a respiratory alkalosis from centrally mediated hyperventilation. As sepsis progresses, patients may have hypoxemia as well as metabolic acidosis and are at high risk to develop respiratory acidosis secondary to a combination of parenchymal lung disease and/or inadequate respiratory effort due to altered mental status. The decision to intubate and ventilate is based on clinical assessment of increased work of breathing, hypoventilation, or impaired mental status. Waiting for confirmatory laboratory tests is discouraged. Up to 40% of CO is used for work of breathing. Therefore, intubation and mechanical ventilation can reverse shock. If possible, volume loading and peripheral or central inotropic/vasoactive drug support is recommended before and during intubation because of relative or absolute hypovolemia, cardiac dysfunction, and the risk of suppressing endogenous stress hormone response with agents that facilitate intubation. High flow devices or even Noninvasive ventilation could be instituted prior to intubation to provide some positive end-expiratory pressure (PEEP) and improve recruitment. The use of nasal prongs or high flow cannulae during intubation prevents hypoxia during the period of apnea in children with low respiratory reserve. Ketamine pretreatment and benzodiazepine post-intubation can be used as a sedative/induction regimen of choice to promote cardiovascular integrity. Atropine

may increase heart rate and could be avoided except in possible high vagal tone. It could be kept as a stand by medication. A short-acting neuromuscular blocker like rocuronium can facilitate intubation (rapid sequence intubation RSI) if the provider is confident she/he can maintain airway patency. All sedatives are cardiodepressive and can unmask shock and lead to profound hypotension and even arrest and hence need to be used with the utmost caution.

If the BP is low, epinephrine (EPI) is the agent of first choice even in peripheral dilution and Dopamine has taken a back seat in the new algorithm. However, the stage of fluid refractory shock is an important defining step as the mortality changes when the patient fails to respond to fluids and first-line vasopressor.

- *Optimize*: Within 6 hours of initial symptoms for septic shock:
  - Apply vasopressors (for hypotension that does not respond to initial fluid resuscitation) to maintain a MAP more than or equal to 65 mm Hg
  - In the event of persistent hypotension after initial fluid administration (MAP < 65 mm Hg/age related) or if initial lactate was more than or equal to 4 mmol/L
  - Re-assess volume status and tissue perfusion and document findings
  - Multimodal monitoring advocated
  - Re-measure lactate if initial lactate elevated.

The bundle is then extended into a further period of optimization of tissue perfusion. The aim here is to optimize the MAP as for age as one marker of tissue perfusion along with lactate and mixed venous oxygen saturation (SVO_2) levels. This is also the period where fluids and vasoactive agents will be titrated and optimized and multimodal monitoring will be used for this process. Whether we use terms like early goal directed therapy as in the Rivers study or any other protocol, the principles of optimizing tissue perfusing and restoring the balance between utilization and delivery of substrate to the tissues remain the goals of therapy.

The continued emphasis is directed to: first hour fluid resuscitation and inotrope drug therapy directed to goals of (i) reducing heart rate to threshold level for age; (ii) getting peripheral pulse to match central pulse volume; (iii) improving mentation; (iv) improving urine output to at least 1 mL/kg/hr; (v) reducing CRT to less than 3 seconds. This assessment is done after each bolus and a quick check for overload in the form of rapid expansion of the liver span, rales and increased work of breathing and enlargement of the cardiac silhouette on Chest X-ray is done.

- *Fluid refractory shock*: If despite of 60 mL/kg of fluid, therapeutic end points like capillary refill less than 2 seconds, threshold heart rate, normal pulses with no differential between the quality of the peripheral and central pulses, warm extremities, urine output more than 1 mL/kg/h, normal mental status, blood pressure more than fifth centile for age, are not met, shock is defined as fluid refractory and child should be shifted to PICU for further monitoring. The patient may still require more fluid boluses with continuous monitoring of clinical parameters to avoid fluid overload. Fluid responsiveness can also be checked using invasive (arterial line) and noninvasive (Doppler echo, USG) methods. These are best described in the chapter on hemodynamic monitoring.
- *Optimizing cardiac output*: Adults have low SVR and tachycardia and maintain their CO by that mechanism. Low CO, not low SVR, is associated with mortality in pediatric septic shock. In 50 children with fluid-refractory catecholamine resistant shock, the majority

(58%) showed a low CO/high SVR state, and only 22% had low CO and low vascular resistance. A reduction in oxygen delivery rather than a defect in oxygen extraction, can be the major determinant of oxygen consumption in children. Unlike adults, a reduction in oxygen delivery rather than a defect in oxygen extraction, can be the major determinant of oxygen consumption in children and hence the recommendation is that a therapeutic goal of cardiac index (CI) 3.3–6.0 L/min/m² may result in improved survival and attainment of the therapeutic goal of oxygen consumption (VO_2) more than 200 mL/min/m² may also be associated with improved outcome. While these parameters may not be easily measurable at various levels of care in our country, certain practice guidelines for manipulation of fluids and inotropes with these in mind as therapeutic goals that would ultimately give clinically apparent endpoints that are easily measurable at the bedside could result in more rational use of fluids, vasoactive drugs, PRBCs, and supportive measures.

If we agree that organ perfusion and substrate delivery is our ultimate aim, then we need to define some perfusion pressure at which this delivery will take place. This will depend on CO, MAP, the CVP, and the SVR. The perfusion pressure being the (MAP – CVP)/SVR. Much of our effort is spent in keeping this equation in balance during the treatment of septic shock. To define it as vasodilatory or vasoconstrictive is to oversimplify the problem as there are overlapping elements and varying CO states between the two conditions in any given patient.

Increased vascular resistance is identified by absent or weak distal pulses, cool limbs, prolonged CRT more than 3 seconds, and narrow pulse pressure with relatively increased diastolic BP.

- *Vasoactive drugs*: In the fluid refractory patient, begin a peripheral inotrope EPI 0.05–0.3 while establishing a central venous line. When administered through a peripheral IV/intraosseous catheter, the inotrope should be infused either as a dilute solution or with a second carrier solution (piggy backing) running at a flow rate to assure that it reaches the heart in a timely fashion. Care must be taken to reduce dosage if evidence of peripheral infiltration/ischemia occurs as alpha adrenergic receptor-mediated effects occur at higher concentrations of dopamine.

Once the central line has been established dopamine, epinephrine, or norepinephrine can be administered as a first line drug as indicated by the hemodynamic state. It is generally appropriate to wait until an effect is observed before stopping the peripheral infusion

- *Titration of vasoactive drugs (Flowchart 1)*: Children with catecholamine resistant shock can present with low CI/high SVR, high CI/ low SVR, or low CI/low SVR shock. There may be mixed types which are confusing and difficult to diagnose. There is no single recipe and no right and wrong but broad principles of management based on clinical and multimodal monitoring parameters. Although children with persistent shock commonly have worsening cardiac failure, hemodynamic states may completely change with time.
- *Shock with low CI ($SCVO_2$ < 70%), normal blood pressure, and high SVR*: This clinical state is similar to that seen in a child with cardiogenic shock in whom afterload reduction is a mainstay of therapy designed to improve blood flow by reducing ventricular afterload and thus increasing ventricular emptying. Dobutamine (5–20 μg/kg/min) or phosphodiesterase inhibitors (PDEIs) like milirinone can be used. Additional volume loading may be necessary to prevent hypotension when loading doses of milrinone are used. Owing to their long half-life, its effects like hypotension and tachyarrythmia or both can be reversed with infusion of norepinephrine or vasopressin.

Flowchart 1: The algorithm from the American College of Critical Care Medicine Clinical Practice Parameters for Hemodynamic Support of Pediatric and Neonatal Septic Shock, 2017.

0 min — Recognize decreased mental status and perfusion. Begin high flow O_2 and establish IO/IV access according to PALS

5 min — If no hepatomegaly or rales/crackles, then push 20 mL/kg isotonic saline boluses and reassess after each bolus up to 60 mL/kg until improved perfusion. Stop for rales, crackles or hepatomegaly. Correct hypoglycemia and hypocalcemia. Begin antibiotics

15 min — **Fluid refractory shock?**

Begin peripheral IV/IO inotrope infusion, preferably epinephrine 0.05–0.3 µg/kg/min. Use atropine/ketamine IV/IO/IM if needed for central vein or airway access

Titrate epinephrine 0.05–0.3 µg/kg/min for cold shock.
(Titrate central dopamine 5–9 µg/kg/min if epinerphrine not available)
Titrate central norepinephrine from 0.05 µg/kg/min and upward to reverse warm shock.
(Titrate central dopamine ≥10 µg/kg/min if norepinephrine not available)

60 min — **Catecholamine-resistant shock?**

If at risk for absolute adrenal insufficiency consider hydrocortione use doppler US, PICCO, FATD or PAC to direct fluid, inotrope, vasopressor, vasodilators goal is normal MAP-CVP, $ScvO_2$ >70%* and CI 3.3–6.0 L/min/m^2

Normal blood pressure cold shock — $ScvO_2$ <70%* / Hb >10 g/dL on epinephrine? → Begin milrinone infusion. Add nitroso-vasodilator if CI <3.3 L/min/m^2 with High SVRI and/or poor skin perfusion. Consider levosimendan if unsuccessful

Low blood pressure cold shock — $ScvO_2$ <70%* / Hb >10 g/dL on epinephrine? → Add norepinephrine to epinephrine to attain normal diastolic blood pressure. If CI <3.3 L/min/m^2 add dobutamine, enoximone, levosimendan, or milrinone

Low blood pressure warm shock — $ScvO_2$ >70%* on norepinephrine? → If euvolemic, add vasopressin, terlipressin, or angiotensin. But, if CI decreases below 3.3 L/min/m^2 add Epinephrine, dobutamine, enoximone, levosimendan

Persistent Catecholamine-resistant shock? — Evaluate pericardial effusion or pneumothorax, maintain IAP <12 mm Hg

Refractory shock? — ECMO

- *Shock with low CI, low blood pressure, and low SVR*: Norepinephrine (NE) (0.04–1 µg/kg/min) can be added to epinephrine to increase diastolic pressure and thereby MAP and SVR. Once an adequate blood pressure is achieved, dobutamine, type III PDEI (particularly enoximone, which has little vasodilatory properties), or levosimendan can be added to norepinephrine to improve CI and $ScvO_2$.
- *Shock with high CI and Low SVR*: When titration of norepinephrine and fluid does not resolve hypotension, then low dose vasopressin 0.0003–0.0008 IU/kg/minute can be helpful in restoring blood pressure; however, these potent vasoconstrictors can reduce CO; therefore it is recommended that these drugs are used with CO/$ScvO_2$ monitoring. It is recommended in a replacement and not a vasopressor dose to avoid its ill effects.

In addition to this and simultaneously in the first 6 hours, it is generally agreed that the application of "Early Goal Directed Therapy" (EGDT) where the following parameters are also fulfilled, leads to a better outcome. What does EGDT try to do? (Box 4).

It restores the balance between delivery and demand quickly by manipulating preload, afterload and contractility using fluids, inotropes, vasodilators to enhance delivery, and PRBCs to deliver more oxygen by increasing O_2 content. Early ventilator support is important as well for complete success and full support, as both oxygen delivery and consumption will then be diverted from the respiratory muscles to more deserving and needy organs and tissues.

> **Box 4:** Early goal-directed therapy (Rivers).
>
> - Normal mean arterial presuure—central venous pressure (CVP) (>60) and mixed venous saturation >70%
> - Urine output >1 mL/kg/hr and cCVP >8–12 cm H_2O
> - All 4 goals to be met for success
> - Done by:
>   – Increasing inotropes/dobutamine and fluids
>   – Sedation and MV to reduce O_2 consumption
>   – Platelet RBCs to keep Hb 10 g/dL

That this could be replicated in a developing country in a crowded busy city like Sao Paulo in Brazil was shown by Oliviera in 2008.

When there is refractory shock: Ask yourself
- Why still hypotensive
- Why not responding
- Other causes of shock
- Check Echo/USG abdomen/source control/bleeding/pneumothorax/cardiac tamponade
- Is abdominal pressure high?
- Is there adrenal failure?

Stabilization: The second phase of optimization is probably the longest and will go into the phase of stabilization.

The emphasis here will be on preventing or reversing organ dysfunction and consolidation of all treatment goals. There will be many balls in the air here and all will have to be juggled simultaneously as laboratory values start to come in and have to be acted upon rationally (Box 5).

Fluid losses and persistent hypovolemia secondary to diffuse capillary leak can continue for days. Fluid therapy is continued with crystalloid or colloid to achieve above goals with continuous monitoring of clinical parameters to avoid fluid overload.

> **Box 5:** Adjustment of parameters during the stabilization phase.
>
> - Antibiotics adjusted as cultures and other values come in
> - Inotropes need constant adjusting
> - *Fluid balance*: Will be time to cut down boluses and reduce even regular fluids
> - *Monitoring*: Multimodal monitoring several times a day for adjustment of fluids and inotropes
> - Ventilation
> - *Oxygenation*: Lactate and $ScVO_2$ to check tissue perfusion
> - *Organ protection*: Nephron and hepatotoxic drugs and substrate delivery
> - Renal function and possible replacement therapy
> - Nutrition for tolerance and calorie delivery
> - Acid–base balance
> - Sedation to minimal levels tolerated and avoiding neuromuscular paralysis

Packed cell transfusion may be given to maintain hemoglobin of more than 10 g/dL if child is hemodynamically unstable and between 7 g/dL and 9 g/dL if shock is controlled. Fresh frozen plasma (FFP) may be used as infusion not as bolus, if international normalized ratio

(INR) is prolonged and bleeding tendency is present. Evidence points to use of FFP when there is bleeding along with deranged coagulation parameters.

Elevated lactate concentration and anion gap measurement can be treated by assuring both adequate oxygen delivery and glucose utilization. Adequate oxygen delivery (indicated by a $ScvO_2 > 70\%$) can be achieved by attaining hemoglobin more than 10 g/dL in a hemodynamically unstable patient (See Flowchart 1).

Steroid therapy: Much debate has been on steroid administration, but recent European multicenter trial in septic adults [the Corticosteroid Therapy of Septic Shock (CORTICUS) trial] showed no benefit of adjunctive hydrocortisone on 28-day mortality. A retrospective study in children using administrative data showed that steroid use was associated with increased mortality and resource utilization. At this point it is only recommended if a child is at risk of absolute adrenal insufficiency or adrenal pituitary axis failure (e.g., purpura fulminans, congenital adrenal hyperplasia, prior recent steroid exposure, hypothalamic/pituitary abnormality) and remains in shock despite adequate fluids with titrated epinephrine and or norepinephrine infusion. Hydrocortisone may be administered as an intermittent or continuous infusion at a dosage which may range from 1 mg/kg every 6 hrly titrated to reversal of shock and tapered once vasopressor support is not required. Recent recommendations are in favor of a single dose.

Glucose and calcium: Glucose delivery rates (GDR) for normal humans are age specific but can be met by delivering a D5-10%-containing maintenance fluid (8 mg/kg/min glucose in newborns, 3-5 mg/kg/min in older children). Hypoglycemia is brain damaging and therefore potentially more lethal in the long and short-term than transient hyperglycemia and must be strictly avoided.

Hyperglycemia is also a risk factor for mortality. Lin and Carcillo reported that children with septic shock, who had hyperglycemia (>140 mg/dL) and acidosis, showed resolution of their anion gap when insulin was added to their glucose regimen.

Insulin requirements usually decrease at approximately 18 hours after the onset of shock. Infusion of insulin and glucose are also effective inotropes. Best outcomes are probably associated with using D5 containing maintaining fluids to ensure glucose delivery and treating hyperglycemia of over 150–180 mg/dL with insulin.

Hypocalcemia contributes to cardiac dysfunction. Calcium replacement should be directed to normalize ionized calcium concentration. Routine calcium levels, even when corrected to albumin levels, are fallacious as the milieu affects the ionized state. Hypercalcemia is also detrimental and overzealous correction should be avoided.

- *De-escalation phase*: This may come after several days. The patient may be fluid overloaded by several liters and on high ventilator settings. The blood pressure may have stabilized and other parameters could be looking better. There are some areas where treatment could be brought down in intensity and some invasive devices could be removed.

Some parameters that would be checked at this stage would be:
- *Echo*: Improved with no systolic or diastolic dysfunction
- SVO_2: >70%
- CVP → 10–12 cm H_2O
- Lactate → <2 mmol/L
- Hb → 9 g/dL
- Inotropes reduced to their minimum

Order of deceleration of inotropes is not etched in stone and depends on the usefulness of each and hemodynamics but as a rule of thumb, the highest doses likely to cause damage could be reduced first:
- Fluid overload is calculated daily by the using the patients admission weight in kg. with a cumulative intake and output in liters. (fluid intake (L)—total output (L))/baseline body weight (in kilograms)] × 100 is the general formula used which does not take into account insensible losses. A positive balance of more than 10% is consider actionable as over 15% is associated with increased ventilator days, hypoxemia and possibly mortality. The choice of fluid removal varies but usually diuretics given as a continuous infusion starting as a low dose of Furosemide and titrating to 1 mg/kg/hr with an eye on potassium levels works.

Principles of removing fluid stepwise:
- Diuresis with infusion of furosemide
- Try other diuretics: metazolone, thiazides, if F does not work
- If diuretic resistant then some form of ultrafiltration
- *Peritoneal dialysis*: weak
- Continuous renal replacement therapy/slow low efficiency dialysis or continuous venovenous hemodialysis→with UF when BP stable
    - *Antibiotics*: As far as possible these need to be de-escalated to the narrowest spectrum possible for the organism obtained. If cultures are sterile, the deescalation could be based on recovery or source patterns. Review every 48 hours.
    (When deciding on the most appropriate antibiotic(s) to prescribe, consider the following factors: recent antibiotic treatment, potential drug interactions, potential adverse effects (e.g. *C. difficile* infection is more likely with broad spectrum antibiotics), consider removal of any foreign body/indwelling device, drainage of pus, or other surgical intervention. For advice on appropriate investigation and management of infections, consult your local infection specialist).
    - Consider removing any indwelling devices that you may not be needed or used. Including urinary catheters. Do not keep a line that you "may need later" or keep intubated "for just one more day". Extubate to a noninvasive device if possible.
    - Consider early feeding and mobilization.
    - Mobilization in bed, out of bed, in a chair are all helpful in prevention of bedsores and infection and expanding the lungs. Gentle limb physiotherapy can be started.
    - Sedative drugs need to be reduced and neuromuscular blocking agents removed or used sparingly as needed only for specifically documented reasons. The earlier these drugs are removed the lesser the chance of critical illness neuromyopathy and prolonged hospital stay. Withdrawal and slow weaning will also be avoided.
    Some patients may take 3-7 days in this de-escalation phase or longer and some like dengue may be in it for only 24-48 hours. The underlying disease and the hemodynamic disturbance will be the determinant of the time frame (Box 6).

Box 6: FAST HUG BID for a daily reminder for all ICU patients.
- Feeding
- Analgesia
- Sedation
- Thromboembolism prophylaxis (not so much in small children)
- Head end up
- Stress ulcer prophylaxis
- Glycemic control
- Bowel clear 2 times per day
- Indwelling lines consider removing
- Descalate antibiotics

Table 3: Modified pediatric RIFLE criteria.

	Serum creatinine criteria	Urine output criteria
Risk	eCCL decreased by 25%	Urine output <0.5 mL/kg/h × 8 hours
Injury	eCCL decreased by 50%	Urine output <0.5 mL/kg/h × 16 hours
Failure	eCCL decreased by 75% or eCCL <35 mL/min/1.73 m²	Urine output <0.3 mL/kg/h × 24 hours, or anuria × 12 hours
Loss	Persistent failure (>4 weeks)	
End-stage kidney disease	End-stage kidney disease (>3 months)	

(eCCL: estimated creatinine clearance); The acronym RIFLE stands for the increasing severity classes—risk, injury, and failure—and the two outcome classes—loss and end-stage kidney disease.

Table 4: Classification using renal failure indices.

	Prerenal	Renal
Urine sediment	Bland	Broad, brownish granular casts
Urine sodium (mEq/L)	<20	>40
Urine osmolality (mosm/L)	>500	<350
Fractional excretion of sodium (Na)	<1%	>2%

(Fractional excretion of Na = Urine/plasma Na divided by urine/plasma creatinine x 100)

RENAL SUPPORT

Renal dysfunction is now well recognized as an independent risk factor for increased morbidity and mortality, particularly when dialysis is needed. It is defined as serum creatinine more than two times the upper limit of normal for age or twofolds increase in baseline creatinine. Intensivists prefer the modified pediatric RIFLE criteria to define and classify acute kidney injury as shown in Table 3. Managing renal dysfunction is simplified by classifying renal failure into prerenal and renal causes by using renal failure indices (Table 4). Fractional excretion of urea (FEurea) can be used by replacing sodium to urea into the same formula if diuretics have been used. Cutoff values for FE urea are less than 35% for prerenal azotemia and greater than 50% for ATN.

The goals of therapy are to prevent further injury by maintaining kidney perfusion with ionotropes or vassopressor and judicious use of fluids to prevent fluid overload and further ischemic damage to the kidney. The nephrotoxic drugs should either be avoided or adjusted as per estimated creatinine clearance.

Schwartz formula $\left[\text{GFR (mL/min/1.73 m}^2\text{)} = k \times \dfrac{\text{height in centimeter}}{\text{serum creatinine}} \right]$ can be used to calculate GFR where k is 0.33 in preterm infants, 0.45 in infants, and 0.55 in older children.

Schwartz formula is not accurate in a sick child with rapidly changing physiological status. Measuring creatinine clearance directly by using the following formula is better estimate of GFR:

$$\frac{\text{urine creatinine} \times \text{volume of urine in mL/min}}{\text{plasma creatinine}} \times \frac{1.73}{\text{body surface area in m}^2}$$

In a sick child with oliguria and kidney injury, it is better to assume GFR less than 10 while dosing. The rise in creatinine occurs well after the injury and drop in GFR.

Monitoring should continue with hourly input/output charting, electrolyte monitoring, and use of early renal replacement once medical therapy fails to correct the complications. The indication for renal replacement therapy are oliguria/anuria with fluid overload refractory to diuretic therapy, persistent hyperkalemia, severe metabolic acidosis, and severe electrolyte abnormality not responding to medical measures.

The choice of dialysis therapy for acute renal failure depends upon clinical circumstances, patient location, and expertise available. This is discussed in the Chapter 23: Basics of RRT in ICU.

HEPATIC DYSFUNCTION

It is defined as total bilirubin of more than 4 mg/dL or alanine aminotransferase twice the normal limit for age as per organ dysfunction criteria Table 2. The Pediatric Acute Liver Failure Study Group defined acute liver failure as follows:
- Biochemical evidence of liver injury
- No history of known chronic liver disease
- Coagulopathy not corrected by vitamin K administration
- International normalized ratio greater than 1.5 if the patient has encephalopathy or greater than 2.0 if the patient does not have encephalopathy.

KEY MESSAGES

- Septic shock in children still constitutes a clinical challenge for healthcare providers, both in the emergency department and the intensive care unit.
- Early diagnosis, allowing rapid therapeutic intervention is essential in improving the outcome of these patients.
- Current treatment includes early fluid resuscitation, tailored use of inotropes and vasopressors, and use of adjuvant treatments, such as low dose hydrocortisone and intravenous immunoglobulin (IVIG) are not known to help.
- Forming a team and following a protocol designed for success within an institution is known to be helpful.

APPENDIX: REFERENCE CHARTS FOR CHILDREN

Normal heart rate by age (beats/minute)		
Age	Awake rate	Sleeping rate
Neonate (<28 d)	100–165	90–160
Infant (1 month–1 year)	100–150	90–160
Toddler (1–2 years)	70–110	80–120
Preschool (3–5 years)	65–110	65–100
School-age (6–11 years)	60–95	58–90
Adolescent (12–15 years)	55–85	50–90

Normal respiratory rate by age (breaths/minute)	
Age	Normal respiratory rate
Infants (<1 year)	30–55
Toddler (1–2 years)	20–30
Preschool (3–5 years)	20–25
School-age (6–11 years)	14–22
Adolescent (12–15 years)	12–18

Normal blood pressure by age		
Age	Systolic blood pressure (mm Hg)	Diastolic blood pressure (mm Hg)
Birth (12 hours)	60–85	45–55
Neonate (96 hours)	67–84	35–53
Infant (1–12 moths)	80–100	55–65
Toddler (1–2 years)	90–105	55–70
Preschooler (3–5 years)	95–107	60–71
School-age (6–9 years)	95–110	60–73
Preadolescent (10–11 years)	100–119	65–76
Adolescent (12–15 years)	110–124	70–79

SUGGESTED READING

1. Akcan AA, Zappitelli M, Loftis LL, et al. Modified RIFLE criteria in critically ill children with acute kidney injury. Kidney Int. 2007;71(10):1028-35.
2. Arikan AA, Zappitelli M, Goldstein, SL, et al. Fluid overload is associated with impaired oxygenation and morbidity in critically ill children. Ped Crit Care Med. 2012;13(3):253-8.
3. Carcillo JA, Pollack MM, Ruttimann UE, et al. Sequential physiologic interactions in cardiogenic and septic shock. Crit Care Med. 1989;17:12-6.
4. Ceneviva G, Paschall JA, Maffei F, et al. Hemodynamic support in fluid refractory pediatric septic shock. Pediatrics. 1998;102:e1.
5. Davis AL, Carcillo JA, Aneja RK, et al. American College of Critical Care Medicine Clinical Practice Parameters for Hemodynamic Support of Pediatric and Neonatal Septic Shock. Crit Care Med. 2017;45(6):1061-93.
6. Han YY, Carcillo JA, Dragotta MA, et al. Early reversal of pediatric-neonatal septic shock by community physicians is associated with improved outcome. Pediatrics. 2003;112:793-9.
7. Kumar A, Roberts D, Wood KE. Duration of hypotension prior to initiation of effective antimicrobial therapy is the critical determinant of survival in human septic shock. Crit Care Med. 2006;34:1589-96.
8. Lin JC, Carcillo JA. Increased glucose/glucose infusion rate ratio predicts anion gap acidosis in pediatric sepsis. Crit Care Med. 2004;32(Suppl 20):A5.
9. Maitland K, Kiguli S, Opaka RO, et al. Mortality after fluid bolus in African children with severe infection. N Engl J Med. 2011;364:2483-95.

10. Pollack MM, Fields AI, Ruttimann UE. Distributions of cardiopulmonary variables in pediatric survivors and nonsurvivors of septic shock. Crit Care Med. 1985;13:454-9.
11. Rivers E, Nguyen B, Havstad S. Early Goal-Directed Therapy Collaborative Group. Early goal-directed therapy in the treatment of severe sepsis and septic shock. N Engl J Med. 2001;345(19):1368-77.
12. Singer M, Deutschman CS, Seymour CW, et al. The Third International Consensus Definitions on Sepsis and Septic Shock. JAMA. 2016;315(8):801.
13. Sprung CL, Annane D, Keh D. Hydrocortisone therapy for patients with septic shock. N Engl J Med. 2008;358(2):111-24.
14. Vincent JL, De Backer D. Circulatory Shock. NEJM. 2013.

Approach to a Comatose Child

17

Manisha Patil, Arun Bansal

LEARNING OBJECTIVES

- To understand the levels of impaired consciousness
- To know the etiopathogenesis of coma
- To learn the management of a comatose child.

INTRODUCTION

Coma is a relatively common medical emergency in pediatrics. Diagnosing and managing a comatose child is a challenging task as the potential causes are numerous. Epidemiological studies generally divide the etiology as traumatic and nontraumatic. The incidence of traumatic coma is 670/100,000 per year and that of nontraumatic coma is 30/100,000 children per year. The incidence of nontraumatic coma is much higher in children as compared to in adults. Central nervous system (CNS) infections are the leading cause of nontraumatic coma in low-income and low-middle income countries.

DEFINITIONS

Consciousness is a state of normal arousal (wakefulness) and awareness of self and environment, thus allowing an individual to perceive, interact, and communicate.

This requires an intact cerebral cortex and reticular activating system. Due to lack of uniformity, various terms used to describe levels of wakefulness such as somnolence, stupor, obtundation, and lethargy are usually avoided.

Coma is a state of sustained, pathologic altered consciousness with loss of both domains (arousal and awareness) lasting for at least 1 hour. It is characterized by no verbal output, response to voice, spontaneous eye opening, and localization to painful stimuli.

It is a type of transitory state that may evolve toward recovery or minimally conscious state or may worsen to a vegetative state or brain death.

The minimally conscious state is a condition in which, though minimal, there is a definite evidence of self or environmental awareness along with altered consciousness as demonstrated by the response to simple commands.

A vegetative state is characterized by complete loss of awareness, i.e., loss of cerebral cortical function with variable preservation of sleep–wake cycle and brainstem function. Hence in this condition, the patient may keep his eyes open without visual fixation or pursuit. It is usually diagnosed if it persists for more than 1 month after the onset of coma.

In brain death, there is the permanent absence of all brain functions, i.e., cortical and brainstem, the patient is irreversibly comatose and apneic with absent brainstem reflexes.

ETIOLOGY (TABLE 1)

Based on the primary site of insult, the causes of coma can be broadly divided into two categories, the CNS causes and non-CNS causes. In non-CNS causes, coma occurs as a manifestation

Table 1: Etiology of coma.

CNS	Non-CNS

A. *Traumatic*
 • Parenchymal injury
 • Intracranial hemorrhage: Subdural, subarachnoid, epidural, intracerebral
 • Diffuse axonal injury
 B. *Nontraumatic*
 • Infections:
   – Bacterial meningitis
   – Viral meningoencephalitis
   – Cerebral malaria
   – Tubercular meningitis
   – Brain abscess
   – Subdural/epidural empyema
   – Rickettsial meningoencephalitis
   – Rabies
   – Toxic encephalopathy (enteric fever, Shigella encephalopathy)
 • *Postinfections/postimmunization*:
   – Acute demyelinating encephalomyelitis
   – Whole cell DPT/Semple rabies vaccine
   – Multiple sclerosis
 • *Vascular*:
   – Arterial ischemic stroke
   – Sinus venous thrombosis
 • *Mass lesions*:
   – Neoplasm
   – Hydrocephalus
 • *Paraoxysmal neurological disorder*:
   – Seizures/status epilepticus
   – Acute confusional migraine
	A. *Metabolic*
	 • Hypoglycemia
	 • Dyselectrolytemia
	 • Diabetic ketoacidosis
	 • Uremia
	 • Hyperammonemia (secondary to Reye's syndrome, hepatic encephalopathy)
	 • *IEM*: mitochondrial, organic acidemia urea cycle disorders
	 • Acute Porphyria
	 B. *Toxic*
	 • *Toxins*: Organophosphates, carbamates, lead poisoning
	 • *Envenomation*: snakebite
	 • *Medications*: Barbiturates, sedatives tricyclic antidepressants
	 • *Illicit substance abuse*: Opioids, alcohol, amphetamines

(DPT: diphtheria/pertussis/tetanus; IEM: inborn errors of metabolism; CNS: central nervous system)

of derangements secondary to toxins or metabolic disorders. Multiple interrelated reasons may be present in a single patient, e.g., a child with bacterial meningitis may be comatose because of hyponatremia secondary to syndrome of inappropriate antidiuretic hormone secretion (SIADH).

EVALUATION OF THE COMATOSE CHILD

Coma is a medical emergency and is usually a manifestation of the life-threatening condition. Hence, the primary aim is to provide immediate life support for initial stabilization followed by a neurological assessment to identify the cause and start specific therapy. This all has to proceed simultaneously to prevent further deterioration or secondary brain injury.

Initial stabilization involves the ABCDE approach:
- *Airway*: In a comatose child due to depressed sensorium and loss of tone in oropharyngeal muscles, tongue falls back and blocks the airway and may also cause pooling of secretions and thereby increase the risk of aspiration. Hence, maintaining an open airway is of utmost importance. This can be done by adequate positioning (head-tilt-chin-lift, jaw thrust in trauma patients) suctioning, inserting nasopharyngeal/oral airway, or endotracheal intubation in patients with poor respiratory drive. Assume cervical injury in every case of trauma and stabilize the cervical spine.
- *Breathing*: Ensure adequate oxygenation by commencing bag and mask ventilation (BMV) in case of inadequate chest movements, poor respiratory efforts, central cyanosis or SpO_2 less than 94%, or poor air entry. Consider endotracheal intubation in raised intracranial pressure (ICP), refractory status epilepticus, hypotensive shock, severe respiratory distress, or failure or prolonged need of BMV.
- *Circulation*: Establish vascular access and maintain adequate perfusion by using fluids or vasoactive drugs to maintain permissive cerebral circulation. Hypertension at presentation can be a consequence of cause or effect of coma.
- *Disability*: Assess neurological status by modified Glasgow Coma Scale (GCS). Treat seizures with IV benzodiazepines followed by IV phenytoin. Identify signs of raised ICP (posturing, unequal pupils, Cushing's triad) and if present, rapidly institute measures to decrease the ICP (manual hyperventilation, osmotherapy). Correct hypoglycemia, hypocalcemia, and hypothermia.
- *Exposure*: Examine for any evidence of trauma, rash, petechiae, purpura. Treat fever/hypothermia appropriately.

Assessment:
- *Focused history*: A detailed history along with a description of events prior to the onset of coma is very crucial to identify the cause of coma.
- *Sudden onset*: Caused by trauma, spontaneous intracranial hemorrhage, seizures, toxin exposure, or envenomation.
- *Slow-progressive conditions*: Expanding mass, hydrocephalus, or indolent infection (TBM).
- *History of fever*: Consider an acute infectious etiology; bacterial meningitis, viral encephalitis, or tropical fever spectrum. But some disorders such as acute disseminated encephalomyelitis, mitochondrial disorders, or Reye's syndrome can also be preceded by a febrile illness.
- *Recurrent episodes*: Suggestive of an inborn error of metabolism, or vascular malformation.

Focused examination: The general physical and neurological examination can provide important clues for identifying the etiology of coma.
- *Temperature*: Both fever and hypothermia may suggest an infective process.
- *Vitals*: Abnormal heart rate, respiratory rate may be caused by fever, shock, or acidosis. Hypotension can be the result of traumatic injury, sepsis, cardiac dysfunction, or toxic ingestion. Features of chronic hypertension (retinopathy, left ventricular hypertrophy) may be present in hypertensive encephalopathy although hypertension can also be a compensatory mechanism (to maintain cerebral perfusion) in raised ICP. Cushing's triad comprising bradycardia, irregular breathing, and hypertension is an ominous sign of brain herniation.
- *Skin examination*: Look for pallor (malaria, intracranial bleed), cyanosis (shock), jaundice (malaria, leptospirosis, hepatitis, enteric fever), petechiae [dengue, disseminated intravascular coagulation (DIC)], or neurocutaneous markers (intracranial malformation).
- The cardiovascular, respiratory, and abdominal examination can point toward the underlying cause.

Neurological examination: The neurological examination helps in localizing the CNS dysfunction and helps in identifying the cause. As the examination requiring patient's cooperation, so cannot be performed, focus on evaluating the level of consciousness, cranial nerves, motor system, brainstem function, and identifying any herniation syndromes.
- *Level of consciousness*: Objective assessment is done by a modified GCS.
- *Examination of cranial nerves*: Evaluates cortical and brainstem control of cranial nerve pathways.
- *Eye examination*: It involves examination of fundus and pupil.
  Signs seen in fundus examination:
  - *Papilledema*: Indicates intracranial hypertension but it takes time to develop, hence, its absence does not rule out raised ICP.
  - *Retinal hemorrhage*: Trauma or disorders of coagulation
  - *Flame-shaped hemorrhages with exudates*: Hypertensive encephalopathy
  - Pupillary examination helps in assessing the brainstem and third nerve function.
  - Examine size, shape, symmetry, and response to light. Pupillary changes usually occur very late in metabolic encephalopathy as compared with structural lesions.
  - Depending on the site of dysfunction, different findings in pupil examination are:
    - *Pontine lesions*: Pinpoint
    - *Midbrain*: Mid-position fixed
    - *Tectal*: Large nonreactive
    - *Metabolic*: Small reactive
    - *Opiate/Organophosphate poisonings*: Pinpoint
    - *Hypoxic-ischemic encephalopathy*: Bilateral fixed dilated
    - *Anticholinergic, sympathomimetic, antidepressant poisoning*: Dilated and fixed.
  Unless proved, unilateral pupillary dilatation in a comatose patient should be considered as an evidence of ipsilateral uncal herniation causing oculomotor nerve compression after excluding mydriatic instillation.
  - *Examination of brainstem function*: Disappearance of roving eye movements in comatose child signifies brainstem dysfunction. In a comatose patient without spontaneous

eye movement, oculocephalic (doll's eye) and oculovestibular reflex assess the midbrain and pons function. The medullary function is evaluated by corneal, gag, and cough reflexes.
- *Lateral gaze palsy*: It is seen in compression of bilateral sixth nerves due to central herniation (raised ICP causing stretching of nerves).
- *Conjugate lateral deviation of eyes*: Indicates a lesion in ipsilateral hemisphere, seizure focus in a contralateral hemisphere or involvement of contralateral parapontine reticular formation (horizontal gaze center).
- *Dysconjugate gaze*: Indicates 3rd, 4th or 6th cranial nerve or extraocular muscle involvement.
- *Tonic upwardgaze*: Seen in bilateral hemispheric damage.
- *Tonic downgaze*: Suggests dorsal midbrain compression.
- *Motor system examination*: Observe trunk and limbs for the position, spontaneous movements, response to stimuli, and examine deep tendon reflexes. Asymmetry in movements and reflexes suggests the involvement of the corticospinal tract. Decorticate or decerebrate posturing signals toward herniation syndromes. Resistance to the extension of the knee when hips are flexed (Kernig sign) or involuntary flexion of the hip when the neck is flexed (Brudzinski sign) suggests meningeal irritation. Identify any involuntary movements as dystonia (extrapyramidal involvement), or myoclonic jerks [subacute sclerosing panencephalitis (SSPE)] which can help in identifying the pathology and etiology.
- *Herniation syndromes*: Whenever there is increased intracranial pressure, there will be displacement of brain tissue from higher to lower pressure giving rise to herniation syndromes (Table 2).

Table 2: Herniation syndromes.

Central herniation: Increased pressure in both cerebral hemispheres causes downward displacement of diencephalon and brainstem compression. It has four stages:

1. Diencephalic stage	Cheyne–Stokes respiration, small reactive pupils with preserved oculocephalic/oculovestibular reflex, withdrawal to pain, and/or decorticate posturing
2. Midbrain–upper pons stage	Hyperventilation, mid-position nonreactive pupils with minimal or absent oculocephalic/oculovestibular reflex, extensor response to pain and/or decerebrate posturing
3. Lower pons–medulla stage	Shallow or ataxic respiration, mid-position nonreactive pupils with no response to oculocephalic/oculovestibular reflex and pain except for withdrawal to plantar stimulation
4. Medullary stage	Slow, irregular respiration, fixed dilated pupils with absent ocular movements, and generalized flaccidity
Uncal herniation: Uncus of temporal lobe displaced	Unilateral fixed dilated pupils with ptosis (3rd nerve palsy) with same-sided hemiparesis
Subfalcine herniation (cingulate)	Paraparesis
Tonsillar herniation (lower brainstem)	Impaired consciousness, lower cranial nerves involvement, respiratory and cardiovascular involvement. Preserved pupillary reflexes and vertical eye movements

Investigations (Box 1)

These can be divided into definite investigations which must be done in all patients with coma and probable investigations which will depend on the etiology.

Definite Tests

- As outlined in initial stabilization, immediate blood glucose, electrolytes (sodium, potassium, calcium, magnesium), complete hemogram, renal function, and liver function tests are a must in all patients.
- If a child is febrile with signs/symptoms (pallor, organomegaly, capillary leak, bleeding, eschar) suggestive of tropical infections, then perform peripheral smear/RDT (malaria), dengue NS1/IgM (dengue, depending on the day of illness), scrub typhus, and leptospira serology.
- Lumbar puncture is a must in any febrile patient unless contraindicated, i.e., intracranial hypertension, hemodynamic instability, focal signs, local site infection, or thrombocytopenia. In such scenario, defer the procedure and treat for suspecting infection. Delay in lumbar puncture should not delay the treatment.
    - Cerebrospinal fluid (CSF) sample should be tested for cell count, protein, glucose, Gram stain, latex agglutination, culture, herpes simplex virus serology, Ziehl-Nelsen stain, acid-fast bacilli (AFB) smear (if symptomatology is for >1 week), and additional tests as per clinical suspicion.
    - Computed tomography (CT) scan should be done in all children with coma after initial resuscitation except in a known metabolic cause; hypoglycemia or diabetic ketoacidosis (DKA). It will detect intracranial bleed, hydrocephalus, cerebral edema, tumor, and meningeal enhancement (infection, brain abscess, or neurocysticercosis). In traumatic coma, CT is indicated if GCS less than 15, 2 hours postinjury, basilar, open or depressed skull fracture, seizures, persistent, or frequent vomiting.

Probable Tests

- *Electroencephalogram (EEG)*: Specific pattern of EEG can help in identifying etiology; periodic lateralized epileptiform discharges are seen in herpes simplex encephalitis, triphasic

---

Box 1: Investigations.

Definite
- Complete blood count
- Blood glucose
- Serum electrolytes (sodium, potassium, calcium, magnesium),
- Renal function test
- Liver function tests
- *If fever*: Peripheral smear for MP/rapid malarial antigen test, dengue NS1/IgM, scrub typhus, leptospira serology, lumbar puncture
- CT scan

Probable
- EEG
- MRI
- Urine toxicology screen
- Blood ammonia levels
- TMS/GCMS, blood carnitine levels
- Urine for porphobilinogen
- ANA, ESR
- TFT, thyroid antibodies

(CT: computed tomography; EEG: electroencephalogram; ESR: erythrocyte sedimentation rate; GCMS: gas chromatography mass spectroscopy; MRI: magnetic resonance imaging; TFT: thyroid function test; TMS: tandem mass spectrometry)

waves in uremic or hepatic encephalopathies, diffuse theta and delta waves along with the absence of faster frequencies in severe encephalopathies. Nonconvulsive status epilepticus in a comatose child is a known phenomenon. Hence, a prolonged EEG can detect subclinical seizures.
- Magnetic resonance imaging (MRI) should be done in patients with unexplained cause of coma or normal/equivocal CT findings. It helps in diagnosing many conditions depending on the characteristic involvement; thalamic hyperintensities in Japanese B encephalitis, asymmetrical hyperintensities in frontotemporal lobe in herpes simplex encephalitis, demyelination in acute disseminated encephalomyelitis (ADEM), or necrotizing lesions in acute necrotizing encephalopathy. It also helps in prognostication, but the benefit must be weighed against the risk of transporting the critically ill patient.
- Urine toxicology screen in patients with no identifiable cause or suspected poisoning.
- Patients presenting with recurrent episodes of encephalopathy should have blood ammonia levels, tandem mass spectrometry/gas chromatography mass spectroscopy (TMS/GCMS) considering the inborn error of metabolism. These tests should be done before stopping feeds and starting treatment to get adequate results.
- In unexplained cases, possibility of CNS vasculitis, porphyria, and Hashimoto's encephalopathy should be kept, and specific investigations [thyroid function test (TFT), thyroid antibodies, urine for porphobilinogen, antinuclear antibody (ANA), erythrocyte sedimentation rate (ESR)] should be done.

TREATMENT

The management of a comatose child should usually proceed along with clinical evaluation and neurological assessment. Treatment should involve supportive and definitive management.

Supportive treatment will be the first-line of treatment to all patients presenting to the emergency department with coma. It involves:
- Initial resuscitation and stabilization (as mentioned earlier).
- Ensure normothermia, normoxia (SpO$_2$ >94%), normovolemia by assessing hydration status (heart rate, pulse pressure).
- Correct hypoglycemia and any electrolyte abnormalities.
- Identify any signs of raised ICP and treat accordingly to prevent herniation and prevent a further rise in ICP.
- General nursing care: Minimal handling, prevent pressure sores by changing positions frequently, and adequate care of eyes to prevent exposure keratitis.
- Monitor vitals, assess neurological status, and identify any new signs of worsening.

Definitive treatment follows the supportive management and will differ depending on the etiology. It involves:
- *Treatment of infections*:
  - In suspected sepsis/meningitis, start broad-spectrum antibiotics (ceftriaxone) immediately.
  - If viral encephalitis is likely, start acyclovir after collecting a sample for HSV PCR.
  - If suspecting tropical infections, start antimalarials (quinine/artesunate) and doxycycline (rickettsial infections).

- *Treatment of poisonings/envenomation*:
  - *Antidotes*: Naloxone in opioid poisoning, atropine in organophosphorus poisoning and flumazenil in benzodiazepine overdose.
  - Antisnake venom in neuroparalytic snakebite
- Steroids in tubercular meningitis, ADEM, or enteric encephalopathy
- Treat specific metabolic causes; renal function in uremia, underlying hepatitis in hepatic encephalopathy, and hyperglycemia in DKA.

PROGNOSIS

Prognosis mainly depends on the severity and etiology of coma. Children who survive infective encephalopathies usually have better outcomes. Poor prognostic factors are young age, lower GCS, and brainstem dysfunction at presentation.

KEY MESSAGES

- Initial stabilization and supportive management is the key to prevent secondary brain injury.
- Identify features of raised ICP and prevent herniation syndromes.
- Identify and treat metabolic causes (hypoglycemia, electrolyte imbalances).
- Commence specific therapy depending on the etiology.
- Etiology and severity of coma helps in prognostication.

SUGGESTED READING

1. McCarthy ML, Serpi T, Kufera JA, et al. Factors influencing admission among children with traumatic brain injury. Acad Emerg Med. 2002;9:684.
2. Shaffner DH, Nichols DG. Chapter Roger Textbook of Pediatric Intensive Care, 5th edition.US: Wolters Kluwer Health; 2015.
3. Sharma S, Kochar GS, Sankhyan N, et al. Approach to the child with coma. Indian J Pediatr. 2010;77:1279-87.
4. Wong CP, Forsyth RJ, Kelly TP, et al. Incidence, aetiology, and outcome of non-traumatic coma: A population-based study. Arch Dis Child. 2001;84:193-9.

Head Injury in Children

18

Soonu Udani

LEARNING OBJECTIVES

- To categorize the severity of head injury
- To consider a stepwise approach to the management of head injury
- To manage increased intracranial pressure
- Treatment

INTRODUCTION

Severe traumatic brain injury (STBI) is a leading cause of mortality and morbidity with a poor chance of intact outcome. The reported mortality in developed countries with excellent emergency medical services that start in the out-of-hospital setting is 9–35%. This has to be much higher in developing countries, where children have poor access to quality health care. Childhood head injuries are the result of domestic accidents, motor vehicle accidents, recreational injuries, and sports mishaps. Non-accidental injuries or child abuse must always be kept in mind when the pattern of injury does not fit the history.

Primary brain injury: This is the direct result of the physical trauma. It may result in uncomplicated concussion with quick recovery and no residual deficit or in serious hemorrhage, contusion or hematomas. Whereas these are all visible on a CT scan, diffuse axonal injury (DAI) can be a severe condition where the initial CT scan may look deceptively benign. Primary injury can only be prevented by prevention of the accidental trauma itself.

Secondary brain injury: Occurs after the primary event due to potentially preventable causes (hypoxia, hypoperfusion, hypercarbia, hematoma) and hence must be prevented as far as possible.

The very events that are thrown into play with the occurrence of the primary injury potentially result in secondary injury. A cycle of metabolic disruption results in loss of regional and finally global autoregulation and cerebral blood flow (CBF). The blood–brain barrier (BBB) is breached and edema ensues. Ischemia leads to regional lactate and glutamate increase, further increasing the potential for neuronal damage and death (Flowchart 1).

Flowchart 1: Primary injury leads to secondary injury.

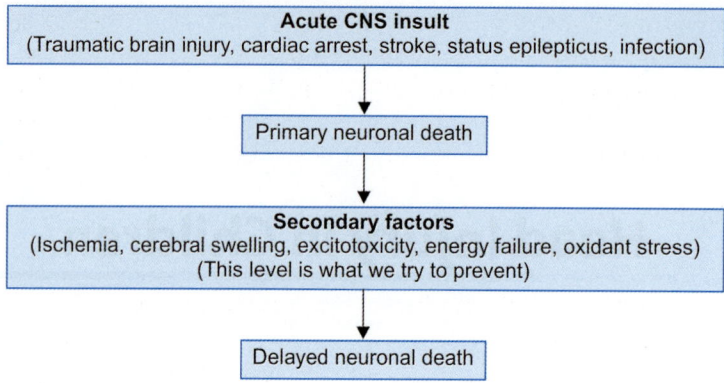

ASSESSMENT

This begins with a history simultaneously with resuscitation.

A doctor not handling the immediate treatment could gather the information:
- The time and mechanism of injury
- What immediate measures were taken
- The neurological condition of the child before examination by the current team.

Seizures: Impact seizures occur immediately or soon after the injury. They may not carry much significance and do not warrant antiepileptic treatment. Focal or multiple seizures with persistent loss of consciousness (LOC) are of significance and should be aggressively treated.

Loss of consciousness: Any period more than 5 minutes warrants imaging and evaluation. Recovery from early LOC with a secondary lapse may be indicative of an extradural hematoma. Children are more likely than adults to have venous extradurals which may develop more slowly. Vomiting after even trivial head injury is not uncommon in children, but observation for this is usually advisable.

Neurological deficit: May be transient after an impact seizure. If the child presents with coma and deficit cannot be assessed, a previous observation of a deficit by the parents or doctor may help in localizing the lesion. Any history of deficit with timing of first appearance should be carefully recorded to be compared with subsequent examinations for improvement or deterioration. It is important to note by history:
- Any change since the trauma
- Is the child improving, deteriorating or stable.

The simplistic AVPU can provide valuable information and can be asked in lay terms to anyone accompanying the child.

A: Alert
V: Responds to verbal commands
P: Responds to pain
U: Unresponsive

A careful written record of the history should be kept for medical as well as medicolegal purposes.

EXAMINATION

Assessment of appearance, work of breathing, and circulation is a quick way of deciding immediate needs as regards circulatory and respiratory support. At no cost should this be delayed in favor of a detailed neurological examination. Neglect in this area will add insult to injury and secondary neuronal death will occur. The neurological examination of the head injured child differs a little from that done for nontraumatic coma or other neurological disorder.

What is the Level of Coma?

This is the most important question of all and may well be the most difficult to answer.

The Glasgow Coma Scale (GCS) was designed to assess depth of coma after head injury in adults and has been used in pediatrics and works well down to the age of 5. In those below that age, the motor and eye opening scales may be used (except that children below the age of 9 months cannot localize pain), but a modification of the verbal scale is needed. The modified scale for pediatrics (see Chapter on Coma) can be consistently reproduced between observers. The response to pain should be examined both with a supraocular stimulus (for localization, flexion, and extension) and with nail bed pressure, for example with a pencil (for withdrawal). There may be a need for flexibility in terms of the overlap between the age groups. Thus, children of any age who are restless and talking unintelligibly have a verbal score of 2 and are therefore deeply unconscious; they are at high risk of further deterioration. At initial presentation, it is preferable to err on the side of recording too low a score, as it is easier to withdraw treatment from a child who is improving than to resuscitate one who deteriorates. An immediate application of the GCS gives a very good idea of the severity of injury.

Classification of head injury using the GCS from 3 to 15 points:
- 13–15: Mild
- 9–12: Moderate
- 3–8: Severe

The clinical picture may fluctuate and the GCS gives a fair estimation of deterioration or improvement when applied at regular intervals. Its point scoring also minimizes inter-observer variation.

Using the GCS and several other parameters in a decision-making algorithm, it is possible to triage the patients. The decision to admit is always easy. It is the decision to discharge a patient that causes concern. The following exclusionary criteria (Box 1) may result in some over-admissions but will almost completely safeguard against sending a potential moderate or severe head injury home too early.

Box 1: Clinical criteria to be met for discharging home/not admitting after minor head trauma.

None of the following:
- Loss of consciousness for more than 5 minutes
- Significant amnesia
- More than 3 episodes of vomiting
- Lethargy or decline in mental status
- No focal neurological deficits
- No post-traumatic seizure including impact seizure
- No spinal fluid otorrhea or rhinorrhea or bleeding
- No shock or other organ involvement that would preclude discharge
- No anticoagulant, anti-inflammatory drug or bleeding diathesis
- No suspicion of child abuse no matter how trivial the injury

Table 1: Assessment of severity of intracranial injury.		
Mild	Moderate	Severe
• Asymptomatic • Loss of consciousness <5 min • GCS 14–15 • Headache • Vomiting <3 episodes	• GCS 9–13 • Loss of consciousness >5 min • Vomiting >3 episodes • Post-traumatic amnesia • Post-traumatic seizures • Serious facial injury • Signs of basal skull fracture • Multiple trauma • Suspected penetrating or depressed skull fracture	• GCS <9 or fall of score by 2 • Focal neurological signs • Penetrating skull injury • Depressed or compound skull fracture

Radiological Criteria for Minor Head Injury

- No intracranial abnormality related to the head injury on CT.
- Skull fractures are acceptable except:
  - Those that cross the middle meningeal artery
  - Those that cross the dural sinuses
  - Those that are depressed more than the thickness of the adjacent skull.

In children fulfilling the above criteria for minor head injury, delayed deterioration is extremely uncommon. These children can be safely discharged home.

Once a child is adjudged to have minor head injury, discharge can be planned immediately or after a short period of observation. The following parameters should be met prior to discharge:

- No hemodynamic instability
- GCS score of 15 at discharge
- No neurological deterioration in the preceding 2 hours
- No focal deficits referable to the head injury
- Able to hold down liquids for at least 30 minutes
- Reliable caretaker who is comfortable with the discharge instructions.

To triage and manage the patient, an assessment of severity in or out of the hospital setting is required. Table 1 and Flowchart 2 can be used as referral points for this.

MANAGEMENT

Initial Management

Post-concussion syndromes: This is another aspect of head injury that the emergency room (ER) physician may have to deal with and triage to a ward, ICU or watch and discharge home. Delayed lethargy, irritability, and behavioral changes may be seen after head injury. This happens in a child where the scan shows nothing and neurological examination is normal, after about 10–30 minutes. Vomiting, sweating, and progressive drowsiness may be seen. If a CT has not already been done, it should be done to rule out an expanding hematoma. Recovery occurs over the next 2–24 hours. No specific treatment is warranted.

Flowchart 2: Triage of head injured patients.

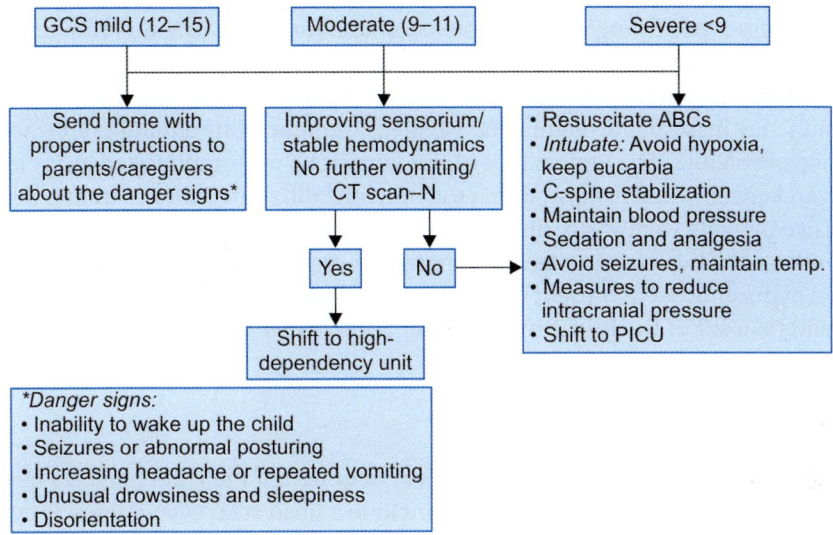

Other transient phenomena: Vomiting, migraine, and cortical blindness can occur. Recovery is the hallmark of post-concussive syndromes.

Tracheal intubation (TI) is indicated for children with severe head injury and coma; GCS less than or equal to 8. Children with multi-trauma, inhalation injury, airway/facial injury and shock with unassessable head injury should also be intubated, especially if at risk for increased intracranial pressure (ICP) from pain and agitation. The cervical spine must be protected and hyperextension of the neck avoided. Orotracheal intubation is preferred as it is quicker and involves less manipulation of the neck. This route also avoids aggravating any anterior basilar skull fracture or introducing infection into the anterior cranial vault.

All patients should be presumed to be on a full stomach. In the initial stabilization, control of the airway—directed to opening, protecting, and maintaining the airway (to prevent hypoxia and the deleterious effects of hypercarbia)—adequate oxygenation, and ventilation are the first priorities. The jaw-thrust maneuver can be performed during bag-mask ventilation. Head tilt and chin-lift maneuvers should be avoided when the status of the cervical spine is not known. Comatose patients need to be tracheally intubated with the rapid sequence intubation (RSI) technique, with due attention to cervical spine stabilization. Common medications used during intubation include thiopental and lidocaine. Etomidate is useful but the problems of adrenal suppression cannot be ignored. It cannot be emphasized enough that even comatose patients must have good sedation and muscle relaxation during intubation to avoid sudden rises in ICP.

Blood Pressure in Head Injury

Hypotension is common and blood loss should never be attributed to the head injury alone. A diligent search should be made for the source of bleeding. Only in children under 2 years can scalp and head trauma cause hypotension. Rapid and aggressive treatment is needed to prevent secondary damage from hypoxic-ischemic injury. A low BP at the time of presentation is associated with a poor prognosis. Hypotension of neurogenic origin is rare and indicates severe brainstem or cervical spine injury. Hypertension as part of the Cushing's triad—hypertension, bradycardia, and hypoventilation—is more common. This indicates raised ICP. This hypertension may mask hypovolemia and BP measurement alone should not be accepted as a sign of normovolemia. The importance of this cannot be overemphasized as is clear from a 1981 study in Lancet where it showed that the outcome differences between hypotensive and normotensive patients were vastly different. If there was no hypotension or hypoxemia—39% had poor outcome, if hypoxemic—59%, if hypotensive at presentation—75%, and if both hypotensive and hypoxemic were present then 100% had a poor outcome. Non-glucose containing fluids should be used in the initial resuscitation and normal saline is the best choice for the first 24 hours.

Imaging

Sometimes, at this point, an imaging study will be required. If the child needs to have a study for any abdominal injury, it is usually wise to include a head scan even if there is no absolute indication. This may prevent a second visit to the scanner and if the child is to undergo surgery on any other part of the body, anesthesia will prevent repeated neurological examinations for several hours. A negative initial scan will help the pediatric intensive care unit (PICU) staff rest easy. There is no role for a skull X-ray in head injury. It gives no additional information besides a possible fracture and is best avoided. Neither should an MRI or ultrasound be ordered. A negative ultrasound cranium in an infant may give a false sense of security as it will miss details. The indications for a CT scan are basically simple. The threshold for ordering a scan is so low that it is not worth elaborating on the indications (Box 2). It is not necessary to repeat a scan at 24–48 hours if there is no clinical deterioration or change in the GCS.

Box 2: Indications for a CT scan.
- Any focal deficit
- Any loss of consciousness for more than a 10 minutes
- GCS persistent <13
- Unable to examine the patient because of sedation, paralysis or intubation for other reasons
- Pupillary inequality
- Cerebrospinal fluid leak
- Depressed skull fracture
- Vomiting more than 3 times

CERVICAL SPINE IMMOBILIZATION

Immobilization with sandbags or a hard collar is essential till instability is ruled out. A quick cross-table lateral X-ray can help visualize at least the top 3 vertebrae and a complete series can be taken later. The cervical spine can also be scanned when and if the child goes for a cranial CT scan. A skeletal survey may be ordered when child abuse is suspected. Here it may be remembered that the cervical spine can be included in the head CT so as to avoid repeated radiation exposure to the neck region.

Once the child is in the PICU and you wish to remove the hard collar even without the check radiology, certain criteria need to be fulfilled:
- The child needs to be awake and cooperative and understand your commands.

- There should be no other distracting injuries causing more pain that outshadow the pain of the spinal injury.
- No sedative, intoxicant or narcotic should be in the system.
- The child should be able to move all the limbs and feel pain and touch everywhere.

Each cervical spinous process is palpated and the child is asked if there is any pain or tenderness. If the answer is no, then the child is asked to gently move the neck up and down and sideways on his/her own volition. The examiner should not perform any passive movement. If there is no pain and movement is free, the spine can be clinically cleared.

Other Associated Injuries

During the process of placing the child on the spine board while log rolling, a person whose hands are free should quickly examine the back, thighs, and legs for bruising, lacerations, crepitus, and obvious fractures. Injuries can be easily missed and 'out of sight is out of mind' once the child is intubated and sedated.

Once the primary survey and initial assessment of severity is done, the patient can be triaged as in Flowchart 2.

The Table 2 shows the clinical signs and correlates for making an anatomical localization of the lesion/s. It is a useful chart to keep in the PICU or ward.

The step-wise management protocol advocated by the Columbia group for ICP is useful as a guide.

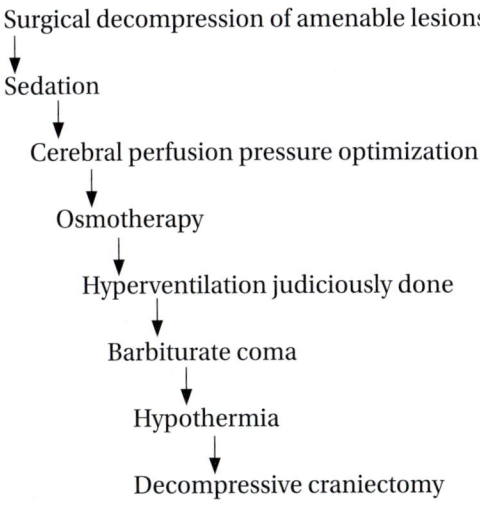

Surgical decompression of amenable lesions
↓
Sedation
↓
Cerebral perfusion pressure optimization
↓
Osmotherapy
↓
Hyperventilation judiciously done
↓
Barbiturate coma
↓
Hypothermia
↓
Decompressive craniectomy

Surgically Amenable Lesions

The following conditions warrant early surgical intervention: (i) All acute extra-axial hematomas of 1 cm or more in thickness; (ii) Subdural or epidural hematomas of more than 5 mm in thickness with midline shift; (iii) Hematomas (>5 mm) with midline shift in patients with moderate brain injury with effacement of the basal cisterns; and (iv) Depressed skull fractures.

Cerebrospinal fluid (CSF) rhinorrhea and otorrhea need conservative care avoiding packing of the ear or nose. Nearly all cases resolve spontaneously over 7–10 days. Less likely

Table 2: General examination.

Site examined	Findings	Interpretation
Scalp, skull	Contusions, lacerations Depression of skull	Underlying brain injury
Face	Periorbital, retroauricular bruising (Blue discoloration will come the next day)	Basilar skull fracture
Ear and nose	Hemotympanum, rhinorrhea, otorrhea	Basilar skull fracture
Fundus	Petechial hemorrhages	Shaken baby syndrome
	Papilledema (Not to be expected in acute phase)	Raised intracranial pressure
	Neurological examination (Secondary survey)	In addition to the GCS which must be done at regular intervals
Transient loss of consciousness	Normal examination or mild drowsiness	Concussion
Dilated pupils	Unilateral fixed dilated +/- contralateral hemiparesis	Transtentorial herniation
	Enlarged nonreactive (Mydriasis)	Mid-brain, III nerve or direct orbital trauma
	Bilateral or fluctuating mydriasis	Ictal or post-ictal phenomena
	Bilateral	Drugs used in cardiopulmonary resuscitation, e.g. adrenaline
Small pupil	Unilateral or Horner's syndrome	Sympathetic chain disruption Common carotid injury Arterial dissection in neck or skull base (May progress to stroke)
Ocular movements	Conjugate tonic eye movement	Ipsilateral frontal lobe injury or Contralateral seizure activity
	Ipsilateral conjugate lateral gaze palsy	Dysfunction of parapontine reticular formation
VII CN	Unilateral lower motor neuron	Nerve injury from basilar skull fracture
V	Corneal reflex absent	Pontine dysfunction
Vestibular caloric	Absent (Normal) - Cold = Opposite Warm = same side (COWS)	Brainstem dysfunction between pontine vestibular nuclei and oculomotor nuclei in mid-brain
IX & X	Gag and cough reflexes	Test integrity of medullary centers
Breathing	Periodic or Cheyne-Stokes	Bilateral hemispheric or upper pontine injury
	Apneustic	Mid-caudal pontine injury
	Ataxic	Medullary respiratory centers

to heal spontaneously are leaks in which CSF rhinorrhea develops days or weeks after surgical or accidental trauma, massive leaks that develop immediately after the surgery, leaks caused by sustained gunshot wounds, or normal-pressure CSF leaks. Antibiotic prophylaxis remains controversial. If there is gross contamination along a fluid pathway, such as with a comminuted fracture of the paranasal sinus resulting from acute trauma, antibiotic prophylaxis does have a role.

INTRACRANIAL PRESSURE

We tend not to think about ICP except in the context of it being raised. All therapies for traumatic brain injury and many for non-traumatic brain injury are aimed at lowering ICP. Hence, an understanding of the pathophysiology of raised ICP starts with an understanding of the physiology.

The intracranial vault is a closed compartment, although with some potential for expansion in the infant. It contains several components, which are essentially in three compartments—the brain, the blood, and the CSF; the tissue component being small. Whenever one compartment expands, another has to reduce its volume proportionately for the pressure in the compartment to remain the same. This is the basis of the Monro–Kellie doctrine (Fig. 1).

Cerebrospinal fluid and blood volume are almost equal. CSF is produced by the choroid plexus in the ventricles at a rate of about 20 mL/hr. It drains into the venous system via the arachnoid villi and granulations in a system of low resistance. Under physiological conditions, this drainage is almost completely dependent on the central/jugular venous pressure. ICP ranges from 3 mm Hg to 15 mm Hg or 5–15 cm H_2O.

Increased volume can be added to the compartment by:
- *Increase in CSF*: Hydrocephalus
- *Increase in brain cell water*: Cytotoxic edema
- *Increase in extracellular water*: Vasogenic edema
- *Mass lesion*: Tumors/hematomas

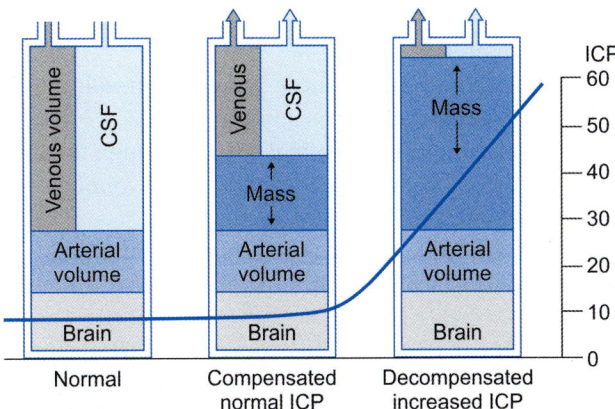

Fig. 1: Monro–Kellie doctrine showing the point of decompensation leading to rise in intracranial pressure.

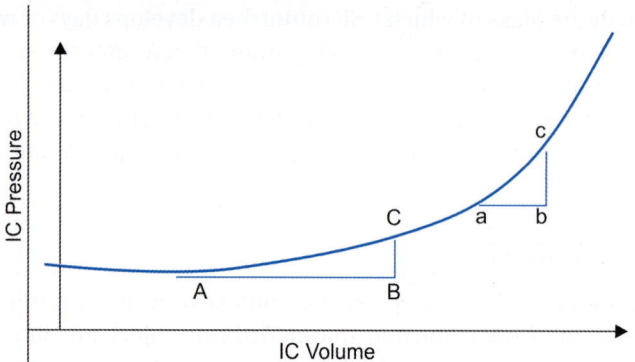

Fig. 2: Schematic diagram of the volume–pressure curve showing the compliant portion A–B where the increase in pressure for a larger volume increase A–B is small (BC). The noncompliant part a–b shows a larger increase in pressure b–c for a small increase in volume a–b.

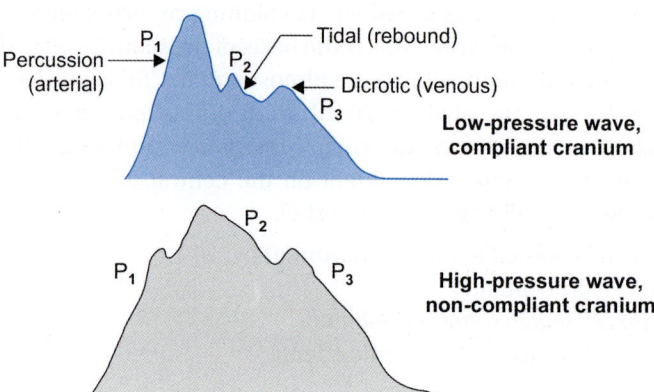

Fig. 3: Intracranial pressure wave forms.

- *Increase in blood flow*: Hyperemia.

To maintain ICP within normal limits, these increases in volume have to be offset by decreases in volume in other compartments.
- CSF is displaced downward into the paraspinal spaces through the foramen magnum.
- Blood is displaced from the intracranial to the extracranial venous system.
- The brain parenchyma is compressed.

After these mechanisms are exhausted, the intracranial compliance (change in pressure per unit volume—$\Delta P/\Delta V$) falls sharply and even small increases in volume cause large increase in ICP. (Figs. 1 and 2).

The compliant brain and the ICP tracing reflect the normal arterial pulsatile waveform. The first picture in Figure 3 shows a wave that looks like an arterial trace. This is changed (second picture in Figure 3) and finally lost when ICP increases. As intracranial compliance falls and the brain gets tighter, the ICP waveform changes (Figs. 3 and 4). The inability to accommodate even small pulsatile changes in cerebral blood volume is reflected in the waveform. The appearance

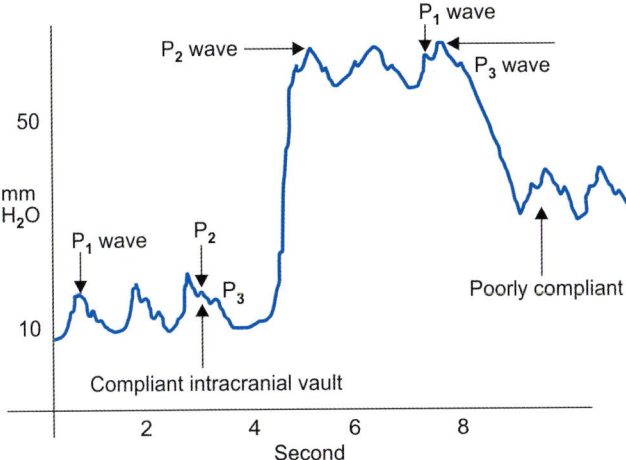

Fig. 4: Plateau waves.

of sinister "A" waves for more than 5 minutes with change in configuration, warrants immediate action to lower ICP.

ICP monitoring waves:
A waves: 40–100 mmHg represent serious rise in ICP. Correlate with decorticate and decerebrate posturing. Lasting over 5 minutes need urgent treatment.
B waves: 0–50 mm Hg. Frequent ill, sustained coughing, irritation
C waves: 0–20 mm Hg. Reflect BP, respiration, coughing and are benign

The recent guidelines for the management of severe brain injury, an update on the 2003 guidelines, have given certain recommendations corresponding to the evidence available and stated these as being from level I–III where level I would be the strongest. These will be referred to in the further text as the 2012 guidelines.

What is the Treatment Threshold for ICP?

Brief increases in ICP for less than 5 minutes are not associated with significant damage. Sustained increases of more than 20 mmHg that do not return to baseline in 5 minutes probably require attention. Most of the evidence in adults and children sets the acceptable high ICP level at 20 mm Hg. In a study by Esparza, an ICP of more than 40 mm Hg was associated with 100% mortality. Those with an ICP of 20–40 had 28% mortality and those with 0–20 had 7% mortality or severe disability.

However, the smaller the child, the less autoregulatory reserve there may be and the ICP may need to be considered for treatment at 15 mm Hg. At best, the answer may lie in individualizing the level for the child. The current recommendation is to attempt to keep the ICP less than 20 mm Hg (Level III in 2012 guidelines).

CEREBRAL PERFUSION PRESSURE

This is a critical determinant of CBF and brain perfusion. Its preservation is the key in ICP management. It is defined as the mean arterial pressure (MAP) minus the ICP,

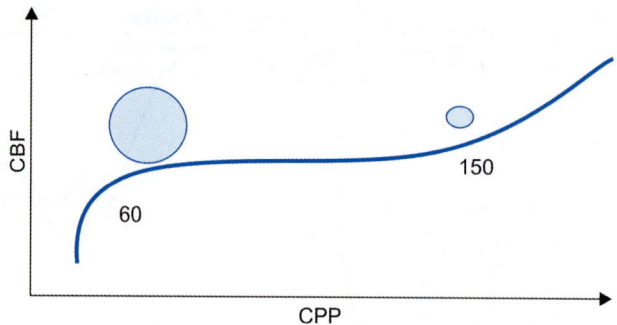

Fig. 5: Change in resistances of blood vessels.
- Cerebral blood flow (CBF) 50 mL/100 g/minute fairly constant
- Cerebral perfusion pressure (CPP) 60–150 mm Hg by cerebral autoregulation

CPP = MAP –ICP. Normally, CBF is autoregulated over a wide range of cerebral perfusion pressure (CPP): 50–150 mm Hg. This is done by arteriolar vasodilation or constriction in response to changes in the CPP (Fig. 5).

Cerebral blood flow is also controlled by changes in $PaCO_2$ and PaO_2, although the responsiveness of the vessels to O_2 is not as great. As $PaCO_2$ rises from 20 mm Hg to 80 mm Hg, so does arteriolar diameter. Therefore, hypercarbia increases blood flow in a more linear fashion. Hypoxemia causes vasodilatation and increases CBF only when PaO_2 falls below 50 mm Hg. This would be an important factor in the ICU patient on controlled ventilation whose CO2 may not fall but who may have inadvertent hypoxic episodes. In order to know the CPP, an ICP monitor and intra-arterial blood pressure monitoring are essential. The pressure transducer used to measure the MAP has to be set at the head level and not the heart level in this case for very accurate results (Fig. 3). Lundberg A waves are the most dangerous kind. They occur suddenly, reach levels of 50–100 mm Hg, and can last from minutes to hours. There is a corresponding drop in the CPP and CBF leading to global hypoxic ischemia. Lundberg B waves are smaller and shorter and not dangerous but harbingers of worse to come. Both the waves end in a termination spike of both ICP and systemic blood pressure.

Proposed model for the pathological cascade of ICP waves:
CPP falls from some drop in MAP or surge in ICP → Vasodilation occurs in order to maintain CBF → Cerebral blood volume increases → Intracranial compartment volume increases → ICP increases → CPP further decreases → vasodilation occurs again and the vicious cycle continues till vasodilation is maximal when the *plateau is reached*. This is a new level of increased CB volume and ICP and decreased CPP and CBF. The plateau ends once CBF is inadequate to maintain tissue oxygenation and ischemia occurs. Reflexly systemic vascular resistance increases and blood pressure increases, MAP rises, and CPP increases. If it is restored to within the autoregulatory range, the blood vessels will return to their original caliber and the CBV and ICP will return to normal. However, if the plateau lasts for too long, ischemia may be permanent and may even lead to severe global neuronal death.

Target for CPP?

The older recommendation was to keep the CPP above 50. Studies showing outcomes at various CPP levels confirm that a higher CPP, usually above 60, is associated with worse outcome.

However, there does not seem to be a significant difference in outcome in CPP values between 40 mm Hg and 60 mm Hg; hence, the recommendation of 40 mmHg as the threshold CPP in the 2012 guidelines.

CPP optimization: This concept is now considered the key to avoiding secondary brain injury. If ICP is greater than 20 cm H_2O and CPP is less than 70 mm Hg, then raising the MAP and thereby the CPP by using a pressor agent such as dopamine, norepinephrine or phenylephrine could lead to reduction in ICP by preventing the cerebral vasodilatation and increased CBF that occurs in response to low perfusion.

There is insufficient data for a level I recommendation. Hence this is a level III recommendation in the 2012 guidelines. Most of the survival studies that showed promising results were considered to be Class III studies. Intracranial pressure of more than 20 may be more commonly found in children who have lack of spontaneous motor function. It is a strong prognostic variable and refractory ICP has a poor outcome. In some studies, there was a clear link between aggressive ICP and CPP management and improved outcome. Targeting these threshold values of ICP 20 mm Hg and CPP 40 mm Hg cannot be done without invasive ICP monitoring and intra-arterial blood pressure monitoring.

Indications for invasive monitoring:
The patient is suspected to be at risk for elevated ICP if the:
- The GCS is less than 8
- STBI + *abnormal CT scan*: 53–63% chance of raised ICP
- STBI + *normal scan*: 35% chance of raised ICP
- Inability to perform CNS examination because of the need for deep sedation even in moderate STBI (GCS 9–12).

The prognosis is such that ICP treatment is indicated and aggressive treatment may be of benefit.

MONITORING DEVICES

Intraventricular Catheters

Continuous monitoring and intermittent drainage when ICP rises makes this a useful method. It is also the gold standard. The risk of infection increases dramatically after 5 days and many consider that prophylactic antibiotics are indicated to lower the risk. CSF drainage: If the ICP rises, 2–3 mL drainage from the IV catheter may help alleviate the rise promptly. Lumbar drainage of CSF should never be undertaken without clear indications and in centers with experience in this process and then under conditions of refractory ICP not amenable to the drainage of the ventricular catheter. There are criteria to be fulfilled before this is undertaken:
- A functioning IV catheter or drain must be in place.
- The cisterns should be open.
- There should be no mass lesion or hemispheric shift.

Intraparenchymal Pressure Transducers

Expensive disposable device at the tip of a fiber optic cable—Camino; or within a strain gauge microsensor—Codman. They are placed in the parenchyma or ventricle. No drainage can be done unless combined with a ventricular drain. New versions (Spieberg device) also give measurements of brain temperature. A third device also gives compliance curves as well as ICP. An oxygen monitoring sensor may also be incorporated.

Subarachnoid and epidural devices are now rarely used.

Noninvasive Measures

Transcranial Doppler (TCD) measures the velocity of blood flow in the cerebral arteries and the character changes with high and low ICP and falling CPP. As CPP falls, diastolic velocity decreases and pulsatility increases, reflecting increased vascular resistance distally. TCD is only sensitive to severe rises in ICP and the best correlations to date have been with changes in regional blood flow as in hemorrhage.

ADVANCED MONITORING

Jugular venous oxygen saturation ($SjVO_2$) and brain tissue PO_2 ($PbtO_2$) are technologies measuring the adequacy of oxygen delivery to the brain directly. $SjVO_2$ or jugular bulb saturation of oxygen, like SvO_2, is an indicator of oxygen extraction of the brain and can be used in a similar manner. A drop in the $SjVO_2$ (<50%) reflects a rise in ICP or a drop in CPP and optimization of CPP can be attempted to bring this back to more than 70. They may, therefore act as surrogate markers of changes in ICP.

Jugular venous oxygen saturation measures the O_2 delivery and extraction much in the way that the SvO_2 does. It is continuously measured at the level of jugular bulb, in the returning blood from the brain, by a fiberoptic O_2 saturation catheter. Intermittent sampling (as done in several centers) is of little value as it may not reflect every small or disastrous rise in ICP and hence delay or deny appropriate intervention.

Brain tissue PO_2 measures regional O_2 tension which will depend on the perfusion pressure. The catheter can be incorporated in the parenchymal catheter for ICP or be separate. A value of less than 15 mm Hg for more than 30 minutes is associated with a poor outcome, hence the threshold target is recommended at 15 mm Hg (Level III).

Near-infrared spectroscopy: It measures regional oxygenation by the ability to penetrate about 4 cm deep and reach the organ under study. Probes are placed over the forehead or over the injured area of the brain.

Steroids have no benefit in head injury as the edema is cytotoxic in nature. This has been emphasized several times.

Hypocapnia reduces CBF by vasoconstriction and hence will reduce ICP. However, it will also reduce CBF to the point of reducing CPP and cause ischemia.

Hyperventilation is not to be employed. Brief periods of less than 10 minutes of hyperventilation to 30 mm Hg, may be employed in the setting of a sudden rise in ICP or impending herniation. This too should be undertaken in the setting of ICP and CPP monitoring as far as possible. Severe hypocapnia by causing severe constriction of cerebral vessels can cause unwarranted ischemia and further exacerbate secondary neuronal damage. The CBF falls below threshold levels worsening neuronal injury. The goal of the therapy is therefore to maintain eucapnia with the $PaCO_2$ at 32–35 mmHg. Never < 30 mm Hg.

We must understand that clinical signs like the Cushing's triad, decerebrate posturing, apnea, and pupillary changes are all signs that come well after the ICP rise has occurred.

Osmotic Diuretics

Mannitol is still the most commonly used agent in the acute situation. It acts in several ways.

It reduces blood viscosity and hence improves cerebral blood flow and prevents stasis. The drop in viscosity results in cerebral vasoconstriction which allows blood flow to be maintained despite a lower blood volume. This action is immediate and lasts about 75 minutes. The later action is by osmotic reduction of brain water. This is from 15 minutes to about 6 hours and requires an intact blood–brain barrier.

It may also deposit in injured brain cells after prolonged use, resulting in rebound edema.

A dose of 0.25–1 g/kg is used and it has been clear from several studies that the low dose is as effective as the high dose and carries less complications of electrolyte imbalance and dehydration. The complications of mannitol therapy like acute tubular necrosis are a result of overzealous dehydration and a serum osmolarity over 320 mmol/L. In today's management of ICP, an euvolemic hyperosmolar state is the target.

Hypertonic Saline

About 3–7% saline has been employed successfully in the treatment of traumatic coma. The hyperosmolar state induced is more sustained and the reduction in ICP tends to be more sustained with fewer peaks requiring intermittent measures. The exact dosage is still unclear and bolus doses from 6.5 mL/kg to 10 mL/kg have been advocated, followed by an infusion of 0.1–2.5 mmol/kg/hr. Serum sodium levels of up to 155+ mmol/L have been reported with no side effects. Patients with a sodium level of more than 180 mmol/L invariably did poorly. Serum osmolarity rather than sodium levels should be monitored for effect, with a target osmolarity of 340–370 mmol/L. Adequate intravascular volume is critical to continue good renal perfusion as transient renal failure may occur. An infusion is given for 48–72 hours and then tapered gradually at about 10% every 6 hours, without causing any abrupt fall in the sodium levels so as to avoid central or extrapontine myelinolysis. Monitoring of the patient's metabolic status at least twice a day is essential. Some evidences say that hypertonic saline (HS) may be useful even in the early resuscitative period as a substitute for normal saline.

There is better evidence and less experience for the use of 3% saline, whereas it is the reverse for mannitol where there is more clinical experience and less evidence. Hence, the current guidelines give a level II recommendation for the use of HS in the acute situation and level III for it as a continuous infusion.

Barbiturates

These act by reducing the metabolic activity of the brain, thereby its oxygen consumption and therefore its demand for supply. The reduced blood flow can now match the reduced demand, preventing substrate starvation and reducing neuronal injury. The doses for this are equivalent to those for general anesthesia, as to really suppress activity, burst suppression is needed on the EEG. The dose has to be titrated to the EEG pattern rather than to the level achieved.

Short-acting barbiturates are used. Thiopental in a loading dose of 4 mg/kg, and as an infusion with 2–4 mg/kg/hr. Significant risks include hypotension in 54% requiring fluids and vasopressors, anergy, pneumonia, sepsis, and hyponatremia. All these singly or in combination increase morbidity and mortality in the head injured patient.

Sedation and Analgesia

Even the most "deeply comatose" patient warrants sedation and analgesia. The perception of pain in such a patient cannot be assessed. The ideal sedative has a short on–off action, does not accumulate in the body, has little or no hemodynamic effect and has anti-convulsant properties. If there is central neurogenic hyperventilation, it may be necessary to sedate and even paralyze the child to control the $PaCO_2$ level. There is no specific outcome data leading to a robust recommendation on which combination of medications work best in reducing ICP. Propofol can cause hypotension and comes with a warning on long-term use in infants and children and etomidate has the danger of suppression of the pituitary adrenal axis. Thiopental, like many others, can cause severe hemodynamic compromise and reduce the CPP causing more harm. In a randomized control trial of 44 patients, Jon Pérez-Bárcena et al. concluded that thiopental appeared to be more effective than pentobarbital in controlling intracranial hypertension refractory to first-tier measures. These findings should be interpreted with caution because of the imbalance in cranial tomography characteristics and the different dosages employed in the two arms of the study. The incidence of adverse effects was similar in both groups.

Hypothermia

Profound and prolonged hypothermia is fraught with complications. Moderate hypothermia with a core temperature of 32–34ºC may be useful. Cooling blankets to both front and back with ice water gastric lavage and pharmacological paralysis to prevent shivering are all needed. Rewarming should always be done at less than 0.5ºC/hr. Sophisticated bedside monitoring and servo-controlled equipment may be required for quality cooling and rewarming. The process should not be undertaken lightly especially in face of the results of the multicenter trial results showing its futility and dangers. There were deaths in 21% of the hypothermia group and in 12% of the normothermia group, but this was not different statistically. Of concern, there was a significant difference in blood pressure between groups, with the hypothermia group experiencing lower blood pressures during the time they were rewarmed. The authors reported that this particular protocol did not improve outcome in children. This should therefore be reserved for children with proven refractory ICP with no treatable lesion and a high risk of death.

Aggressive Treatment of Seizures

Seizure activity, even if not overt, is known to increase the cerebral metabolic demand result in relative ischemia. Most units administer phenytoin prophylactically, especially if the patient is to be sedated and paralyzed. If there is suspected activity as seen by nystagmoid eye movements, subtle twitches or fluctuations in consciousness, an EEG will identify true seizures.

Seizures

As seizures do worsen ICP and the seriously head injured patient has a high incidence of early symptomatic seizures, prophylactic medication like fosphenytoin, valproate or levetiracetam should be administered (See Chapter on status epilepticus).

Management of raised ICP begins in the emergency room with RSI avoiding drugs that would raise ICP or drop CPP. Premedication with lidocaine and induction with propofol or pentothal (if BP is stable) and rocuronium is preferred. Adequate oxygenation, eucapnia (an end tidal CO_2 is useful in this), and good analgesia and sedation is mandated. Transient rises in ICP caused by noxious stimuli like suctioning can be prevented by the use of IV or tracheal lidocaine.

Immediate post-traumatic seizures: These may follow even minor trauma. Immediate seizure may occur immediately on impact or within the first 24 hours. Most appear within the first 3 hours, are short-lived, generalized and not associated with any CT scan findings. They do not predict future epilepsy, require no treatment and bear a good prognosis for future outcome. If the nature of the seizure is complex, prolonged or focal; further observation and treatment may be warranted.

DECOMPRESSIVE CRANIECTOMY

A neurosurgeon should be involved right from the beginning for any STBI even if there is no immediate intervention required. When and if ICP becomes refractory, a decision to surgically decompress the cranium may be the difference between life and death and amount of permanent deficit the patient may suffer.

Decompressive craniectomy (DECRA) for severe brain injury and medically refractory intracranial hypertension in children lowers ICP and may improve outcome. Ideal candidates for decompressive craniectomy would be those satisfying the following criterion: (i) Diffuse cerebral swelling on cranial CT imaging; (ii) Within 48 hours of injury; (iii) No episodes of sustained ICP more than 40 mm Hg before surgery; (iv) GCS more than 3 at some point subsequent to injury; (v) Secondary clinical deterioration; (vi) Evolving cerebral herniation syndrome.

The dura is opened and the bone flap kept out, either in the abdominal wall or preserved. While studies in adults have questioned the long-term outcome of DECRA as leading to life with severe disability on the Glasgow Outcome Scales (GOS), in children outcomes appear to be better and this could be not only lifesaving but also provide a fair quality of life.

Other conditions that raise ICP:
- *Unrecognized seizures*: Prophylactic phenytoin should be considered, especially if an intraventricular catheter is placed.
- *Fever*: ICP rises by several points for each degree of fever. For this reason, hypothermia is being investigated as a possible modality of treatment with encouraging results. Indomethacin may be the ideal antipyretic. It has been shown to reduce cerebral blood flow and ICP in STBI. Prostaglandin inhibition and vasoconstriction may be the mechanisms of action.
- *Full bladder*: Adequate drainage by an indwelling catheter is preferred.
- Constrictive cervical collars or large bore internal jugular lines obstructing venous flow should be avoided.
- Recumbent posture is to be avoided and the head should be elevated at 30° not more.
- *Environmental stimulation*: All unnecessary touch, rough handling, moving, noise should be controlled or kept to a minimum. Sedation is overlooked as fighting against physical restraints, asynchrony with the ventilator, and suctioning, can all increase ICP. Even when

Table 3: Some specific injuries.

Injury	Features	Treatment
Subgaleal hematomas	Collection of blood above periosteum	No needling. Watch hematocrit
Cephalhematoma	Subperiosteal. Limited by suture line	No treatment required
Skull fractures	Linear, diastatic or depressed	Only depressed may require urgent elevation
Basilar skull fractures	CSF otorrhea or rhinorrhea (β_2 transferrin distinguishes CSF from nasal secretions)	Expectant management. No packing of ear, no prophylactic antibiotics. 85% spontaneously seal. 4% meningitis. If leak persists, ENT repair
Epidural hematoma	Lucid interval in only 33%	Urgent evacuation if mass effect
Subdural hematoma	Underlying brain injury common. Cortical bridging vein tear. If chronic, think of child abuse	Evacuate if large or causing mass effect
Intraparenchymal injury	Focal contusions, diffuse axonal injury, hematomas	Neurosurgical intervention usually not helpful. Decompressive craniectomy with or without lesionectomy

comatose, these patients can feel pain. Propofol is a hypnotic with no analgesic properties and hence an opioid must be used in combination. Muscle relaxants may be needed, especially for shivering but should never be used without adequate analgesia and sedation.

Nutrition: Hunger may or may not be perceived but after the first 24–48 hours enteral nutrition must be started. There is no evidence to suggest that any specific diet is needed. Glycemic control should follow the usual parameters of the treating ICU which would not allow severe hyperglycemia (over 180 mg/dL) but never allow any degree of hypoglycemia (Table 3).

There are many advances in neuromonitoring but these are infrequently used in routine ICU care of the brain injured patient hence we will just list them (Box 3).

Box 3: Further cerebral monitoring.

1. *Electrophysiological monitoring*:
   i. Electroencephalography
   ii. Evoked potentials
   iii. Bispectral (BIS) index monitoring
2. *Invasive*:
   i. Intracranial pressure (ICP) monitoring
   ii. Jugular venous O_2 saturation ($SjVO_2$)
   iii. Cerebral microdialysis
   iv. Laboratory markers and brain microdialysis
3. *Noninvasive*:
   i. Near-infrared spectroscopy (NIRS)
   ii. Transcranial Doppler (TCD)
   iii. Magnetic resonance spectroscopy (MRS)

KEY MESSAGES

Decrease intracranbial pressure—threshold 20 mm Hg:
- Evacuate mass-occupying hemorrhages.
- Consider ICP monitoring and draining CSF with ventriculostomy when possible.
- Hyperosmolar therapy with HS rather than mannitol.

- Be mindful of keeping a good CPP threshold 40 mm Hg.
- Mid-line neck, elevated head not more than 30º.
- Treat pain and agitation—consider pre-medication for nursing activities, +/- neuromuscular blockade (only when needed).
- Careful monitoring of ICP during nursing care, cluster nursing activities, and limit handling when possible.
- Suction (strong correlation to sudden rises in ICP) only as needed, limit passes, pre-oxygenate/ +/- pre-hyperventilate ($PaCO_2$ not < 30)/use lidocaine IV or IT when possible.
- After careful preparation of visitors, allow calm contact.
- No hyperventilation less than 30 mm Hg.
- No steroids.
- Decompressive craniectomy.
- Hypothermia.
- Avoid hyperglycemia (early).
- Decrease cerebral metabolic rate.
- Prevent seizures.
- Avoid hyperthermia.
- Thiopental for refractory conditions.

SUGGESTED READING

1. Adelson PD, Bratton SL, Carney NA, et al. Guidelines for the acute medical management of severe traumatic brain injury in infants, children and adolescents. Ped Cit Care Med. 2003; 4(3suppl):S1-75.
2. Chestnut RM, Marshall LF. Treatment of abnormal intracranial pressure. Neurosurg Clin N Am. 1991;22(2):267-84.
3. Cruz J. The first decade of continuous monitoring of jugular bulb oxyhemoglobin saturation: management strategies and clinical outcome. Crit Care Med. 1998;26:344-51.
4. Guidelines for the acute medical management of severe traumatic brain injury in infants children and adolescents, 2nd edition. Chapter 5. Ped Crit Care Med. 2012;13(1Supp).
5. Hahn YS, McLone DG. Risk factors in the outcome of children with minor head injury. Ped Neurosurg. 1993;19:135-42.
6. Hutchison JS, Ward, RE, Lacroix J, et al. Hypothermia therapy after traumatic brain injury in children. N Engl J Med. 2008;358:2447-56.
7. Lang EW, Chestnut RM. Intracranial pressure monitoring and management. Neurosur Clin N Am. 1994;5(4):573-605.
8. McHugh GS, Engel DC, Butcher I, et al. Prognostic value of secondary insults in traumatic brain injury: results from the IMPACT study. J Neurotrauma. 2007;24(2):287-93.
9. Muizelaar JP, Marmarou A, Ward JD. Adverse effects of prolonged hyperventilation in patients with severe head injury: a randomized control trial. J Neurosurg. 1991;75:731-9.
10. Muizelaar JP, wei EP, Kontos HA. Mannitol causes compensatory vasoconstriction and vasodilation in response to blood viscosity changes. J Neurosurg. 1983;59:828.
11. Qiu W, Zhang Y, Sheng H, et al. Effects of therapeutic mild hypothermia on patients with severe traumatic brain injury after craniotomy. J Crit Care. 2007;22(3):229-35.
12. Tatman A, Warren A, Williams A, et al. Development of a modified paediatric coma scale in intensive care practice. Arch Dis Child. 1997;77:519-21.

19
Status Epilepticus

Soonu Udani

LEARNING OBJECTIVES

- Early management of seizure
- Management of status and refractory status
- Accelerated management options

INTRODUCTION

Epilepsy has been recognized since prehistoric times with reference to cave paintings, in records of ancient civilizations from the Mayan and Incan paintings and in Biblical references. Ancient Indian medical texts had prescribed cures for the disease and even today many of our patients seek alternative medicinal cures as adjuncts to what we prescribe.

Convulsive, generalized status epilepticus (SE) is one of the most common emergencies faced, both in office as well as in intensive care situations. Prompt management is effective in terminating seizures as well as in stabilizing vital signs and preventing secondary organ and brain damage. While most episodes will terminate spontaneously, requiring follow-up care, for the intensivist, it is the acute care of continued seizure activity that poses a challenge, especially when there is poor response to initial treatment.

DEFINITIONS

With recognition of the requirement for treatment urgency, the standard definition of SE, "a 30 min seizure with no recovery of consciousness" has been abandoned for practical treatment. In 2015, The International League Against Epilepsy (ILAE) favored a shorter time window (e.g., >5–10 min of continuous seizures) particularly for generalized convulsive seizures. This changed the definition and incorporated two time frames, t1 and t2 of 5 and 30 min, respectively.

- t1 (5 min) = When the seizure either fails to naturally terminate or cannot be medically terminated *urgent treatment should be initiated*
- t2 (30 min) = Long-term damage may result if this is allowed to continue and treatment needs to be accelerated.

For treatment purposes, it is easier to define SE by the treatment time frame when there is poor response.

The definitions beyond SE are not standardized and when used in the literature are generally defined as per the author using the term. Generally, refractory status epilepticus (RSE) is the term used when there is failure to respond to the first two lines of medication and seizures have lasted well beyond the regular doses of drugs used, which by convention would be two to three drugs after 1 h in time. The time frame for this is ill defined. It is rather the escalation of treatment that defines this term and the subsequent phase of super refractory status epilepticus (SRSE), where the patient fails to respond after 24 h and in some references, even to general anesthesia. The American Epilepsy Society (AES) has defined these phases by management.

Stabilization phase 0–5 min = ti (ILAE)
Initial treatment phase 5–20 min = t2 (ILAE)
Second therapy phase 20–40 min
Third therapy phase >40 min.

PATHOPHYSIOLOGY

Glutamate is the major amino acid excitatory neurotransmitter in the brain. Some affected individuals have prolonged seizures thought to be caused by excessive activation of excitatory amino acid receptors. Other excitatory neurotransmitters that contribute to SE include aspartate and acetylcholine. There are possibly many mechanisms involved, both in starting and stopping seizures and when the normal mechanisms that limit the spread of seizures become ineffective, SE ensues.

Gamma-aminobutyric acid (GABA) is the main inhibitory neurotransmitter in the brain, and antagonists to it may contribute to SE. Many drugs used in SE are GABA agonists. Antiepileptic drugs are also tailored toward the blockage of several other receptors like the N-methyl-D-aspartate (NMDA).

The principles of treatment would therefore be to use drug combinations that would target different receptors and work in tandem to suppress the excitatory activity that is RSE.

ETIOLOGY

Febrile SE remains the most common cause of SE. This often terminates with first-line medication but many conditions that cause SE are associated with fever. Most children are normal prior to the onset of SE unless they have a premorbid neurological condition showing the first manifestation of epilepsy. Virtually any cause of epilepsy may have a first presentation with SE.

For the intensivist, SE in children can be broadly classified into categories based on etiology:
- *Symptomatic*: acute/remote/progressive
  - Acute symptomatic SE may also be an acute symptom of medical or neurologic disease.
    - Central nervous system infections (meningitis, encephalitis)
    - Acute hypoxic ischemic insult [cardiopulmonary resuscitation (CPR), drowning, hypotension]
    - Metabolic disease (e.g., hypoglycemia, inborn error of metabolism)

- Electrolyte imbalance (hyponatremia)
- Traumatic brain injury
- Drugs, intoxication, poisoning
- Cerebrovascular event (infarcts, bleeds)
- Remote symptomatic epilepsy/seizures → caused by an insult early in life:
  - Perinatal hypoxic–ischemic injury
  - Trauma
  - Infection
  - Congenital brain malformation
- Progressive → brain tumors:
  - Progressive myoclonic epilepsy
  - Syndromic epilepsies
  - Inherited disorders
- Unknown or cryptogenic—no known or identifiable cause.

SYSTEMIC EFFECTS DURING STATUS EPILEPTICUS

Initially, there is an outpouring of catecholamines, resulting in tachycardia and raised blood pressure (BP). The danger of hypoxia here is from respiratory depression or choking.

Blood glucose too is usually elevated, unless hypoglycemia is the cause.

If SE remains unchecked, compensatory mechanisms may get exhausted and with hypoxia, bradycardia occurs. Hypotension and hypercarbia will further complicate the situation. Cerebral perfusion which may be high in the beginning will start falling and intracranial pressure is known to rise during SE. Hypoxia and muscle activity will increase lactic acidosis and in extreme situations, rhabdomyolysis may also occur.

Hence, the emphasis in management is not only on drugs but also on good supportive care of airway breathing and circulation aimed at prevention of hypoxia and hypotension.

MANAGEMENT

Out of hospital treatment: Since seizures beget seizures and if not terminated within 5 min, tend to last longer, rapid termination is the aim. Treatment delay has been found to have poor treatment response. Five caretakers need to be taught how to manage and terminate episodes at home prior to transport to the nearest health care facility. Rectal diazepam (DZ) is useful but has now been replaced by the more socially acceptable and easier to use buccal or intranasal midazolam (MDZ), especially in older children. MDZ stopped 75% of the seizures and DZ 59%.

Initial assessment: At first contact, simultaneous efforts at seizure termination with assessment and stabilization need to be done. If alone, it is best to call an extrahand in early.
- Brief physical examination should assess respiratory and circulatory status. An adequate airway should be established immediately if there is respiratory compromise supportive therapy (e.g., oxygen, mechanical ventilation) instituted as needed.
- Intravenous (IV) catheter should be placed for blood sampling and administration of medications.

- Ongoing monitoring of vital signs should be initiated.
- Rapid neurologic examination
- Preliminary classification of the type of status epilepticus (SE)
- History obtained from a witness may help determine the cause of the seizures.

Laboratory studies: Blood and urine for:
- Glucose by finger stick
- Serum electrolytes, calcium, and magnesium levels
- Arterial blood gases
- A complete blood count (CBC)
- Urine and blood toxicology (if suspected)
- Serum drug levels
- Others as per clinical profile.

Subtherapeutic levels are found in almost one-third of children presenting in SE and dosing can be rationalized once the levels are known.

The AES has recently published guidelines (2016) for adults and children which break up the management into four phases.

Firstline initial therapy phase (5–20 min of seizure activity): Benzodiazepines (BZDs) remain the first-line treatment for SE because they can rapidly control seizures. The three most commonly used BZDs used here are DZ, lorazepam (LZ), and MDZ. For first-line IV therapy, LZ is preferred. In a study of 273 children (aged 3 months to 18 years) with convulsive SE were randomly assigned to receive LZ (0.1 mg/kg IV) or DZ (0.2 mg/kg IV). There was no difference in time to seizure termination without recurrence at 30 min or rate of ventilation.

Although the time from injection to LZs maximum effect can be as long as 2 min. The effective duration of action, as long as 4–6 h, is longer than DZ because of its less pronounced redistribution into adipose tissue. This vitiates the need to add on an additional drug like phenytoin to prevent recurrence of seizure should the effect wear off in a situation of simple febrile status.

Diazepam's action can be seen in 2–3 s as it is highly lipid soluble and it immediately crosses the blood-brain barrier. It is also stable at room temperature and is therefore popular for travel kits and emergency situations.

Lorazepam 0.1 mg/kg IV up to a maximum of 4 mg by slow IV push over 1 min and its effect assessed over the next 5–10 min or DZ 0.2 mg/kg IV (maximum dose 8 mg)

If seizures continue after 5 min, additional doses of LZ or DZ can be given. The risk of respiratory depression increases if more than two doses of BZDs are administered.

Second therapy phase: If seizures continue for 10 min after at least two doses of BZDs most protocols begin treatment with fosphenytoin at a dose of 20 mg phenytoin equivalents (PE)/kg IV and a rate of 3 mg PE/kg/min (maximum rate 150 mg PE/min). Alternatively, a higher initial dose of 30 mg PE/kg IV of fosphenytoin can be used.

If seizures persist, an additional half dose can be given 10 min after the loading dose. Another option is to administer a weight-based dose of IV valproate, phenobarbital, or levetiracetam.

This is now the stage of initial RSE as two or more primary drugs have failed and over an hour would have elapsed.

When this stage fails to control seizures, additional second and third line therapy adds only marginal benefit (2.3–5%). Here intermediate steps are waste of precious time with limited benefit and a change to an *"accelerated protocol"* has been proposed. Where the *second therapy phase* described above can be skipped and coma induction with MDZ, pentobarbital, or propofol [all with continuous electroencephalogram (EEG) monitoring] should be started. Thus, the patient directly enters into the *third therapy phase* saving 15-25 min of time. The application of such treatment has to be balanced with available expertise and infrastructure.

Third therapy phase: Prior to initiating this stage, it would be important to maximize existing medication by rechecking levels and reloading existing drugs if levels are suboptimal MDZ is the most widely used agent for coma induction. After the loading dose (Table 1), the incremental doses need to be done every 10-15 min or when repetitive clinical or electrographic seizures are seen. The end point is unclear. Further escalation of doses beyond 0.6-0.8 mg/kg/h may not have any added benefit if the GABA receptors are saturated or internalized. When MDZ was used as the initial agent for RSE, the rate of clinical seizure control was 76%, which was achieved on average 41 min after starting the infusion. When MDZ was used in conjunction with continuous EEG, the time to seizure control was much longer and the mean dose required for seizure control was 10.7 µg/kg/min compared with a lower dose (2.8 µg/kg/min) in the studies not using this form of monitoring, suggesting that continuous EEG provided additional targets for treatment. In this analysis, the only study that showed a shorter time to seizure control deviating from the mean of 41 min was by Singhi et al. where seizure control was achieved in 16 min.

Table 1: Coma inducing agents.

Drugs	Loading dose	Maintenance dose	Side effects
Midazolam	0.2 mg/kg	0.2–1 mg/kg/h	• Hypotension • Respiratory depression • Tolerance

Propofol	2 mg/kg	1–5 mg/kg/h	• Hypotension
			• Respiratory depression
			• PRIS monitor lactate, TG (>400), CPK, K
			• Avoid in infants
			• Evidenced by:
			  – Rhabdomyolysis
			  – Shock
			  – Metabolic acidosis
			  – ↑Risk with ketogenic diet

Thiopental	2–4 mg/kg	1–5 mg/kg/h	• Hypotension • Respiratory depression • Tolerance
High-dose phenobarbital Avoid in NCS and epilepsia partialis	30 mg/kg	Repeat 10–20 mg/kg/day over 4–5 days	• Hypotension • Respiratory depression

(NCS: nonconvulsive status; PRIS: propofol infusion syndrome; TG: triglycerides; CPK: creatine phosphokinase)

Thiopental, pentobarbital: The act of enhancing the action of the GABA receptors may have the additional advantage of being neuroprotective (Table 1). They exhibit zero-order kinetics and due to rapid redistribution have a profound tendency to accumulate resulting in a long half-life in anesthesia and thus long recovery time.

Hemodynamics can be supported so hypotension itself is not a reason to discontinue therapy unless it is refractory to support or poses a threat to cerebral perfusion pressure.

Profound suppression of brain activity may have a protective effect and "break the cycle" of seizures, thus reducing the chance of seizure recurrence upon tapering of medications.

Debate continues regarding the recommended length of the periods of EEG suppression (the interburst interval) and how long the burst suppression pattern should be maintained (Fig. 1).

As many of these drugs act via the GABA receptors, which get exhausted or internalize during SE, seizures that become refractory to coma inducing therapies could now be considered "super-refractory" (Figs. 2A and B).

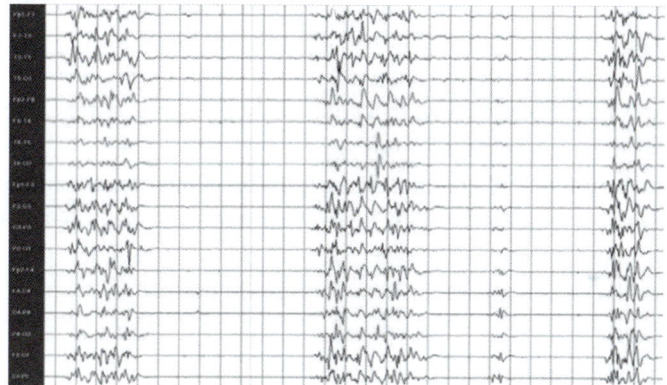

Fig. 1: Burst suppression on electroencephalogram. Three bursts per page.

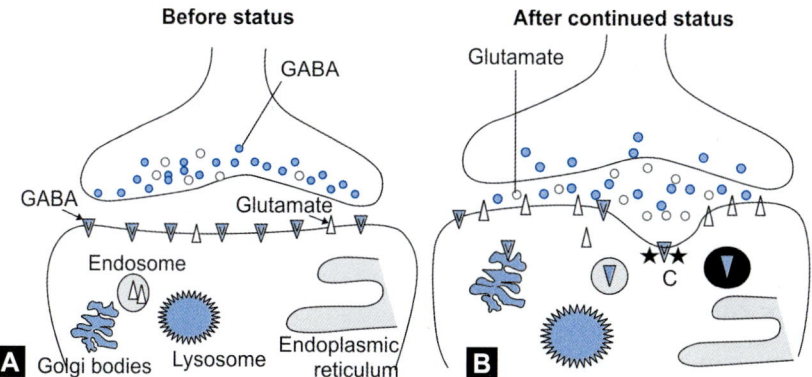

Figs. 2A and B: (A) GABA receptors lined up to receive GABA; (B) As GABA gets released, the receptors are fewer and some are in the cell so the excitation continues.
(GABA: Gamma-aminobutyric acid)

Other therapies in combination need to be applied at this stage.
- *Among them is the ketogenic diet.* Induces a state of controlled ketosis.
- Mechanism: alter brain-energy metabolism
- Increases the synthesis of GABA
- Reduces synthesis of reactive oxygen species.

This can be started in the very initial phase by removing all glucose containing solutions from the management, including syrups. It is then started with tube feeds at 3:1 or 4:1 fat : nonfat ratio, with fats consisting of animal fat, vegetable oils, or medium chain triglycerides. Supplements with vitamins, calcium, phosphorous, bicarbonate, and laxatives are sometimes needed. Short-and long-term complications include: diarrhea, feed intolerance, constipation (12–50%) growth failure, hypoglycemia, acidosis, renal stones (3–7%). This is started along with other adjuvant drugs that may help in controlling SE and usually before going to general anesthesia.

In the largest case series, isoflurane and desflurane were used in seven patients, six of whom had not responded to previous therapy with MDZ, propofol, and pentobarbital. Anesthesia was maintained for a mean (range) of 11 (2–26) days.

The action is by the potentiation of postsynaptic GABAergic currents thalamocortical pathways. Isoflurane 1.5–2.5% is used with a good gas scavenging system. The skill of the team and monitoring has to be stepped up for this step.

Weaning should be longer with IV anesthesia (pentobarbital) than volatile anesthetics, and it is reasonable to wean over 24 h (but may be much longer with pentobarbital).

During repeat cycles, wean after 3–5 days. A multidisciplinary process is useful in maintenance of good overall support for organ and brain perfusion.

PICU care includes:
- 1:1 Nursing care. With multimodal monitoring
- Mechanical ventilation
- Inotropes
- Continuous EEG monitoring
- Temperature
- Arterial line for BP monitoring and maintenance
- Central line as many drugs cannot be given for long periods peripherally
- Indwelling urinary catheter for good output monitoring.

During the period of coma induction and burst suppression, there may be some uncoupling of electrographic and clinical seizures. Thus, many seizures designated as RSE may occur during weaning from coma-inducing medications, and may be solely electrographic.

ADJUNCTIVE DRUGS

Because of the pathophysiological changes in SE, there is a tolerance to the first and second line as well as the coma inducing drugs as described earlier. The reasons are outlined in Box 1.

The need therefore arises for additional drugs that may choose to act by other pathways. These drugs are of little value alone but may have added benefit when used in conjunction with the drugs already on board. As it would be the purview of the pediatric neurologist to guide this therapy, only brief mention will be made of these.

> **Box 1:** Causes for tolerance development.
>
> - Loss of GABA-mediated inhibition
> - Downregulation of GABA-A receptors
> - Upregulation of NMDA and glutamate receptors
> - Alteration of ion channels
> - Altered neuropeptide expression (substance P and neuropeptide Y)
> - DNA methylation, micro-RNA regulation and altered gene expression.
>
> (DNA: deoxyribonucleic acid; GABA: gamma-aminobutyric acid; NMDA: N-methy-D-asparate; RNA: ribonucleic acid).

Lacosamide: Slow inactivation of voltage-gated sodium channels results in stabilization of hyperexcitable neuronal membranes and inhibition of neuronal firing with reduction of long-term channel availability without affecting the physiologic function. Only six case reports and series were published, all of which employed a retrospective design. Overall, data from 36 pediatric SE patients are available with success rates in terminating SE of 45–78%.

Topiramate (TPM): It acts through voltage-gated sodium channels and high-voltage-activated calcium channels as well as the GABA-A receptors, α-amino-3-hydroxy-5-methyl-4-isoxazolepropionic acid (AMPA)/kainate receptors, carbonic anhydrase isoenzymes. It may alter the activity of its targets by modifying their phosphorylation state instead of by a direct action. Among 71 episodes, 17 (23.9%) were treated with TPM. This may not be a very effective treatment for RSE.

Immunity and inflammation in SE and its sequelae: Routine use of intravenous immunoglobulin (IVIG) for pediatric RSE cannot be recommended at this time and should be considered experimental.

NOVEL THERAPIES

Steroids and immunotherapy: Inflammation appears to play a determinant role in ongoing seizures and their long-term consequences independently of infection or autoimmunity. Secondary to discovery of certain antibodies mediating RSE [anti-NMDA, anti-voltage gated potassium channel (VGKC)] a proposed role of steroids and IVIG has taken root in the management of SE.

Electrical, deep brain, and vagal nerve stimulation and magnetic stimulation therapy: It is postulated that these can alter the synchronization of epileptic discharges, increase the refractory period of neuronal discharge or alter membrane or neurotransmitter function.

Cannabinoids are now used in serious refractory epilepsies. These need to be under strictly monitored and approved conditions.

Hypothermia: It reduces the cerebral metabolic rate, oxygen utilization, adenosine triphosphate (ATP) consumption, glutaminergic drive, mitochondrial dysfunction, calcium overload, free radical production and oxidative stress, permeability of the blood–brain barrier, and proinflammatory reactions.

Electroconvulsive therapy: Its antiepileptic effects are proposed to be due to the increased presynaptic release of GABA and prolonged refractory period after a seizure. To cause a formed convulsion, electroconvulsive therapy has to be given when the anesthetic is reversed and the anticonvulsant drugs discontinued, as the anesthetics and antiepileptic drugs massively reduce cortical excitability.

Epilepsy surgery: In selected situations, mainly where there is a clearly definable radiological lesion and/or electrophysiological evidence of a focal onset, emergency surgical resection has been used as a "last-resort" treatment of SRSE. The different types—focal cortical resection, lobar and multilobar resection, anatomic and functional hemispherectomy, corpus callosotomy, and multiple subpial transaction.

Neuroimaging: Most children will get some imaging done in the course of their SE. A computed tomography (CT) scan will usually not yield much and magnetic resonance imaging (MRI) is needed to look for infective or treatable etiologies. In a study by Yoong found 80 children after suffering from chronic solvent induced encephalopathy (CSE) for a mean of 31.2 days, structural abnormalities were found in 31%. Abnormal neurological examination at assessment, CSE that was not a prolonged febrile seizure, and a continuous rather than an intermittent seizure, was all predictive of an abnormal scan. Hence in the first episode of SE, an MRI is recommended, although SE itself can produce changes in the MRI and atrophy or changes of hypoxic ischemic injury may confuse the picture.

KEY MESSAGES

- Status epilepticus is a common pediatric as well as critical care emergency.
- Good supportive care goes hand in hand with prompt seizure termination.
- Attention to oxygenation and BP will prevent further brain damage.
- Optimization of doses before adding new drugs should be attempted.
- Every unit must make its own implementable protocol within available guidelines (Table 2).
- A multidisciplinary approach is needed in RSE with high-level monitoring.
- There should be no hesitation to transfer if optimal care cannot be delivered.

SUGGESTED READING

1. Chamberlain JM, Okada P, Holsti M, et al. Lorazepam vs diazepam for pediatric status epilepticus: A randomized clinical trial. JAMA. 2014;311(16):1652-60.
2. Glausser T, Shinnar S, Gloss D, et al. New guideline for treatment of prolonged seizures in children and adults. AES Epilepsy currents. Jan-Feb 2016;48-61.
3. Hanhan UA, Fiallos MR, Orlowski JP. Status epilepticus. Pediatr Clin North Am. 2001;48(3):683.
4. Kofke WA, Young RS, Davis P, et al. Isoflurane for refractory status epilepticus: A clinical series. Anesthesiology. 1989;71:653-9.

Table 2: Status epilepticus protocol.

Stage	Management
Impending SE, 0–5 min AES stabilization stage	No IV access/casualty Consider buccal midazolam (MDZ) or rectal diazepam Benzodiazepines Lorazepam, 0.1 mg/kg IV (maximum, 5 mg) over 1 min Allow 5 min to determine whether seizure terminates Give oxygen. Stabilize airway, respiration, and hemodynamics as needed Obtain IV access Check bedside glucose Begin ECG monitoring
Established SE, 5–10 min AES Initial therapy stage	Repeat benzodiazepine administration Administer fosphenytoin PE30 mg/kg IV at 2–3 mg/kg/min (maximum, 150 mg/min) If the patient's age is <2 years, consider pyridoxine 100 mg IV push *Testing*: Bedside glucose CBC cultures Electrolytes, calcium, magnesium, phosphate, LFT, toxicology, if indicated (serum, urine preserve till further clarity) AED levels, PT, PTT urgent neuroimaging if treatable cause is suspected. MRI is preferred Support airway, respiration, hemodynamics as needed Continuous vital sign and ECG monitoring Consult neurology service
Initial refractory SE AES secondary therapy stage	If seizure continues 10 min after fosphenytoin infusion, repeat 10 mg/kg dose of FosPh Wait 10 min Administer levetiracetam 60 mg/kg IV at 5 mg/kg/min (maximum, 3 g) If contraindication to levetiracetam and no specific concern regarding liver/metabolic/mitochondrial disease, then administer valproate 40 mg/kg at 5 mg/kg/min
Established RSE	If seizure continues 5 min after levetiracetam or valproate, administer phenobarbital 20–30 mg/kg IV at 2 mg/kg/min (maximum rate, 60 mg/min) Admit to PICU. Or go to accelerated protocol—MDZ directly Prepare to secure airway, mechanically ventilate, and obtain central venous access and continuous hemodynamic monitoring through arterial line After clinical seizure terminates, will likely need EEG monitoring to assess for subclinical seizures
Coma induction AES third therapy stage SR SE	If seizure continues 10 min after completion of phenobarbital infusion, then initiate coma with MDZ 0.2 mg/kg bolus (maximum, 10 mg) over 2 min, and then initiate infusion at 0.1 mg/kg/h If clinical seizures persist 5 min after initial MDZ bolus, then administer additional MDZ bolus of 0.2 mg/kg bolus. Continue infusion If clinical seizures persist after another 5 min, then administer another MDZ bolus of 0.2 mg/kg, and increase MDZ Repeat as needed. If seizures persist at maximum MDZ (generally, 2 mg/kg/h) or MDZ infusion is not tolerated Intubate secure ABP and CVP line. prepare inotrope on standby *Start*: Thiopental 4 mg/kg load and 1–2 mg/kg/h. Increase only on advise of consultant and EEG for burst suppression according to neuro service

Contd...

Contd...

Stage	Management
Coma phase	Continue pharmacologic coma for 24 h after last seizure, with EEG goal of burst suppression Continue EEG monitoring with at least t.i.d reviews Continue initial medications (phenytoin goal level, 20–30 µg/mL; phenobarbital goal level, 40–50 µg/mL) Daily phenobarbital and free phenytoin levels. Consider high dose phenobarbital therapy instead of thiopental Continue levetiracetam at 40–80 mg/kg IV, divided every 6 h (maximum, 3 g)
Weaning phase	Reduce MDZ by 0.05 mg/kg/h every 3 h, with frequent EEG review If no clinical or electrographic seizures, then wean until off Continue EEG for at least 24 h after end of infusion, to evaluate for recurrent electrographic seizures
Repeat coma phase	If clinical or subclinical seizures occur, reinstitute coma with MDZ for 24 h Similarly for thiopental NB: MDZ does not cause burst suppression, the end point is loss of seizure activity
Repeat weaning phase	Reduce MDZ by 0.06 mg/kg/h every 3 h If seizure persists, then manage as guided by neurology consultation

Source: Glausser T et al. (2016).

(ABP: arterial blood pressure; ACTH: adrenocorticotropic hormone; AED: anticonvulsant; AES: American Epilepsy Society; b.i.d.: twice daily; CBC: complete blood count; CVP: central venous pressure; ECG: electrocardiography; EEG: electroencephalogram; EKG: electrocardiogram; IV: intravenous; LFT: liver function tests; MEG: magnetoencephalography; Mg: magnesium; MRI: magnetic resonance imaging; NG: nasogastric; Ph: phosphorus; PICU: pediatric intensive care unit; PT: prothrombin time; PTT: partial thromboplastin time; RSE: refractory status epilepticus; SE: status epilepticus; t.i.d.: three times daily)

5. Lehtimäki K, Långsjö JW, Ollikainen J, et al. Successful management of super-refractory status epilepticus with thalamic deep brain stimulation. Ann Neurol. 2017;81(1):142-6
6. Mpimbaza A, Ndeezi G, Staedke S, et al. Comparison of buccal midazolam with rectal diazepam in the treatment of prolonged seizures in Ugandan children: A randomized clinical trial. Pediatrics. 2008 Jan;121(1):e58-64.
7. Scott PM, Holt PJ, Sladky JT. Topiramate Loading for refractory status epilepticus in children. Epilepsia. 2006;47(6):1070-71.
8. Scott RC, Besag FM, Neville BG. Buccal midazolam and rectal diazepam for treatment of prolonged seizures in childhood and adolescence: A randomised trial. Lancet. 1999 Feb 20;353(9153):623-6.
9. Shinnar S, Berg AT, Moshe SL, et al. How long do new-onset seizures in children last? Ann Neurol. 2001;49(5):659.
10. Singhi S, Murthy A, Singhi P, et al. Continuous midazolam versus diazepam infusion for refractory convulsive status epilepticus. Neurol. 2002;17(2):106-10.
11. Strzelczyk A, Zollner PJ, Willems LM, et al. Lacosamide in status epilepticu: Systematic review of current evidence. Epilepsia. 2017;(11):1-18.

12. Trinka E, Cock H, Hesdorffer D, et al. A definition and classification of status epilepticus--Report of the ILAE Task Force on Classification of Status Epilepticus. Epilepsia. 2015;56(10):1515.
13. Wasterlain CG, Baxter CF, Baldwin RA. GABA metabolism in the substantia nigra, cortex, and hippocampus during status epilepticus. Neurochem Res. 1993;18(4):527.
14. Wilkes R, Tasker RC. Intensive care treatment of uncontrolled status epilepticus in children: systematic literature search of midazolam and anesthetic therapies. Pediatr Crit Care Med. 2014;15(7): 632-9.
15. Yoong M, Madari R, Martinos M, et al. The role of magnetic resonance imaging in the follow-up of children with convulsive status epilepticus. Dev Med Child Neurol. 2012;54:328.

End-of-life Care in the Pediatric Intensive Care Unit

20

Bala Ramachandran

LEARNING OBJECTIVES

- Understand what is end-of-life care (EOLC)
- Learn the modalities of EOLC
- Learn how to communicate effectively with the family, document EOLC decisions, and implement the same
- Briefly understand the legal framework in India regarding EOLC
- To introduce the key components of providing EOLC, along with practical guidelines on how to implement them.

INTRODUCTION

End-of-life care (EOLC) is an often misunderstood concept by both physicians and hospital administrators. It is an essential component of the continuum of care and can make the difference between comfort during the last moments of life and a prolonged, tortuous dying process.

BACKGROUND

"Death can be a peaceful event or a great agony when it is inappropriately sustained by life support".
—Roger Bone

"Death is not extinguishing the light; it is putting out the lamp because the dawn has come".
—Rabindranath Tagore

Death is an inevitable part of life but is often an unwelcomed topic for discussion, especially in the ICU. However, just as physicians have an obligation to work toward cure of the patient, they also have a similar obligation to make the process of dying comfortable when cure is no longer possible. In the USA and Europe, some kind of withholding or withdrawing of care precedes death in as many as 90% of patients who die in the ICU. This occurs even in 40–60% of neonates and children. However, the rates in India are much lower. In one study, about 34% of patients in four major hospitals in Mumbai had some form of end of life decisions. In the Quality of Death Report published by the Economist Intelligence Unit, India has been rated in both 2010 and 2015 as having the poorest EOLC. The barriers in India are many—there is a lack of awareness among the public about EOLC and a culture of "fighting to the end", physicians are not trained in how to discuss EOLC and maintain a focus only on a curative intent; there is a lack of clarity regarding the legality of EOL decisions and physicians are afraid of either being accused of providing substandard care or legal repercussions. The end result is that patients with very poor prognoses are admitted to the ICU in their last days of life, subjected to multiple painful technologies and suffer. The family bears the psychological and financial burden of such inappropriate and expensive prolongation of death.

ETHICAL PRINCIPLES FOLLOWED IN END-OF-LIFE CARE

- Autonomy refers to the patient's right to make decisions regarding his own medical treatment and incorporates the concept of informed consent. A patient has to consent to any form of medical therapy. Similarly, he has the right to refuse a therapy or intervention. In the case of children, the parents or guardians make the decisions on the patient's behalf.
- Beneficence is the principle that the doctor has to protect the welfare of the patient. The needs of the patient come before the needs of family, society or other patients. In a treatable condition, this means providing good curative care. However, when the condition is terminal, it may be in the patient's best interests to forego therapy. In these circumstances, it would also be in the patient and family's best interests to protect them from social and financial harm, when these wishes are clearly expressed.
- Nonmaleficence refers to the principle that no harm should come to the patient as a result of the physician's actions. This is also referred to "primum non nocere" and serves to protect the patient. It requires the physician to constantly balance the benefits versus risks of treatment. Harm includes both physiological/psychological and social/financial harm. The patient and family must be given an opportunity to prepare for death in a suitable and comfortable environment.
- Justice refers to the ideal that all patients suffering from the same condition should get similar treatment. This is also known as distributive justice and ensures fairness of treatment. It is especially relevant to developing countries where resources are scarce, costs high, and patient affordability poor. Subjecting the patient to expensive futile therapies goes against this principle.

GUIDELINES FOR PROVIDING END-OF-LIFE CARE

What is End-of-life Care?

End-of-life care is the provision of multidisciplinary holistic care to a patient who has an advanced, progressive, incurable disease or other life-limiting condition so that they can have the best quality of life before dying. The care is not just to the patient but includes the entire family and healthcare providers.

Objectives of EOLC

The objectives of EOLC are to achieve a "good death", for anyone who is dying. The key is to ensure good quality of life and death, rather than focusing on curative therapies. The first step is to recognize that death is approaching. EOLC should aim to control physical symptoms by providing adequate pain relief relieving discomfort. It should also cater to the emotional needs of the patient and the family. The goal is not to prolong life unnecessarily by artificial means, but to allow the patient to die with dignity. Just as every patient has the right to receiving high quality medical care; he also has the right to good EOLC when he can no longer be cured.

Guidelines for the EOLC Process

Recognition of Futility

The first step is to recognize that the patient can no longer be cured and is dying. This is not always straightforward. In pediatrics, limitation of care may be justified in four situations: (i) permanent vegetative state; (ii) "no chance" situation; (iii) "no purpose" situation; and (iv) "unbearable" situation. Common conditions where futility may occur include catastrophic illness with severe organ dysfunction not responding to therapy, irreversible coma in the absence of brain death, chronic severe neurological conditions with severe cognitive and/or functional impairment, progressive metastatic malignancy that has failed to respond to treatment, or a postcardiac arrest state with severe neurological damage.

Consensus among Caregivers

It is extremely important that the entire medical team agrees that the patient is dying, and further care is futile. If there are any differences of opinion, then EOLC discussion should be postponed until consensus can be arrived at. One well-known source of dissatisfaction among families is the provision of conflicting information by various healthcare providers. The senior physician-in-charge of the patient should be responsible for communicating the patient's condition to the entire team.

Disclosure to the Family

The team leader should make an honest, accurate, and early disclosure of the patient's poor prognosis to the family. He or she should explain that further aggressive care is futile, and it would be in the patient's best interests to allow him to die naturally. It is best if all the concerned family members are addressed jointly by the healthcare team so that inconsistencies caused by communicating at different times by different people are avoided.

Discussion of the Modalities of EOLC to the Family

Families often misunderstand what is meant by EOLC and therefore the physician should clearly explain what are the various modalities available. He should emphasize that the overall goal is not to save or prolong life but to keep the patient comfortable.

There are three standard options for limiting life support:
Do not resuscitate (DNR): This means that resuscitation will not be attempted in the event of significant deterioration in the patient's cardiorespiratory status. DNR orders are used all over

the world, including India. In India, there is no legal standing for such an order, and therefore each hospital has to decide its own policies. Families sometimes interpret the term DNR and think that it is possible to resuscitate the patient, but the physician is unwilling to do so. Therefore, this is gradually being replaced by the term do not attempt resuscitation (DNAR). DNR does not mean "do not treat"—families often feel abandoned once they have signed a DNR form. These patients and families require even more time and effort on the part of the healthcare team. DNR orders must clearly state what interventions can and cannot be carried out. The family must also understand that the order can be rescinded at any time.

Withholding of life support: This means that new life support therapies will not be started, and existing supports not escalated. These could be invasive mechanical ventilation, vasoactive drugs, renal replacement, etc. The family must understand that this may lead to the death of the patient.

Withdrawal of life support: This means stopping a treatment once it has already been started. Withholding and withdrawing life support is very common in developed countries but in India, only a small percentage of families opt for this option. In addition, the legal status and methodology of limitation of life support is not clearly understood by most clinicians. Therefore, they are afraid to limit care because of fear of being accused of not treating the patient properly or of legal repercussions. Physicians are often more comfortable with withholding care rather than withdrawing. However, legally and ethically there is no difference between the two. The family and the entire healthcare team must understand that care is never withdrawn, but only an individual therapy. The patient should continue to receive palliative care and kept comfortable.

Other modalities, such as physician-assisted suicide and euthanasia are not legal in India.

- *Shared decision-making*: The traditional pattern of providing medical care through paternalism (where the physician makes all the decisions) is giving way to shared decision-making all over the world, including India. Therefore, all efforts must be made to engage the family effectively, explain the patient's condition accurately, and then jointly decide on the course of action. This respects the patient/family's autonomy to make informed decisions, while simultaneously providing beneficent care. In case of any conflict with the family or if they are unable to decide, all supportive measures must be continued while efforts are made to come to an acceptable consensus. This may take multiple meetings and discussions with various family members. Though life supportive measures should be continued, the physician is not obligated to introduce additional therapies if it is medically inappropriate and not in the patient's best interests, even if the family demands it.
- *Transparency and accountability through accurate documentation*: The entire process of deciding upon and implementing EOLC should be accurately and completely documented in the case sheet. Since these decisions have major impact on the patient, at least one other physician should be involved in the decision-making process. The notes should include details of the discussion, the final decision, the specific therapies that will be withdrawn or withheld, and what comfort strategies are planned. The notes should also mention who were present from the medical team and the family during the discussion. Though a signature from the family is not compulsory, it is preferable to have the form signed by the surrogate decision maker and a member of the medical team.

- *Implementing the process of withholding or withdrawing life support*: This is an extremely important, but often incorrectly implemented step. Specialists in palliative care are usually better placed to keep the patient comfortable and their assistance should be sought when available. The goals are now to keep the patient comfortable, provide privacy, and allow him to die with dignity. He should ideally be shifted into a single room. He should be positioned comfortably, and all unnecessary monitoring devices removed. Blood investigations should not be ordered and medicines other than what are needed for comfort stopped, within the confines of what has been agreed with the family. Family members should be allowed to visit without restriction and any religious or cultural rituals allowed. Once he has been made comfortable, life supportive measures, such as mechanical ventilation and vasoactive drugs, etc. are withdrawn, depending on what has been discussed with the family. At all times, steps must be taken to ensure that the patient is kept comfortable. Fluids and/or nutrition are usually continued.

Doctrine of Double Effect: Patients at the end of life may require aggressive analgesia and sedation to relieve pain and discomfort. However, it is not uncommon for healthcare providers to refuse or limit such therapy because they are afraid that sedatives and opioid drugs can themselves lead to respiratory depression and may therefore hasten death. Because of this, the patient has to suffer unnecessary pain and agitation. Actions at this stage should be guided by the Doctrine of Double Effect. This states that when an action (medication or therapy) has two effects, one good and the other bad, the action is justifiable provided certain conditions are met. These conditions are as follows:
- The action in itself must be good, or at least morally neutral.
- The agent must be given in order to provide the good and not the bad effect. For example, when fentanyl is given to a child with metastatic malignancy, it must be to provide analgesia and not suppress respirations.
- The good effect must be the result of the action itself, and not as a result of the bad effect. For example, giving rocuronium to an unventilated patient can cause death, thereby ending pain and suffering. The bad effects here (death) results in the good effect (pain relief)—this is an unacceptable means to an end.
- The good effect must be proportionally stronger than the bad effect.

The key difference is the intent of the physician. As long as the action is done to relieve pain and suffering, it is permissible, even if the drug can cause adverse effects such as respiratory depression that may hasten death. However, if the intent is to kill the patient, then the action becomes euthanasia, which is not permissible.
- *Compassionate family support*: Effective EOLC is much more than simply removing from the ventilator and providing analgesia. The patient and family's wishes must be respected as much as possible. Healthcare providers accustomed to providing curative care are often uncomfortable in dealing with dying patients and their families. As a result, they hesitate to go into the rooms and the family feels neglected and abandoned. Every effort must be made to provide moral support, carrying out their cultural and religious requests. After the patient's death, they must be guided on what are the next steps to be taken and assistance offered as needed. This may include providing an ambulance to take the body home. The requisite documentation, legal and billing formalities must be completed expeditiously so that the family does not have to wait long. Bereavement support must be provided through

trained social workers or other personnel, as required. Some families may wish to come back at a later date to discuss their child's illness and death. This should be seen not as a waste of the physician's time, but as an extension of the care provided while the child was alive. Families will appreciate and remember simple acts of kindness.

CURRENT LEGAL FRAMEWORK IN INDIA REGARDING END-OF-LIFE CARE

There is considerable confusion in the medical community regarding the exact legal position regarding EOLC issues, such as withdrawing life support, DNR orders, etc. The law in India, as everywhere else, is slowly evolving. In the Transplantation of Human Organs Act in 1994, the Government of India gave permission to declare a person brain dead and then harvest organs. However, there was no mention of what should be done in the case of brain dead patients who were not going to be organ donors.

In the Aruna Shanbaug case, the Court mentioned that "Brain death is death". It also ruled that life support could be withdrawn or withheld in some situations, such as persistent vegetative state, but the process of obtaining permission was too cumbersome to be of practical use.

A petition was filed by an NGO "Common Cause" to declare the right to die with dignity a fundamental right. The Indian Society of Critical Care Medicine (ISCCM) was also a party respondent in this petition. The Supreme Court of India gave its verdict in the case of "Common Cause vs. the Union of India" in March 2018. It ruled that every individual has the right to die with dignity and upheld the practice of passive euthanasia—the removal of life support from persons who have slipped into a persistent vegetative state. It also laid down detailed procedural guidelines on how this is to be implemented. It allowed Advanced Directives and Living Wills, which are instructions spelled out in advance by a competent living person as to what should be done in terms of medical support if he should become terminally ill. It also specified that if a person had not issued Advance Directives, then consent from the surrogate decision maker would substitute for the Advance Directive, subject to close supervision by and concurrence of trained medical personnel. Though these developments are welcome, the procedures laid down are still very cumbersome. For implementing an EOLC decision, a lengthy procedure has to be followed at two levels—a medical board of the hospital and the district collector. Such procedures are unworkable in situations where decisions have to be made within hours or days.

COMMUNICATION—HOW TO BREAK BAD NEWS

Though many clinicians are excellent in their management of the patient, they are not necessarily effective communicators. Therefore, families often do not get a good understanding of the patient's condition and cannot make good decisions. This is even more important when bad news has to be told—many doctors are uncomfortable discussing bad news and therefore may not communicate effectively. Good communication skills are developed over time and the following steps will help perfect these:
- Recognize your own personal biases and value judgements. Do not allow these to cloud your advice—be nonjudgmental.
- Find a quiet, comfortable area and minimize disturbances—this is an extremely important time for the families, who may have been waiting many hours for the opportunity.

- Avoid interruptions such as telephone calls—shutting off your phone will send a message to the family that you consider them important and help improve trust.
- Allow the family to bring support persons. Parents find being seated next to the door more comfortable since they do not feel "boxed in". Ask the patient's nurse to attend but limit the number of other healthcare providers.
- Everyone should be seated. Introduce the team members by name and make eye contact with the family. Know the child's name.
- Ask open ended questions, such as "What is your understanding of your child's condition?" or "What are you hoping for?".
- Speak in simple language and avoid medical jargon. Give information in small chunks and periodically review the family's understanding.
- Reflect back the parents' views.
- Talk less and listen more—allow the family to express their thoughts and emotions. The physician should spend 75% of his time listening and only 25% in talking. Show empathy with the family's emotions and give them enough time to overcome these—unless this is done, it is impossible to proceed.
- Summarize the conversation at the end.

CONCLUSION

End-of-life care is an often confusing and daunting situation that is, nevertheless, extremely important in intensive care. Healthcare providers must familiarize themselves with the process of providing compassionate, ethical EOLC so that patients who cannot be cured can be allowed to die without pain and suffering. Learning how to communicate effectively is one of the most important steps in this process. The dismal situation regarding availability of palliative care in India will improve only if all concerned persons, including healthcare providers, take it upon themselves to not only learn how to provide curative care, but also to provide care to a dying patient. Every person has both the right to live and also the right to die with dignity.

KEY POINTS

- End-of-life care issues are extremely important in intensive care.
- The modalities of EOLC are DNR, withholding and withdrawing support.
- There is no difference between withholding and withdrawing support.
- Analgesia and sedation should not be withheld due to fear of side effects.
- Good communication skills are paramount to the success of discussions with the family.

SUGGESTED READING

1. Chakravarty A, Kapoor P. Concepts and debates in end of life care. Ind J Med Ethics. 2012;9(3): 202-6.
2. Gursahani R, Mani RK. India: not a country to die in. Ind J Med Ethics. 2016;NS(1):30-5.
3. Mani RK, Amin P, Chawla R, et al. Guidelines for end-of-life and palliative care in Indian Intensive Care Units: ISCCM consensus Ethical Position Statement. Ind J Crit Care Med. 2012;16(3):166-81.
4. Mani RK. Constitutional and legal protection for life support limitation in India. Ind J Palliat Care. 2015;21:258-61.

5. Mishra S, Mukhopadhyay K, Tiwari S, et al. End of life care: Consensus statement of the Indian Academy of Pediatrics. Ind Pediatr. 2017;54(10):851-9.
6. Myatra SN, Salins N, Iyer S, et al. End of life care policy: an integrated plan for the dying. Ind J Crit Care Med. 2014;18(9):615-35.
7. Reportable In The Supreme Court of India Civil Original Jurisdiction. Common Cause vs. the Union of India. Writ Petition (Civil) No. 215 of 2005. [online] Available from https://www.sci.gov.in/supremecourt/2005/9123/9123_2005_Judgement_09-Mar-2018.pdf [Accessed December 2018].
9. Yadav M. End of life care support: Ethical and legal scenario in India. J Ind Assoc Forensic Med. 2006;28(3):971-3.

Diabetic Ketoacidosis in Children

21

Vijai Williams, Jayashree Muralidharan

LEARNING OBJECTIVES

- Diagnose diabetic ketoacidosis especially in a new onset diabetes
- Assess dehydration and correct with appropriate fluid therapy
- Arrest ketogenesis with insulin therapy
- Anticipate complications and treat them
- Look for precipitating causes

INTRODUCTION

Diabetic ketoacidosis is a pathological state of severe high anion gap (AG) metabolic acidosis (HAGMA) caused by insulin deficiency leading to accumulation of ketoacids far exceeding the normal buffering capacity of the body. T1DM is one of the common chronic conditions of childhood with an incidence of about 3% worldwide. DKA can be the initial presentation in about 15–70% children of T1DM and in about 1–10% of previously diagnosed diabetic children. DKA requires careful monitoring during fluid and insulin therapy and is a common indication for pediatric intensive care unit (PICU) admissions.

DEFINITION AND PATHOPHYSIOLOGY

The definition for DKA has remained the same over the years. It is defined by the biochemical criteria as shown in Box 1. DKA occurs due to an interplay between insulin (deficiency) and counterregulatory hormones (CRHs) (excess). Insulin is the key regulator of glucose and fatty acid metabolism and helps in maintaining a balance between catabolism and anabolism. Insulin deficiency leads to hyperglycemia and

Box 1: Diagnostic criteria for diabetic ketoacidosis (DKA) [International Society for Pediatric and Adolescent Diabetes (ISPAD) 2018).

- Hyperglycemia with random blood glucose (BG) > 200 mg/dL
- Venous pH <7.3 or bicarbonate <15 mmol/L
- Ketonemia (>3 mmol/L) and ketonuria (>2+)

(Rarely DKA can present with normal glucose values especially if the patient is partially treated or is severely malnourished.)

ketosis. The former is a result of both decreased glucose storage and utilization in the peripheral tissues. The latter results from lipolysis and release of free fatty acids and underutilization of ketones in the peripheral tissues, thus resulting in both an overproduction as well as underutilization of ketones. The hyperglycemia is further aggravated by CRHs (epinephrine, cortisol, and growth hormone) released in response to stress, which block the action of insulin and enhance the release of glucagon, resulting in increased glycogenolysis in the liver. Early during the course of diabetes, peripheral utilization defect predominates over defect in hepatic gluconeogenesis thus manifesting only as postprandial hyperglycemia. During the later course as insulin deficiency worsens, fasting hyperglycemia appears. When blood glucose (BG) levels exceed renal threshold (180 mg/dL), glycosuria occurs and leads to osmotic diuresis and dehydration. Vomiting secondary to ketosis aggravates dehydration and acidosis stimulating release of CRHs. The CRH released in response to dehydration, activate lipase in adipose tissue causing lipolysis and ketoacidosis resulting in a vicious cycle.

Metabolic acidosis leads to shift of intracellular potassium to plasma in exchange of hydrogen ion thus causing normal serum values; however, a total body deficiency of potassium occurs. Similar mechanism results in phosphate depletion. Therefore, electrolyte deficits of up to 3–5 mEq/kg of potassium and 0.5–1.5 mmol/kg of phosphate can occur in DKA.

CLINICAL FEATURES

The presentation may vary from subtle malaise to severe altered mentation. Most of the manifestations are related to osmotic diuresis and volume loss. Ketoacidosis leads to tachycardia, deep and rapid (Kussmaul's) respiration, a fruity odor of the breath, nausea, and vomiting. Abdominal pain mimicking an acute abdomen is a very common manifestation of DKA. Confusion and drowsiness are common; progressive worsening of consciousness is seen with delayed presentation and is an ominous sign. Fever is uncommon, and if present, is usually indicative of an underlying infection.

In children with DKA, there is poor correlation between clinical features and severity of acidosis and dehydration assessment. Hence, children suspected to have DKA should be considered critically ill until evaluation proves otherwise. Severity is graded as shown in Table 1. There are several risk factors that precipitate DKA in a child as listed in Table 2.

Table 1: Severity of diabetic ketoacidosis.

Parameter	Arterial pH	Serum bicarbonate (mmol/L)	Level of consciousness
Mild	7.3–7.2	10–15	Alert
Moderate	7.2–7.1	5–10	Alert/drowsy
Severe	<7.1	<5	Stupor/coma

Table 2: Risk factors for DKA.

New onset T1DM	Known T1DM
• Younger age (<2 years) • Delayed diagnosis • Lower socioeconomic status • Infection	• Insulin omission • Insulin pump failure • Previous episodes of DKA • Poor metabolic control • Puberty and adolescence • Psychiatric (including eating) disorders • Infection

(DKA: diabetic ketoacidosis; T1DM: type 1 diabetes mellitus)

DIFFERENTIAL DIAGNOSIS

Hyperglycemic hyperosmolar state (HHS) associated with diabetes/non-diabetes is a close differential for DKA. In contrast to DKA, there is usually enough insulin to suppress ketogenesis, but not to control BG. Typically, these children present with disproportionately high BG with mild or no ketosis. The diagnostic criteria for HHS is shown in Box 2.

Box 2: Diagnostic criteria for hyperglycemic hyperosmotic state.

- Blood glucose (BG) >600 mg/dL
- Arterial pH >7.30; venous pH >7.25
- Serum bicarbonate >15 mmol/L
- Mild ketonuria, absent to small ketonemia
- Effective serum osmolality >320 mOsm/kg in presence of stupor, coma or seizures.

MANAGEMENT

Diabetic ketoacidosis requires aggressive protocol-based management to achieve end points and prevent complications as highlighted below. Unlike the West, where timely treatment is sought, most children with DKA in India reach late due to delayed health seeking behavior and lack of awareness about symptoms. Poor socioeconomic status, poor adherence to therapy, associated malnutrition, comorbidities like sepsis, and inadequate treatment at first contact healthcare facility puts our children at higher risk for severe and complicated DKA.

Goals of Therapy

- Assess and appropriately correct dehydration to restore renal perfusion and facilitate peripheral glucose utilization.
- Arrest ketogenesis with insulin therapy.
- Anticipate and replace ongoing fluid and electrolyte losses.
- Assess and treat precipitating cause (e.g. infection).
- Anticipate and intervene rapidly if complications occur [e.g. cerebral edema (CE)].

Immediate Steps of Stabilization in an Emergency Room

Acute management should follow the general principles of advanced life support.
- Airway measures (basic and advanced) may be needed in children with DKA who are deeply comatose with features of CE.
- Continuous nasogastric aspiration is essential to decompress a hugely dilated stomach.
- Two peripheral lines must be secured for fluids and insulin infusion.
- Hypotension is rare in DKA; if present, indicates either severe uncorrected hypovolemia or associated septic shock. Volume resuscitation will be required in children with shock.
- All children must be under continuous cardiac monitoring.
- Bladder catheterization may be required in children with low Glasgow coma scale (GCS).
- Consider antibiotics in a febrile child after obtaining appropriate cultures.

Fluid Therapy

Rationale

Volume depletion in DKA activates the renin–angiotensin–aldosterone and CRH axis. These hormones act toward preserving the intravascular volume, but at the same time increase insulin resistance. Fluid resuscitation expands intravascular, interstitial and intracellular volume, corrects dehydration, enhances renal glucose clearance (following improved renal perfusion), causes decline in CRH, and augments insulin sensitivity.

Hydration alone has been shown to reduce glucose concentration by 17–80% during a period of 12–15 hours, which represents an average plasma glucose reduction rate of 25–50 mg/hr. Slow and even rehydration without major osmolar shifts is the key.

Assessment of Dehydration

Clinical assessment of dehydration in DKA is difficult and unreliable; decreased skin turgor, dry oral mucosa, sunken eyes, capillary refill time more than 2 seconds, and altered neurological status were found to be poor predictors of fluid deficit in DKA. Reduced skin turgor are absent as children have preserved intravascular volume due to hyperosmolarity. The assumed deficits in a range of 6.5–8.5% have been seen in several studies. A median absolute measure of dehydration as calculated by body water estimation was found to be 8.7%. This estimate was the best fit to avoid risks of overhydration as well as underhydration. DKA is one clinical condition where the "one size fits all" policy seems more appropriate.

Fluid Calculation

Children in shock (poor perfusion associated with or without hypotension) require volume expansion with 20 mL/kg bolus of isotonic saline over 30–60 minutes. In compensated shock, the rate of bolus can be slow over 1 hour followed by slow correction as described below.

In hemodynamically stable children, deficit for dehydration correction is taken as a rough estimate of 6.5–8.5% (A). This is added to the 36–48 hours maintenance fluid (B).

Hence, the total fluid requirement for a child in DKA would be = (A + B) − C
- Deficit calculation (A): % dehydration assumed × body weight.

Table 3: Fluid requirement based on weight.

Weight	Fluid (mL/kg)
<10 kg	100
10–20 kg	1,000 mL + 50
< 20 kg	1,500 mL + 20

- *Maintenance fluid calculation (B)*: From the Holliday–Segar equation which roughly estimates fluid requirement based on weight (Table 3).
- All isotonic fluid boluses (C), if received during resuscitation, need to be subtracted from the total volume.
- Total fluid requirement is calculated for 36–48 hours and hourly infusion rate is obtained.
- Urine output monitoring may not be reliable, as the child may have polyuria due to glycosuria, and urinary losses need not be replaced routinely.
- If any child develops CEs during therapy, fluid should be tailored to suit needs of raised increased intracranial pressure (ICP) management.
- Strict assessment of fluid balance is essential in all children.

Type of Fluid to be Used

- Isotonic saline is used for initial resuscitation and may be continued for the initial 4–6 hours before replacing it with N/2 saline (0.45%).
- This switch is determined by the serum sodium and osmolality levels and more importantly the availability of plain N/2 saline (without dextrose). In case of nonavailability, isotonic saline can be continued.
- A recent randomized controlled trial (RCT) comparing slower versus rapid fluid administration using either 0.45% saline or 0.9% saline failed to show any significant differences in the frequency of either altered mental status or CE and long-term neurocognitive outcomes.
- Continued use of large volumes of normal saline (NS) can however cause hyperchloremic metabolic acidosis due to their high chloride content which has now been shown to be associated with acute kidney injury (AKI) and delayed resolution of acidosis.
- Balanced fluids (containing lower chloride) have been found to be better in preventing kidney injury; however, further studies are needed before they can be adopted as standard of care.

Rate of Fluid Correction

Rate of fluid correction is another area of debate. Many centers prefer a slow and even correction spaced over 36–48 hours, as this has been shown to reduce the risk of CE. The rate of correction is determined by the initial BG levels, serum osmolality, corrected sodium, severity of acidosis, presence of AKI, and depth of altered sensorium. Slower correction is recommended for children with severe DKA and those having very high BG, osmolality, and corrected sodium.

Insulin Therapy

Rationale

Insulin replacement is the mainstay of therapy in T1DM. It facilitates glucose utilization and halts ketosis. Goal is to decrease hyperglycemia and arrest ketosis.
- Start insulin after first hour of fluid therapy as incidence of CE was more in children who received insulin within first hour of starting fluids.
- No role of bolus insulin administration.
- Regular insulin is preferred at an infusion at a rate of 0.1 U/kg/hr. This is known as standard dose.
- Lower dose (0.05 U/kg/hr) as continuous infusion has been tried and found to be as effective as standard low dose regimen (0.1 U/kg/hr). The authors' unit follows the 0.05 U/kg/hr regimen after a RCT conducted in the unit which showed similar time to resolution of DKA as compared to standard therapy, and lesser incidence of hypoglycemia.
- Fresh insulin in appropriate dilution has to be given through separate intravenous access.
- The entire line has to be adequately flushed with the insulin solution. Insulin tends to adhere to the tubing and may not be delivered appropriately, unless flushed prior to the start of the infusion.
- If there is nonresponse to insulin one has to confirm the checklist (Box 3).

> **Box 3:** Checklist before escalating dose or changing insulin.
> - Patency of intravenous (IV) cannula
> - Insulin preparation, storage, and expiry date
> - Appropriateness of dilution
> - Lines are flushed adequately
> - Insulin dose can be hiked if all above parameters are checked and found correct.

Type and Route of Insulin

Regular insulin by intravenous route is the preferred modality at present. Prospective RCTs have tried newer rapid acting insulin analogs in place of intravenous regular insulin, and have found them to be safe and effective and safely delivered through subcutaneous route. They were more cost-effective in patients without major comorbidities admitted to the intensive care unit (ICU). Their use in moderate-to-severe DKA, however, still needs further evaluation.

Electrolyte Imbalance

Hypokalemia

It is a common and dangerous complication of DKA. Osmotic polyuria excretes potassium along with ketoanions. With insulin therapy, potassium is driven into the intracellular compartment resulting in plummeting of potassium levels during therapy. The complication tends to be severe in malnourished children due to poor potassium stores. Anticipate hypokalemia if serum potassium level is normal or low in presence of severe acidosis and in all with malnutrition. Goal of therapy is to maintain serum potassium between 4 mEq and 5 mEq/L. If the child is hypokalemic at admission, potassium correction is to be started immediately along with addition of maintenance potassium at 40 mmol/L after ensuring adequate urine output. Administration of insulin may be delayed in severe hypokalemia and may be started after fluid and potassium replacement.

Phosphate

Hypophosphatemia is secondary to osmotic polyuria. Whole body phosphate depletion is a hallmark of poorly controlled diabetes, but typically remains asymptomatic. Routine supplementation is not recommended. Replacement is indicated in those with anemia, cardiac dysfunction, respiratory depression, muscle weakness or in children with serum phosphate lower than 1–1.5 mg/dL. One-third of potassium replacement may be administered as potassium phosphate either as intravenous or as phosphate enema.

Chloride

Ongoing loss of bicarbonate from renal tubules leads to retention of chloride. Excessive infusion of chloride containing fluids (NS) can add to the brunt. The resultant normal AG metabolic acidosis (NAGMA) though self-limiting may be erroneously interpreted as nonresolution of ketoacidosis, if careful AG estimation is not done at bedside. Balanced fluids with lower chloride content may decrease this complication and are being increasingly studied.

Bicarbonate

Loss of bicarbonate from renal tubules can occur during excretion of ketoacids. However, correction with bicarbonate is not routinely recommended except in severe DKA with pH less than 6.9 associated with life-threatening hyperkalemia or compromised cardiac function.

Monitoring during Therapy

Clinical and Biochemical

All children during treatment need continuous cardiac monitoring. Complete neurological examination with special emphasis on pupils, GCS, and deep tendon reflexes (DTRs) anticipating CE during therapy is mandatory. Hourly BG monitoring is essential. Fluid balance needs to be calculated periodically.

Laboratory Tests

- Blood glucose, blood gases, serum electrolytes, urea, creatinine, and hematocrit should be repeated 2–4 hours or more frequently, depending on clinical need.
- Blood beta-hydroxybutyrate (blood ketones) concentrations, if available, every 2 hourly. Urinary ketones may be used instead if blood ketones are not available. Remember urinary ketones only help in diagnosis, but not in deciding resolution of DKA as commercially available kits generally measure acetoacetate, which continues to appear even after resolution of DKA.
- Lipids and triglycerides can be grossly elevated causing the blood sample to show a visible rim of lipids.
- Severity of extracellular fluid contraction can be assessed by serum urea and hematocrit.
- Anion gap estimation [$AG = Na - (Cl + HCO_3)$; normal 8–12] helps in monitoring; closure of AG indicates correction of ketoacidosis.

- Corrected sodium = measured Na + 2 [(plasma glucose − 5.6)/5.6] mmol/L or measured Na + 1.6 [(plasma glucose − 100)/100] mg/dL is a better indicator of sodium variation when corrected for glucose.
- Effective osmolality (mOsm/kg) = 2 × (plasma Na) + plasma glucose mmol/L, needs to be maintained at optimal level without allowing wide fluctuations.

Targets for Gradual Reduction of Effective Serum Osmolality

- Desired rate of fall of BG is 50–100 mg/dL/hr after starting insulin.
- The pH is expected to increase by 0.03/hr.
- Serum sodium increases by 0.5 mmol/L for each 1 mmol/L decrease in BG with least variability in corrected sodium.
- Rate of fall of serum osmolality should be 3–8 mOsm/kg/hr for HHS and for DKA, a more gradual fall is found to reduce CE.

Persistent Acidosis

Persistent acidosis is defined as bicarbonate less than 10 mEq/mL despite 8–10 hours of therapy for DKA. The first step before proceeding further is to calculate the AG.

High Anion Gap Acidosis

- Improper insulin dose, dilution, and rate of infusion
- Incorrect administration; flush the intravenous line completely before starting insulin
- Rarely, this may be secondary to lactic acidosis/renal compromise.

Normal Anion Gap Acidosis

Hyperchloremia due to chloride containing fluids such as NS.

End Points of Therapy

- Normal sensorium with good oral tolerance
- Resolution of acidosis, pH more than 7.3 or bicarbonate more than 15 mmol/L
- Closed anion gap.
  There is considerable variability in the definition of end-points used in different studies.

Transition to Subcutaneous Insulin

Once the acidosis is passive and oral acceptance and tolerance is good, a subcutaneous insulin regimen can be initiated at 1 U/kg/day of regular insulin in four divided doses. This can be later changed to basal bolus or spilt mix regimen. There should be an overlap of 1–2 hours between the first dose of subcutaneous insulin and intravenous insulin infusion to prevent a precipitous drop in serum insulin levels and consequent hyperglycemia and ketoacidosis. In a known TIDM on home insulin regimen, their home dose of insulin may be restarted and titrated for desired BG levels.

COMPLICATIONS

Cerebral Edema

Children have higher incidence of symptomatic CE as compared to adults, particularly in those with new onset diabetes. It remains a major contributor to DKA related deaths (10–25%). The current model proposed for CE in DKA is the two hit hypothesis. First hit is before DKA therapy is initiated wherein the dehydration and cerebral hypoperfusion cause ischemia-related cerebral injury. Second hit occurs after fluid therapy is started and is due to reperfusion injury. Akin to other hyperosmolar states, "idiogenic osmoles" are generated in the brain cells to protect them against intracellular dehydration and shrinkage. Rapid decrease in extracellular osmolality draws fluid into the intracellular compartment favoring development of CE. This may be secondary to rapid reduction of BG, too vigorous fluid replacement with failure of corrected sodium to rise with therapy and bicarbonate use.

Cerebral edema usually occurs few hours after start of DKA therapy with varied symptomatology, ranging from headache to abrupt neurological deterioration and coma. A high index of suspicion for CE is therefore needed and should be considered in patients with impaired sensorium persisting despite improvement in acidosis and in those with early subtle neurological signs. It may be too late to react at the time of profound neurological depression and respiratory arrest.

When CE is suspected, close monitoring of BG and electrolytes is essential to avoid osmotic disequilibrium. Mannitol may be used to counter CE. Fluid volume administered should be curtailed, and other antiraised ICP measures should be initiated.

Hypoglycemia

Hypoglycemia as a therapy related complication in the West has decreased considerably with use of low-dose insulin infusion. However, the incidence in LMIC despite standard dose insulin is still high due to associated malnutrition. Hourly monitoring of BG and early addition of dextrose (when BG reaches 250 mg/dL) to fluid regimen, especially in malnourished children, is recommended. This allows for continuation of insulin till ketosis is reversed and prevents hypoglycemia. It is advisable to have a two-bag system containing 10% dextrose (first bag) and no dextrose (second bag) so that there is a smooth transition to varying dextrose concentration.

Acute Respiratory Distress Syndrome

Noncardiogenic pulmonary edema is a result of reduced colloidal oncotic pressure in pulmonary capillaries due to exclusive crystalloid replacements in DKA. In hypoxemic patients with increased pulmonary alveolar-arterial gradient, one should suspect pulmonary edema. It can be avoided by judicious fluid replacement.

Acute kidney Injury

Acute kidney injury is a common complication encountered during DKA management. Retrospective analysis in the authors' unit revealed an incidence of 35% AKI in children with

DKA. Elevated chloride levels were an independent predictor of AKI. This study again suggests a possible beneficial role of balanced solutions in preventing this morbidity.

PREVENTION IS BETTER THAN CURE

Sick-day Rules

Since the principal reason for DKA recurrence is omission of insulin, most cases can be avoided by proper patient education. Clear guidelines must be issued to patients on sick-day management; not stopping insulin, monitoring BG and urine ketones regularly, ensuring usual carbohydrate intake with plenty of fluids, and seeking early medical help. These measures will help prevent the occurrence of DKA.

SUMMARY

Diabetic ketoacidosis (DKA) is a preventable life-threatening complication of type 1 diabetes mellitus (T1DM). DKA is quite common in children, with about one-fourth of new onset diabetes presenting for the first time as DKA. Prompt recognition of subtle symptoms is important as diagnosis in these children is not always apparent. Immediate treatment includes fluids replacement, parenteral insulin combined with careful clinical, and biochemical monitoring. In low-middle income countries (LMIC), DKA is associated with higher incidence of complications due to delayed presentation, poor compliance to therapy, and higher comorbidities like malnutrition and sepsis. DKA in children warrants a multidisciplinary approach both during and after an episode. Since parents play a key role in the day-to-day management, sustained parental education is paramount to prevent recurrence.

SUGGESTED READING

1. Dhochak N, Jayashree M, Singhi S. A randomized controlled trial of one bag vs. two bag system of fluid delivery in children with diabetic ketoacidosis: Experience from a developing country. J Crit Care. 2018;43:340-5.
2. Duck SC, Wyatt DT. Factors associated with brain herniation in the treatment of diabetic ketoacidosis. J Pediatr. 1988;113(1 Pt 1):10-4.
3. Edge JA, Dunger DB. Variations in the management of diabetic ketoacidosis in children. Diabet Med J Br Diabet Assoc. 1994;11(10):984-6.
4. Edge JA, Hawkins MM, Winter DL, et al. The risk and outcome of cerebral oedema developing during diabetic ketoacidosis. Arch Dis Child. 2001;85(1):16-22.
5. Fisher JN, Kitabchi AE. A randomized study of phosphate therapy in the treatment of diabetic ketoacidosis. J Clin Endocrinol Metab. 1983;57(1):177-80.
6. Glaser N, Barnett P, McCaslin I, et al. Risk Factors for Cerebral Edema in Children with Diabetic Ketoacidosis. N Engl J Med. 2001;344(4):264-9.
7. Glaser NS, Ghetti S, Casper TC, et al. Pediatric diabetic ketoacidosis, fluid therapy, and cerebral injury: the design of a factorial randomized controlled trial: Pediatric DKA fluid therapy randomized trial. Pediatr Diabetes. 2013;14(6):435-46.
8. Glaser NS, Wootton-Gorges SL, Marcin JP, et al. Mechanism of cerebral edema in children with diabetic ketoacidosis. J Pediatr. 2004;145(2):164-71.
9. Inward CD. Fluid management in diabetic ketoacidosis. Arch Dis Child. 2002;86(6):443-4.

10. Jayashree M, Sasidharan R, Singhi S, et al. Root cause analysis of diabetic ketoacidosis admissions at a tertiary referral pediatric emergency department in North India. Indian J Endocrinol Metab. 2017;21(5):710-14.
11. Koves IH, Neutze J, Donath S, et al. The Accuracy of Clinical Assessment of Dehydration During Diabetic Ketoacidosis in Childhood. Diabetes Care. 2004;27(10):2485-7.
12. Michael P. Poirier, David Greer, et al. A Prospective Study of the "Two-Bag System" in Diabetic Ketoacidosis Management. Clin Pediatr (Phila). 2004;43(9):809-13.
13. Moulik NR, Jayashree M, Singhi S, et al. Nutritional status and complications in children with diabetic ketoacidosis. Pediatr Crit Care Med. 2012;13(4):e227-33.
14. Nallasamy K, Jayashree M, Singhi S, et al. Low-Dose vs Standard-Dose Insulin in Pediatric Diabetic Ketoacidosis: A Randomized Clinical Trial. JAMA Pediatr. 2014;168(11):999-1005.
15. Puttha R, Cooke D, Subbarayan A, et al. Low dose (0.05 units/kg/h) is comparable with standard dose (0.1 units/kg/h) intravenous insulin infusion for the initial treatment of diabetic ketoacidosis in children with type 1 diabetes-an observational study. Pediatr Diabetes. 2010;11(1):12-7.
16. Umpierrez GE, Cuervo R, Karabell A, et al. Treatment of diabetic ketoacidosis with subcutaneous insulin aspart. Diabetes Care. 2004;27(8):1873-8.
17. Vehik K, Hamman RF, Lezotte D, et al. Childhood growth and age at diagnosis with Type 1 diabetes in Colorado young people. Diabet Med J Br Diabet Assoc. 2009;26(10):961-7.
18. Williams V, Jayashree M. Fluid and Electrolyte Management in Diabetic Ketacidosis. Indian J Pract Pediatr. 2018;20(1):12.
19. Wilson HK, Keuer SP, Lea AS, et al. Phosphate therapy in diabetic ketoacidosis. Arch Intern Med. 1982;142(3):517-20.
20. Wolfsdorf J, Craig ME, Daneman D, et al. Diabetic ketoacidosis in children and adolescents with diabetes. Pediatr Diabetes. 2009;10:118-33.
21. Yuen N, Anderson SE, Glaser N, et al. Cerebral Blood Flow and Cerebral Edema in Rats with Diabetic Ketoacidosis. Diabetes. 2008;57(10):2588-94.
22. Zeitler P, Haqq A, Rosenbloom A, et al. Hyperglycemic hyperosmolar syndrome in children: pathophysiological considerations and suggested guidelines for treatment. J Pediatr. 2011;158(1):9-14.

Basics of Renal Replacement Therapy

22

Nisha Krishnamurthy, Uma Ali

LEARNING OBJECTIVES

- To understand the various modalities available for renal replacement therapy (RRT)
- To understand the mechanisms and application of the modalities
- To be able to form prescription plans for various conditions.

INTRODUCTION

Acute kidney injury (AKI) is commonly encountered in critically ill children, where it may be present at the time of admission to the pediatric intensive care unit (PICU) or develop subsequently in the course of the underlying critical illness. The indications for renal replacement therapy (RRT) include the traditional ones like hyperkalemia, refractory metabolic acidosis, pulmonary edema, uremia, and fluid overload. In these critically ill children, fluid restriction alone may not be sufficient to tide over fluid overload, as they need various medications like vasoactive drugs, sedatives, continuous flushes, antibiotics, electrolyte replacements over and above their nutrition requirements. The increasing need for RRT is due to an increasing recognition and incidence of AKI in critically ill children as more survive the early phase due to enhanced care.

The various modalities available for renal replacement are:
- Peritoneal dialysis (PD)
- Intermittent hemodialysis (IHD)
- Sustained low efficiency dialysis (SLED)
- Continuous renal replacement therapy (CRRT).

Each of these modalities has its own advantages and disadvantages and they are to be selected in a given patient judiciously depending on the indication and feasibility of performing the therapy.

MECHANISMS OF SOLUTE AND FLUID REMOVAL

The different modes of dialysis operate on the basis of the physical principles that govern the movement of solutes and fluid across a semipermeable membrane. The solute removal mainly occurs via diffusion, convection, adsorption or a combination of these. Fluid removal is mainly by ultrafiltration.

Diffusion

It is the process where the solutes move from an area of higher concentration to the area of lower concentration across a semipermeable membrane. This movement depends on the difference in the concentration gradient, with greater transfer when the gradient is higher. It also depends on the surface area of the membrane used and the size of the molecule. Diffusion is more effective in the removal of small-sized molecules like urea or creatinine. The modes of dialysis where dialysate fluid is used depend on diffusion for solute removal. The dialysate is run countercurrent to blood flow and at a higher flow rate than the blood flow rate so as to maximize the concentration gradient.

Convection

It is the movement of solute across the semipermeable membrane due to solvent flux as ultrafiltration due to the pressure gradient. This movement of the solute across the membrane is independent of its concentration gradient, but dependent on the porosity of the membrane. The positive pressure needed for this ultrafiltration is created by increasing either the blood flow rate, the hydrostatic pressure in the blood compartment or by increasing the negative pressure in the dialysate compartment by decreasing the oncotic pressure of plasma by predilution. This method is effective for removal of fluid and middle-size molecules.

Adsorption

Adsorption is the adherence of solutes like peptides and proteins to surfaces of extracorporeal circuit. It occurs to a certain extent in all CRRT circuits, and adds to removal of large molecules. Adsorption of a substance becomes less effective over a period of time due to saturation of the membrane.

Ultrafiltration

It is the movement of water across a semipermeable membrane because of the transmembrane pressure gradient. It depends on the membrane surface area, its hydraulic permeability and trans-membrane pressure gradient. Convection occurs with ultrafiltration, so higher rates of ultrafiltration will cause greater removal of small and middle-size molecules, as allowed by the membrane. A membrane's effectiveness to ultrafiltrate fluid is measured by its ultrafiltration coefficient, which is the volume of ultrafiltrate per unit time, divided by the pressure gradient across the membrane.

Sieving Coefficient (SC)

It is the ratio of the concentration of solute in ultrafiltrate to that in plasma. A high sieving coefficient is desirable for middle-size molecules but not for albumin-size molecules.

SC = 1 indicates complete permeability (e.g. urea, creatinine)
SC = 0 indicates complete impermeability

Sieving coefficient of a solute determines the extent to which a solute crosses the semipermeable membrane under the pressure forces which are driving this movement. The major factors affecting the sieving coefficient are the solute's molecular size, its protein binding and the membrane porosity. The sieving coefficient for a particular solute may decline over the duration of treatment as plasma proteins that are too large to cross the membrane, accumulate along the membrane surface. This phenomenon of protein concentration polarization can potentially change the charge of the pores and restrict access to them.

MODES OF RENAL REPLACEMENT THERAPY

Peritoneal Dialysis

A mode where dialysis occurs using the peritoneal cavity and its surface as the semipermeable membrane, allowing for exchange of fluid and solutes between the dialysis fluid and capillary blood, where dialysate is instilled at a variable volume and dwell time. The advantages of peritoneal dialysis are outlined in Box 1.

Box 1: Advantages of peritoneal dialysis.

- Easy to initiate
- Can be done in a low resource setting
- No need for highly trained/skilled personnel
- No need to establish vascular access
- No need for expensive equipment
- No need for extracorporeal circulation
- No need for anticoagulation
- Minimal blood loss, if at all
- Especially beneficial in children with heart failure, hemodynamic instability, bleeding diathesis
- Is a form of continuous renal replacement therapy
- Possible less negative impact on renal function recovery

Mechanisms

The three-layered peritoneum consists of mesothelium, interstitium, and capillary wall with a continuous layer of non-fenestrated endothelial cells supported by a basement membrane. This capillary wall is permeable to water through aquaporins, water, and small solutes can be transported through small pores and the macromolecules are transported through the sparsely located large pores passively. In this mode, diffusion, absorption and convection mechanisms play a role in dialysis. Dialysate fluid contains electrolytes to allow for correction of electrolyte imbalances and to maintain acid–base balance. Glucose, lactate or bicarbonate diffuse from higher concentration dialysate fluid into the lower concentration in capillary blood, whereas uremic solutes and potassium move in the opposite direction into the dialysate fluid. Diffusion depends on factors like the concentration gradient of the solute between the capillary blood and instilled dialysis fluid, the effective surface area of the peritoneum recruited for dialysis based on the fill volume used, the molecular weight of the solute, and the intrinsic resistance of the peritoneal membrane.

Ultrafiltration occurs due to the osmotic gradient between the capillary blood and dialysis fluid, where the high concentration of glucose (or other osmotic agent like codextrin) in the dialysis fluid creates the oncotic pressure gradient needed to draw out fluid from the blood compartment into the peritoneal space. Also, the higher hydrostatic pressure in the blood vessels aids in formation of ultrafiltrate. This ultrafiltration contributes to solute removal via convection. There is a constant rate (1.0–2.0 mL/min) of fluid absorption from the peritoneal space via the lymphatics, which reduces the efficiency of fluid and solute removal by peritoneal dialysis. This absorption is greater in the presence of higher intraperitoneal pressure as seen with a sitting position as compared to supine or standing position and if the fill volume is large. The fill volume at initiation of peritoneal dialysis is usually around 10–20 mL/kg and gradually increased up to 40–50 mL/kg. Development of respiratory distress with increasing fill volume, leakage from catheter insertion site, appearance of hernia are some of the complications to be monitored for this period. The dwell time initially should be around 30 minutes, to be increased to 60 minutes, where shorter cycles allow better solute clearances. Outflow is aided by gravity and takes not more than 20–30 minutes; hence each cycle is to be completed within 1–2 hours.

Peritoneal dialysis prescription: PD orders to include, e.g. in a 10 kg child:
- Planned duration of the PD: 72 hours
- % glucose solution to be used: 1.5 %
- Fill volume per cycle: To begin with 200 mL, up to maximum of 400 mL/cycle
- Dwell time per cycle: 20–30 minutes
- Number of rapid cycles: 3–6 cycles after catheter insertion
- Dwell time per cycle (after rapid cycles)
- Outflow time: Maximum 20 minutes (by gravity)
- Total duration of each cycle (inflow + dwell + outflow): Not to exceed 1 hour
- Heparin to be added to PD fluid: 500 u/L
- Other additions to fluid (Potassium, etc.): As needed
- Balance per cycle: Depending on hemodynamic status and need for fluid removal
- Cumulative balance: Recording/charting to be maintained
- Tests to be done: 6 hourly-electrolytes, venous blood gas (VBG); 24 hourly—blood urea nitrogen (BUN), creatinine
- To monitor vital parameters, change in outflow volume and appearance, to monitor ease of inflow and outflow, to monitor for any discomfort/pain, if persistent positive balance in two or more consecutive cycles.

Modifications can be made to further optimize peritoneal dialysis, such as increasing the glucose concentration of the dialysis fluid by addition of 50% glucose at a fixed volume. Also a high bicarbonate concentration can be made, to be used in cases where the metabolic acidosis is refractory to therapy with the regular dialysis fluid.

Intermittent Hemodialysis

An extracorporeal mode of RRT, using the dialyzer which acts as the semipermeable membrane, across which occur fluid and solute clearance by diffusion and ultrafiltration.

In IHD, blood is drawn through a vascular access at the rate of 3–10 mL/kg/min (up to a maximum of 400 mL/min), passes through a blood pump which generates the positive pressure and into the dialyzer. Here, the dialysate runs countercurrent to the blood flow, at a rate of 400–500 mL/min for children less than 20 kg and 600–700 mL/min for children more than 20 kg. When the blood and dialysate fluid flow in the same direction (concurrent), solute concentration in the blood will begin to fall along with simultaneous rise in solute concentration in the dialysate fluid due to diffusion. Diffusion will stop when solute concentration is similar on both sides. In countercurrent flow, blood and dialysate fluid flow in opposite directions. This is advantageous and promotes continuous clearance of solutes by maintaining an adequate diffusion gradient throughout. During dialysis, a high concentration gradient can be maintained by increasing either blood flow rate or dialysate flow rate. Optimal solute clearance occurs when the dialysate flow rate is twice the blood flow rate.

Hollow fiber dialyzers are used in proportion to the body surface area (dialyzer/BSA = 0.7–1). The transfer of solutes depends on blood flow rate, dialysate flow rate, the solute concentration gradient, dialysate composition, surface area of the dialyzer and its permeability.

Regarding the extracorporeal circuit, which includes the tubing and the dialyzer, if the total blood volume of the circuit is greater than 10% of the estimated total blood volume (TBV), a circuit prime with 5% albumin or blood is recommended. The total blood volume is approximately equal to 100 mL/kg body weight in neonates and 80 mL/kg for infants and children. As a general rule blood prime is used if the patient is anemic. To avoid the risk of clotting the circuit, priming with packed red blood cells diluted with normal saline or 5% albumin to achieve a final hematocrit of 30–35% is suggested.

The duration of the session, for the first session is to be calculated to achieve a 30% drop in blood urea nitrogen level, subsequently increased stepwise to 4 hours sessions, over a period of 3 days. The vascular access for short-term dialysis is usually the dual lumen, appropriate-sized catheter, placed in the internal jugular vein (IJV) or femoral vein and for chronic use it is a tunneled cuffed dual lumen catheter placed in the IJV. Arteriovenous fistula or an arteriovenous graft can also be used for chronic dialysis.

Anticoagulation of the extracorporeal circuit is usually used, but not mandatory, depending on the risk of bleeding against the risk of the dialyzer clotting. In children, unfractionated heparin is preferred, however, low-molecular-weight heparin and citrate may be used as well. The initial dose of heparin is given as a loading dose, followed by maintenance every hour, stopped 30 minutes prior to stopping the session.

The commonly seen complications on IHD are:
- Dialysis disequilibrium syndrome (DDS) due to osmolarity changes, causing shift of water from extracellular to intracellular space across the blood–brain barrier. It presents as nausea, vomiting, seizures, altered sensorium, hypertension, and muscle twitching. These symptoms occur during or immediately after the dialysis session and are generally self-limiting, although recovery may take a few days. It can be prevented by structuring the dialysis to achieve a targeted decrease in blood urea nitrogen levels, using dialyzers with smaller surface area, setting lower blood and dialysate flow rates. If fluid overloaded, then isolated ultrafiltration is followed by dialysis.
- Intradialytic hypotension, due to imbalance between ultrafiltration and vascular refilling and paradoxical decrease in sympathetic activity.
- Nausea, vomiting, muscle cramps, etc.

Prescription of IHD

To include, e.g., in a 10 kg child, body surface area approximately 0.5 m^2:
- *Dialyzer surface area*: 0.5 m^2 (0.8–1.0 x patient's BSA) (volume approximately 30 mL) (Table 1)
- *Tubing size/volume*: 75 mL (Pediatric), 127 mL (Adult)

Table 1: Effective surface area of dialyzers.

Dialyzers	Effective surface area (m²) [Suitable for range of body surface area]
F3	0.4 [0.4–0.55]
F4	0.7 [0.7–1.0]
F5	0.9 [0.9–1.3]
F6	1.3

- *Blood flow rate (mL/min) (3–8 mL/kg/min)*: 30 mL/min up to maximum of 80 mL/min
- *Dialysate flow rate (mL/min)*: Up to 300–500 mL/min for less than 20 kg
- *Maximum allowed extracorporeal (dialyzer + tubing)*: 80 mL volume [Not to exceed 10% of total blood volume (TBV), where TBV for children = weight in kg x 80 mL]
- *Priming volume, if needed (mL)*: 5% albumin, normal saline or packed red blood cells. As total extracorporeal volume is 30 mL + 75 mL, priming volume will be 25–30 mL.
- Solution to be used as prime (Blood/Albumin/Normal saline)
- *Duration of session*: 4 hours once IHD established
- *Anticoagulation*: Heparin
- *Loading and maintenance doses*: Loading 20-50 u/kg bolus and 10 u/kg/hr
- *Ultrafiltration targeted per hour (maximum 10–12 mL/kg/hr)*: Maximum 480 mL/4 hours session
- *Isolated ultrafiltration, if needed (maximum 20–25 mL/kg/hr)*: 250 mL/hour maximum
- Sodium profiling, if needed
- Drugs to be administered during HD
- HD catheter lock
- Investigations, if any, to be sent pre-HD
- Monitoring chart for heart rate/respiratory rate/blood pressure/saturation, every 15 minutes
- Adverse events, if any, during HD
- Intervention made.

Sustained Low-efficiency Dialysis

It is a hybrid therapy which acts as an intermediate between IHD and CRRT. The aim of SLED is to combine the advantages offered by the CRRT and IHD modes, such as a lower ultrafiltration rate for better hemodynamic stability, low efficiency of solute removal with lower chances of DDS, increased duration per session of SLED to compensate for the lower efficiency to still achieve adequate solute clearance, with net clearances even better than IHD. SLED being a prolonged intermittent type of dialysis, allows flexibility in terms of time for other diagnostic and therapeutic procedures that may be needed.

The machine and the extracorporeal circuit used is the same as that used for IHD. The difference being in the lowered blood and dialysate flow rates (making it low in efficiency) to 100–200 mL/min or 10–20 mL/kg/min and 300 mL/min, respectively, and prolonged duration up to 8–12 hour sessions. However, longer durations of SLED up to 15–24 hours have also been used. The ultrafiltration per hour is limited to not more than 4–5 mL/kg/hr in view of the preexisting hemodynamic instability in the critically ill children.

The complications of SLED, similar to those in IHD, but also include hypokalemia, hypophosphatemia, and hypomagnesemia which may need supplementation. Also hypotension is a major concern during SLED.

Drug dosing is to be carefully monitored and adjusted while the child is undergoing SLED, as with solute removal, drug removal during SLED is quite high. There is a paucity of data, especially in children, regarding the adjustments to be made, especially for antibiotics, while on SLED. Data available for a few drugs like meropenem, where additional doses, over a longer duration of infusion are recommended.

The modes of SLED that have been used are:
- *SLEDD*: Sustained low-efficiency daily dialysis
- *SLEDD-f*: It is a modification of SLEDD, where hemofiltration is added, thereby providing the additional benefit of convective clearance to the existing diffusion clearance. This is achieved by using replacement fluid to offset the fluid losses. This mandates the need for ultrapure water, dry sterile powder concentrates, high-flux dialyzer and replacement fluid.
- *SLEDD-c*: Sustained low-efficiency daily continuous dialysis. This is a process where SLEDD is run continuously for as many days as needed.

The advantages of SLED are that it can be done with conventional HD machines, lower cost of dialysis sessions as compared with CRRT and the dialysis technicians and nurses are familiar with the procedure.

Continuous Renal Replacement Therapy

It is an extracorporeal therapy designed to suit the needs of treatment of AKI in critically ill children, with fluid overload, where the facility and expertise are available. CRRT allows for greater precision in ultrafiltration volume control, fluid balance, lower blood flow rates suitable to critically ill children. As the procedure is carried out over a prolonged duration and provides a steady and slow removal of fluid and solutes, it is better tolerated hemodynamically by the critically ill child. The advantage over peritoneal dialysis, being in the ability to control the ultrafiltration.

The varieties of CRRT are based on the primary mode of solute/fluid removal. The CRRT machine, different from the conventional hemodialysis machine, has a blood pump, dialysate pump, pre-blood pump for prefilter replacement fluid delivery when heparin anticoagulation is used or for citrate delivery during citrate anticoagulation, replacement fluid pump, effluent pump for net fluid removal along with blood leak detectors and deaeration chamber.

Slow Continuous Ultrafiltration

Slow continuous fluid removal is useful in fluid overload states like cardiac failure. There is no component of dialysis and the rate of fluid removal is low therefore the solute clearance by this method is poor. The transmembrane pressure allows for fluid movement into effluent. No dialysate or replacement fluid is used in this method.

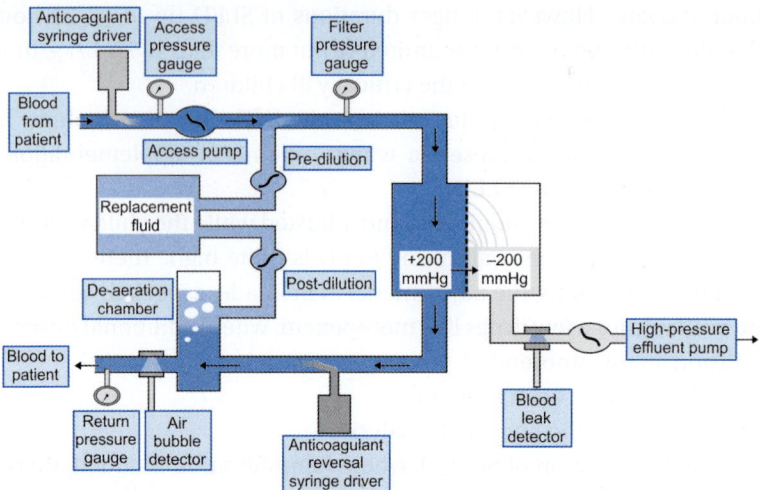

Fig. 1: Continuous venovenous hemofiltration.
Source: Image adapted from Gambro Prismaflex brochure.

Continuous Venovenous Hemofiltration (CVVHF) (Fig. 1)

It is the closest mimic of the naturally occurring glomerular filtration. The main component of fluid and solute removal is convection, dependent of large volume of ultrafiltration provided by replacement fluid used either prefilter or postfilter. The fluid moves across the semipermeable membrane under a transmembrane pressure, taking with it the solutes by convection. The rate of solute removal depends on rate of ultrafiltration. Hence for good solute removal, the ultrafiltration rate needs to be high leading to fluid removal that is far in excess of body's volume needs. As large amounts of fluid transfer occur during ultrafiltration, replacement fluid is needed to maintain fluid balance and prevent hypovolemia. The net fluid removal is the difference between the ultrafiltration rate and replacement fluid rate. No dialysate fluid is used.

Continuous Venovenous Hemodialysis (CVVHD) (Fig. 2)

It is similar to conventional hemodialysis, but done at a much slower rate. The mode of solute clearance is diffusion as in conventional hemodialysis. However, it is different from IHD in that the dialysate flow rate is very low and the blood flow rates of 10 mL/kg/min in infants up to 200 mL/min in adolescents are used. No replacement fluid is used, only dialysate fluid used.

Continuous Venovenous Hemodiafiltration (CVVHDF) (Fig. 3)

It is a combination of CVVHF and CVVHD, thereby using both modes, diffusion and convection for solute and fluid removal. Hence both replacement and dialysate fluid are used.

The dialyzers used for conventional dialysis differ from the filters for hemofiltration. In the pore size and structure, the hemofilters have larger pores with straight wide channels in their support structure, with less resistance to fluid flow. They do not need much pressure for fluid removal and can remove small and middle molecules well. These hemofilters are of a greater permeability, hence the high flux.

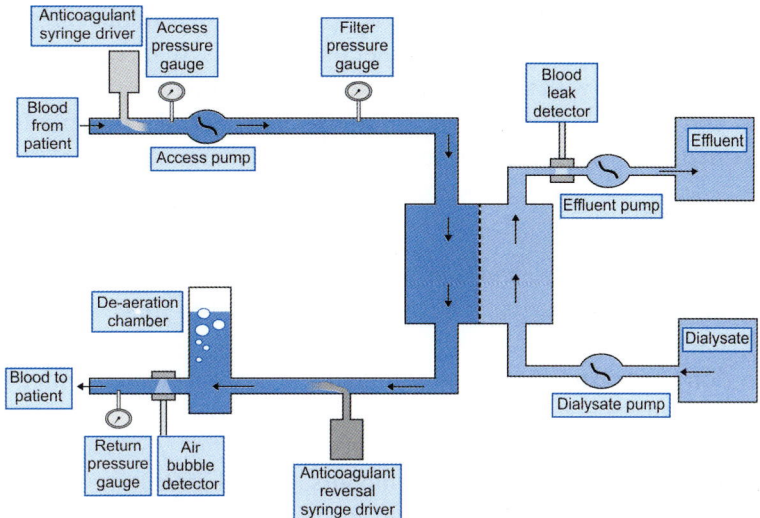

Fig. 2: Continuous venovenous hemodialysis.
Source: Image adapted from Gambro Prismaflex brochure.

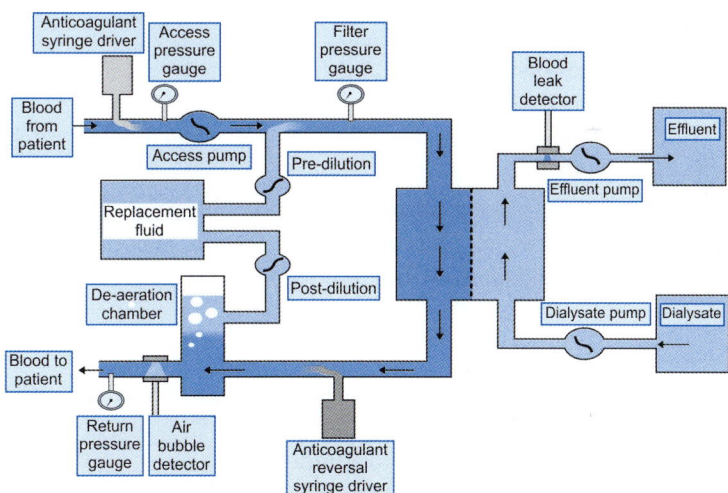

Fig. 3: Continuous venovenous hemodiafiltration.
Source: Image adapted from Gambro Prismaflex brochure.

Dialysate fluid is commercially available sterile crystalloid fluid, which contains levels of sodium, chloride, and magnesium same as blood. They are either lactate based or bicarbonate based fluids. The replacement fluid can be normal saline, or its combination with calcium chloride, magnesium sulfate or sodium bicarbonate. The replacement fluid can be added to extracorporeal circuit either before blood reaches the filter or after blood has passed through the filter and before it is returned to the patient via vascular access.

Advantages of CRRT are that it is a continuous process, closely mimicking the glomerular function of native kidney and it does need a water purification system. Disadvantages being, it needs a dedicated machine with several pumps to control blood flow, dialysate flow, fluid replacement pre- and post-fluid with effluent rate and technician and staff expertise of handling the machine, with therapy being more expensive than the other modalities of dialysis.

Prescription of CRRT

- Patient parameters: Height/weight/age/body surface area/vitals
- Fluid overload status (i.e. excessive fluid volume expected by weight increase or calculation of fluid balance)
- Hourly infusion rate (vasoactive drugs/antibiotics/blood and blood products/nutrition)
- Native urine output
- Filter/dialyzer and tubings
- Priming volume, and solution to be used (blood/saline/albumin)
- *CRRT modality*: CVVHF/CVVHD/CVVHDF
- *Blood flow rate*: In neonates—10–12 mL/kg/min, in children—4–8 mL/kg/min, in adolescents—2–4 mL/kg/min
- *Dialysate flow rate(DFR)*: In CVVHD—25–35 mL/kg/hr, CVVHDF-DFR + Fluid replacement rate (FRR) = 2 L/m^2/hr
- FRR usually 25–35 mL/kg/hr
- Patient fluid removal rate—usually 1–2 mL/kg/hr
- Anticoagulation—heparin/citrate
- Monitoring of vitals, temperature, intake-output balance, electrolytes, calcium, phosphorus, and magnesium levels.

The common complications seen during CRRT are bleeding, thrombosis, hemolysis, hypothermia, hypokalemia, hypophosphatemia, hypocalcemia, hypomagnesemia, metabolic alkalosis, citrate intoxication, and altered drug removal.

KEY POINTS

- Dialysis in the intensive care setting should be jointly undertaken by the ICU and Nephrology team
- No mode has been proven to be superior to another
- Unstable patients need slow, careful dialysis

SUGGESTED READING

1. Alkandari O, Eddington KA, Hyder A, et al. Acute kidney injury is an independent risk factor for pediatric intensive care unit mortality, longer length of stay and prolonged mechanical ventilation in critically ill children: a two-center retrospective cohort study. Crit Care. 2011;15:R146.
2. Askenazi DJ, Goldstein SL, Koralkar R, et al. 2013 Continuous renal replacement therapy for children ≤10 kg: a report from the prospective pediatric continuous renal replacement therapy registry. J Pediatr. 2013;162:587-92.
3. Deep A, Goldstein A (Eds). Textbook of Critical Care Nephrology and Renal Replacement Therapy in Children. Springer. 2018.

4. Foland JA, Fortenberry JD, Warshaw BL, et al. Fluid overload before continuous hemofiltration and survival in critically ill children: a retrospective analysis. Crit Care Med. 2004;32:1771-6.
5. Gillespie RS, Seidel K, Symons JM. Effect of fluid overload and dose of replacement fluid on survival in hemofiltration. Pediatr Nephrol. 2004;19:1394-9.
6. Hayes LW, Oster RA, Tofil NM, et al. Outcomes of critically ill children requiring continuous renal replacement therapy. J Crit Care. 2009;2009:394-400.
7. Kiessling SG (Ed). Textbook of Pediatric Nephrology in the ICU. Springer. 2009.
8. Marshall MR, Ma T, Galler D, et al. Sustained low-efficiency daily diafiltration (SLEDD-f) for critically ill patients requiring renal replacement therapy: towards an adequate therapy. Nephrol Dial Transplant. 2004;19(4):877-84.
9. Sutherland SM, Zappitelli M, Alexander SR, et al. Fluid overload and mortality in children receiving continuous renal replacement therapy: the prospective pediatric continuous renal replacement therapy registry. Am J Kidney Dis. 2010;55:316-25.

23. Gastrointestinal Tract Bleed

Abhishek Bansal

LEARNING OBJECTIVES

- Suspect Gastrointestinal Tract (GIT) bleed in children
- Make a list of differential diagnosis based on history and clinical examination with respect to age.
- Plan detailed investigation; stabilize hemodynamic instability
- Explain role of endoscopic interventions and newer medical therapies in GI bleed.

INTRODUCTION

A gastrointestinal tract (GIT) bleed could potentially be a serious acute or chronic situation and may need hospitalization and urgent attention; at the same time, it is a frightening experience for the family and child. GIT bleed can take place from oral cavity to anus, virtually from any part of the GIT system. Minor episodes of GIT bleeding could be self-limiting but serious bleeds may pose a threat to life. Depending on the clinical presentation, GIT bleeding can be classified into acute, chronic, and obscure. The ligament of Treitz divides the anatomical location of the bleed into coming from the upper and lower tract if it is proximal or distal to it respectively. An accurate diagnosis is crucial for directing proper investigations and prompt management which include initial risk assessment, resuscitation and specific interventions.

EPIDEMIOLOGY

Gastrointestinal tract bleed is an uncommon occurrence in the general pediatric population. In pediatric intensive care units (PICUs), 6–20% of patients develop upper GIT bleed (UGITB), but the incidence of lower GIT bleeding in not well documented. One US-based study revealed 0.5% of total discharged patients from hospital had a diagnosis of a GIT bleed. Male gender, older children (children >11 years) were more likely to bleed; 11–15- year-old children had the highest incidence of bleed (84.2 per 10,000) and less than 1 year the least (24.4 per 10,000). The mostcommon site of bleeding documented was a rectal bleed (17.6 per 10,000) followed by hematemesis (11.2 per 10,000). The highest mortality in GIT bleeding was associated with intestinal perforation (8.7%) and esophageal perforation (8.4%).

BLOOD OR BLOOD MIMICKING SUBSTANCES

There are foods and drugs which may mimic fresh or altered blood in emesis or stool. It is important to decide at the time of initial evaluation that what appears to be blood is actually blood; wrong identification may lead to unwarranted investigations and interventions and can create panic. Foods that may impart red color to vomitus or stool are beet, red toffees and candies, fruit punch and among medication is rifampicin. A black color could be due to iron containing medications, charcoal, bismuth, and foods like blueberries and spinach. Fortunately, blood can easily be differentiated from all other substances by a widely available test—guaiac test, which changes its color in the presence of hemoglobin. Test kits are also available commercially to test blood in stool or emesis like Hemoccult (HCT) and Gastroccult.

ACUTE (OVERT) VS CHRONIC (OCCULT) VS OBSCURE GIT BLEED

Given the potential life threatening nature and a wide variety of underlying pathological causes and consequently based on various different therapeutic approaches, it is prudent to define bleed on the basis of clinical features.

As per the rate of blood loss, GIT bleed can be classified in three forms: acute (overt), chronic (occult) or obscure. GIT bleed may manifests in the form of hematemesis (vomiting of fresh blood or altered coffee colored material), melena (dark tarry stool), or hematochezia (fresh blood *per rectum*). Low grade or occult GIT bleed is not appreciable to the parents or patients and present as positive occult blood in stool or iron deficiency anemia. Obscure GIT bleeding is GIT bleed with an unidentified source even after upper gastrointestinal (GI) endoscopy and colonoscopy. However, it usually originates from the small intestine. Patients with obscure bleed usually present with positive fecal occult blood test (FOBT) or iron deficiency anemia. Obscure bleeding may be either overt or occult.

UPPER VS LOWER GIT BLEED

Upper GIT bleeds include bleeding anywhere from oral cavity, esophagus, stomach, and duodenum till ligament of Treitz which is located at duodenojejunal flexure. A lower GIT bleed occurs distal to it. Recently, anatomical classification has redefined bleeds as per endoscopic accessibility of the intestine.
- Upper GIT bleed is considered—till ampula of Vater, which is within reach of an upper GI endoscope.
- *Lower GIT bleed*:
  - Mid-GIT from ampulla of Vater to ileocecal junction.
  - Lower GIT from ileocecal junction to the colon.

In patients with GIT bleed, many a times, the site of bleed is obvious by clinical presentation itself. UGITB, sometimes, could be due to swallowed blood from epistaxis; or in newborns it may represent the swallowed maternal blood. Both upper and lower GIT bleed can lead to melena, but occasionally massive UGITB may manifest as hematochezia.

ETIOLOGY OF GIT BLEED

Though there is a substantial overlap among the causes, still etiologies can be categorized as upper and lower GIT bleed in newborns, infants, 1–5 years old and older children.

Table 1: Causes of upper GIT bleed as per age.

Newborns	1–12 months	1–5 years	>5 years
Swallowed maternal blood	GER-induced esophagitis	Erosive esophagitis	Esophageal varices
Stress gastritis	Gastritis secondary to stress, NSAIDs, Zollinger–Ellison syndrome, Crohn's disease	Esophageal varices	Portal hypertension gastropathy
Trauma of the feeding tube		Caustic ingestion	Gastritis due to *Helicobacter pylori*, NSAIDs
Vitamin K deficiency		Mallory–Weiss syndrome	
Sepsis	Caustic ingestion	Peptic and duodenal ulcers	Caustic ingestion
Cow milk protein allergy	Foreign body ingestion	Foreign body	Mallory–Weiss syndrome
Indomethacin therapy		NSAIDs use	Vasculitis; HSP
			Hemobilia
			Eosinophilic gastroenteritis

(GER: gastroesophageal reflux; GIT: gastrointestinal tract; HSP: Henoch–schönlein purpura; NSAIDs: nonsteroidal anti-inflammatory drugs)

Upper GIT Bleed in Children (Table 1)

For ascertaining a differential diagnosis, a detailed clinical history along with a general physical examination is supplemented with laboratory tests and diagnostic procedures. In neonatal hematemesis, maternal blood can be easily differentiated from baby's blood by the alkali denaturation test (Apt–Downey test) as fetal hemoglobin is resistant to alkali. In infants and older children presenting with hematemesis, if there is a history of epigastric pain, chest pain, heart burn, or repeated regurgitation, it may point toward acid peptic disease, peptic/duodenal ulcers, or erosive esophagitis. History of intake of drugs like nonsteroidal anti-inflammatory drugs (NSAIDs) can be a major cause of hematemesis. Patients in the ICU can develop UGITB secondary to stress ulcers or trauma caused by a nasogastric (NG) tube. The presence of violent vomiting or retching before hematemesis causes a mucosal tear at the gastroesophageal junction (Mallory–Weiss syndrome). Bleeding in association with severe abdominal pain, palpable purpuric rashes of lower limbs may suggest Henoch–Schonlein purpura.

Lower GIT Bleed in Children (Table 2)

Lower GI bleed is usually a self-limiting condition. 80% of cases get treated in the outpatient department (OPD) or discharged from emergency department, however, melena caused by varices and Meckel's diverticulum may be life-threatening emergencies; sometimes massive UGITB can masquerade as lower GIT bleed.

The causes of lower GIT bleeding are listed in Table 2. In infants, episodic cramping abdominal pain suggested by unexplained episodes of excessive crying associated with red currant jelly stool indicates intussusception; milk protein allergy may manifest as a cranky baby with increased frequency of blood in the stool but not diarrhea. Volvulus and gangrenous bowel present as vomiting, often billious and acute abdomen with ileus and Hirschsprung's present as constipation with abdominal distension.

Table 2: Causes of lower GIT bleed as per age.

Newborns	1–12 months	1–5 years	>5 years
Anal fissure NEC Vit K deficiency Volvulus Hirschsprung enterocolitis CMPA Sepsis Coagulopathy Indomethacin therapy Intussusception	Anal fissure Intussusception Milk protein allergy Volvulus Gangrenous bowel Hirschsprung's disease Bowel duplication Bleeding diathesis	Infective colitis Polyp Anal fissure Meckel's diverticulum IBD Intussusception Hemolytic–uremic syndrome Lymphonodular hyperplasia HSP	Infective colitis Polyp IBD Lymphonodular hyperplasia HSP Angiodysplasia Hemolytic uremic syndrome

(CMPA: cow's milk protein allergy; GIT: gastrointestinal tract; HSP: Henoch-Schönlein purpura; IBD: inflammatory bowel disease; NEC: necrotizing enterocolitis)
Source: Wolfram W. Pediatric Gastrointestinal Bleeding: Background, Etiology, Epidemiology [Internet]. Emedicine.medscape.com. 2018 [cited 7 September 2018]. Available from: https://emedicine.medscape.com/article/1955984-overview#showall.
Romano C, Oliva S, Martellossi S, et al. Pediatric gastrointestinal bleeding: Perspectives from the Italian Society of Pediatric Gastroenterology. World J Gastroenterol. 2017; 23(8):1328-37.

In children of 1–5 years age group, the common causes are listed in Table 2 and Box 1. Profuse watery diarrhea with bleeding per rectum could be a sign of infective colitis. Rampant use of antibiotics is associated with *Clostridium difficile* colitis. Children with inflammatory bowel disease (IBD) usually have their diagnosis established well before bleeding episode occurs, bleeding is more common in the ulcerative colitis than Crohn's disease.

Box 1: Causes of painless rectal bleeding.
- Colonic polyps.
- Bleeding diathesis
- Meckel's diverticulum
- Intestinal duplication
- Vascular malformation

During the initial encounter with a patient of lower GIT bleed, the focus is on differentiating patients who may need surgical intervention. In any infant or child who is ill looking, a surgical cause like intussusception, volvulus, necrotizing enteritis, or perforation should be suspected. If bleeding is significant and presents as both bright red and dark red stool, at all ages Meckel's diverticulum is a strong possibility. In older children with severe disease, hemolytic–uremic syndrome, Henoch–Schonlein purpura, and IBD could be the cause of bleeding.

Painless rectal bleeding with normal stool habits indicates polyps, bleeding diathesis, vascular malformations, Meckel's diverticulum, and eosinophilic colitis. Constipation and hard stool are often associated with anal fissures which lead to pain and bleeding during defecation.

Obscure GIT Bleed in Children

It is defined as GIT bleed of unknown source which persists or recurs even after normal initial evaluation including upper GI endoscopy and colonoscopy. It may or may not have apparent blood in stool, thus obscure GIT bleed could be overt or occult. Occult obscure GIT bleed is usually suspected after an incidental finding of positive occult stool blood or iron deficiency anemia. Etiology depends on the age of the child and location of bleeding; in some cases, location can be identified by upper GIT endoscopy or colonoscopy. Common causes are intestinal polyps, Meckel's diverticulum, vascular malformation, Crohn's disease, and intestinal duplication (Box 2). As in adults, combined acute and chronic obscure GIT bleed is seen in 5% of GI bleed cases in pediatrics. Almost in 75% of cases of obscure GIT bleed the cause is finally found in the small intestine.

Box 2: Causes of occult GIT bleed.
• Gastritis
• Acid peptic disease/peptic and dudenal ulcers
• Esophagitis
• IBD
• Vascular malformation
• Eosinophilic gastroenteritis
• Polyp
• Vascular malformation

(GI: gastrointestinal tract; IBD: inflammatory bowel disease)

INITIAL EVALUATION

On first encounter, a thorough but rapid evaluation is mandatory. The child's airway, breathing, circulation, and neurological status should be assessed and determined whether there has been any significant blood loss or any active ongoing bleeding. Comorbid conditions like bleeding diathesis [idiopathic thrombocytopenic purpura (ITP), hemophilia, etc.], liver disease may be present. If the clinical condition is unstable, it suggests significant blood loss and resultant circulatory failure, and requires immediate intervention to support the deteriorating condition of the child based on short, focused history. If the child is found to be stable clinically, then a detailed history and physical examination can be undertaken before initiating management (Box 3).

Box 3: Initial evaluation of GIT bleed.
• ABCD assessment
• Estimation of blood volume loss
• Active bleeding
• Comorbid conditions
• Detailed history
• Physical examination

(ABCD: airway, breathing, circulation, disability; GIT: gastrointestinal tract)

History should be sought from parents or available attendants/care givers. The time passed since bleeding started, source or location of bleeding, extent of bleeding (how many cloths soaked in blood) should be inquired. Any past history of bleeding episodes, bleeding diathesis, liver disease, intestinal disease, any medications (NSAIDs, anticoagulants, antibiotics), alcohol consumption are some of the critical points to note.

A physical examination can determine seriousness and urgency. Simultaneously, it aids in establishing a diagnosis. Altered vital signs, anemia, and orthostatic change suggest large volume blood loss. The presence of jaundice, ascites with pain in the right hypochondrium, raised serum glutamic pyruvic transaminase (SGPT) and serum glutamic–oxaloacetic transaminase (SGOT) levels may indicate a liver disorder and a risk of portal hypertension leading to variceal bleeding. History of umbilical vein catheterization can be a clue to portal vein thrombosis.

Maternal blood ingestion is the most common cause of suspected GI bleeding in neonates. Two sources of swallowed blood are: (i) mother's blood ingested by baby during birth and (ii) blood from cracked nipples ingested during breastfeeding (Table 3).

Table 3: Physical examination of child with GIT bleed.

Vital signs
- Heart rate
- Pulse volume
- Perfusion
- Respiratory rate
- Blood pressure
- Orthostatic change
- Oxygen saturation
- Temperature

Rectal examination
- Gross blood, red current jelly
- Melena
- Fissure, polyp, hemorrhoids, prolapse

Head and neck
- Pallor
- Jaundice
- Oral bleeding

Abdomen
- Distension
- Ascites
- Tenderness
- Abnormal vessel on the skin

Weight of the child

MANAGEMENT

Strategies for management depend on the initial evaluation of the child with GIT bleeding. As discussed above, circulatory compromise takes precedence over everything else and warrants aggressive resuscitation.

Early consultation with pediatric gastroenterologist and pediatric surgeon are valuable and should be sought.

Complete blood counts, liver functions including coagulogram, liver enzymes, bilirubin, albumin; renal function, arterial blood gas and cross match. The placement of NG tube is recommended to confirm the UGITB, simultaneously gastric lavage can also be done if upper GI endoscopy is planned. This helps determine the location of the bleed in cases of melena due to heavy UGITB. The presence of fresh blood in the NG aspirate indicates fresh ongoing bleeding. Continued bleeding from varices is not a contraindication for NG placement.

Volume resuscitative guidelines remain the same for GI bleeds and blood products should be used early for replacement.

Bacterial sepsis is a possible complication in patients with chronic liver disease with variceal bleeding. Increased white cells with polymorphonucleocytosis may suggest sepsis and hence early initiation of broad spectrum antibiotics is recommended after taking appropriate cultures. Short-term use of antibiotics has shown to improve survival.

Coagulopathy and thrombocytopenia should be corrected, if present, by using fresh frozen plasma and platelet concentrate respectively. Platelets should be maintained above 50,000/mm^3. Altered prothrombin time (PT) and international normalized ratio (INR) suggests disseminated intravascular coagulation or significant liver disease, deranged activated partial prothrombin time (aPTT) point toward hemophilia or coagulopathy. Parenteral vitamin K 1–2 mg, fresh frozen plasma 10–20 mL/kg or cryoprecipitates are to be provided to the patient. Nonetheless, coagulopathy may not correct in spite of transfusing blood products in the presence of significant liver disease. In such children, recombinant factor VIIa can be used and also in patients who are at risk of developing fluid overload.

High blood urea nitrogen (BUN) may indicate UGIB, where the body reabsorbs the intraluminal blood and this leads to rise in BUN, expect massive GIT bleed and significant blood loss. Request for packed red blood cell and transfuse the child to maintain hematocrit.

After initial evaluation and emergency management, when the child is stabilized, further investigations are initiated to pin point the cause and location of GIT bleeding (Flowcharts 1 to 5).

Flowchart 1: Algorithm for upper GIT bleed.

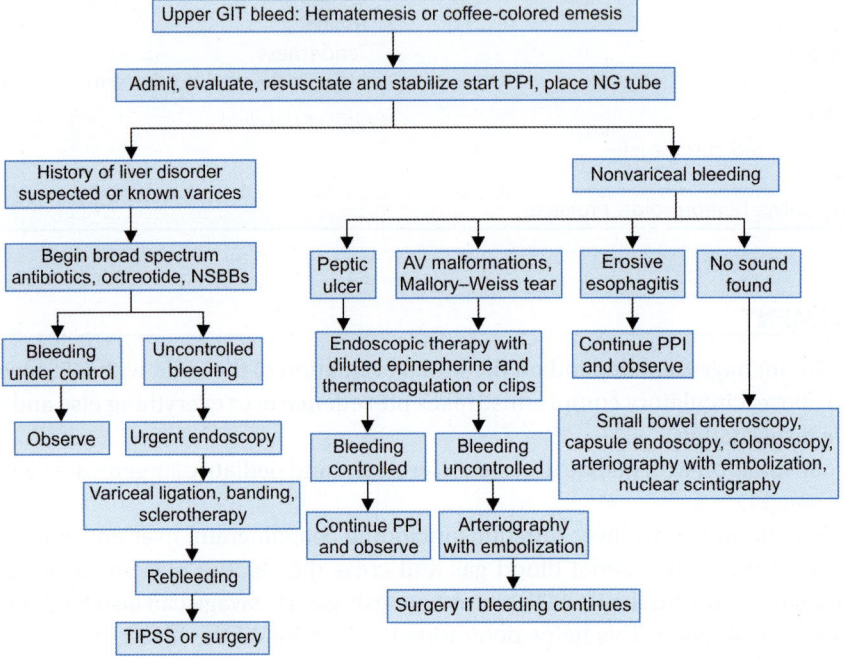

(GI: gastrointestinal; NG: nasogastric; NSBB: nonselective beta blocker; PPI: proton pump inhibitor; TIPSS: transjugular intrahepatic portosystemic shunt)

Flowchart 2: Algorithm for lower GIT bleed.

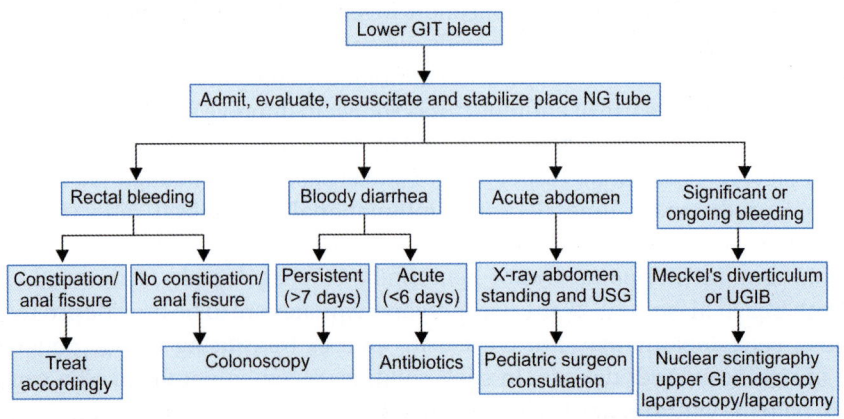

(GI: gastrointestinal; NG: nasogastric; UGITB: upper GIT bleed; USG: ultrasonography)

Flowchart 3: Algorithm for acute overt GIT bleed.

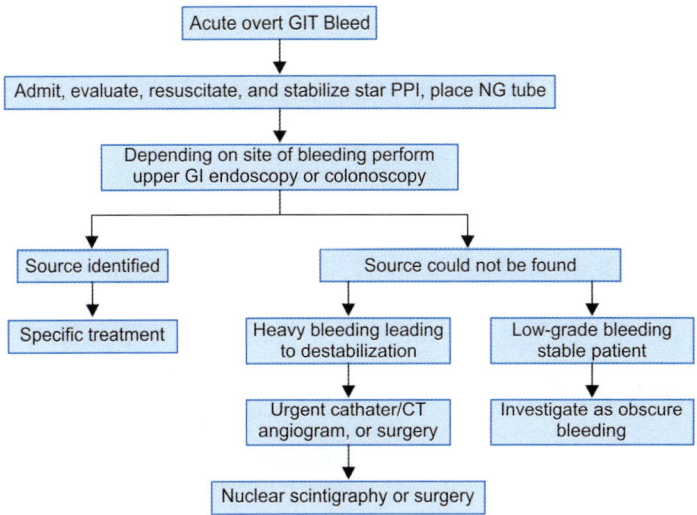

(CT: computed tomography; GI: gastrointestinal; NG: nasogastric; PPI: proton pump inhibitor)

Flowchart 4: Algorithm for chronic occult GIT bleed.

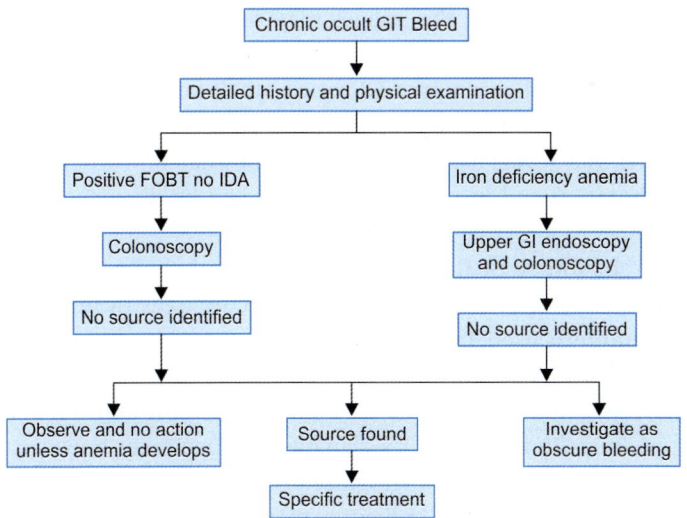

(GI: gastrointestinal; FOBT: fecal occult blood test; IDA: iron deficiency anemia)

Radioimaging has unequivocal place in the evaluation of GIT bleed. Ultrasonography and magnetic resonance imaging (MRI) are preferred and common first-line imaging as they do not have ionizing radiation. All patients with GIT bleed probably do not need abdominal radiograph but patients with suspected obstruction should undergo plain abdominal

Flowchart 5: Algorithm for obscure GIT bleed.

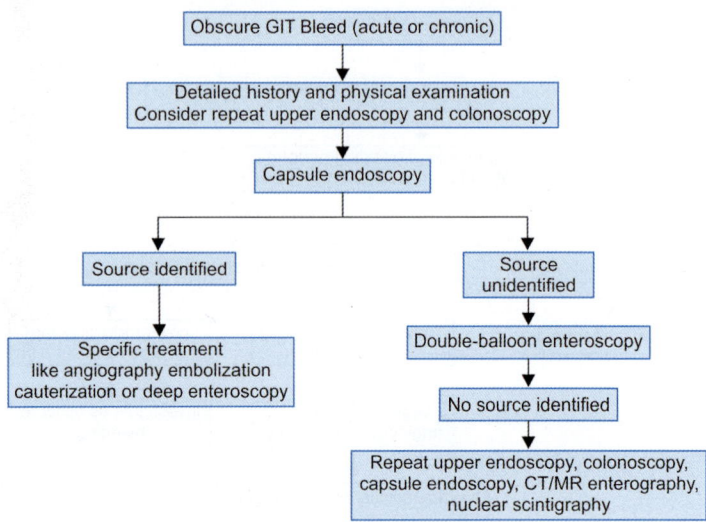

(CT: computed tomography; GI: gastrointestinal; MR: magnetic resonance)

radiography. Abdominal radiography may also be helpful in neonates in whom necrotizing enterocolitis (NEC) is a possibility; the images may show free air, pneumatosis intestinalis, or portal air. In nonemergency GIT bleed situation, imaging studies may begin with barium contrast studies (barium swallows, upper GI series, small bowel follow-throughs, or barium enemas) to figure out foreign bodies, esophagitis, IBD, or polyps. Malrotation with midgut volvulous in neonates may reveal itself as "corkscrew" of small bowel or a "bird's beak" on oral contrast study. Malrotation and intussusception both can be diagnosed with color Doppler ultrasound.

To locate the exact source of the bleed, nuclear scintigraphy (Meckel's scan, which is performed using 99 mTc pertechnetate to highlight the ectopic gastric mucosa); (Figs. 1A and B) and selective angiography is used, but these techniques are generally employed after negative endoscopic studies or in very sick patients who are not expected to tolerate surgery. Nuclear scintigraphy is more sensitive but less specific then angiography and can detect bleeding at a rate as low as 0.1 mL/min. Though Meckel's scan has low specificity, however, it serves as a fair guide for determining site of selective angiography, figure out requirement for wireless video capsule endoscopy (VCE) or give some indication to perform exploratory laparotomy and look for the etiology and site of hemorrhage. Selective arteriography can diagnose bleeding at rate of 0.5 mL/min and extravasation of contrast is confirmatory of GIT bleed in angiography. When a persistent or life threatening bleeding is identified, percutaneous transcatheter therapy with selective intra-arterial vasopressin infusion for vasoconstriction and embolization can be done by an interventional radiologist. Bowel infarction is a possible serious complication of this technique.

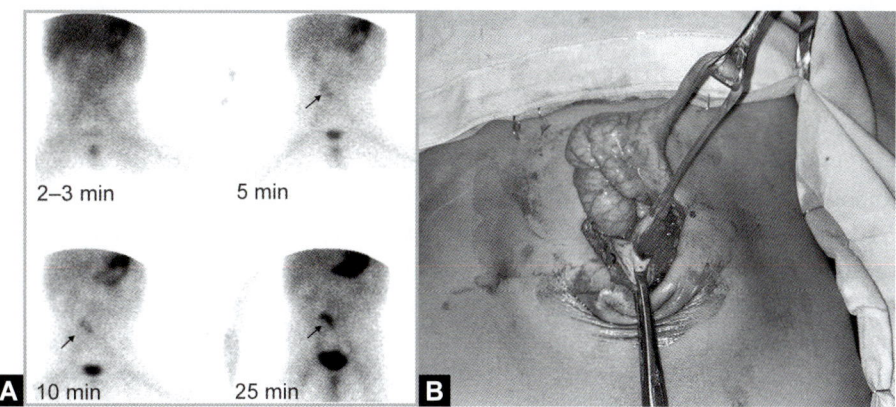

Figs. 1A and B: (A) Meckel's scan.
(*Courtesy*: Dr LP Kashyap. (B) Meckel's diverticulum—intraoperative).
(*Courtesy*: Dr Sumit Kumar)

Medical Management

Medical management involves two approaches:
1. Acid suppression
2. Manipulation of blood flow

Two class of acid suppression drugs are available, H_2 antagonists and proton pump inhibitors (PPIs). They have shown to be of benefit in treatment of ulcer bleeding or UGITB and PPIs are superior to H_2 antagonists. Out of five PPIs available commercially, omeprazole, pantoprazole, rabiprazole, lansoprazole, and esomeprazole. There is no difference in outcome.

Dosing of these drugs has been extrapolated from adults, and recommendations are: Pantoprazole intravenous route, 1–3 mg/kg over 1 h infusion and then 0.2 mg/kg/h to maintain gastric pH more than 6 during episodes of active bleeding. Studies have shown that PPI treatment reduces risk of rebleeding, requirement of surgery, need for transfusion, and is associated with lesser duration of hospital stay. PPIs were also demonstrated to reduce bleeding induced by NSAIDs.

Manipulation of blood flow employs two different approaches, (i) vasoactive drugs and (ii) nonselective beta blockers (NSBBs).

The first vasoactive drug used for GIT bleed was Vasopressin. Other drugs are somatostatin, octreotide, and terlipressin. Vasopressin decreases splanchnic blood flow by vasoconstriction of splanchnic arteries, thus reducing portal blood flow and bringing down portal pressure, consequently decreasing variceal bleeding. Octreotide is a synthetic analog of somatostatin, is a selective splanchnic vasoconstrictor, and reduces portal flow, resulting in decreased variceal bleeding. It is used in the doses of 1 µg/kg bolus and then 1–5 µg/kg/h as continuous infusion. Taper the dose by 50% when no active bleeding occur for 24 h and stop the infusion if no fresh bleeding takes place even on 25% of initial dose of octreotide. Though octreotide is more commonly used for variceal bleeding, it has also been used successfully for nonvariceal peptic ulcer bleeding before the endoscopy or when the endoscopy is unsuccessful or contraindicated. There is limited data on efficacy and safety of octreotide for chronic GIT bleed patients.

Terlipressin has generalized systemic arterial vasoconstrictive effect which is more pronounced on splanchnic arteries. It produces long lasting (up to 4 h) decrease in portal venous blood flow. Several studies have shown terlipressin to confer survival benefits to variceal patients. In adults, terlipressin is considered the first choice; octreotide and somatostatin being second choice of drugs. Studies in children still have not shown superiority of terlipressin over other vasoactive drugs but Erkek et al. reported a single-child experience of its use for successful management of severe nonvariceal UGITB. Terlipressin has good safety profile but hyponatremia and seizures have been reported in pediatric patients, thus serum sodium levels should be monitored in patients placed on terlipressin.

Nonselective beta blockers like propranolol, nodalol, and carvedilol are extensively studied and used in adults. They have been shown to reduce portal pressure and blood flow by decreasing cardiac output and producing splanchnic vasoconstriction by blockade of β_1 and β_2 receptors. Out of all three, carvedilol proved to be the most effective in reducing portal blood flow. There are no published randomized control trials evaluating safety and efficacy of NSBBs in pediatric population. The most appropriate dose is also not known, currently propranolol being used in range of 2–8 mg/kg/day and carvedilol 0.1–0.7 mg/kg/day in two divided doses. The published experience in pediatric patients is limited to primary and secondary prevention of variceal bleeding. There are currently no indications recommended to start NSBBs to prevent formation of varices; thus, data in literature are also limited on prevention of first variceal bleed.

Endoscopy

The objective of endoscopy is to identify the source of bleeding, stop it, and prevent rebleeding, serving diagnostic as well as therapeutic purposes. Usually, endoscopy is done when patient is stabilized hemodynamically, preferably within the first 24 h. There are various therapeutic interventions possible using endoscopy like injection therapy, mechanical therapy, ablation therapy for GIT bleed; the choice depending on bleeding characteristics. Each of these techniques has been modified for upper, lower, and deep endoscopy (Table 4).

Table 4: Endoscopic therapy techniques.

Injection therapy	Ablation therapy	Mechanical therapy
• Diluted epinephrine injection • Sclerosant injection	• *Contact methods*: Thermocoagulation heater probe Electrocoagulation • *Noncontact method*: Argon plasma coagulation	• Band ligation • Hemoclips

Upper Endoscopy

Upper GI endoscopy is performed for hematemesis, melena, hematochezia, and obscure GIT bleed. This serves both diagnostic and therapeutic purpose. It can diagnose the cause and source of bleeding like esophagitis, esophageal varices, peptic ulcers, duodenal ulcers, etc. Clinician can differentiate between fresh and old bleeding by noting the presence of clots and cherry red spots. It is desirable to perform gastric lavage and aspiration of stomach contents through an NG tube before upper GI endoscopy, as it improves visualization. Preferably the tube should be removed after endoscopy due to the potential risk of causing mucosal injury. The presence of varices is not a contraindication to placement of an NG tube. Semielective endoscopy is safer as this gives time to stabilize the child for sedation. Emergency endoscopy is performed only when heavy bleeding continues despite optimal medical management and significant transfusion requirement remains. Management of GIT bleed using upper endoscopy can be divided into two broad headings, (i) variceal bleed and (ii) nonvariceal bleed.

Variceal bleed: Sclerosant injection [endoscopic sclerotherapy (EST)] and endoscopic variceal band ligation (EBL) are used to control variceal bleeding. Several sclerosants are used for this purpose like absolute alcohol, 5% sodium morrhuate, 5% ethanolamine oleate, and sodium tetradecyl sulfate. Sclerotherapy produces esophageal ulcers in up to 90% of patients within a day and in 70% by 7 days. The risk of bleeding from these ulcers is 20%, and other complications include dysphagia, esophageal stricture, esophageal perforation, mediastinitis, pericarditis, peritonitis, and increased risk of bleeding from portal gastropathy. EBL in another method to control bleeding which results in thrombosis and necrosis of the mucosa finally sloughs leaving an ulcer. The ulcer heals in due course of time and thus varix is obliterated. Esophageal ulcers develop in 90% of treated individuals in a week and all complications mentioned above can happen in EBL, though at lower incidence. Uncontrolled or recurrent bleeding despite above measures may necessitates use of balloon temponade which stops bleeding in many patients, but these is risk of esophageal perforation, pressure necrosis of mucosa, and risk of rebleeding after deflation of balloon. Another technique in cases of uncontrolled bleeding from varices to achieve hemostasis is transjugular intrahepatic portosystemic shunt (TIPS). However, the strongest indication for TIPS placement is secondary prevention of esophageal variceal bleeding. In TIPS, angiographically a side-to-side communication is created between hepatic and portal veins, which works as portosystemic shunt and deflate the portal pressure allowing blood to flow from the portal to systemic circulation. Conditions where systemic venous pressure rises are contraindication for TIPS. Absolute contraindications to TIPS placement include severe pulmonary hypertension (mean pulmonary pressure >45 mm Hg), severe tricuspid regurgitation, congestive heart failure, severe liver failure, and polycystic liver disease. Also, no patients with active sepsis should undergo TIPS. Gastric varices can also be treated using ESL, EBL, and TIPS.

After achieving hemostasis of variceal bleeding, pharmacotherapy is employed to prevent rebleeding. NSBBs and spironolactone are used to reduce the portal pressure there by decreasing the probability of bleeding from the treated varices.

Nonvariceal bleed: The causes of nonvariceal UGITB are peptic and duodenal ulcers, Mallory-Weiss tear, erosive gastritis and duodenitis, esophagitis, esophageal ulcers, and vascular malformations. Lesions at high risk of rebleeding are called stigmata of recent hemorrhage (SRH) and include actively bleeding ulcers, nonbleeding visible vessels (NBVVs), and adherent clots. These require aggressive management to reduce the risk of rebleeding and its associated 5–16-fold increased risk of death.

Various techniques are in use for the treatment of SRH. Diluted adrenaline injection either alone or in combination with other techniques is a traditional method of hemostasis. Injection of diluted epinephrine is successful in controlling nonvariceal bleeding in almost 80% of cases, but multiple meta-analysis have shown that combination therapy (epinephrine injection plus ablation or banding) is even superior and controls bleeding in 90% of patients, reducing risk of rebleeding to 10%. Other methods are stainless steel hemostatic clips, loops to tie polyps, compression of artery using heat. Noncontact heating devices are argon plasma coagulation (APC) and Nd:YAG laser, while thermal contact techniques are bipolar electrocoagulation (BPE) and heater probe thermocoagulation (HPT).

Colonoscopy

Colonoscopy is lower GI endoscopy; it is undertaken in children with fresh blood per rectum and in cases of positive occult stool blood where upper GI endoscopy failed to find the etiology. Colonoscopy needs proper bowel preparation, thus most of the time it is elective or semi-elective, but rarely urgent colonoscopies are undertaken.

All the diagnostic and therapeutic techniques described in upper GI endoscopy are possible to perform in colonoscopy and are used to stop bleeding.

When radionuclide studies, such as angiography and endoscopy fails to diagnose and locate bleeding, and in obscure GIT bleeding cases, another option is push enteroscopy or double-balloon endoscopy. Alternatively, VCE can be used which works wirelessly but not able to take biopsy sample is its main limitation. Double-balloon enteroscopy has the advantage of diagnostic as well as therapeutic characteristics. Its ability to diagnose the cause of obscure bleeding is as high as 70–100%, especially when performed after positive VCE. When nothing helps and everything fails, laparoscopy and intraoperative endoscopy can be performed using an endoscope inserted in the mid-ileum by a small incision made in the intestine. Exploratory laparotomy is the last option when other methods cannot find the cause of GIT bleeding.

Consultation with pediatric surgeon is to be sought in cases of bleeding not responding to medical management and endoscopy. Surgical intervention could be lifesaving in conditions like Meckel's diverticulum, fulminant colitis, and familial adenomatous polyposis.

KEY MESSAGES

- Medical management is first-line treatment in variceal bleed; octreotide, somatostatin, terlipressin, NSBBs, and PPI are the mainstay. PPI has a major role to play in nonvariceal UGITB.
- Rectal examination should not be missed in fresh rectal bleed; as anal fissure is a common cause.
- Endoscopy is the most preferred method of study in GI bleed, and should be undertaken after stabilization of patient, preferably in 24 h.

- Endoscopy serves both purposes, identification of site of bleeding and etiology; and treatment of bleeding.
- Recurrent of persistent iron deficiency anemia despite adequate treatment with iron is a sign of obscure GI bleed. Video capsule endoscopy is the investigation of choice.

SUGGESTED READING

1. Balachandran B, Singhi S. Emergency management of lower gastrointestinal bleed in children. Indian J Pediatr. 2013;80:219-25 [PMID: 23355012 DOI: 10.1007/s12098-012-0955-x].
2. Bull-Henry K, Al-Kawas FH. Evaluation of occult gastrointestinal bleeding. Am Fam Physician. 2013;87:430-6 [PMID: 23547576].
3. Cappell MS. Therapeutic endoscopy for acute upper gastrointestinal bleeding. Nat Rev Gastroenterol Hepatol. 2010;7:214-29 [PMID: 20212504 DOI: 10.1038/nrgastro.2010.24] 55.
4. Cardile S, Martinelli M, Barabino A, et al. Italian survey on nonsteroidal anti-inflammatory drugs and gastrointestinal bleeding in children. World J Gastroenterol. 2016;22:1877-83 [PMID: 26855547 DOI: 10.3748/wjg.v22.i5.1877].
5. Copelan A, Kapoor B, Sands M. Transjugular intrahepatic portosystemic shunt: Indications, contraindications, and patient work-up. Semin Intervent Radiol. 2014;31(3):235-42 [DOI:10.1055/s-0034-1382790].
6. Erkek N, Senel S, Hizli S, et al. Terlipressin saved the life of a child with severe nonvariceal upper gastrointestinal bleeding. Am J Emerg Med. 2011;29:133.e5-133.e6 [PMID: 20825884 DOI: 10.1016/j.ajem.2010.02.010].
7. Hiorns MP. Gastrointestinal tract imaging in children: Current techniques. Pediatr Radiol. January 2011;41(1):42-54.
8. Laine L, McQuaid KR. Endoscopic therapy for bleeding ulcers: An evidence-based approach based on meta-analyses of randomized controlled trials. Clin Gastroenterol Hepatol. 2009; 7:33-47; quiz 1-2 [PMID: 18986845 DOI: 10.1016/j.cgh.2008.08.016].
9. Moustafa MH, Taylor M, Fletcher L. "My two-week-old-daughter is throwing up blood". Acad Emerg Med. 2005;12(8):775-7.
10. Neidich GA, Cole SR. Gastrointestinal bleeding. Pediatr Rev 2014;35:243-53; quiz 254 [PMID: 24891598 DOI: 10.1542/ pir.35-6-243].
11. Pant C, Sankararaman S, Deshpande A, et al. Gastrointestinal bleeding in hospitalized children in the United States. Curr Med Res Opin. 2014;30(6):1065-9.
12. Romano C, Oliva S, Martellossi S, et al. Pediatric gastrointestinal bleeding: Perspectives from the Italian Society of Pediatric Gastroenterology. World J Gastroenterol. 2017; 23(8):1328-37.
13. Ünal F, Çakır M, Baran M, et al. Application of endoscopic hemoclips for nonvariceal upper gastrointestinal bleeding in children. Turk J Gastroenterol. 2014;25:147-51 [PMID: 25003673 DOI: 10.5152/tjg.2014.3419].
14. Wolfram W. Pediatric Gastrointestinal Bleeding: Background, Etiology, Epidemiology [Internet]. Emedicine.medscape.com. 2018 [cited 7 September 2018]. Available from: https://emedicine.medscape.com/article/1955984-overview#showall
15. Yokoyama K, Yano T, Kumagai H, et al. Double-balloon enteroscopy for pediatric patients: Evaluation of safety and efficacy in 257 cases. J Pediatr Gastroenterol Nutr. 2016;63:34-40 [PMID: 26628449 DOI: 10.1097/MPG.0000000000001048].

24. Acute Liver Failure

Maninder Dhaliwal, Veena Raghunathan

LEARNING OBJECTIVES

- To understand the terminology associated with acute liver failure (ALF)
- To understand the etiopathogenesis and diagnostic approach to ALF
- To understand the acute management of ALF.

INTRODUCTION

Acute liver failure (ALF) is a term used to describe sudden and severe life-threatening liver injury in a previously healthy person. Although rare, it must be recognized early and appropriate treatment initiated, without which chances of survival are very low. The manifestations of liver failure are not limited and are multisystemic. Cerebral edema, coagulation disturbances, and immune deficiencies are some of the multiorgan abnormalities that accompany ALF. The management of ALF is essentially supportive; specifically targeted at each of the associated organ dysfunctions with the objective of maintaining the patient till spontaneous regeneration of the diseased liver. However, in some cases of catastrophic illness, supportive medical management may not suffice, in which cases liver transplantation becomes the only option for survival. In these cases too, medical management has to be meticulous, with focus on prevention/treatment of sepsis and neurocritical monitoring till recovery from the transplant.

DEFINITION OF PEDIATRIC ACUTE LIVER FAILURE

The definition of ALF has evolved with time. The initial term used was "fulminant" hepatic failure coined by Bernuau et al. in 1986; however, this has been replaced by the more widely accepted term "acute liver failure." ALF in adults is classically defined as onset of encephalopathy within 8 weeks of jaundice in a patient with no history of preexisting liver disease. However, this adult definition is not appropriate for defining pediatric ALF (PALF) because of multiple reasons:
- Hepatic encephalopathy (HE) may not necessarily be present in children with ALF. Also, when present, it is difficult to recognize especially in younger children and infants. Hence unlike adults, hepatic encephalopathy is not essential of PALF.

- Coagulopathy not corrected by Vitamin K is the most important and consistent feature of PALF. It may or may not be accompanied by hepatic encephalopathy. In adults, when uncorrected coagulopathy is present without hepatic encephalopathy, it is known as acute liver injury, not ALF. However, this does not hold true in children.
- As neonatal ALF is a well-documented condition, the time limit of 8 weeks in the adult definition becomes irrelevant.
- Clinical presentation of ALF may actually be the initial manifestation of a metabolic condition, e.g., Wilson disease, which can have underlying obscure changes of chronic liver disease. So unlike adults, ALF in children can occur in presence of underlying chronic liver disease.

Due to these discrepancies, the definition of PALF was developed by the Pediatric Acute Liver Failure Study Group and is now the most widely accepted definition. The following criteria are used in the same:

- Biochemical evidence of acute liver injury
- No evidence of a known chronic liver disease
- Presence of coagulopathy that is not corrected by parenteral administration of vitamin K
- International normalized ratio (INR) greater than 1.5 in a patient with encephalopathy or greater than 2 without encephalopathy.

In adults, ALF is further subdivided into hyperacute liver failure, ALF, and subacute liver failure based on the temporal evolution (Table 1). This classification has some clinical relevance as it can provide cues to the underlying etiology and has prognostic value as well. Essentially a short time span from jaundice to encephalopathy (e.g., Hepatitis A-induced ALF/paracetamol-induced ALF) implies a greater chance of spontaneous recovery; however, risk of cerebral edema is higher. A longer jaundice-to-encephalopathy interval is usually associated with non-Hepatitis A-E etiology. Such patients have a lesser incidence of cerebral edema; however, chances of survival by spontaneous recovery are lower.

The term "acute on chronic liver failure" is sometimes used. However, there is no clarity on its definition. It is generally used to describe rapid deterioration of a preexistent chronic liver disease which is associated with high short-term mortality.

Table 1: Subdivisions of acute liver failure (ALF).

O'Grady et al.	Depending on jaundice to hepatic encephalopathy (HE) interval • Hyperacute liver failure: 0–7 days • ALF: 8–28 days • Subacute liver failure: 29–72 days • Late-onset ALF: 56–182 days
International Association for the Study of the Liver	ALF: Occurrence of HE within 4 weeks after onset of symptoms Subclassification • ALF—hyperacute: within 10 days • ALF—fulminant: 10–30 days • ALF—not otherwise specified Subacute liver failure–development of ascites and/or HE from 5 to 24 weeks after onset of symptoms

Table 2: Age-wise etiologies of pediatric acute liver failure (PALF).

	Infectious disease	Cardiovascular	Drugs/Toxins	Metabolic/Immune
Infant	Herpes simplex Adenovirus Parvovirus B19 Hepatitis B Echovirus Measles HHV-6 VZV	Birth asphyxia Congenital heart disease and cardiac surgery Myocarditis	Paracetamol Overdose Valproate TMP/SMX	Galactosemia Tyrosinemia Fatty acid defects Mitochondrial defects Neonatal hemochromatosis HFI
Child	Hepatitis A,B,C,D,E Leptospirosis, EBV, Dengue fever	Cardiomyopathy Budd–Chiari, syndrome Myocarditis	Rifampicin, TMP/SMX, Valproate, Halothane, Paracetamol overdose	Autoimmune disease Wilson's disease Leukemia Hemophagocytic syndrome Mitochondrial defects
Adolescent	Hepatitis A,B,C,D,E Dengue fever	Congestive heart failure Heat stroke Shock	Acetaminophen, MAO inhibitor, Tetracycline, Mushroom poisoning	Wilson's disease Autoimmune disease Fatty liver of pregnancy Niemann–Pick type C

(HHV-6: human herpes virus 6; MAO: monoamine oxidase; TMP/SMX: trimethoprim-sulfamethoxazole; VZV, varicella-zoster virus)

ETIOLOGY

The causes of ALF can be broadly classified into: Infective, metabolic, toxic, autoimmune, malignancy-induced, vascular-induced, and indeterminant. The most common cause worldwide of PALF is indeterminate. In India, according to various large center studies, the commonest cause is hepatitis A either by itself or in combination with other infective viruses. The etiology of PALF varies according to age (Table 2).

Infections

Hepatitis A in 0.5% of cases can cause ALF. Other viral causes of ALF include: Epstein–Barr virus (EBV), parvovirus 19, echovirus. Dengue can lead to severe liver involvement including ALF. Certain viruses like herpes simplex and varicella zoster can affect an immunocompromised host leading to ALF. In about 15% of PALF, the cause is presumed infectious: non-hepatitis A-G, hence classified as "indeterminate." Leptospirosis is an important bacterial cause of ALF. In the setting of severe sepsis with multiorgan involvement, liver may be severely affected. In such cases of multiorgan dysfunction syndrome (MODS), it may, sometimes, be difficult to distinguish between infection and ALF as the primary inciting factor for MODS.

Metabolic Diseases

Most metabolic diseases present early in life, usually in infancy itself. Clinical presentations can vary according to the underlying disorder. While galactosemia and tyrosinemia present as jaundice with encephalopathy the mitochondrial respiratory chain defects may present as a multisystem disorder with coagulation defects, ketotic hypoglycemia, lactic acidosis, and encephalopathy even in the absence of jaundice. Reye's syndrome presents beyond infancy with a fulminant anicteric hepatitis. Fulminant Wilson's disease usually presents in children more than 7 years old with autoimmune hemolytic anemia, icterus, and encephalopathy. This diagnosis must be rigorously pursued in this setting.

Toxins/Drugs

Drugs or toxins can lead to dose-dependent or idiosyncratic hepatotoxic response. Paracetamol is a dose-related hepatotoxic drug and symptoms occur within 48 hours of ingestion. Paracetamol is metabolized to reactive metabolites, which is then detoxified by conjugation in glutathione pathway. In paracetamol overdose, the glutathione stores are depleted and these metabolites combine with the cysteine group on proteins and form hepatotoxic products.

Idiosyncratic reactions to drugs tend to occur later after exposure. Drugs which may cause ALF are anticonvulsants, inhalational anesthetic agents, and antitubercular drugs. Sodium valproate causes ALF in 1 in 5,000 children in the first 6 months after the start of therapy. Carbamazepine, dilantin and phenobarbitone are all potential causes of ALF. Of the antitubercular drugs isoniazid (INH), rifampicin, and pyrazinamide are all potentially hepatotoxic.

Mushroom poisoning with the species Amanita phalloides and recreational drugs like "ecstasy" are known to cause liver failure.

Autoimmune

Autoimmune hepatitis (AIH) is one of the causes of ALF which responds very well to medications (steroids and immunosuppressants). Hence, it is important to identify it correctly.

Vascular

Hepatic vein occlusion or thrombosis, Budd–Chiari syndrome, and veno-occlusive diseases of the liver may lead to liver dysfunction and present rarely with ALF.

PATHOGENESIS OF ACUTE LIVER FAILURE

Irrespective of etiology, hepatocellular injury is fundamental to pathogenesis of ALF. The original insult and ensuing cytokine release eventually cause necrosis/apoptosis of the hepatocytes. Hepatocellular injury leads to impaired glucose homeostasis, increased lactate production, impaired coagulation factor production and reduced ability to metabolize certain drugs and toxins.

In addition to this, the inflammatory cytokines released in the liver spread into the systemic circulation. Decreased endotoxin clearance leads to a systemic inflammatory response syndrome (SIRS). There is also general loss of Kupffer cell function. The compensatory anti-inflammatory response syndrome (CARS)—mediated by anti-inflammatory cytokines ensues aimed to counter the inflammatory response; however, it is insufficient and predisposes to bacterial and fungal sepsis during evolution of ALF.

The pathogenesis of HE in ALF is complex and multifactorial. Ammonia is a potent neurotoxin which has a direct inhibitory action on GABA (gamma-aminobutyric acid) receptors and activates inhibitory neuronal pathways. Increased ammonia levels in the brain leads to increased glutamine production in the astrocytes which predisposes to the movement of water into the cells (via osmotic effect) leading to cerebral edema. Hyperammonemia in ALF develops rapidly unlike subacute/chronic liver failure, where osmotic compensatory mechanisms are functioning. This probably explains why cerebral edema is more common in the acute setting. This has been further supported by studies where higher arterial ammonia levels have been found to be predictive of higher mortality and associated with more number of complications: cerebral edema (ammonia serum levels > 124 µmol/L), seizures, and cerebral herniation (ammonia serum levels >150–200 µmol/L) in ALF, but this correlation does not exist in subacute or chronic liver failure. Apart from hyperammonemia, increased levels of false neurotransmitters and neuroinhibitory GABA along with various other cytokines and chemicals are also believed to contribute to cerebral edema and dysregulation of metabolism in the brain leading to HE.

CLINICAL FEATURES

Acute liver failure is a dynamic condition; hence, clinical features may show rapid evolution. Detailed history and physical examination is important for initial assessment. Clinical examination is carried out with two aims: first to pinpoint the etiology of ALF and second to determine various organs involvement including renal, cerebral, hepatic, cardiovascular, respiratory, and acid-base balance. In ALF of viral etiology, initial symptoms such as fever, myalgia, and nausea precede onset of jaundice. As jaundice worsens, liver enzymes rapidly increase and prothrombin time increases usually before HE appears. Initial symptoms may be obscure and nonspecific in infants, sometimes, only related to vomiting, altered general condition, and jaundice may develop subsequently. A rapidly shrinking liver with falling liver enzymes and rising bilirubin, suggests massive hepatocellular necrosis and is a poor prognostic indicator. Ascites is usually not a feature of ALF except in cases of Budd–Chiari syndrome.

As discussed earlier, HE may be absent in spite of severe liver dysfunction in children. When it develops, it may do so within hours to days to weeks. HE is classified into four grades using a modification of the West Haven criteria in children (Tables 3 and 4). The pediatric patient with ALF should be clinically assessed multiple times during the day for every component of the HE score, as progression can be very quick.

DIAGNOSTIC WORKUP

Laboratory tests can be broadly divided into:
- General investigations for assessment of major organ systems and sepsis screening
- Specific investigations for etiology
- Serial liver assessment.
  General investigations are elaborated in Table 5.
  Etiological tests should be carried out according to age and clinical presentation (Table 6). Among the various etiologies, fulminant Wilson's disease is challenging to diagnose. Low ceruloplasmin, which is a feature of Wilson disease, does not help to distinguish as it can

Table 3: Stages of hepatic encephalopathy.

	Stages			
	I	II	III	IV
Symptoms	Periods of lethargy, euphoria; reversal of day-night sleeping; may be alert	Drowsiness, inappropriate behavior, agitation, wide mood swings, disorientation	Stupor but arousable, confused, incoherent speech	Coma; IVa responds to noxious stimuli; IVb no response
Signs	Trouble drawing figures, performing mental tasks	Asterixis, fetor hepaticus, incontinence	Asterixis, hyperreflexia, extensor reflexes, rigidity	Areflexia, no asterixis, flaccidity
Electroencephalogram (EEG)	Normal	Generalized slowing, θ waves	Markedly abnormal, triphasic waves	Markedly abnormal bilateral slowing, δ waves, electric-cortical silence

Adapted from the West Haven criteria.

Table 4: Stages of hepatic encephalopathy for infant and child less than 4 years.

	Stages			
	I	II	III	IV
Symptoms	Inconsolable crying, inattention to tasks, Child is not acting like self to parents		Stupor, somnolence, combativeness	Coma; IVa responds to noxious stimuli; IVb no response
Signs	Normal or hyper-reflexic. Other neurological signs are difficult to test		Hyperreflexia, extensor reflexes, rigidity	Areflexia, flaccidity, decerebrate or decorticate posturing
Electroencephalogram (EEG)	Difficult to test and interpret		Markedly abnormal, triphasic waves	Markedly abnormal bilateral slowing, electric-cortical silence

be low in any patient with ALF. Kayser–Fleischer (KF) rings are also not always consistently present, and it is often difficult to carry out slit-lamp examination for the same in a sick bed-bound patient. Serum and urine copper levels take several days to process. Certain laboratory investigations have been studied to be useful in supporting the diagnosis of Wilson disease in the setting of ALF. These include:
- Very low serum alkaline phosphatase or uric acid levels
- Combining ratios: Ratio of serum alkaline phosphatase to total bilirubin less than 4 and aspartate to ALT more than 2.2 can be used as a reliable markers
- Presence of Coombs negative hemolytic anemia.

Table 5: General investigations.

Systems	Laboratory investigations
Hematological	Complete blood cell count PT, INR, aPTT, fibrinogen, D-dimer, blood group, cross-match
Metabolic and electrolytes	Blood glucose, lactate, arterial ammonia, serum osmolarity. Blood gas with pH, sodium, potassium, calcium, magnesium, bicarbonate, creatinine
Sepsis	Procalcitonin, urinalysis, and microscopic analysis, blood cultures, urine cultures, tracheal cultures (if intubated)
Imaging and other testing	Chest radiograph, electrocardiogram, abdominal ultrasound with Doppler
CNS	EEG, fundus for papilledema, ONSD, ICP monitor?

(aPTT: activated partial thromboplastin time; CNS: central nervous system; EEG: electroencephalography; ICP: intracranial pressure; INR: international normalized ratio; ONSD: optic nerve sheath diameter; PT: prothrombin time.)

Table 6: Specific diagnostic tests to evaluate etiology of acute liver failure.

Cause	Test
Hepatitis A infection	Anti-HAV antibody (IgM)
Hepatitis B infection	HbsAg, anti-core antibody (HbcAb IgM)
Hepatitis D infection	Anti-hepatitis D virus antibody (IgM)
Hepatitis C infection	Anti-hepatitis C virus antibody (IgM)
Other infections	CMV; EBV; VZV; echovirus; parvovirus B19; malaria; dengue; leptospirosis
Autoimmune hepatitis	Autoantibodies ANA, ASMA, anti-LKM1, immunoglobulins IgG
Hemophagocytic lymphohistiocytosis	Bone marrow aspiration (typical cells), raised ferritin, raised triglycerides, low/absent NK cell activity
Neonatal hemochromatosis/congenital alloimmune hepatitis	Buccal mucosal biopsy, raised ferritin, high transferrin saturation
Veno-occlusive disease/malignancies	Doppler ultrasonography/venography imaging (computed tomography/magnetic resonance imaging) and histology
Toxicology screen and drug panel	Acetaminophen, opiates, barbiturates, cocaine, alcohol
Metabolic liver disease	
Galactosemia	Galactose-1-phosphate uridyl transferase assay (provided child not received blood transfusion in last 3 months)
Tyrosinemia	Urinary succinylacetone
Wilson's disease	Urinary copper (>100 µg/day), Kayser–Fleischer ring, Coombs negative hemolytic anemia, low serum ceruloplasmin
Urea cycle defect	Plasma aminoacidogram, orotic acid estimation in urine to diagnose supplementation OTC deficiency
Fatty acid oxidation defect	Carnitine—acyl carnitine profile
Mitochondrial hepatopathies	Muscle and liver biopsies for quantitative assay of respiratory chain enzymes, tandem mass spectroscopy

(ANA: antinuclear antibody; anti-LKM: anti liver, kidney microsome; ASMA: antismooth muscle antibody; CMV: cytomegalovirus; EBV: epstein-Barr virus; HAV: hepatitis A virus; HbsAg: hepatitis B surface antigen; NK: natural killer; OTC: ornithine transcarbamylase.)

Liver tests: Serial measurement of liver function tests especially bilirubin (total and direct), serum aminotransferases along with prothrombin time, partial thromboplastin time, ammonia, and lactate help to assess if liver function is improving/deteriorating. Rapidly decreasing serum aminotransferases need to be interpreted with caution as if associated with increasing bilirubin and worsening coagulopathy, it indicates worsening liver status not improvement. Arterial ammonia sampling is recommended as venous levels may often be higher due to extraction of ammonia across the skeletal muscles. Low levels of factor V, VII, and fibrinogen indicate synthetic dysfunction of liver. Factor VIII level helps to differentiate between coagulopathy due to ALF versus disseminated intravascular coagulation (DIC). Factor VIII level will be normal in ALF and low in DIC. Liver ultrasound with Doppler is an essential investigation in all cases of ALF. It gives information regarding liver parenchymal echotexture, presence of splenomegaly, portal hypertension, and documents patency of hepatic artery and portal and hepatic veins.

MANAGEMENT

The mortality in ALF has reduced over time due to better understanding of the disease process and various advances in critical care medicine. The three dreaded complications in ALF which mainly contribute to mortality include: cerebral edema, MODS, and sepsis. The main principles of management include:
- Monitoring and support of various organ systems
- Treatment of complications
- Maintain optimal conditions to maximize chances of spontaneous recovery and/or best post-transplant survival.

Transport of a Child with Encephalopathy

Due to rapidity of disease progression, the patient should be managed in a facility which has expertise for mechanical ventilation, renal replacement therapy, equipment for intracranial pressure (ICP) monitoring, and importantly prompt availability of blood products. Typically all this level of support is available in a transplant center, where if needed, emergency liver transplantation (ELT) can be performed as an ultimate life-saving measure. Planning for transfer to a transplant center should begin in patients with grade I or II encephalopathy because they may worsen rapidly. Early transfer is important as the risks involved with patient transport may increase or even preclude transfer once stage III or IV encephalopathy develops.

Any child who has more than grade II encephalopathy should be preferably intubated and airway secured before the transport. The transport team should have facilities for adequate monitoring and management of the hemodynamic state en route depending upon the severity of illness. Prompt and accurate communication with the teams involved is critical.

Various Aspects of Management

Electrolytes and Sugar

- It is important to monitor blood sugar regularly (1–2 hours) in patients with ALF as there is a high risk of hypoglycemia. Hypoglycemia is detrimental to the brain and can cause rapid worsening of hepatic encephalopathy. Continuous glucose infusion rate of at least 6–8 mg/kg/min is recommended in such patients. Dextrose concentrations more than 12.5% cannot be given by peripheral venous cannula and require central line (jugular/femoral) for administration. Apart from sugars, other electrolytes especially potassium, phosphorus, and magnesium should be regularly monitored and maintained in normal range. The target sodium should be 145–155.

Fluids and Hemodynamic Considerations

The aim is to maintain adequate intravascular volume and renal function. Excessive fluid should be avoided to decrease risk of cerebral edema and fluid overload. The practice of two-thirds maintenance restriction is ok only if patient is hemodynamically stable. However, children are frequently hypovolemic due to poor fluid intake and vomiting/diarrhea and fluid restriction can be detrimental in such cases.

Acute liver failure is usually a vasoplegic state with significant arterial vasodilatation due to increased levels of systemic endogenous vasodilators (e.g., nitric oxide). This leads to a hyperdynamic circulation with low systemic vascular resistance and wide pulse pressure (similar to sepsis). This hemodynamic state should be treated with fluids followed by vasopressor agent. Norepinephrine is the preferred drug for this state; to be administered through a central line. Although well documented in adult literature, pediatric data on use of norepinephrine is scant. However, it remains the logical choice even in pediatric population. Bedside echocardiography is very useful to assess volume status and can guide fluid therapy. Arterial line insertion is useful in patient with hemodynamic instability or in patients when ICP monitoring is being planned. This is a role of hydrocortisone in patients with refractory hypotension as adrenal insufficiency can be seen in ALF.

Respiratory System and Ventilation

Indications of intubation are:
- More than grade II encephalopathy
- Raised intracranial pressure
- Rapidly deteriorating course
- Respiratory failure
- Cardiovascular collapse.

Oral intubation is preferred by modified RSI (rapid sequence intubation), with a cuffed endotracheal tube, due to risk of bleeding and aspiration. Proprofol can be used intermittently for sedation. Aim to oxygenate (SpO_2 >90%) and maintain normocarbia ($PaCO_2$ 35–45 mm Hg).

Excessive hyperventilation should be avoided and must not be used as a prophylactic measure, but only as a transient maneuver to control surges of ICP, as it may paradoxically compromise the cerebral perfusion pressure (CPP). Partial pressure of CO_2 ($PaCO_2$) less than 30 mm Hg must be avoided.

Mechanical ventilation exposes patient to a spectrum of ventilator-associated complications such as pneumonia and acute respiratory distress syndrome (ARDS). Protective lung strategy is the gold standard to manage acute lung injuries, but with a careful balancing act as high positive end-expiratory pressure (PEEP) with low tidal volume can adversely affect cerebral edema.

Effective sedation before tracheal suction is essential to prevent ICP surges.

Cerebral Edema and Intracranial Hypertension

The foremost PALFSG database of 348 patients reported that hepatic encephalopathy was common and occurred in 55% of children. Of these, 75% of patients had grade I/II encephalopathy, 17% had grade III and 7% had grade IV encephalopathy. The most important aspects of management of cerebral edema in ALF are early recognition and minimizing aggravating conditions for ICP surges. The key points in management are:

- The patient should be nursed in a quiet surrounding and unnecessary disturbances/painful stimuli must be avoided.
- Maintain patient head in midline. Head-end elevation by 20–30° (provided no shock) to optimize jugular venous outflow. Avoid neck flexion.
- Aggressive treatment of fever as high temperature can lead to increase in ICP.
- Close monitoring and maintenance of mean arterial pressure for age along with adequate oxygenation and normocarbia.
- Lowering endogenous nitrogen intake (by limiting bleeding and controlling infection) or exogenous nitrogen intake [avoiding unjustified fresh-frozen plasma (FFP) administration].
- Lactulose was previously recommended by some groups in early stages of encephalopathy but there is presently insufficient evidence to support the use of nonabsorbable disaccharides (lactulose and lactitol) for HE in ALF. The adverse effects of lactulose include abdominal distension, ileus, microulcers, and osmotic diarrhea leading to dyselectrolytemia.
- No role of neomycin and L-ornithine L-aspartate/L-ornithine phenyl acetate at present.
- Ornithine aspartate and sodium benzoate have been proposed to decrease serum ammonia, in Reye's syndrome and in urea cycle defects, but hemofiltration remains the main treatment of acute hyperammonemia. Large trials in adults have shown no benefit of ornithine aspartate in ALF.
- Patients with ALF can go through waxing and waning levels of consciousness. They sometimes get very agitated and are at risk of harm to themselves. Sedation in them is tricky, as any sedation would interfere in their neurological assessment. A short-acting sedative like propofol (1–2 mg/kg) is preferred for restraint or short procedures. Opiates can be used judiciously. Benzodiazepines should be avoided.
- *Osmotic therapy*: Mannitol and hypertonic saline are used to raise blood osmolarity, thereby reducing astrocyte swelling in brain. About 20% mannitol given as repeated 2 mL/kg boluses is useful as first-line therapy provided serial serum osmolality is below 320 mOsm/L. Mannitol cannot be used continuously as the equilibrium in osmolality will make it ineffective. Apart from exerting hyperosmolar effect, mannitol increases cerebral blood flow, which explains the rapidity of its action. However, it cannot be used in presence of shock/significant kidney injury. In such situations, hypertonic saline is advantageous and can be used as a prophylactic measure with few side effects, with a goal of achieving sodium of 145–155 mEq/L, provided serum osmolality remains below 360 mOsm/L.

Treatment Considerations for Advanced (Grade III/IV) Encephalopathy

- *Intubation and ventilation*: Any patient with encephalopathy which has progressed beyond grade II should be managed by controlled intubation and ventilation to avoid further ICP surges. Adequate sedation and analgesia are of utmost importance in such cases. Propofol

and fentanyl are suggested combination; benzodiazepines should be avoided. Propofol has two additional advantages: It decreases cerebral blood flow, therefore, decreases ICP and decreases risk of seizure activity. However, propofol can cause hypotension in hemodynamically unstable patients and its use beyond 24 hours in children is not generally recommended due to risk of propofol infusion syndrome.
- If osmotic therapies fail to adequately control ICP, other adjunctive measures to reduce ICP include: transient hyperventilation (only if signs of impending herniation), moderate hypothermia (32–33°C), and barbiturate coma.
- *ICP monitoring*: The aim of managing cerebral edema in ALF is to maintain ICP less than 20 mm Hg or cerebral perfusion pressure (CPP) more than 50–60 mm Hg. Use of invasive ICP monitoring in children as well as adults is controversial. Risk of intracranial bleed and absence of evidence of survival benefit are the main reasons against routine use. The importance of close clinical monitoring in hepatic encephalopathy cannot be undermined; however, this is difficult once patient has progressed to advanced encephalopathy (grade III/ IV). Noninvasive methods such as near-infrared spectroscopy, transcranial Doppler examination, and optic nerve sheath diameter are new emerging tools to identify and monitor ICP.
- *Seizures*: Phenytoin or levetiracetam is useful for treatment of seizures in ALF. Prophylactic antiepileptics in ALF are not recommended. Continuous electroencephalogram (EEG) monitoring is advisable especially in high-risk patients. EEG changes occur very early in HE, even before physiological or biochemical disturbances.

Infectious Disease Consideration

As described in pathogenesis, patients with ALF have impaired immune function. Additionally presence of indwelling catheters, bed-bound state, use of H2 receptor blockers, etc. all predispose to the development of infections in these patients. Sepsis leads to worsening of hepatic encephalopathy and overall poor prognosis hence must be treated promptly.

The indications for empirical antibiotic therapy in ALF include:
- Positive surveillance cultures
- Advancing hepatic encephalopathy (stage III/IV)
- Persistent hypotension
- Systemic inflammatory response syndrome
- Patients listed for liver transplant (LT).

The antibiotic (s) chosen must be broad-spectrum covering both gram-positive and gram-negative organisms and must also take into consideration local flora of the hospital. Third-generation cephalosporins/piperacillin-tazobactam + teicoplanin are generally used. Nephrotoxic drugs such as aminoglycosides/vancomycin should be avoided. Once an organism is identified, the antibiotic therapy can be specifically tailored based on sensitivity. Oral nonabsorbable antibiotics used for selective gut decontamination do not appear to improve survival in patients receiving systemic antibiotics.

Prophylactic systemic antifungal therapy should be considered in:
- Patients listed for LT
- Patients having renal failure
- Rapidly advancing encephalopathy (stage III/IV)
- Poor response to antibacterial therapy.

Hematologic Failure: Dealing with Coagulopathy

Overt bleeding is not as common as is believed to be in patients with ALF. ALF is, in fact, a rebalanced hemostatic state where there is loss of hepatically derived both procoagulant factors (Factor V, VII) as well as anticoagulant factors (Protein C/S, antithrombin III). Thus, deranged INR is by itself NOT an indication for prophylactic FFP transfusion. FFP transfusion will interfere with serial assessment of liver function (prothrombin time monitoring). Also unnecessary FFP transfusion contributes to fluid and protein overload and hyperviscosity syndrome. The only scenarios in which FFP transfusion may be warranted include if any invasive procedure is planned (central line/ICP monitor) or if patient is listed for LT. The general targets for INR and platelet count in such cases would be INR less than 1.5 and platelet count more than 50,000/mm^3. In case of a patient with bleeding manifestation though, FFP should be administered. Cryoprecipitate should also be administered for a bleeding patient with fibrinogen less than 100 mg/dL. There is an emerging role for thromboelastography according to newer studies to guide blood product therapy. If FFP fails to normalize INR, recombinant factor VIIa (rFVIIa) can be considered.

Gastrointestinal Hemorrhage

Gastrointestinal bleeding is common in PALF and can be life-threatening. Stress ulceration, coagulopathy, and preexisting portal hypertension may all contribute. GI bleed may worsen encephalopathy. Patients with PALF should receive prophylactic H2 antagonists (Ranitidine 1–3 mg/kg) or proton pump inhibitors (pantoprazole 0.5–1.0 mg/kg/day up to 20 mg for children < 40 kg) to reduce risk of stress-related GI bleeding. When GI bleeding occurs, both thrombocytopenia and coagulopathy should be corrected. Packed blood cell, FFP, and platelet transfusion must be given as needed promptly. Intravenous vitamin K 5–10 mg should be administered; but can be avoided in patients with G6PD deficiency due to hemolysis risk. Octreotide (splanchnic vasoconstrictor) infusion (0.5–1 µg/kg/min) can be given in case bleeding is profuse.

Acute Kidney Injury

Acute kidney injury (AKI) occurs in ALF with an incidence of 30–85% depending on the etiology. As ALF is a hyperdynamic state with low blood pressure, the renal autoregulation curve is shifted to the right, thus it becomes pressure dependent and at risk for development of acute tubular necrosis. Other precipitating factors for AKI in ALF include:
- Gastrointestinal bleeding
- Septicemia and dehydration
- Nephrotoxic drugs (e.g., aminoglycosides should be avoided).

Urine output of more than 1 mL/kg/hr is a good marker of renal perfusion and all children with ALF should be catheterized to strictly monitor the same. The aim is to maintain optimal circulating blood volume and ensure good urine output. If a patient develops oliguria, early fluid challenge should be administered followed by a diuretic (only if patient is hemodynamically stable). Dopamine prophylaxis for renoprotection is no longer recommended. Tubular nephropathy is frequently observed and results in low blood phosphate, magnesium, and potassium. Poor urine output leads to fluid accumulation which is overall detrimental in ALF.

In such cases where positive fluid balance is rising, continuous renal replacement therapy (CRRT) should be considered. CRRT has two advantages in this setting: fluid balance control and additionally clearance of toxic substances which accumulate in ALF including ammonia and lactate. ALF is one condition in which CRRT can be considered for certain purely nonrenal conditions including hyperammonemia more than 200 micromoles/L, grade III/IV encephalopathy with high ammonia, metabolic disarray, and fluid overload (before AKI sets in). Continuous rather than intermittent RRT is advisable in ALF, because of the reduced shifts in blood pressure associated with its use and subsequently less shifts in ICP.

Nutrition

Acute liver failure is a catabolic state and hence there is a need for proper nutritional supplementation in ALF. There is no need for protein restriction in stage I and II encephalopathy; normal intake is recommended. In hepatic encephalopathy beyond grade II, restricted protein up to 0.5–1 g/kg per day is recommended. Enteral route is preferred wherever feasible. Calorie dense feeds are better as they avoid excess water and hypo-osmolarity which can be detrimental to cerebral edema. Higher caloric density feeds are preferred to avoid excessive free water and hypo-osmolality, which may exacerbate cerebral edema. When enteral feeding is not possible, parenteral nutrition can be provided via a dedicated port of a central line (35–40 kcal/kg per day). Metabolic liver disease requires a special mention, as they require unique modified diet; early identification and implementation of appropriate nutrition plan can be lifesaving.

Etiologyspecific Treatment (Table 7)

It is given in detail in Table 7.

Table 7: Target-specific therapy of underlying acute liver failure (ALF).

Cause	Treatment
Acetaminophen poisoning	Activated charcoal 1 g/kg orally
	N-acetylcysteine 150 mg/kg IV in 15 minutes, then maintenance dose 50 mg/kg over 4 hours, followed by 100 mg/kg administered over 16 hours
HSV	Acyclovir 10 mg/kg 8 hourly or 150 mg/m^2/day IV
Neonatal hemochromatosis	Deferoxamine 30 mg/kg/day IV in 3 doses Selenium 2–3 mcg/kg/day IV N-acetyl-cysteine 140 mg/kg, then 70 mg/kg orally or IV tocopherol polyethylene glycol succinate 20 UI/kg/day orally
Mushroom poisoning	Penicillin G 300,000–1 million units/kg/day IV Silymarin 30–40 mg/kg/day IV or orally
Acute Hepatitis B	Interferon - α - 2b for children > 1 year of age and older Lamivudine or entecavir for children > 2 years of age and older
Autoimmune hepatitis	Methylprednisolone 1–2 mg/kg IV (max 60 mg) Azathioprine may be added to steroids

Liver Support Systems

There is lot of ongoing research on extracorporeal support systems to support the acutely failing liver till spontaneous recovery or as a bridge to transplant. The ideal support system must be capable of detoxification as well as performing all the metabolic and synthetic functions of liver. A variety of systems have been tested to date, with no certain evidence of efficacy. Currently available liver support systems are not recommended outside of research trials.

Role of N-acetyl Cysteine (NAC)

N-acetyl cysteine is an antioxidant and has an established role in paracetamol-induced hepatocellular failure. When used early as an antidote after a single, intentional acetaminophen overdose, NAC is extremely effective at replenishing hepatic glutathione stores and preventing severe N-acetyl-p-benzoquinone imine-induced hepatotoxicity and liver failure. N-acetyl cysteine has been increasingly considered for use in ALF of other causes because of its complex antioxidant, immunological effects, which results in improved tissue oxygenation and good safety profile. However, a recent pediatric randomized controlled trial did not support its broad use in nonacetaminophen pediatric ALF. The optimal duration of NAC therapy in these patients is unclear, some say till reversal of encephalopathy or till resolving liver enzymes or standard 3-7 days protocol. The route IV is preferred for NAC in ALF and dose for nonacetaminophen ALF is 100-150 mg/kg/day; diluted in 5-10% dextrose.

Emergency Liver Transplantation

Emergency liver transplantation remains the only treatment for poor prognosis group in ALF. The decision to transplant or to wait remains fraught with uncertainty; although a number prognostic scores have been described. The most commonly used transplantation criteria are those developed at King's College in London and Beaujon's Hospital in Paris (Table 8). However, these criteria fail to be adequate in children, mainly due to a very weak negative predictive value. Based on studies in children (nonacetaminophen ALF) INR more than 4 or factor V concentration of less than 25% as the best available criteria for listing for LT in the present era. Although prognostic scoring systems help in predicting course of a patient, the final decision to transplant or not must be based on clinical judgment. LT is contraindicated in presence of metastatic malignant disease, lymphohistiocytosis, and systemic metabolic or systemic mitochondrial respiratory chain disorders. Other contraindications are brain herniation, uncontrolled sepsis, and severe respiratory failure.

King's College Hospital and Clichy liver transplantation criteria for ALF are used in PALF (see chapter on Liver Transplantation)

CONCLUSION

PALF can occur due to various etiologies. In India, infections remain the most common cause. It is a complex but treatable syndrome and requires multidisciplinary approach, advanced intensive care management and available option of emergency liver transplant. Cerebral edema is common and can be fatal unless identified early and aggressively managed. Multiorgan dysfunction and sepsis also contribute to mortality. Early referral to tertiary centers has contributed to decreased mortality. Liver transplantation is the only life-saving option when spontaneous recovery is unlikely and should be timely offered.

KEY POINTS

- Acute liver failure is a complex disease and should be managed in an experienced intensive care facility for best outcomes.
- Infection is the most common cause of ALF in India.
- Presence of encephalopathy is not an essential criteria in PALF; coagulopathy is crucial.
- Coagulopathy (INR) is the key criteria in diagnosing PALF. Serial INR monitoring is a dynamic indicator of disease progression.
- Fresh frozen plasma should be avoided as long as no active bleeding is present.
- Liver transplantation is the only definitive treatment in rapidly deteriorating cases and must be given timely consideration in each case; prognostic scoring systems are available to guide the same.
- There is an increasing role for supportive therapy to support the failing liver and other organs pending liver transplantation—early aggressive treatment of sepsis, extensive neuromonitoring and neuroprotection and early use of CRRT.

SUGGESTED READING

1. Acharya SK, Bhatia V, Sreenivas V, et al. Efficacy of L-ornithine L-aspartate in acute liver failure: A double-blind, randomized, placebo-controlled study. Gastroenterology. 2009;136:2159-68.
2. Agarwal B, Wright G, Gatt A, et al. Evaluation of coagulation abnormalities in acute liver failure. J Hepatol. 2012;57:780-6.
3. Aggarwal S, Brooks DM, Kang Y, et al. Noninvasive monitoring of cerebral perfusion pressure in patients with acute liver failure using transcranial Doppler ultrasonography. Liver Transpl. 2008;14:1048-57.
4. Alba L, Hay JE, Angulo P, et al. Lactulose therapy in acute liver failures. J Hepatol. 2002;36:33.
5. Arora NK, Nanda SK, Gulati S, et al. Acute viral hepatitis types E, A, and B singly and in combination in acute liver failure in children in north India. J Med Virol. 1996;48:215-21.
6. Auzinger G, Wendon J. Intensive care management of acute liver failure. Curr Opin Crit Care. 2008;14:179-88.
7. Bernal W, Hall C, Karvellas CJ, et al. Arterial ammonia and clinical risk factors for encephalopathy and intracranial hypertension in acute liver failure. Hepatology. 2007;46:1844-52.
8. Bernuau J, Goudeau A, Poynard T, et al. Multivariate analysis of prognostic factors in fulminant hepatitis B. Hepatology. 1986;6:648-51.
9. Bernuau J, Rueff B, Benhamou JP. Fulminant and subfulminant liver failure: Definitions and causes. Semin Liver Dis. 1986;6:97-106.
10. Bhatia V, Batra Y, Acharya SK. Prophylactic phenytoin does not improve cerebral edema or survival in acute liver failure—a controlled clinical trial. J Hepatol. 2004;41:89-96.
11. Bhowmick K, Mammen A, Moses PD, et al. Hepatitis A in pediatric acute liver failure in southern India. Indian J Gastroenterol. 2005;24:34.
12. Clemmesen JO, Larsen FS, Kondrup J, et al. Cerebral herniation in patients with acute liver failure is correlated with arterial ammonia concentration. Hepatology. 1999;29:648-53.
13. Davenport A. The management of renal failure in patients at risk of cerebral edema/hypoxia. New Horiz. 1995;3:717-24.
14. Ede RJ, Gimson AE, Bihari D, et al. Controlled hyperventilation in the prevention of cerebral oedema in fulminant hepatic failure. J Hepatol. 1986;2:43-51.

15. Ellis AJ, Wendon JA, Williams R. Subclinical seizure activity and prophylactic phenytoin infusion in acute liver failure: A controlled clinical trial. Hepatology. 2000;32:536-41.
16. Hawker F. Liver dysfunction in critical illness. Anaesth Intensive Care. 1991;19:165-81.
17. Korman JD, Volenberg I, Balko J, et al. Screening for Wilson disease in acute liver failure by serum testing: A comparison of currently used tests. Hepatology. 2008;48(4):1030-2.
18. Kumar R, Shalimar, Sharma H, et al. Persistent hyperammonemia is associated with complications and poor outcomes in patients with acute liver failure. Clin Gastroenterol Hepatol. 2012;10:925-31.
19. Larsen FS, Strauss G, Knudsen GM, et al. Cerebral perfusion, cardiac output, and arterial pressure in patients with fulminant hepatic failure. Crit Care Med. 2000;28:996-1000.
20. Leber B, Spindelboeck W, Stadlbauer V. Infectious complications of acute and chronic liver disease. Semin Respir Crit Care Med. 2012;33:80-95.
21. Lee WM, Hynan LS, Rossaro L, et al. Intravenous N-acetylcysteine improves transplant-free survival in early stage non-acetaminophen acute liver failure. Gastroenterology. 2009;137:856-64.
22. Lee WM, Squires Jr RH, Nyberg SL, et al. Acute liver failure: Summary of a workshop. Hepatology. 2008;47:1401-15.
23. Liu J, Gluud L, Als-Nielsen B, et al. Artificial and bioartificial support systems for liver failure. Cochrane Database Syst Rev. 2004;1:CD003628.
24. Mitchell A, Daul AE, Beiderlinden M, et al. A new system for regional citrate anticoagulation in continuous venovenous hemodialysis (CVVHD). Clin Nephrol. 2003;59:106-14.
25. Murphy N, Auzinger G, Bernel W, et al. The effect of hypertonic sodium chloride on intracranial pressure in patients with acute liver failure. Hepatology. 2004;39:464-70.
26. Narkewicz MR, Dell Olio D, Karpen SJ, et al. Pattern of diagnostic evaluation for the causes of pediatric acute liver failure: An opportunity for quality improvement. J Pediatr. 2009;155:801-6e1.
27. O'Grady JG, Alexander GJ, Hayllar KM, et al. Early indicators of prognosis in fulminant hepatic failure. Gastroenterology. 1989;97:439-45.
28. O'Grady JG, Schalm SW, Williams R. Acute liver failure: Redefining the syndromes. Lancet. 1993;342:273-5.
29. Pereira SP, Rowbotham D, Fitt S, et al. Pharmacokinetics and efficacy of oral versus intravenous mixed micellar phylloquinone (vitamin K1) in severe acute liver disease. J Hepatol. 2005;42:365-70.
30. Plauth M, Cabré E, Riggio O, et al. ESPEN guidelines on enteral nutrition: Liver disease. Clin Nutr. 2006;25:285-94.
31. Roberts E, Schilsky ML. A practice guideline on Wilson disease. Hepatology. 2008;47:2089-111.
32. Sarin SK, Kedarisetty CK, Abbas Z, et al. Acute-on-chronic liver failure: consensus recommendations of the Asian Pacific Association for the Study of the Liver (APASL). Hepatol Int. 2009;3(1):269-82.
33. Shanmugam NP, Dhawan A. Selection criteria for liver transplantation in paediatric acute liver failure: The saga continues. Pediatr Transplant. 2011;15:5-6.
34. Shubin NJ, Monaghan SF, Ayala A, et al. Anti-inflammatory mechanisms of sepsis. Contrib Microbiol. 2011;17:108-24.
35. Squires Jr RH, Shneider BL, Bucuvalas J, et al. Acute liver failure in children: The first 348 patients in the pediatric acute liver failure study group. J Pediatr. 2006;148:652-8.
36. Squires RH Jr, Schneider BL, Bucuvalas J, et al. Acute liver failure in children: The first 348 patients in the pediatric acute liver failure study group. J Pediatr. 2006;148:652-8.
37. Squires RH, Dhawan A, Alonso E, et al. Intravenous N-acetylcysteine in pediatric patients with non-acetaminophen acute liver failure: A placebo-controlled clinical trial. Hepatology. 2013;57:1542-9.
38. Stravitz RT, Kramer AH, Davern T, et al. Intensive care of patients with acute liver failure: Recommendations of the US Acute Liver Failure Study Group. Crit Care Med. 2007;35:2498-508.
39. Stravitz RT, Kramer DJ. Management of acute liver failure. Nat Rev Gastroenterol Hepatol. 2009;6:542-53.

40. Stravitz RT, Lisman T, Luketic VA, et al. Minimal effects of acute liver injury/acute liver failure on hemostasis as assessed by thromboelastography. J Hepatol. 2012;56:129-36.
41. Sundaram SS, Alonso EM, Narkewicz MR, et al. Characterization and outcomes of young infants with acute liver failure. J Pediatr. 2011;159:813-8e1.
42. Tandon BN, Bernauau J, O'Grady J, et al. Recommendations of the International Association for the Study of the Liver Subcommittee on nomenclature of acute and subacute liver failure. J Gastroenterol Hepatol. 199;14:403-4.
43. Trey C, Davidson C. The management of fulminant hepatic failure. In: Popper H, Schaffner F, eds. Progress in Liver Diseases, Vol 111. New York, NY: Grun and Stratten; 1970. pp. 282-98.
44. Vaquero J, Polson J, Chung C, et al. Infection and the progression of hepatic encephalopathy in acute liver failure. Gastroenterology. 2003;125:755-64.
45. Walsh TS, Wigmore SJ, Hopton P, et al. Energy expenditure in acetaminophen-induced fulminant hepatic failure. Crit Care Med. 2000;28:649-54.
46. Whitington PF, Alonso AE. Fulminant hepatitis and acute liver failure. In: Kelly DA, ed. Paediatric Liver Disease. Oxford: Blackwell; 2003. pp. 107-26.
47. Wijdicks EFM, Nyberg SL. Propofol to control intracranial pressure in fulminant hepatic failure. Transplant Proc. 2002;34:1220-2.

Pre- and Postoperative Management of a Liver Transplant Patient

25

Aoyon Sengupta, Rajappan Pillai

LEARNING OBJECTIVES

- Whom to transplant—indications, contraindications
- How to select transplant recipients?
- When to list patients for transplant?
- How allocate organs and prioritize recipients?
- Pretransplant evaluation and management of donor and recipient
- Post-transplant care
- Complications and their management.

INTRODUCTION

Over the last few decades, liver transplant has become an accepted treatment modality for the management of end-stage liver disease in adults as well as children. An increasing refinement of surgical techniques, better pre- and postoperative management, and availability of more potent immunosuppressive therapy with lesser adverse effects have significantly contributed to improved outcomes. Data from the US Organ Procurement and Transplantation Network (OPTN)/Scientific Registry of Transplant Recipients (SRTR) puts the 1-year patient survival rate at 83–91% and the 5-year patient survival at 82–84%. The Studies of Pediatric Liver Transplantation (SPLIT) registry database, a cooperative research network of pediatric transplantation centers in the United States and Canada, which studies trends in transplant indications, techniques and outcomes, also reveals 1-year survival rates of 91.4% and 5-year survival rates of 86.5%.[1] Over the last two decades, there has been a steady increase in the number of liver transplantations being conducted in India, with most centers placing the 1-year survival at 85–90%.[2]

EVOLUTION OF LIVER TRANSPLANT

Dr Thomas E Starzl who is often referred to as the "Father of modern transplantation," performed the first liver transplant on a 3-year-old child with biliary atresia in 1963 at the University of Colorado Health Sciences Center. Although the child did not survive the procedure and died due to surgical difficulties and excessive bleeding, he continued with his efforts to refine the procedure. In 1967, he performed the first successful liver transplant on a 1-year-old child with hepatocellular carcinoma.

The outcome of the transplants in the initial years was poor in view of the complex procedure, physiologically decompensated patients, inadequate pre- and postoperative care, and nonavailability of potent immunosuppression.

The introduction of cyclosporin for immunosuppression proved to be an important milestone in the field of solid organ transplant. Better immunosuppression along with continuous innovations in surgical techniques and rapid improvements in pre-, intra-, and postoperative care resulted in improved outcomes, and in 1983, the National Institute of Health recognized liver transplantation as an accepted treatment modality for end-stage liver disease.

In India, the passage of the Human Organ Transplantation Act in 1994 paved the way for the initiation of transplant programs in a regulated manner. The first successful liver transplant was conducted in 1998 and since then the program has taken giant strides and India has emerged as one of the leading centers for live donor liver transplant in the world.

As liver transplantation comes of age as a lifesaving measure, there has been a rapid expansion of transplant programs worldwide and many new conditions have found their way into the list of indications leading to an acute shortage of donor organs. This has emerged as the key limiting factor in optimal exploitation of this therapeutic modality and methods, viz., live donors, split grafts, extended criteria donors are being utilized to circumvent the issue.

INDICATIONS FOR PEDIATRIC LIVER TRANSPLANT

Advances in surgical and supportive management, development of potent immunosuppressants, and better understanding of the underlying disease processes have increased the scope of liver transplantations.

Hepatic failure is the primary indication for a liver transplant and can be consequent to:
- Primary progressive liver diseases, viz., extra- or intrahepatic cholestasis
- Acute decompensation of the existing liver disease
- Acute liver failure, not amenable to maximal medical management
- Metabolic diseases involving the liver
- Primary hepatic malignancies.

Extrahepatic biliary atresia has emerged as the most common indication for pediatric liver transplant based on the studies conducted at different centers worldwide,[1,3,4] sometimes numbering up to 50% of all cases performed. Liver transplant is recommended for all children with biliary atresia who have undergone hepatoportoenterostomy and yet develop complications of chronic liver disease or recurrent cholangitis. The American Association for the Study of Liver Diseases (AASLD) practice guidelines recommend that all children with biliary atresia who have undergone hepatoportoenterostomy and have a total serum bilirubin of >6 mg/dL at 3 months postprocedure should be urgently referred to a liver transplant. Evaluation for transplant should be initiated for those with bilirubin levels between 2 and 6 mg/dL.[5] Transplant is also indicated in other progressive liver disorders, viz., alpha 1-antitrypsin deficiency, progressive familial intrahepatic cholestasis, primary sclerosing cholangitis, etc.

Nonprogressive primary liver diseases, viz., Alagille syndrome, have significant morbidity and debilitating symptoms leading to impaired quality of life. Although deranged synthetic function, portal hypertension, and encephalopathy are rare, complications, such as severe cholestasis, intractable pruritus, failure to thrive, hypercholesterolemia, and osteodystrophy have prompted consideration for liver transplant in such cases. However, the decision for transplant also rests on the severity of other organ involvement and the expected benefit to the patient.[5]

Liver transplant has emerged as a lifesaving therapeutic modality in acute liver failure progressing to end-stage liver disease and accounts for 7–8% of all liver transplants and about 11% of pediatric liver transplants.[6,7] The criteria for the diagnosis of pediatric acute liver failure include: (i) the absence of a known or chronic liver disease, (ii) coagulopathy that is not responsive to parenteral vitamin K, and (iii) international normalized ratio (INR) between 1.5 and 1.9 with encephalopathy or ≥2.0 without encephalopathy. The outcome in acute liver failure can range from complete recovery of liver function to progression to end-stage liver disease, multiorgan failure and death, depending on the extent of damage to hepatocytes. Establishing the etiology, institution of appropriate treatment modalities and early referral to a transplant center for multidisciplinary care, dynamic monitoring of prognosticating criteria and transplant if indicated are important in improving outcomes. However, the results of transplant for acute liver failure are inferior to that of transplants performed for other indications with 1-year survival ranging from 74 to 84%.[6,8] A data review from the United Network for Organ Sharing (UNOS) reveal that the survival of children undergoing transplantation for acute liver failure is significantly lower than for biliary atresia. There is an increased pre-transplant mortality in children with acute liver failure when compared to other causes of end-stage liver disease.[9]

An increasing number of children are now undergoing liver transplant due to hepatic malignancies. Hepatoblastoma is the most common primary hepatic malignancy in children followed by hepatocellular carcinoma and complete resection with chemotherapy as the treatment of choice. However, children with nonresectable tumors or lesions showing poor response to chemotherapy should be offered total hepatectomy and liver transplantation as viable therapeutic options.[10,11] Transplant can also be offered to children with hepatoblastoma who have pulmonary metastasis provided the metastatic lesions are no longer visible in computed tomography (CT) scan after chemotherapy or a surgical resection has removed the lesion completely and tumor free margins are demonstrated.[5] For children with hepatocellular carcinoma, transplant should be offered in the absence of radiological evidence of extrahepatic disease or vascular invasion, irrespective of the size or number of lesions.

Liver transplant is being used as a treatment modality to benefit patients suffering from metabolic disorders. The transplant may be curative in certain conditions, viz., urea cycle defect, maple-syrup urine disease, glycogen-storage disorder type 1. If it does not result in complete cure, it can still improve the quality of life of the affected individual and mitigate symptoms depending on the level of extrahepatic manifestations and severity of the disease.[12] A review of the Studies of Pediatric Liver Transplantation (SPLIT) registry database from 1995 to 2008 reveals that 14.9% of transplant recipients had metabolic disorder as the primary indication with urea cycle defects being the most common condition listed.[13] For conditions which are curable with transplant, urgent referral is recommended to prevent or minimize damage to other organs (Box 1).

Box 1: Indications for pediatric liver transplant.

Cholestatic diseases
- Extrahepatic biliary atresia
- Progressive familial intrahepatic cholestasis (Byler disease)
- Idiopathic neonatal hepatitis
- Alagille (bile duct paucity) syndrome
- Sclerosing cholangitis
- Parenteral nutrition-induced liver injury

Acute liver failure
- Infectious—HAV, HBV, herpes viruses, EBV, sepsis
- Drugs—acetaminophen, valproate, isoniazid, carbamazepine, halothane
- Toxins—amanita phalloides, zinc phosphide
- Metabolic—Wilson's disease
- Autoimmune hepatitis

Metabolic diseases
- Alpha-1 antitrypsin deficiency
- Tyrosinemia type 1
- Wilson disease
- Neonatal hemochromatosis
- Cystic fibrosis
- Crigler-Najjar syndrome type I
- Ornithine transcarbamylase deficiency
- Maple syrup urine disease
- Familial hypercholesterolemia
- Glycogen storage disease types I, III, and IV
- Crigler-Najjar syndrome type I
- Urea cycle defects
- Primary hyperoxaluria
- Organic acidemia

Malignancies
- Hepatoblastoma
- Hepatocellular carcinoma
- Hemangioendothelioma

Miscellaneous
- Budd–Chiari syndrome
- Noncirrhotic portal hypertension
- Caroli's disease
- Factor VII deficiency
- Protein C deficiency

(HAV: hepatitis A virus; HBV: hepatitis B virus; EBV: Epstein–Barr virus)

Box 2: Contraindications to pediatric liver transplant.
• Overwhelming sepsis due to bacterial, fungal, or viral infection outside the liver
• Acquired immunodeficiency syndrome
• Extrahepatic malignancies which are incurable
• Severe extrahepatic disease—irreparable damage to CNS, CVS, lungs due to any cause
• Niemann–Pick disease type C—does not halt progression of neurological derangements
• Valproate-induced liver injury—causes multisystem mitochondrial injury
• Markedly dysfunctional psychosocial environment

(CNS: central nervous system; CVS: cardiovascular system)

CONTRAINDICATIONS TO PEDIATRIC LIVER TRANSPLANT

Although over the last few decades the contraindications to liver transplant have steadily decreased, attempts should still be made to identify patients in whom the underlying disease process would preclude improved survival or an enhanced quality of life, thus rendering the entire process futile (Box 2).

SELECTION CRITERIA FOR TRANSPLANT RECIPIENTS

A patient with chronic liver disease is put on the transplant list once manifestations of decompensation of liver functions appear. The liver functions can be broadly categorized into four groups, including synthetic functions, elimination of toxins, biliary clearance, and maintaining glucose homeostasis through gluconeogenesis, glycogenesis, and glycogenolysis. An impaired synthetic function leading to coagulopathy or ascites, deranged glucose homeostasis leading to hypoglycemia, progressively increasing jaundice, portal hypertension, evidence of variceal bleed, encephalopathy, growth failure, and severe malnutrition are important signs of decompensated chronic liver disease in children. A useful guide to the timing of transplant may be provided by laboratory parameters like. (i) a persistent rise in total bilirubin, (ii) prolonged prothrombin time (PT) and INR, and (iii) persistent decrease in serum albumin levels. A serial evaluation of nutritional parameters helps in identifying early hepatic decompensation. Progressive reduction of fat as measured by triceps skinfold or subscapular skinfold or protein stores as measured by the mid-arm circumference, despite aggressive nutritional support is a reasonably accurate indicator of hepatic decompensation. An important consideration in children with chronic liver disease is that their social and motor development is invariably delayed. For children with chronic liver disease, it is imperative that the transplant is performed before the disease progresses to an extent that transplant is no longer feasible, before quality of life is significantly impaired and growth and development is irreversibly retarded.

In acute liver failure, appropriate selection and listing of patients for transplant still remains a challenge and the selection criteria are far from perfect. Several prognostication systems using a wide range of variables have been used worldwide in an effort to identify patients at high risk of mortality. When evaluating the accuracy of a system to identify patients with high risk of mortality without a transplant, one should consider the positive and negative predictive

> **Box 3:** King's College Criteria.
>
> *Acetaminophen-induced ALF*
> - Arterial blood pH <7.30 (irrespective of grade of encephalopathy) or All of the following
> - Prothrombin time >100 sec (INR >6.5)
> - Serum creatinine >3.4 mg/dL
> - Grade III or IV hepatic encephalopathy
>
> *Nonacetaminophen-induced ALF*
> - Prothrombin time >100 sec (INR >6.5) (irrespective of grade of encephalopathy) or Any three of the following (irrespective of the grade of encephalopathy)
>   - Age <10 or >40 years
>   - *Etiology*: non-A/non-B hepatitis, drug-induced
>   - Duration of jaundice to encephalopathy >7 days
>   - Prothrombin time >50 sec (INR > 3.5)
>   - Serum bilirubin >17.5 mg/dL

(ALF: acute liver failure; INR: International normalized ratio)

values. The importance of the positive predictive value is that a positive prognostic test should accurately predict mortality without transplant, whereas the importance of the negative predictive value is that it should identify patients who will survive without it.

Since their introduction in 1989, the Kings College Criteria has been widely used for identifying patients with acute liver failure in need of a transplant. There are different sets of criteria for acetaminophen and non-acetaminophen induced acute liver failure (Box 3).

The Kings College Criteria uses readily available parameters and has been widely used with a fair degree of accuracy since its introduction to identify patients with acute liver failure, who will not survive without a transplant. It has been validated to different degrees in several studies over the years. Studies have demonstrated that the King's College Criteria has a high positive predictive value although the negative predictive value is lower. Therefore, it can be said that the King's College criteria will identify patients requiring transplant with reasonable accuracy. However, the drawbacks are that the criteria will select some patients for transplant, who might have survived without it and more importantly, not meeting the criteria does not ensure survival without a transplant, especially in non-acetaminophen cases.

Other prognosticating systems like the Clichy criteria, Model for End-Stage Liver Disease (MELD) Score, and Acute Liver Failure Study Group Index have been used with varying degrees of accuracy but none have proven to be conclusively superior to the King's College Criteria. A few other parameters have been studied and found be of value in predicting the need for transplant. Notable among them has been lactate levels after fluid resuscitation. Addition of lactate to King's College Criteria has increased the accuracy of prediction, especially in acetaminophen-induced acute liver failure. Low serum phosphate, extent of necrosis on liver biopsy, liver volume assessed by CT, serum alpha fetoprotein, serum Gc-globulin, apoptosis, and necrosis markers like M65 have been reported to carry prognostic value. There have been few studies with small patient groups; hence further work is required to assess the utility of these in prognosticating outcome either alone or in conjunction with other criteria.

REFERRAL TIMING

It is imperative to refer a patient with acute or irreversible liver failure to a transplant center at the earliest. The referral may not always result in a transplant, but it gives the patient the opportunity to be cared for by a multidisciplinary team in a center equipped to handle such cases. Accurate diagnosis, institution of appropriate therapy, and supportive care along with intensive monitoring may eliminate the need for a transplant. However, if the patient does go on to receive a transplant, the outcomes are significantly better, if the recipient has been referred early, pretransplant care has been optimized and complications handled effectively.

ORGAN ALLOCATION AND PRIORITIZATION

Organ allocation is a complex procedure which in the initial days of transplantation was done primarily on the basis of time spent on the waiting list. However, due to an unacceptably large number of deaths on the waiting list, there has been a shift toward a disease severity-based approach for organ allocation. Since 2002 onward the MELD Score for adults and children ≥ 12 years and the Pediatric End-Stage Liver Disease (PELD) Score for children <12 years have been used in North America to stratify patients based on their disease severity and risk of mortality or intensive care unit (ICU) admission within three months of listing. In 2006, Eurotransplant, which oversees organ allocation in seven European countries, namely, Austria, Belgium, Croatia, Germany, Luxemburg, the Netherlands, and Slovenia, adopted the MELD scores. The National Health Service (NHS) in the UK uses the UK End-Stage Liver Disease (UKELD) scores, developed in 2008, for this purpose.

The MELD Score is calculated based on: (i) bilirubin—a measure of the excretory function, (ii) INR—a measure of the synthetic function, and (iii) creatinine—a measure of other organ involvement as is common with severe liver disease. Since 2016, serum sodium—a measure of the severity of portal hypertension is being used to recalculate the MELD score if the initial score is >11. Scores range from 6, which indicates less severe illness to 40, which implies a critically sick patient. The UKELD score is calculated using bilirubin, creatinine, INR, and sodium levels.

The PELD score, which is based on data derived from the SPLIT registry, uses parameters such as (i) bilirubin, (ii) albumin, (iii) INR, (iv) age <1 year, and (v) growth failure. The PELD score can be higher or lower than the MELD score. The MELD and the PELD scoring is repeated several times at regular intervals after listing and may go up or down based on the severity of the disease at the time when the scoring is done. This repeated assessment ensures that the graft is made available to a recipient who needs it the most.

This system is however not without its drawbacks. The PELD score does not take into account complications arising from decompensated liver disease which may increase the risk of mortality and neither does it account for the presence of metabolic liver disease or primary hepatic malignancies. This has been addressed by introducing PELD exceptions, wherein the PELD score is adjusted higher by assigning points for the presence of failure to thrive, intractable ascites, pathologic bone fractures, refractory pruritus, hemorrhage due to complications associated with portal hypertension, hepatorenal syndrome, hepatopulmonary syndrome, or portosystemic shunting.[5] PELD exceptions are also applicable to transplant recipients with metabolic diseases and primary hepatic malignancies. Transplant recipients with urea cycle defect or organic acidemias should be assigned a PELD/MELD score of 30 on listing. If such recipients do not receive an organ within 30 days, they are listed as Status 1B. A similar method of listing is also applicable for patients with hepatoblastomas, although the 30-day waiting period before escalation to Status 1B is not required for them.

The Status 1 category was introduced to include recipients who should be accorded maximum priority for organ allocation as they are at risk of imminent death. This was further subdivided into 1A and 1B with those with the maximum risk being placed in 1A (Box 4).[14]

In India, given the poor organ donation rate leading to a scarcity of deceased donor organs and the absence of a national policy or database on organ donation and allocation, the process of allocation of organs is very different and varies from state to state based on their individual policies.

> **Box 4:** Criteria for inclusion as Status 1A and 1B.
>
> *Status 1A*
> - Fulminant liver failure in the ICU plus at least one of the following:
>   - On mechanical ventilation
>   - Renal failure requiring dialysis
>   - INR >2.0
> - Primary graft nonfunction diagnosed within 7 days of transplant with the presence of two of the following:
>   - ALT >2000 IU/L
>   - INR >2.5
>   - Total bilirubin >10 mg/dL
>   - Or acidosis, with arterial pH <7.30 or venous pH <7.25 and/or lactate >4
> - Hepatic artery thrombosis in a transplanted liver diagnosed within 14 days of transplant
>
> *Status 1B*
> - Chronic liver disease admitted in the ICU with MELD/PELD score >25 and fulfilling one of the following criteria:
>   - Mechanical ventilation
>   - Gastrointestinal bleed
>   - Renal failure requiring some form of renal replacement therapy
>   - Glasgow coma score <10
>
> (ICU: intensive care unit; INR: International normalized ratio; MELD: model for end-stage liver disease; PELD: pediatric for end-stage liver disease)

Organs from deceased donors in India are allocated based on: (i) the presence of a super urgent listing, i.e., a patient with acute liver failure, who gets priority in most state policies; (ii) availability of in-house recipient; and (iii) waiting time on the transplant list. Some states also allocate organs by rotation among institutes performing transplants within the state. Therefore, except patients with acute liver failure, organs are not allotted based on medical urgency as is the case in other parts of the world.[15]

PRETRANSPLANT EVALUATION AND MANAGEMENT

A thorough evaluation of a transplant recipient by a multidisciplinary team after referral or listing for transplant is an important prerequisite to ensure optimum outcomes.

The aims of the pretransplant evaluation are manifold and can be summarized as below:
- Confirmation of the diagnosis
- Assessment of the degree of decompensation of liver functions and the urgency for the transplant procedure
- Assess the level of comorbidities and degree of involvement of other organs

- Look for availability of treatment options which do not entail transplant
- Rule out contraindications to transplant
- If a transplant is inevitable, formulate a plan for management and optimization of ongoing treatment till the transplant is performed
- Look into the availability of an appropriate donor
- Look at the immunization status and formulate a strategy to complete pending immunizations
- Assess the psychosocial and economic status of the recipient and family
- Anticipate complications and develop a management plan including immediate postoperative support and long-term treatment.

Diagnostic Evaluation

It is important to have a definitive diagnosis before embarking upon a transplant as it not only has a bearing on the outcome, but in some of the conditions, viz., primary sclerosing cholangitis, autoimmune hepatitis, bile salt excretory pump defects, there is a possibility of recurrence in the transplanted liver. Children with extrahepatic biliary atresia should be diagnosed much in advance. Children with other chronic liver diseases should also undergo extensive evaluation to identify structural, genetic, metabolic, or immune-mediated conditions and have a confirmed diagnosis. Acute liver failure should be evaluated to rule out infective etiologies, autoimmune conditions, or drugs and toxins as the cause of the acute liver failure. In spite of a thorough evaluation, in some cases of acute liver failure, the diagnosis may remain indeterminate.

Assessment and Management of Hepatic Decompensation

A thorough clinical evaluation along with a detailed assessment of the synthetic, excretory, and metabolic functions of the liver is mandatory. Signs of decompensation, viz., ascites, portal hypertension, and its associated complications like esophageal varices need to be looked for. Malnutrition, vitamin deficiencies, delayed growth, and development need to be identified.

Ascites is a common finding in end-stage liver disease and can be attributed to hypoalbuminemia, portal hypertension, or hyperaldosteronism. The presence of ascites may lead to significant morbidity by impairing respiration, decreasing renal perfusion, and acting as a nidus for infection. Although no clear guidelines for the initiation of therapy for ascites exist, treatment for clinically detectable ascites may be initiated with aldosterone antagonists. In the presence of hypoalbuminemia, albumin infusion along with a diuretic may be attempted. Large volume ascites, not amenable to medical management and leading to respiratory embarrassment, may require repeated paracentesis or a transjugular intrahepatic portosystemic shunt. Caution should be exercised while using loop diuretics for aggressive diuresis due to the risk of precipitating hepatorenal syndrome. All children routinely undergo a CT scan of the abdomen as part of pretransplant workup. Practices regarding evaluation and management of varices vary widely between institutions. Patients with documented upper or lower gastrointestinal (GI) bleeding should undergo upper or lower GI endoscopy to look for and treat varices.

Assessment of Cardiopulmonary Status

Transplant recipients with end-stage liver disease may also be suffering from cardiopulmonary issues. Children with Alagille syndrome often have associated cardiac defects. Cirrhotic cardiomyopathy, characterized by increased cardiac output, impaired diastolic function, and myocardial hypertrophy is commonly associated with biliary atresia. Children with inborn errors of metabolism, viz., glycogen storage disease or mitochondrial disorders may also have associated cardiomyopathy. Hepatopulmonary syndrome and portopulmonary hypertension, both consequences of portosystemic shunting are potentially fatal complications and can affect outcomes. An echocardiography with Doppler should be performed in all patients awaiting transplant to diagnose any cardiac issues which may have a bearing on transplant outcomes.

Children with cystic fibrosis progressing to end-stage liver disease may have significant impairment of respiratory function which may influence the post-transplant course. Hence, a thorough evaluation of pulmonary function is essential as part of pretransplant evaluation.

Assessment of Renal Function

Impairment of renal function is often present in children suffering from end-stage liver disease. Conditions, such as primary hyperoxaluria, congenital hepatic fibrosis, alpha-1-antitrypsin deficiency, and Alagille syndrome have associated renal dysfunction. Hence, evaluation of renal function using the Pediatric Risk, Injury, Failure, Loss, End Stage Renal Disease (pRIFLE) criteria which combines the estimation of creatinine clearance by the Schwartz method and urine output to categorize the extent of renal impairment done in all recipients of liver transplant.

Assessment of Neurological Status

Delayed development, especially in the gross motor and language domains, have been demonstrated in children suffering from chronic liver disease, more so in children with biliary atresia. Poor nutrition in these children leads to severe calorie deficits and vitamin deficiencies, especially the fat-soluble ones. In children with severe intellectual and developmental delay, pretransplant may have a significant adverse impact on neurocognitive development and post-transplant procedure may no longer be a viable option.

A thorough neurological assessment with emphasis on cognition and developmental aspects is conducted on all recipients with the aim to identify deficits and institute nutritional and other therapies to minimize the developmental delay and optimize neurological outcomes post-transplant.

Assessment of Nutritional Status and Management

A majority of children with chronic liver disease are severely malnourished. This can be attributed to malabsorption along with a hypermetabolic state and poor oral intake. Deficiency of fat-soluble vitamins is a common occurrence. Adequate nutritional rehabilitation prior to transplant has been found to improve graft survival and neurocognitive development post-transplant.

The assessment of nutritional adequacy should be done by serial monitoring of the triceps skin-fold thickness and mid-arm circumference. Weight may not be an accurate measure as it may overestimate the nutritional status.

Aggressive nutritional support should be instituted in all children where a liver transplant is being contemplated. The enteral route is preferred if there are no contraindications to its use. Medium chain triglycerides are preferred in patients with cholestasis and adequate protein intake of 2–3 g/kg/day is ensured in the absence of hyperammonemia. Fat-soluble vitamins and vitamin B complex should be supplemented in adequate doses. If oral intake is insufficient, nasogastric feeds may be a viable alternative to improve calorie intake. Occasionally parenteral nutrition may be required to ensure adequate nutrition and growth in severely malnourished children and those with feed intolerance to improve post-transplant outcomes.

Assessment of Immunization Status

Vaccine preventable diseases may cause significant morbidity and mortality in recipients of liver transplant, both before and after transplant. Therefore, a review of the immunization status of the child and a strategy to complete the immunization process is an important part of pretransplant workup. Most children with chronic liver disease have not completed their vaccination schedules.

The safety and uptake of vaccines has been found to be better before the onset of end-stage liver disease and an accelerated schedule may be followed in children listed for transplant in order to complete the immunization prior to transplant. It is important to remember that although inactivated vaccines may be administered post-transplant, the efficacy has been found to be less than if administered pretransplant and live vaccines cannot be administered post-transplant. Live vaccines should be given a minimum of 4 weeks before the transplant is scheduled.

Healthcare workers and close contacts of transplant recipients should be immunized against all vaccine preventable diseases so that there is no risk of exposure to the recipient. Healthcare workers and family members should receive all indicated vaccines, including live attenuated vaccines except oral polio vaccine, as paralytic polio has been described in contacts of oral poliovirus vaccine (OPV) recipients. The live attenuated vaccines should preferably be administered to the contacts at least 4 weeks prior to transplant.

Influenza infection in patients with chronic liver disease and transplant recipients causes a more severe disease with increased incidence of decompensation pretransplant and a heightened risk of graft rejection post-transplant. It is recommended that all transplant recipients and their immediate contacts be administered the seasonal inactivated influenza vaccine yearly (Table 1).

Assessment of Dental Hygiene

Dental caries are a frequent finding in children with end-stage liver disease and there have been reports of post-transplant sepsis from dental infections. Assessment by a pediatric dentist to rule out the presence of caries and infections is routinely done as a part of pretransplant evaluation.

Table 1: Vaccination in transplant recipients.

Vaccine	Type	Pretransplant	Post-transplant
BCG	Live	Yes	No
Diphtheria	Inactivated	Yes	Yes
Pertussis	Inactivated	Yes	Yes
Tetanus	Inactivated	Yes	Yes
Haemophilus influenzae	Inactivated	Yes	Yes
Inactivated polio virus	Inactivated	Yes	Yes
Hepatitis B	Inactivated	Yes	Yes
Measles	Live	Yes	No
Mumps	Live	Yes	No
Rubella	Live	Yes	No
Varicella	Live	Yes	No
Rotavirus	Live	Yes	No
Hepatitis A	Inactivated	Yes	Yes
Conjugated pneumococcal	Inactivated	Yes	Yes
Polysaccharide pneumococcal	Inactivated	Yes	Yes
Rabies	Inactivated	Yes	Yes
Human papillomavirus	Inactivated	Yes	Yes
Neisseria meningitides	Inactivated	Yes	Yes
Influenza	Inactivated	Yes	Yes

(BCG: bacillus Calmette–Guérin)

Psychosocial Assessment

A recipient of liver transplant needs to adhere to long-term treatment plans and regular follow-up schedules which have a significant bearing on the outcome of transplant. The recipient and the caregivers should be made aware of this and its importance needs to be stressed upon the recipient and/or the family. An assessment of the understanding of the family about the procedure and the ability to ensure adherence to the treatment protocol is an important part of pretransplant evaluation.

LIVE DONOR LIVER TRANSPLANT

Increasing indications for liver transplant has resulted in more patients being listed and this has led to a scarcity of organs from deceased donors with organ donation rates having plateaued over time, resulting in large number of deaths while on the waiting list. This led to the introduction of live donor liver transplants, wherein a segment of the liver from a compatible living donor is transplanted in a recipient. The impetus for live donor transplant has come from two areas, one of which is pediatric liver transplants, where there is a lack of deceased donors of appropriate size and an inordinately high mortality on the waiting list. The other being regions with extremely low organ donation rates has made live donor transplants being the only viable option. To consider a live donor liver transplant, the transplant should be the only available therapeutic option in circumstances of nonavailability of a deceased donor organ.

There are a few distinct advantages associated with a live donor liver transplant, viz., (i) a short waiting period, (ii) possibility of a transplant before severe decompensation, (iii) a planned surgery with possibility of a better outcome, (iv) a better probability of receiving a healthy graft which may also help improve outcome, and (v) a decreased cold ischemia time which improves graft quality. Studies have shown improved survival in children receiving live donor transplants when compared to deceased donor transplants.

Donor Selection

As mandated by law, the donor has to be a close family member, who can be either be the spouse, parents, grandparents, siblings, children, grandchildren, or other close relatives. This clause has been put in place to prevent trade in human organs.

In addition, the donor must be (i) blood group compatible, (ii) between 18 and 55 years of age, (iii) having a liver large enough to provide adequate volume for the recipient and the donor, and (iv) in good physical and mental health as demonstrated through a thorough medical and psychological evaluation. The donor should fully comprehend the risks involved and there should be no evidence of coercion (Table 2).

Donor Evaluation

The first step in donor evaluation is to ascertain blood group compatibility. Once blood group matching is confirmed, the donor is subjected to further evaluation. A thorough history is taken and a clinical examination is done, followed by blood tests to check the cell counts, renal function, liver function, and screen for transmissible viruses like hepatitis B, hepatitis C, human immunodeficiency virus (HIV), etc. The donor also undergoes CT/magnetic resonance imaging (MRI) to assess the volume of the liver, the biliary architecture, and the adequacy of vascular structures, which aid in the surgical planning. A few centers perform a liver biopsy routinely as a part of donor workup. The donor undergoes a chest X-ray and electrocardiography (ECG) to rule out any pulmonary or cardiac abnormality which may

Table 2: Blood group compatibility.

Donor blood group	Recipient blood group
O	O, A, B or AB
A	A or AB
B	B or AB
AB	AB

make the donor unfit for surgery. Once the donor is deemed to be physically fit, his mental health is assessed through a psychological evaluation, to ascertain their understanding of the procedure, the associated complications, their willingness to voluntarily donate the organ and their mental stability to go ahead with it.

INNOVATIONS TO INCREASE GRAFT AVAILABILITY

Certain innovations in transplant techniques have been introduced over time to help patients who need a transplant and may not have a suitable living donor and are unlikely to get a deceased donor in time.

ABO Incompatible (ABOi) Transplant

With increasing numbers on the waiting list and availability of suitable living or deceased donors being a limiting factor, ABO incompatible transplants are being performed with improving results. With refinement in treatment leading to lesser incidence of complications and better outcomes, it has gained acceptance as a feasible option, when a compatible graft may not be available in time. Although protocols vary among centers, Institution of immunosuppression pretransplant, perioperative use of plasmapheresis to reduce antibody titers and post-transplant use of intravenous immunoglobulin (IVIg) and aggressive immunosuppression using up to four agents has resulted in improving outcomes of ABO incompatible transplants. This modality has an important bearing for pediatric recipients as young children with immature immune systems and fewer antibodies have been found to tolerate ABO incompatible transplants better without having acute rejection.

Swap Transplant

If a patient does not have a suitable donor amongst his family but there is a suitable donor for another patient requiring a transplant and if there is a family member of the second patient who is suitable for the first patient then the two families can exchange donors and provide grafts for both patients. This exchange can save two lives and is referred to as swap transplant.

Dual-lobe Transplant

Studies have shown that at least 50% of the liver volume of the recipient is essential to maintain basic liver functions and sustain life. It is sometimes seen that the donor graft volume is insufficient to meet the functional demands of the recipient and a larger area of resection from the donor may be required, which may in turn jeopardize the safety of the donor. As in any live donor transplant the safety of the donor is paramount, such donors are deemed unfit and hence rejected thereby depriving a recipient of a chance of survival. To alleviate the problem of small for size grafts, two lobes are harvested from two different donors and grafted in a single recipient to serve the dual purpose of maintaining donor safety and recipient survival. The procedure is technically challenging and places two donors at risk for the sake of one recipient. However, in situations where there is a severe shortage of deceased donors and non-availability of appropriate living donors, it provides a patient an opportunity to get a lifesaving transplant.

Partial/Reduced Size Liver Grafts

Split liver transplant is when the liver of a deceased donor is split into the left and right lobes either in situ or after extraction of the graft and the smaller left lobe is transplanted in a child while the larger right lobe is transplanted in an adult. In this manner by splitting a single organ graft, availability can be increased and waiting time decreased.

Reduced size transplants are when a full graft is obtained from a deceased donor and reduced in size to match the recipient and then transplanted. This technique is generally used in pediatric liver transplants when the graft from an adult deceased donor may be too large to fit in the child.

Studies have demonstrated similar outcomes for whole and partial grafts among children but the survival is decreased among adults with partial grafts when compared to whole grafts.

KEY POINTS

- Liver transplant is a viable option in liver failure
- Possible candidates for transplant should be identified early and moved to a "liver unit"
- Pre-transplant care needs to be meticulous to prevent the patient from becoming a non-transplant candidate.

SUGGESTED READING

1. Adam R, Karam V, Delvart V, et al. Evolution of indications and results of liver transplantation in Europe. A report from the European Liver Transplant Registry (ELTR). J Hepatol. 2012;57:675-88.
2. Austin MT, Leys CM, Feurer ID, et al. Liver transplantation for childhood hepatic malignancy: A review of the United Network for Organ Sharing (UNOS) database. J Pediatr Surg. 2006;41(1):182-6.
3. Baliga P, Alvarez S, Lindblad A, et al. Posttransplant survival in pediatric fulminant hepatic failure: The SPLIT experience. Liver Transplant. 2004;10(11):1364-71.
4. Germani G, Theocharidou E, Adam R, et al. Liver transplantation for acute liver failure in Europe: Outcomes over 20 years from the ELTR database. J Hepatol. 2012;57:288-96.
5. Kamath BM, Olthoff KM. Liver transplantation in children: Update 2010. Pediatr Clin North Am. 2010;57:401-14.
6. Kaur S, Wadhwa N, Sibal A, et al. Outcome of live donor liver transplantation in Indian children with bodyweight <7.5kg. Indian Pediatr. 2011;48:51-4.
7. McDiarmid SV, Anand R, Lindblad AS. Studies of pediatric liver transplantation: 2002 update. An overview of demographics, indications, timing, and immunosuppressive practices in pediatric liver transplantation in the United States and Canada. Pediatr Transplant. 2004;8:284-94.
8. McDiarmid SV, Goodrich NP, Harper AM, et al. Liver transplantation for Status 1: The consequences of good intentions. Liver Transplant. 2007;13:699-707.
9. Mendizabal M, Silva MO. Liver transplantation in acute liver failure: A challenging scenario. World J Gastroenterol. 2016 Jan 28;22(4):1523-31.
10. Meyers RL, Tiao GM, Dunn SP, et al. Liver transplantation in the management of unresectable hepatoblastoma in children. Front Biosci (Elite Ed). 2012;4:1293-302.
11. Nagral S, Nanavati A, Nagral A. Liver transplantation in India: At the crossroads. J Clinical Exp Hepatol. 2015;5(4):329-40.
12. Narasimhan G. Living donor liver transplantation in India. Hepatobiliary Surg Nutr. 2016;5(2):127-32.

13. Oishi K, Arnon R, Wasserstein MP, et al. Liver transplantation for pediatric inherited metabolic disorders: Considerations for indications, complications, perioperative management. Pediatric Transplant. 2016;20(6):756-69.
14. Shneider BL, Vockley J, Mazariegos GV. Trading places: Liver transplantation as a treatment, not a cure, for metabolic liver disease. Liver Transplant. 2011;17:628-30.
15. Squires RH, Vicky Ng, Romero R, et al. Evaluation of the pediatric patient for liver transplantation: 2014 Practice Guideline by the American Association for the Study of Liver Diseases, American Society of Transplantation and the North American Society for Pediatric Gastroenterology, Hepatology and Nutrition. Hepatol. 2014;60:362-98.

Nutrition in Critically Ill Children

26

Madhumati Otiv, Umesh Vaidya

LEARNING OBJECTIVES

- Understand the goals of nutrition in critically ill child
- Know type of nutrition in different pathologic conditions
- Importance of early nutrition in critically ill
- Methods of nutrition delivery

INTRODUCTION

Nutritional support refers to enteral or parenteral provision of calories, proteins, electrolytes, trace elements, vitamins, and minerals along with sufficient fluids. Acute critical illness is characterized by catabolism exceeding anabolism. Nutrition supports the demands of the catabolic and anabolic states and also ongoing growth of the children.

GOALS OF NUTRITION

To meet the metabolic needs in order to mitigate the breakdown of muscle protein and to provide substrate for the anabolic state during recovery.

ENERGY EXPENDITURE IN CRITICALLY ILL CHILDREN

Critical illness in children is associated with hypercatabolic state resulting into muscle wasting. This is due to release of inflammatory mediators such as interleukin 1, tumor necrosis factor, and cytokines resulting into generation of catecholamines, glucocorticoids, glucagons, aldosterone, and antidiuretic hormone causing increased protein breakdown and negative nitrogen balance. Energy expenditure (EE) increases further by pain, anxiety, fever, muscular effort, increased work of breathing, and shivering.

Evidence has shown that the EE may vary with the underlying disease. For instance, children with burns, sepsis, trauma and elective surgery are likely to have EE in the decreasing order which may vary from lower to higher EE with passage of time. This was observed on the basis of indirect calorimetric measurements that calculate EE on the basis of respiratory quotient (RQ = CO_2 eliminated/O_2 consumed) which is 1 and 0.7 for energy generated by burning carbohydrates and fats, respectively. A nutritionally deprived child will preferably metabolize fats and thus will have RQ of 0.7, while a child who is overfed may have RQ of 1 due to predominant carbohydrate utilization. Indirect calorimetry is currently available only in the research setting.

To calculate energy requirements in critically ill children:
While the energy requirements of normal children are well known, for the reasons mentioned above, it is difficult to clinically predict the EE (PEE) of critically ill children. Many methods based on various formulae/equations using weight and height of the children along with adjustments for stress factors (e.g. Harris Benedict formula, Talbot formula, Schofield's equations, adjusting with stress factor, etc.) have been tried. Most of these formulae are not validated for critically ill children and have poor agreement with indirect calorimetry, however of all these, Schofield's equation for calculation of EE has been frequently used in critically ill children as shown below:

- EE for more than 3 years: 0.167W + 15.174H—617.6
- EE for 3–10 years: 19.59W + 1.303H + 414.9
- EE for 10–18 years: 16.25W + 1.372H + 515.5
- EE for 18–30 years: 15.057W—0.1H + 705.8
  (W: weight; H: height)

RECOMMENDATION FOR FEEDING IN PICU

Since there is no satisfactory formula for calculation of PEE, and unavailability of indirect calorimetry, it is reasonable to keep caloric target 20% above usual requirement (accounting for stress factor), to be achieved over 4–5 days. A ratio of 70/30 (%) calories derived from carbohydrate to fat is reasonable in most circumstances. Protein requirement for 0–2 years, 2–13 years, and above 13 years is 2–3 g/kg, 1.5–2 g/kg, and 1.5 g/kg, respectively.

Feeding in Special Situations

Patients with burn, need above 200 kcal/kg, but calories derived from fat should be less than 15%, as lipolysis induced by burns increases free fatty acid load and impair immunity. Acute liver disease requires protein restriction to 0.5 g/kg (to step up cautiously) to restrict ammonia production. Acute and chronic renal disease requires appropriate restriction of fluids and potassium and caloric dense feeds. Acute stage of fatty acid oxidation defects, and inborn errors of protein metabolism (organic acidemia, hyperammonemia) require fat-free and protein-free diet, respectively along with more concentrated forms (>10%) of dextrose infusions in order to force the patient to use carbohydrate alone as a source of energy.

Overfeeding and Underfeeding

Both underfeeding and overfeeding are detrimental and may increase the ventilator requirements due to muscle wasting or increased CO_2 production, respectively. Underfeeding is more common as compared with overfeeding in ICU. Overfeeding increases the chances of steatosis, cholestasis, risk of infection, and hyperglycemia which is associated with worse outcomes. BSL monitoring is required in all the critically ill children. Underlying diseases such as liver failure, protein–energy malnutrition, malaria, and diabetes are vulnerable for hypoglycemia. In children optimum blood sugar targets are between 140 mg% and 180 mg% and lower values for tighter glucose control are not recommended.

Enteral Versus Parenteral Nutrition

Enteral nutrition is easy to administer, cheaper, and decreases the susceptibility to nosocomial infection by preserving mucosal integrity, gut immune function, stress ulcers, and reduction of inflammation in critically ill patients if provided early in the course of critical illness. Even 7 days of fasting may lead to mucosal atrophy which is a known cause of transmucosal migration of pathogenic organisms. Even a small amount of enteral nutrition may promote intestinal secretion and preserve the mucosal integrity. Parenteral nutrition is expensive, associated with higher incidence of infections requiring expert teams, and special infrastructure.

NUTRITIONAL ASSESSMENT

Clinical Examination

The assessment of nutrition in a critically ill child is challenging. Usual interpretation of anthropometry is not appropriate in presence of edema, fluid retention, hypoproteinemia, anemia etc. Care must be taken to identify associated vitamin and mineral deficiency. Recent evidence shows that vitamin D deficiency is both common among critically ill children and associated with greater severity of critical illness.

Laboratory Examination

Despite immense efforts in search of biochemical methods of assessing nutritional status; parameters like albumin, prealbumin, transthyretin, and inflammatory mediators like interleukin and C-reactive protein (CRP) do not seem to reflect either catabolic or anabolic state. Albumin gets adversely affected in liver disease and sepsis and also does not reflect acute changes due to longer half-life. Prealbumin, even though has a shorter half-life, decreases in liver disease and inflammation and increases in renal failure due to poor clearance. Some preliminary evidence seem to be accumulating in favor of transthyretin. The studies on interleukin are still inconclusive and it is not clear if fall of CRP itself permits rise of prealbumin.

Methods of Establishing Enteral Nutritional Support

Early feeding, (< 48 hours after admission) is beneficial, and strongly recommended.

Nasogastric vs. post-pyloric: Nasogastric feeding is easy to administer while post-pyloric feeding requires expertise and monitoring. Post-pyloric feeding may not prevent gastroesophageal reflux, but in some patients where gastric feeding has failed, post-pyloric may be used to achieve nutritional targets by continuous feeding protocols.

Continuous vs. intermittent: Continuous tube feeding does not offer advantages of smaller gastric residual volume, number of vomiting or diarrheal episodes, however, it may help to achieve nutritional targets during post-pyloric feeding.

Hurdles in establishing enteral nutrition: Causes of inadequate feeding in PICU setting are delayed initiation, suboptimal prescription, fluid restrictions and frequent interruption (elective procedures, diagnostic tests, unplanned intervention, feeding intolerance), etc. Many causes amongst these are avoidable by meticulous planning, communication, specifying exact time of the procedure, avoiding postponement of planned procedures, and also unnecessary long fasting. Other causes of feed interruptions are high gastric residual volume, abdominal discomfort, and diarrhea. Extremely judicious use of pharmacotherapy such as metoclopramide, peri-colace, erythromycin lactobionate, and enema can help in establishing feeding. Protocolized feeding, staff education, ICU nutritionist can help in optimizing nutrition goals by avoiding arbitrary interruptions in feeding.

Contraindications: Absolute contraindications to enteral nutrition are bowel obstruction, severe ileus, major GI bleeding, intractable vomiting or diarrhea, a high output fistula, and new anastomosis at a risk of dehiscence. Unstable child with poor perfusion or on pressor drugs such as noradrenaline, high-dose adrenaline, and vasopressin may be not tolerate enteral nutrition. Mere absence of peristaltic sound is not a contraindication for feeding and sometimes feeding itself can initiate intestinal propulsion.

Ideal enteral feed: The ideal commercial formula is isotonic with caloric density of 1 kcal/mL preferably lactose free, with protein content of 40 g/1,000 mL, with nonprotein calorie to nitrogen ratio of 150 [(carbohydrate calories + fat calories × 6.25)/(proteins in g)] and should be a mixture of simple and complex carbohydrates with adequate amounts of long-chain fatty acids, essential vitamins, minerals, and micronutrients.

Predigested formulae: Predigested formulae comprises of hydrolyzed protein, less complex carbohydrates, lesser fats and more medium chain triglycerides. Predigested formulae are indicated in thoracic duct leak, chylothorax, or chylous ascites, malabsorptive syndromes (unresponsive to pancreatic enzymes), and failure to tolerate standard enteral nutrition.

Immunonutrition: Some studies have shown Cu, Se, Zn in higher doses may reduce infections, and enhance wound healing. However, in patients with acute respiratory distress syndrome (ARDS), omega-3 fatty acids, alpha linolenic acid, and antioxidant supplementation are harmful and associated with significantly higher mortality. In severe burns, glutamine supplementation may improve the outcome but requires more research.

Total Parenteral Nutrition

Total parenteral nutrition (TPN) is recommended only when enteral nutrition cannnot be administered. It is costlier and requires special infrastructure and a well-trained dedicated team. It is prepared in 10% dextrose with 1–3 g/kg of amino acids (through bacterial filter) and fats on day one (to step up slowly) with appropriate quantity of Na, K, Mg, and Ca under aseptic precautions. A dedicated central IV access is required for lipids. TPN is associated with higher incidence of nosocomial infections, azotemia, acidosis, dyselectrolytemia, cholestasis, thrombocytopenia, hemolysis, and eosinophilia. Clinical monitoring in the form of weight, input–output, and laboratory monitoring (BSL, liver functions, kidney functions, Ca, Mg, P, electrolytes, triglycerides, proteins) is required. Contraindications to TPN include hyperosmolality, severe hyperglycemia, severe electrolyte abnormalities, volume overload, and inadequate attempts to feed enterally. Sepsis or SIRS is a relative contraindication to parenteral nutrition.

Refeeding Syndrome

This is characterized by shock, cardiorespiratory failure, altered sensorium due to metabolic disturbances that occur as a result of reinstitution of nutrition to patients who are starved or severely malnourished. During prolonged fasting, body derives its energy from fats by generating ketones. While fasting results into suppressed insulin secretion and increased glucagon secretion, there is a reversal during refeeding in response to increased glycemia. This leads to anabolic process with increased synthesis of glycogen, fat, and proteins associated with increased consumption of phosphates, magnesium, and potassium followed by depletion of intracellular ATP and 2,3-diphosphoglycerate in red blood cells, cellular dysfunction with inadequate oxygen delivery to the body's organs. Intracellular movement of electrolytes occurs along with a fall in the serum electrolytes including phosphate, potassium, and magnesium. Glucose and levels of the thiamine may also fall. Cardiac arrhythmias are the most common cause of death from refeeding syndrome, with other significant risks including confusion, coma and convulsions, and cardiac failure.

SUGGESTED READING

1. Botrán M, LópezHerce J, Mencía S, et al. Relationship between energy expenditure, nutritional status and clinical severity before starting enteral nutrition in critically ill children. Brit J Nutr. 2011;105:731-7.
2. Mehta N, Compher and ASPEN. Board of Directors. ASPEN Clinical Guidelines: Nutrition Support of the Critically Ill Child. JPEN. 2009;33; 260-76.
3. Mehta N, McAleer D, Hamilton S, et al. Challenges to optimal enteral nutrition in a multidisciplinary pediatric intensive care unit. JPEN. 2009:1-7.
4. Petrillo-Albarano T, Pettignano R, Asfaw M, et al. Use of a feeding protocol to improve nutritional support through early, aggressive, enteral nutrition in the pediatric intensive care unit. Ped Crit Care Med. 2006;7:340-4.
5. Rice TW, Wheeler AP, Thompson BT, et al. Enteral omega-3 fatty acid, gamma-linolenic acid, and antioxidant supplementation in acute lung injury. JAMA. 2011;14:1574-81.

Dengue in Pediatric Intensive Care Unit

27

Javed Ismail, Jhuma Sankar

LEARNING OBJECTIVES

- Epidemiology of dengue and severe dengue. How does it spread?
- The pathophysiology of dengue illness.
- To recognize dengue clinically. What are the warning signs of severe dengue? Are there any atypical presentations of dengue?
- To differentiate from other tropical infections at the bedside
- To manage dengue with or without warning signs and severe dengue.

CASE

A 7-year-old boy presented with complaints of high-grade intermittent fever for past 3 days. He also had three episodes of nonbilious vomiting, periumbilical abdominal pain and diffuse body aches for past 1 day. He did not have bleeding from any site or rash over the body. On admission to the emergency, he was in cold hypotensive shock. Examination revealed mild periorbital puffiness, decreased breath sounds on right hemithorax suggestive of right pleural effusion; and mild tenderness over right hypochondrium. With possibilities of severe dengue, scrub typhus, or septic shock he was resuscitated with fluid bolus of 20 mL/kg normal saline and then was started on infusion of Ringer's lactate at 7 mL/kg/hour. The child was shifted to pediatric intensive care unit (PICU) for further management. During PICU stay, the fluid infusion rate was tapered over next 12 hours to 3 mL/kg/hour and then stopped. Child had seizures followed by altered sensorium requiring mechanical ventilation for 5 days. Subsequently, he was extubated and discharged from the PICU.

EPIDEMIOLOGY

The global incidence of dengue is on an increasing trend, since past two decades, with increase in number of reported cases from 2.2 million in 2010 to 3.2 million in 2015 in three World Health Organization (WHO) regions. About 500,000 people require hospitalization of which about 2.5% die each year with dengue. It has become an endemic disease in more than

100 countries and is characterized by explosive outbreaks. Southeast Asia and the Western Pacific regions contribute to about 75% of the global dengue burden. In India, it occurs as outbreaks predominantly in urban areas now spreading rapidly to rural areas too. In the past 5 years (2010–2015), the incidence has increased by 2.6 folds compared to previous years. The reported proportion of severe cases among laboratory confirmed Indian studies is about 29% and a case fatality ratio varying between 0% and 25%.

PATHOPHYSIOLOGY

Dengue is caused by single-stranded ribonucleic acid (RNA) virus belonging to genus *Flavivirus* and family *Flaviviridae*. Four serotypes (DEN-1, 2, 3, 4) of dengue virus (DENV) have been identified and each of them have been found to cause epidemics of dengue fever of varying severity. The infection caused by one serotype offers lifelong immunity against that specific serotype and transient cross immunity against the other 3 serotypes. It is transmitted by the bite of two common vectors *Aedes aegypti* and *Aedes albopictus*. These are anthropophilic, day biters, and can feed on multiple hosts. Their predominant breeding sites are stagnant water around household and construction areas. Transmission of dengue is seasonal occurring immediately after the monsoon when the humidity and temperature are optimal for rapid vector breeding. Following the bite of an infected host during the viremic phase, the virus enters the vector and replicates in the epithelial cells of midgut, infects its salivary glands and the mosquito remains infected for life. When this vector bites the other host, the clinical features appear after an incubation period of 4–10 days (intrinsic incubation period). The vector also demonstrates transovarian transmission and the eggs remain viable for many months in the absence of water.

The clinical manifestation of dengue infection is a spectrum varying from mild undifferentiated fever to severe bleeding, shock, or organ dysfunctions. The evolution of clinical course and outcome is often unpredictable. Majority of primary infection is either asymptomatic or manifests as undifferentiated fever, whereas the secondary infection by another serotype may manifest with a severe disease. Secondary infection results in an antibody dependent enhancement of viral replication, overwhelming host immune response, cytokine storm, endothelial dysfunction which in turn results in increased vascular permeability, capillary leak, hemoconcentration and shock (which are the hallmarks of severe dengue). This endothelial dysfunction is transient and predominantly functional, resuming back to normal within next 24–48 hours. Thrombocytopenia occurs as a result of alteration in megakaryocytopoieses due to infection of hematopoietic cells, increased peripheral destruction, increased consumption and impaired aggregation. Bleeding tendencies are secondary to abnormalities in hemostasis resulting from many causes like hypoxia, acidosis, shock, low-platelet count, platelet dysfunction, coagulopathy, endothelial dysfunction, and disseminated intravascular coagulation. Higher viral loads have been demonstrated in severe cases suggesting its correlation with disease severity. The viral strain (DENV-2 > DENV-3) and the sequence of viral strain also determines the severity of illness with DENV-1 or DENV-2 carrying the highest risk of severe dengue. Children with coexisting chronic diseases, such as diabetes mellitus, congenital heart disease, nephrotic syndrome, and asthma may have a greater risk of developing severe dengue.

CLINICAL PRESENTATION

Dengue illness begins abruptly and has three clinically recognizable phases, namely: (i) febrile; (ii) critical; and (iii) recovery phase (Fig. 1).

Febrile Phase

- This phase starts with sudden onset high-grade fever lasting 2–7 days.
- It is often accompanied by facial flushing, skin erythema, generalized body ache, myalgia, arthralgia, retro-orbital pain, headache, congestion of throat, eyes, flushing of palms and soles, nausea, vomiting, and anorexia.
- Clinical examination may reveal tender hepatomegaly.
- We should look for hemorrhagic manifestations like petechiae or mucosal bleeding and evidence of other coinfections.
- Tourniquet test done during this stage maybe positive indicating increased capillary fragility
- Total white cell count may show a progressive decline.
- Patient should be advised to watch for warning signs of severe dengue.

Tourniquet test: Mark a square inch over the ventral aspect of forearm just an inch away from the cubital crease. Keep the blood pressure cuff inflated between systolic and diastolic pressure for 5 minutes. Meanwhile note the appearance of petechiae over the marked square inch. If the number of petechiae is more than or equal to 10 per square inch, the test is considered to be positive and it predicts the diagnosis of dengue with an area under curve of 0.7.

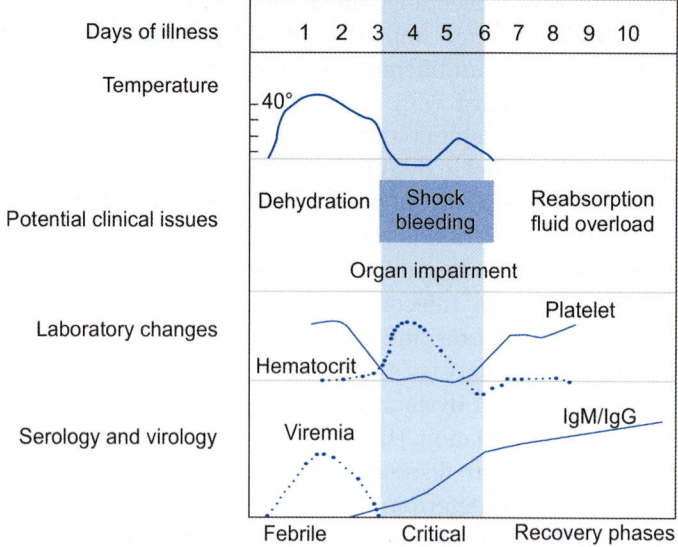

Fig. 1: Course of dengue illness.
Source: Adapted from WHO handbook for clinical management of dengue.

Critical Phase

This phase typically begins between day 3 and day 7 of illness, starting with defervescence and appearance of warning signs. Majority of patients recover without going into this critical phase.
- During this phase, plasma leakage occurs; severity of which predicts the rapidity of progression of illness.
- Increase in hematocrit—one of the earliest signs of plasma leakage.
- Clinically, warning signs like abdominal pain, persistent vomiting, mucosal bleeds, lethargy, restlessness, hepatomegaly, clinical fluid accumulation like ascites or pleural effusion are observed.
- Persistent vomiting and severe abdominal pain are early signs which could be misdiagnosed as acute cholecystitis or renal colic and can delay treatment in the lines of dengue.
- Often accompanied by rapid decline in platelet counts.
- This phase lasts for 24–48 hours, and may extend up to 72 hours.
- Some patients may not follow this typical progression to critical phase with defervescence and may manifest with severe dengue during the febrile phase itself.
- The plasma leakage may progress and can manifest as hypotension and shock.
- Typical presentation like cold clammy extremities, tachycardia, silent tachypnea, weak pulses and a narrow pulse pressure (≤20 mm Hg) with or without hypotension.
- Children with compensated shock may be conscious, alert with normal systolic blood pressure and thus the severity can be misjudged unless other signs of shock are looked for.
- In contrast, during the fever episodes, as a normal physiological response there can be tachycardia, vasoconstriction, and cool peripheries, which can be misinterpreted as shock.
- This tachycardia and peripheral vasoconstriction should be interpreted with other signs such as peripheral and central pulse volume.
- Hypotension being a late sign of shock in children, it signals imminent cardiorespiratory arrest.
- If the shock is profound or prolonged it may be accompanied by progressive multiorgan dysfunction and severe metabolic acidosis.
- Administration of intravenous fluids titrated to offset this hemoconcentration along with close monitoring of the hematocrit is the crux in treatment of this phase.
- Many patients improve as the plasma leakage ceases spontaneously after 48–72 hours.
- However, some may progress to severe dengue with multiorgan dysfunction despite adequate intravenous fluids.
- Most dengue deaths occur in patients with profound or prolonged shock complicated by severe bleeding manifestations.

Some patients present with bleeding manifestations like epistaxis, gum bleeds, puncture site bleeds. An ongoing occult severe bleeding may manifest as shock with sudden drop in hematocrit. Prolonged shock, hypoxia may trigger disseminated intravascular coagulation (DIC) further worsening the bleeding manifestations. Patients on nonsteroidal anti-inflammatory drugs (NSAIDs) or steroids or those with peptic ulcers may have increased tendency to bleed.

Recovery Phase

Those patients improving from the plasma leakage enter into this phase of resorption of leaked fluid. There may be associated diuresis, sinus bradycardia and hypertension usually lasting about 48–72 hours.
- Some patients may manifest with features of hypervolemia like pulmonary edema, congestive heart failure especially in those who have received overzealous intravenous fluids.
- Diffuse maculopapular rash with significant pruritus is common during this phase.
- Also, the general well-being and appetite improves. Leukopenia and thrombocytopenia gradually improve over time.

Atypical Manifestations

Severe organ dysfunctions without significant plasma leakage (like myocarditis, encephalitis, hepatitis) or due to coinfections or due to high-risk host factors (like infants, underlying comorbidities like diabetes mellitus, congenital heart disease, nephrotic syndrome, and asthma) constitute "***Expanded Dengue Syndrome***". Most common atypical manifestations are gastrointestinal like hepatitis, pancreatitis, acalculous cholecystitis. Cardiac manifestations like myocarditis, heart block, pericarditis have been reported prior. Encephalitis like presentation, seizures, encephalopathy, or acute disseminated encephalomyelitis (ADEM) or Guillain–Barre syndrome are rare manifestations.

To aid in early clinical recognition of patients, a revised classification of dengue was proposed by WHO in 2009 (Table 1).

Table 1: Dengue case classification (WHO 2009).

Dengue ± warning signs		Severe dengue

Probable dengue:
• Fever and 2 of the following criteria:
  – Nausea, vomiting
  – Rash
  – Aches and pains
  – Tourniquet test positive
  – Leukopenia
  – Any warning sign
	Warning signs:
	• Abdominal pain or tenderness
	• Persistent vomiting
	• Clinical fluid accumulation
	• Mucosal bleed
	• Lethargy, restlessness
	• Liver enlargement >2 cm
	• Bleeding (coffee ground vomitus, black-colored stools)
		Severe plasma leakage:
		• Shock
		• Fluid accumulation with respiratory distress
		Severe bleeding
		Severe organ impairment
		• Liver: AST or ALT ≥1,000
		• CNS: impaired consciousness
		• Heart and other organ involvement

Laboratory-confirmed dengue (important when there is no sign of plasma leakage)	Increase in Hct concurrent with rapid decrease in platelet count	
(ALT: alanine aminotransferase; AST: aspartate aminotransferase; CNS: central nervous system; Hct: hematocrit)		

Differentiating from Other Tropical Infections

The differentials commonly considered are:
- Malaria, scrub typhus, leptospirosis and other hemorrhagic viral infections such as chikungunya, nipah, etc.

For a patient presenting to the doctor with undifferentiated fever, the presence of a diffuse erythematous rash, retro-orbital pain, diffuse myalgia, hepatomegaly, ascites, pleural effusion bleeding manifestations are clinical clues suggestive of dengue.

MANAGEMENT

Laboratory

Initial Investigations

A complete blood count should be done at the first visit to the hospital and should be repeated periodically. Leukopenia is common during febrile phase and precedes the onset of critical phase. A rising hematocrit and falling platelet count suggests the development of hemoconcentration during the critical phase. Prothrombin time and partial thromboplastin time may also be prolonged. In the absence of hemorrhagic tendencies, these parameters need not be corrected.

Hematocrit: A simple but perhaps one of the most useful tests, serial hematocrit evaluation helps in identifying the degree of capillary leak and intervening appropriately. If available in the bed side laboratory, a microcentrifuge often guides the fluid therapy. Blood may be collected into a capillary tube after a finger prick and centrifuged in the microcentrifuge. This method saves time and avoids the need for multiple intravenous pricks (Fig. 2).

Diagnostic Tests

Specific diagnostic investigations are aimed at confirming the diagnosis of dengue, to diagnosis coexisting infections. These may not be mandatory for acute management of patients.

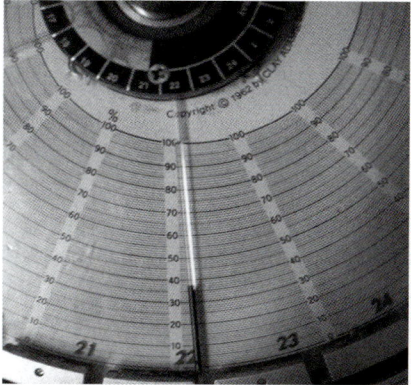

Fig. 2: Microcentrifuge. Useful in bedside evaluation of hematocrit using capillary tubes.

Dengue diagnosis: Commonly available test employs detection of viral components [nonstructural protein 1 (NS1) antigen, viral genome or the virus] and serological response (IgM or IgG antibodies) to dengue infection.
- During the *febrile phase* of illness (first 5 days after onset of fever): Viremia is detectable. NS1 antigen can be detected using enzyme-linked immunosorbent assay (ELISA) or rapid card tests.
- After 5 days (during *critical or convalescent phase*): Dengue specific IgM antibody is the best marker of recent infection. Both rapid card test and ELISA are available for detecting the same. Serum IgG levels help identify whether the child is having primary or secondary infection. High IgG levels with low IgM are characteristic of secondary infection.
- *Confirmed dengue infection*: Either of positive NS1Ag or seroconversion from negative to positive IgM or a fourfold increase in IgG titers on paired sera denote confirmed dengue infection.
- *Probable dengue*: IgM positivity (on single serum sample) detected after day 5 of clinical symptoms denotes *probable dengue*. Other virus isolation techniques, genome detection, histochemical staining of tissue samples are less commonly used.

Tests for organ function assessment: Raised hepatic enzymes are suggestive of hepatic involvement in dengue (levels in thousands are not uncommon). Furthermore, coinfections and paracetamol overdosage can also contribute to liver impairment. Serum glucose, electrolytes, blood gases, bicarbonate, calcium, and renal parameters must also be monitored. Hyponatremia, hypocalcemia, and hypoglycemia are common during the critical phase. Echocardiography and continuous electrocardiogram (ECG) monitoring may be required to detect myocardial dysfunction.
- *Imaging*: Presence of pleural fluid and/or ascites suggests the presence of capillary leak. Gallbladder wall edema has also been noted.
- *Urine analysis*: It may reveal microscopic hematuria in about 40% of patients. Hemoglobinuria may occur in patients with concomitant hemoglobinopathies.

Coinfections: In patients with atypical manifestations or with additional clinical signs, such as splenomegaly, jaundice, high-grade fever, or eschar, etc., specific tests should be done to rule out typhoid, malaria, leptospirosis, and scrub typhus.

CLINICAL ASSESSMENT AND GRADING OF SEVERITY

Brief history including symptoms, past medical history, any comorbidities, physical examination for signs of organ dysfunction, shock and simple laboratory tests like hematocrit should be done. In addition to the routine, history should include total duration of illness, fluid intake, and approximate urine output per day, history of warning signs, any alteration in mental state, history of recent travel and similar symptoms in neighborhood. Physical examination should specifically include examination for rash, bleeding manifestations, detailed assessment for shock, assessment of hydration status, and a tourniquet test. Basic laboratory investigations like hematocrit (preferably done using microcentrifuge), platelet counts, and total leukocyte counts should be done.

Based on the findings in history, examination and initial lab investigations, patients should be graded in severity as in Table 1.

Probable Dengue without Warning Signs and with Warning Signs

Children *not having any warning signs* presenting to the hospital with either clinical and or laboratory evidence may be managed at home. An overview of management of dengue with and without warning signs is given in Flowchart 1.

Severe Dengue (Severe Plasma Leakage, Severe Bleeding, Organ Dysfunctions)

All patient with severe dengue should be admitted in a healthcare setting with adequate manpower and facility for close monitoring preferably an intensive care unit. Intravenous fluids titrated appropriately for the plasma leakage (monitored with trends of hematocrit) with close monitoring are the sole intervention required.

Severe plasma leakage—Shock: Shock in dengue primarily occurs due to plasma leakage resulting in intravascular hypovolemia. Thus, fluids are the cornerstone of treatment. Unlike septic shock, the duration of plasma leakage is usually short-lasting. So, smaller volumes of isotonic fluids are infused over longer periods of time to maintain intravascular volume meanwhile preventing fluid overload. *Isotonic fluids given in quantities just adequate to maintain the effective circulating volume is the best strategy* in managing shock. Supplemental oxygen is provided in a nonthreatening manner as in any case of shock. Baseline hematocrit is estimated before the start of fluid therapy.

Compensated shock (Flowchart 2):
- Start intravenous isotonic fluids at 10–20 mL/kg/hour for 1 hour. Continue monitoring the patient for decrease in hematocrit and resolution of signs of shock.
- If the shock improves, continue fluid infusion rate at 10 mL/kg/hour over first 1–2 hours, then decrease the infusion rate to 7 mL/kg/hour for next 2 hours.
- If the clinical improvement is sustained, decrease the infusion rate further to 5 mL/kg/hour for next 4 hours. Subsequently, fluid rate can be tapered to 3 mL/kg/hour for next 24–48 hours and then stopped as the oral fluid intake improves. The total duration of intravenous fluid infusion is usually 48 hours.
- If at any point, the shock resurfaces or worsens, increase the fluid infusion rate back to 10–20 mL/kg/hour and continue monitoring for signs of shock resolution.
- If the hematocrit continues to be high with persistent shock, try a bolus of colloid (5% albumin) at 10–20 mL/kg/hour. If there is improvement, continue with crystalloids at 7–10 mL/kg/hour for 1–2 hours and then further reduce as above.
- If there is a sudden fall in hematocrit, from the baseline value with persistence or worsening of shock, it indicates ongoing occult bleeding. Arrange for cross-matched fresh whole blood or packed red cells and transfuse, if there is evidence of ongoing bleeding.

Signs of shock resolution
- Decrease in tachycardia
- Well-felt central and peripheral pulses
- Warm and pink peripheries
- Capillary refill time less than 2 seconds
- Improving or normal consciousness
- Urine output at least 0.5 mL/kg/hour
- Resolution of metabolic acidosis and normalization of lactate.

Flowchart 1: Overview of management of dengue.

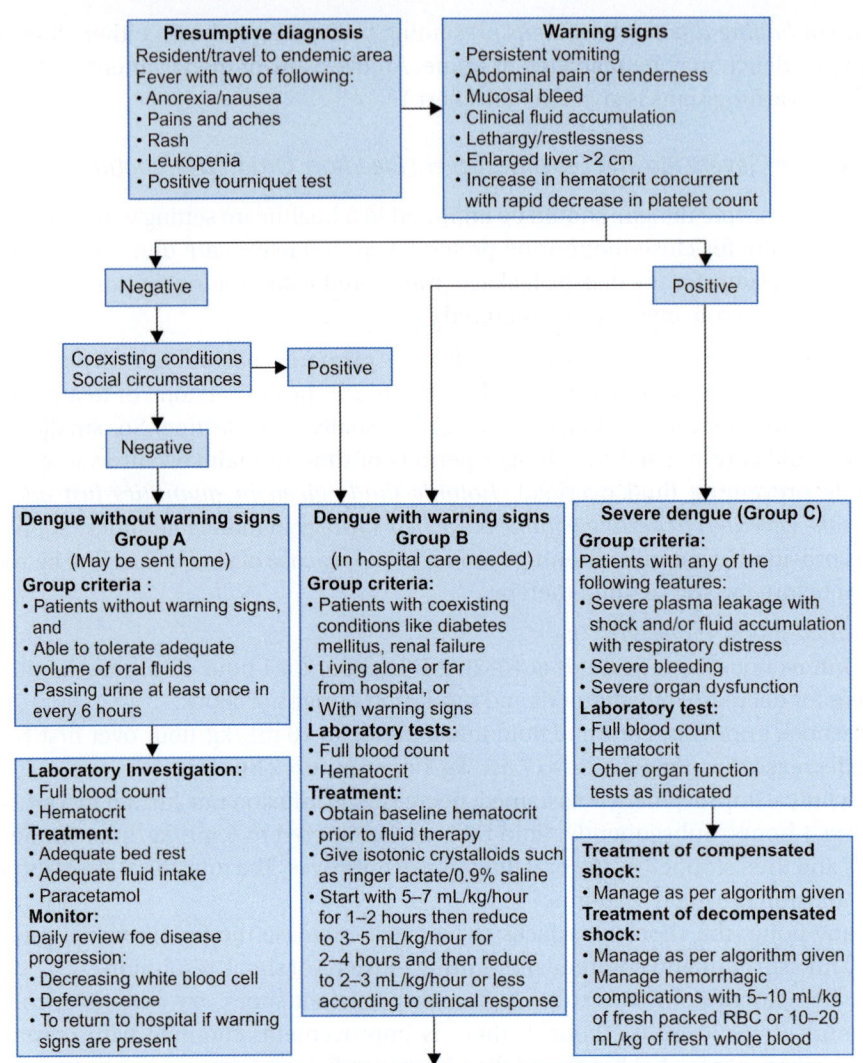

Flowchart 2: Management of dengue with compensated shock.

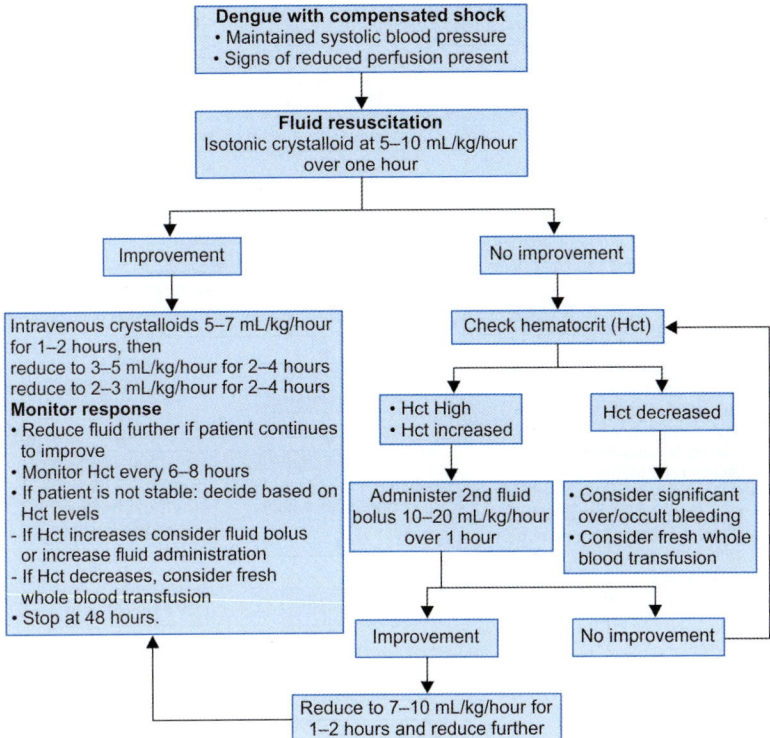

Hypotensive shock
The management of dengue with hypotensive shock is given in Flowchart 3. Hypotensive shock is managed aggressively with initial bolus of 20 mL/kg of isotonic crystalloids (0.9% saline, Ringer's lactate) or colloids (5% albumin) administered as rapid as possible, using a 3-way pull-push or pressure bag technique, meanwhile monitoring for resolution of shock or appearance of pulmonary edema.
- *Colloids are indicated in*:
  - Patients with prolonged shock or severe ongoing plasma leakage (as indicated by persistently high hematocrit despite fluid resuscitation)
  - Patients with clinical signs of fluid overload (like puffiness of eyes, anasarca, respiratory distress). Among colloids dextran-40, Gelatin, or 5% albumin are preferred.
- On reassessment, if hypotension persists, a second bolus of 10 mL/kg of crystalloid or colloid should be infused over 30 minutes to one hour. If blood pressure stabilizes, the fluid infusion rate is decrease to 10 mL/kg/hour for 1 hour followed by 5–7 mL/kg/hour for 2 hours and tapered gradually as in the case of compensated shock.
- If blood pressure (BP) fails to stabilize, compare the baseline hematocrit with current hematocrit.

Flowchart 3: Management of dengue with hypotensive shock.

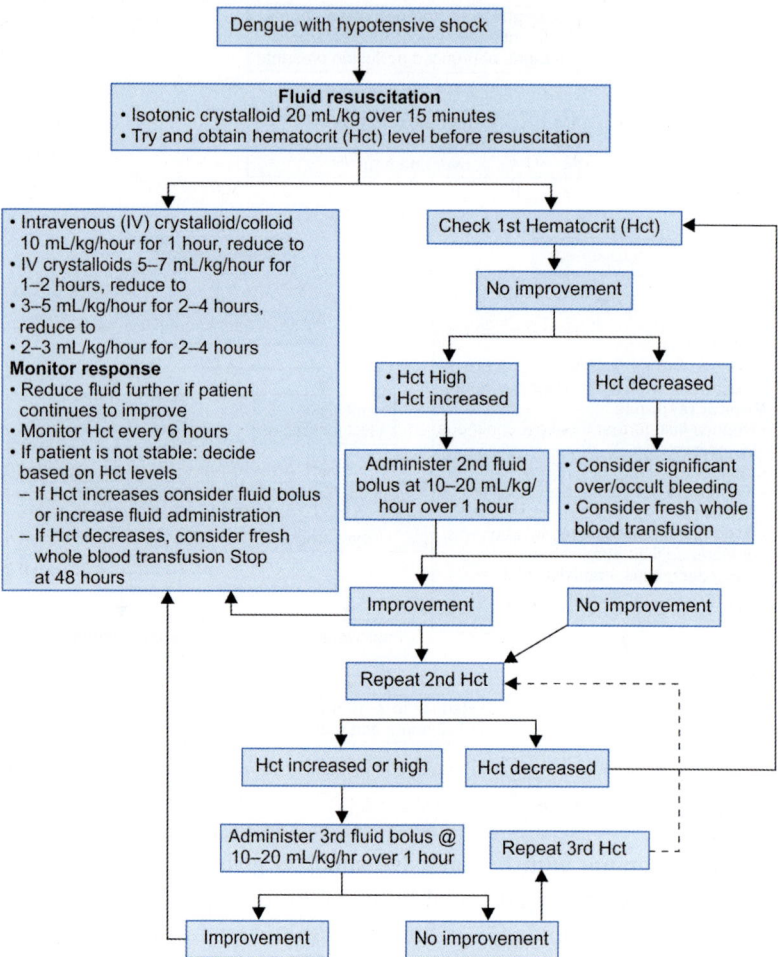

- If the hematocrit is same or increasing, one more bolus of crystalloid or colloid of 10–20 mL/kg is administered over one hour. If the clinical condition improves, decrease the rate of infusion to 7–10 mL/kg/hour for next 2 hours and further as in case of compensated shock.
- If the hematocrit has decreased significantly from the baseline (infants <30–35%, children <35–50%), it may be implying ongoing occult bleeding. Examine the patient for the same and arrange for fresh whole blood or packed red cells. If there is no bleeding, administer one more bolus of 10–20 mL/kg of colloid over 30 minutes and titrate the fluid infusion rate according to the hematocrit change.
- The clinical condition is dynamic and may deteriorate any time after stabilization. So, the patient should be monitored continuously for the same.

- Fluids being the main crux of treatment in dengue shock, vasoactive infusions are not preferred. If patient continues to be hypotensive and *intravascular hypovolemia is ruled out* after giving adequate volume (40–60 mL/kg over 1–2 hours) or by ultrasound measured dynamic changes in vena cava diameter, the mechanism of shock in such a patient may be accompanying myocardial dysfunction. Echocardiography can confirm the diagnosis. Low dose inotropic agents like epinephrine or dopamine can be initiated, if patient is hypotensive. Milrinone is preferred in patients with myocardial dysfunction and compensated shock. Due to the inherent risk of bleeding, invasive monitoring is reserved for patients with refractory hypotensive shock and generally avoided in patients with compensated shock.

Indications for switching from intravenous to oral fluids:
- Stable hemodynamics—shock resolved
- No warning signs
- Adequate urine output
- Stable or decreasing hematocrit in presence of good pulse volume.

Severe plasma leakage—fluid accumulation with respiratory distress/failure: Respiratory distress during critical phase of dengue, may be due to following causes:
- Massive pleural effusion or ascites causing lung collapse during the critical phase
- Acute pulmonary edema due to myocardial dysfunction or fluid overload during convalescent phase where resorption of leaked fluid occurs
- Severe metabolic acidosis due to uncorrected shock
- Pulmonary hemorrhage
- Acute respiratory distress syndrome (ARDS).

The goal of treatment in any case is to improve the gas exchange. Noninvasive ventilation (NIV) can be initially tried in milder cases of respiratory distress especially in cooperative children. NIV is preferred as it preserves the spontaneous respiratory efforts which are essential to maintain venous return to right heart during a state of hypovolemia. Early respiratory support offloads the workload on the respiratory muscles, thus improving perfusion to the vital organs during states of shock. The decision regarding timing of intubation and invasive mechanical ventilation is purely clinical and has to judged case to case basis.

- In patient with significant pleural or ascites causing respiratory distress NIV can be tried.
- Therapeutic drainage of the effusions is indicated only when high ventilator pressure settings are needed to achieve adequate gas exchange. Since, there is risk of bleeding, coagulopathy should be corrected prior to pleural tap.
- Patients with pulmonary edema due to fluid overload (presenting with clinical features like periorbital edema, puffiness of face, anasarca, elevated jugular venous pressures, dilated vena cava on ultrasound) would have received large volumes of fluid during critical phase, or have received hypotonic fluids, blood products or may have comorbid conditions like renal failure.
- Fluid restriction, diuretic infusion, positive pressure ventilation, early renal replacement therapy (in cases of oliguric renal failure or fluid overload refractory to medical management) are effective strategies in patients with pulmonary edema due to fluid overload.
- Acute respiratory distress syndrome due to dengue infection can occur as an atypical manifestation and if severe may require invasive ventilation.

- Serum potassium levels should be monitored and treated to prevent complications of severe hypokalemia induced by diuresis.
- High-positive end-expiratory pressure (PEEP) may be needed in the presence of chest wall edema, ascites, pleural effusion, or pulmonary edema.

Acute respiratory distress syndrome is a well-described atypical manifestation of severe dengue occurring without clinical signs of fluid overload or a massive pleural effusion. Severe plasma leakage in to the alveoli and the cytokine storm related to endothelial dysfunction seems the likely cause. Management remains ventilation strategy similar to other cases of ARDS, with more emphasis on fluid titration according to hematocrit. Rare cases of severe ARDS requiring extracorporeal membrane oxygenation (ECMO) support have been reported.

Severe Bleeding

A wide spectrum of bleeding manifestations extending from minor mucosal bleed, such as epistaxis, skin bruises at intravenous site to massive gastrointestinal bleed like hematemesis, bleeding per rectum and bleeds following bladder catheterization or peritoneal dialysis have been reported.

Management of bleeding: Minor mucosal bleed without hemodynamic abnormalities is considered a minor bleed. Major bleeds are gastrointestinal bleed or bleeding per vaginum or occult bleed (intra-abdominal) with associated shock. Refractory shock is the major risk factor for severe bleeding. Other common risk factors are severe or persistent metabolic acidosis, renal or liver failure, NSAID usage, and anticoagulant therapy.

Clinical features that help recognize a major bleed include the following clinical scenarios:
- Obvious blood loss
- Rapid fall in hematocrit in a shocked child
- Refractory shock not responding to fluid bolus of 40–60 mL/kg
- Hypotensive shock associated with low or normal hematocrit prior to fluid resuscitation
- Abdominal distension with tenderness associated with or without metabolic acidosis in a shocked child.

Since, bleeding in dengue, is a consequence of severe hypoxia, shock, and acidosis, it has been hypothesized that improvement in 2,3-DPG (diphosphoglycerate) levels would reduce the tendency to hemorrhage by enhancing oxygen delivery to the tissues. Transfusion of 10–20 mL/kg of *fresh whole blood or fresh packed red cells are the first choice* and they are rich in 2,3-DPG. If shock persists and hematocrit continues to be low, a second fresh blood transfusion should be considered. The volume of transfusion depends on the estimated volume of bleeding. Fresh frozen plasma (FFP) or platelet transfusions do not improve the coagulopathy or thrombocytopenia, rather may contribute to coagulopathy and hence should be considered only if bleeding persists despite two fresh whole blood transfusions. Platelet transfusions in a non-shock patient may be considered only when significant thrombocytopenia exists and an invasive procedure is being planned.

Severe Organ Dysfunction

Myocardial dysfunction: Cardiac manifestations of dengue are:
- Cardiogenic shock (diastolic and systolic dysfunction)

- Myocarditis
- Pericardial effusion
- Arrhythmias (such as supraventricular tachycardia, ventricular arrhythmias)
- Conduction blocks.

During the critical phase, majority of the patients have an asymptomatic myocarditis. Both diastolic and systolic dysfunction can occur in severe cases and should be managed accordingly with lusiotropic and inotropic agents. Serial echocardiographic studies done in severe dengue reveal an early diastolic wall motion abnormality and decreased left ventricular systolic function especially during active plasma leakage. Cardiac function correlated with severity of dengue with function being poorest in dengue shock compared to dengue hemorrhagic fever and undifferentiated dengue fever. Cardiac function as estimated only by ejection fraction (EF) may be falsely low due to hypovolemia and it may normalize as the plasma leakage settles or with fluid resuscitation as in majority of the patients. Among the various echocardiographic parameters like Tei index, EF and $E/E'-E/E'$ was sensitive and specific to identify cardiogenic shock whereas Tei index identifies subclinical myocardial dysfunction. Myocardial involvement may be associated with transient elevation of troponin (T) and creatine kinase-MB (CK-MB) levels. Direct infection of myocytes with dengue virus have been demonstrated. Autopsy findings reveal mononuclear cell infiltrate in the myocardium on immunohistochemistry suggestive of myocarditis. Patients in the convalescence phase may present with features of pulmonary edema and decreased left ventricular systolic function due to resorption of leaked fluid.

Neurological complications: Common manifestations are seizures and encephalopathy. They commonly occur due to:
- Impaired cerebral perfusion during plasma leakage
- Intracranial bleeding
- Acute liver failure resulting in toxic encephalopathy
- Raised intracranial pressure
- Demyelination: ADEM
- Electrolyte disturbances
- Rarely encephalitis, meningitis
- Myelitis—transverse myelitis or longitudinally extensive transverse myelitis
- Ischemic stroke (due to dengue vasculitis).

Dengue virus being non-neurotropic, direct viral invasion presenting as encephalitis or meningitis is rare. During an outbreak or in endemic regions, patients presenting with only neurological manifestations can be due to atypical dengue infection. The serological tests and other hematological parameters may help in identifying these patients. Management of these patients involves stabilizing the airway, breathing, and circulation followed by neuroimaging which helps in identifying the most plausible pathogenesis.
- High dose steroids have been used in patients with ADEM or transverse myelitis with good recovery
- Control of bleeding—fresh whole blood transfusion, FFP transfusion to correct coagulopathy

- Increased intracranial pressure (ICP) to be checked in patients with significant cerebral edema
- Identifying and treatment of bacterial coinfection in patients with meningitis
- Supportive measures to optimize circulation, correction of electrolyte disturbances in all patients and liver supportive measures in patients with acute liver failure.

Peripheral nervous system manifestations like Guillain-Barre syndrome (GBS), neuritis, and cranial nerve palsies have been reported. In patients with GBS, plasma exchange and intravenous immunoglobulin infusion are effective.

Hepatitis: Moderate elevation of transaminases occurs in majority of patients with severe dengue. The mechanism of liver injury includes:
- Direct viral invasion of hepatocytes
- Dysregulated immune response
- Secondary—ischemic injury due to shock, hypoxia and acidosis
- Coinfection with hepatitis A, E
- Hepatotoxic drugs—acetaminophen overdose or decreased excretion.

Clinically, they present with hepatomegaly, right hypochondriac tenderness, jaundice or bleeding tendencies with laboratory elevation of transaminase and alkaline phosphatase levels. These abnormalities are much severe and frequent among patients with severe dengue compared to probable dengue. Dengue virus is one of the common cause of acute liver failure to in endemic regions and during outbreaks and case fatality is high (60–70%) in severe cases of liver failure. These patients develop multiorgan dysfunction requiring intensive monitoring, fluid management, close monitoring for hypoglycemia, bleeding, encephalopathy, hyperammonemia, and electrolyte abnormalities. They should also be worked up for coinfection with other hepatotrophic viruses. Liver biopsy studies report massive hepatic necrosis with dengue virus demonstrated in the hepatocytes.

Renal failure: Dengue fever can result in acute kidney injury (AKI) especially in severe cases. Microvascular injury due to hypoxia, rhabdomyolysis, hemolysis causing pigmentary nephropathy and prerenal AKI are the common mechanisms attributed to AKI. In Thailand, severe dengue caused AKI in about 0.9% (25/2,893) of admissions, with a high mortality rate of 64.0%. This entity should be differentiated from renal failure of prerenal etiology. Fluid management, modification of drug doses for glomerular filtration rate (GFR), avoidance of nephrotoxic medications, monitoring of electrolytes, early institution of renal replacement therapies are the priciples in management. Anticoagulants should be cautiously used in patients undergoing extracorporeal renal support like continuous venovenous hemofiltration (CVVH). Peritoneal dialysis though carries a risk of bleeding; it can be done if CVVH is not available.

Other Intensive Care Issues

Fluid Overload

Prevention: Although, fluid overload occurs as a consequence of capillary leak, overzealous administration of intravenous fluids (IVF) or giving hypotonic fluids can predispose to this complication. Administration of IVF in the febrile phase or in dengue without warning signs or prolonged administration even after resolution of shock or during the recovery phase must be avoided. In addition, administration of hypotonic fluids such as 5% dextrose, half normal saline or Isolyte P can cause accumulation of free water and interstitial fluid over load. Colloids can be used during resuscitation of hypotensive shock thereby reducing the need for large volumes of crystalloids to maintain the intravascular volume.

Treatment of fluid overload:
- *Fluid overload without shock or respiratory distress*: Discontinuation of fluids is sufficient in these children. Diuresis occurs spontaneously or can be augmented with furosemide infusion during the recovery phase.
- *Fluid overload with respiratory distress without shock*: Noninvasive respiratory support with supplemental oxygen should be provided. Diuretics should be administered at low infusion rates of 0.05–0.1 mg/kg/hour to enable gentle diuresis without compromising hemodynamic stability. Careful monitoring of urine output and perfusion is mandatory.
- *Fluid overload with respiratory distress and shock*: Requires intensive care monitoring with invasive lines, ventilator support either invasive or noninvasive and initiation renal replacement therapy for ultrafiltration.

Abdominal Compartment Syndrome

Aggressive fluid resuscitation and severe plasma leakage are the main risk factors for abdominal compartment syndrome (ACS). Worsening shock, acidosis, progressive oliguria despite fluid resuscitation points towards development of ACS. If left untreated may lead on to refractory shock and established AKI. Intra-abdominal pressure should be monitored using Foley's catheter in-situ in patients receiving fluids more than 30 mL/kg in first 3 hours.

Treatment of abdominal compartment syndrome:
- Optimize sedation and analgesia
- Decompress gastrointestinal tract
- Decrease the ventilator pressures (PEEP) as feasible
- Prefer colloids for correcting ongoing shock
- Neuromuscular paralysis should be reserved for severe cases
- Drainage of ascites should be slow and controlled with close monitoring for bleeding and worsening shock. Colloid infusion can be given along with drainage to treat worsening shock.

Hemophagocytic Lymphohistiocytosis

Hemophagocytic lymphohistiocytosis (HLH) should be strongly suspected in dengue patients persistent high grade fever, bicytopenia, hyperferritinemia with worsening coagulopathy despite stabilization of shock. Ferritin levels are often elevated to the tune of 10,000 µg/L. Bone marrow may show evidence of hemophagocytosis. However, a negative bone marrow should not preclude a diagnosis of HLH, if other HLH 2004 criteria is satisfied. In a systematic review of 122 cases of dengue HLH following criteria were present: fever in 97%, splenomegaly in 78%, hepatomegaly in 70%, anemia in 76%, thrombocytopenia in 90%, coagulopathy in 91%, and serum ferritin is more than 500 µg/L in 97%.

Treatment of dengue HLH: Evidence regarding treatment of secondary HLH due to dengue is limited to case series and reports. Majority of the authors have used monotherapy unlike the standard HLH 2004 protocol. Various regimens that have been reported are:
- *Monotherapy:*
  - Corticosteroids
    - Dexamethasone at 10 mg/m^2/day for initial 5 days followed by tapering over 4–8 weeks
    - Methyl prednisolone 2 mg/kg/day for initial 5 days followed by tapering
  - Intravenous immunoglobulin (IVIG) 2 g/kg over 5 days or over 2 days.

Combination of corticosteroids and IVIG each of various doses as described above have been used. Few authors have used cyclosporine and or etoposide along with IVIG or steroids. Some patients with dengue present in the early febrile phase or in the critical phase with a significant isolated hyperferritinemia (>10,000 mg/L). In such cases, prior to treatment, other criteria to suggest worsening organ dysfunction (mainly liver dysfunction–transaminases, coagulopathy) should be looked for in addition to criteria for HLH.

Coinfections

Dengue being a tropical disease, coinfection has been described with other common diseases like scrub typhus, leptospirosis, enteric fever, respiratory syncytial virus, cytomegalovirus, Epstein Barr virus, Hepatitis A, B, C, E, and malaria. In addition, patient may develop health care associated infection anytime during the hospital stay. High index of suspicion should be kept in patients with dengue serological positivity with atypical manifestations to identify coinfections.

KEY MESSAGES

- Dengue should be considered in any child presenting with acute short febrile illness during an outbreak.
- Children with warning signs should be meticulously monitored with clinical and laboratory parameters for complications during defervescence.
- Shock, severe bleeding, severe organ dysfunctions are manifestations of severe dengue
- Atypical presentations are relatively common during an outbreak
- Fluid therapy in severe dengue should be titrated just adequate to maintain intravascular volume with total duration not exceeding 24–36 hours.
- Intensive care monitoring, organ support therapies, anticipation and treatment of complications are the strongholds in managing patients with multiorgan involvement.

SUGGESTED READING

1. Directorate General of Health Services, Government of India, New Delhi. (2008). Guidelines for clinical management of dengue fever, dengue hemorrhagic fever and dengue shock syndrome.
2. Ganeshkumar P, Murhekar MV, Poornima V, et al. Dengue infection in India: A systematic review and meta-analysis. PLOS Negl Trop Dis. 2018;12(7):e0006618.
3. Jalac LRS, de Vera M, Alejandria MM. The use of colloids and crystalloids in pediatric dengue shock syndrome: A systematic review and meta-analysis. Philippine J Microbiol Infect Dis. 2010;39:14-27.

4. Kalayanarooj S. Choice of colloidal solutions in dengue hemorrhagic fever patients J Med Assoc Thai. 2008;91(Suppl 3):S97-103.
5. Kamath SR, Ranjit S. Clinical features, complications and atypical manifestations of children with severe forms of dengue hemorrhagic fever in South India. Indian J Pediatr. 2006;72.
6. Laoprasopwattana K, Pruekprasert P, Dissaneewate P, et al. Outcome of dengue hemorrhagic fever-caused acute kidney injury in Thai children. Pediatr. 2010;157(2):303-9.
7. Laoprasopwattana K, Pruekprasert P, Dissaneewate P, et al. Outcome of dengue hemorrhagic fever-caused acute kidney injury in Thai children. J Pediatr. 2010;157(2):303-9.
8. Lye DC, Lee VJ, Sun Y, et al. Lack of efficacy of prophylactic platelet transfusion for severe thrombocytopenia in adults with acute uncomplicated dengue infection. Clin Infect Dis. 2009;48:1262-5.
9. Narayanan M, Aravind MA, Thilothammal N, et al. Dengue fever epidemic in Chennai – A study of clinical profile and outcome. Indian Pediatr. 2002;39:1027-33.
10. Premaratna R, Liyanaarachchi E, Weerasinghe M, et al. Should colloid boluses be prioritized over crystalloid boluses for the management of dengue shock syndrome in the presence of ascites and pleural effusions? BMC Infect Dis. 2011;11:52
11. Smart K, Safitri I. What treatments are effective for the management of shock in severe dengue? Int Child Health Rev Collab. 2009.
12. Tantracheewathorn T. Risk factors of dengue shock syndrome in children. J Med Assoc Thai. 2007;90(2):272-7.
13. Varatharaj A. Encephalitis in the clinical spectrum of dengue infection. Neurol India. 2010;(58):585-91.
14. World Health Organization and the Special Programme for Research and Training in Tropical Diseases. Dengue Guidelines for Diagnosis, Treatment, Prevention and Control. New edition, 2009.

Management of a Child with Polytrauma

28

Bharat Mehra, Suresh Gupta

LEARNING OBJECTIVES

- Mechanisms of injuries
- Assessment of severity
- Management of polytrauma.

INTRODUCTION

Injury is a major, preventable public health problem in terms of morbidity, premature mortality, and disability. Worldwide, an estimated 6 million people die due to injuries annually and this figure is expected to rise to 8 million in 2020. Injury and violence are major killers of children throughout the world, responsible for approximately 9,50,000 deaths annually in those under the age of 18 years. From an Indian perspective, injury is the second leading cause of morbidity and mortality among children.

Mortality in trauma patients has an immediate, early, and late trimodal distribution. Fifty percent of patients have immediate death at the scene due to fatal injuries. No trauma care can reduce this mortality except for preventive strategies. Early death (30%) can occur within an hour of injury and late death (20%) can happen days after the injury due to sepsis and multiorgan failure. Early and late deaths are preventable by good trauma care at specialized centers.

Children with multiple injuries carry a very high risk of morbidity and mortality. Management of such children requires timely resuscitation and care by the pediatric critical care team. This chapter outlines the principles of management of children with multiple injuries except head and cervical spine injuries.

MECHANISM OF INJURY

Mechanism of injury is an important determinant for the severity and prognosis of injury. Blunt injuries are the most common type of injuries seen in the pediatric cohort while penetrating injuries are less compared with adult population. Certain common mechanisms of injuries include:

- *Injuries due to fall*: Fall from a height is the major cause of head injury in Indian children. Falling from a significant height (>10 ft or >3 times of the height) can result in long bone fractures, intrathoracic and intra abdominal injuries.
- *Pedestrian injury*: A walking child hit by a moving vehicle may result in Waddell's triad of a fractured femur due to the leg striking the bumper of a vehicle, abdomen with upper chest injury caused by the hood, and contralateral head injury from falling on the ground after being hit.
- *Bicycle injury*: Injuries range from minor abrasion to major blunt abdominal contusion. Children without helmets are more prone to head injuries. Knee and elbow injuries can be prevented with pads.
- *Motor vehicle occupant injury*: This is a common cause of injury during childhood. Children without restraint are likely to have penetrating injuries due to ejection from the automobile windows while those with restraint get only head and neck injuries. Lap belts can cause contusion and injury to intra-abdominal organs.

MEASUREMENT OF PEDIATRIC INJURY SEVERITY

There are several scoring systems for field triage and injury severity. Each trauma score has its own advantages and disadvantages and none can be considered ideal. The most commonly used are the Pediatric Trauma Score (Table 1) and Revised Trauma Score (Table 2). The Pediatric

Pediatric trauma score	+2	+1	–1
Weight	>20	10–20 kg	<10 kg
Airway	Patent	Maintainable	Not maintainable
Systolic BP	>90 mm Hg	50–90 mm Hg	<50 mm Hg
CNS	Awake	+ LOC	Unresponsive
Fractures	None	Closed or suspected	Multiple, closed, or open
Wounds	None	Minor	Major, penetrating, or burns

Table 1: Pediatric trauma score (PTS).

(CNS: central nervous system; LOC: loss of consciousness)
Minor trauma is PTS 9–12, use local guidelines/protocols.
Potentially life threatening is PTS 6–8, suggests need for trauma center.
Life threatening is PTS 0–5, need for trauma center.

Glasgow coma scale (GCS)	Systolic blood pressure (SBP)	Respiratory rate (RR)	Coded value
13–15	>89	10–29	4
9–12	76–89	>29	3
6–8	50–75	6–9	2
4–5	1–49	1–5	1
3	0	0	0

Table 2: Revised trauma score (RTS).

The RTS range is 0–12. In START triage, a patient with an RTS score of 12 is labeled delayed, 11 is urgent, and 10–3 is immediate. Those who have an RTS below 3 are declared dead and should not receive definite care because they are highly unlikely to survive without a significant amount of resources. A coded form of the RTS is used for quality assurance and outcome prediction. RTS = 0.9368 GCS + 0.7326 SBP + 0.2908 RR. Values for the code RTS range 0 to 7.8408. (0 = dead 7.8408 = normal).

Trauma Score has been shown to be a better predictor for emergency department disposition, whereas the Revised Trauma Score has a better predictive value for overall outcome.

UNIQUE ASPECTS OF PEDIATRIC TRAUMA

Pediatric trauma usually carries certain unique features which are important from the management point of view. These are:
- Blunt injuries are more common while penetrating injuries predominate in adults.
- Head injuries are very common in children due to a relatively larger percentage of body mass. Head injury accounts for one-third of trauma mortality in children.
- The cervical spine is at a higher risk of injury due to a relatively large head and weak neck muscles of a child.
- Abdominal contents are prone to damage because of the smaller cavity, weak musculature, and little fat pad covering, while intrathoracic injuries can occur without any external rib fractures.
- Long bone fractures commonly involve growth plates. Greenstick and buckle type of fracture are unique to this age group.
- Trauma in children has a developmental and psychological aspect also.

MANAGEMENT OF A CHILD WITH POLYTRUAMA

Team Approach

Management of a child with multiple injuries requires a multidisciplinary approach involving the pediatric emergency physician, trained paramedical staff, pediatric surgeons, pediatric orthopedic surgeons, neurosurgeon, and pediatric intensivist. Plastic surgeons may also be needed. The management begins at the event site with pediatric life support along with transport the child to a trauma center.

In the Field

Pediatric trauma resuscitation should begin as early as possible following the injury. The main emphasis of pre-hospital trauma care is maintaining vital function through aggressive resuscitation in the *platinum half hour* or the *golden hour*. Pediatric transport teams can follow a "scoop and run" or "stay and play" approach depending on the condition of the child at the trauma site. In both approaches, getting the child to the emergency department should be the priority.

Initial Assessment

Guidelines for the evaluation and management of trauma victims have been well established by the American College of Surgeons. Priorities for the management of trauma victims are similar to those of any other sick child in the emergency room. This initial stabilization includes a primary survey, resuscitation, secondary survey, and subsequent triage. If any life-threatening condition is identified in the primary survey, it should be addressed immediately before progressing to the next step. For example, if tension pneumothorax is identified during the primary survey, it should be relieved immediately. Airway, breathing, circulation,

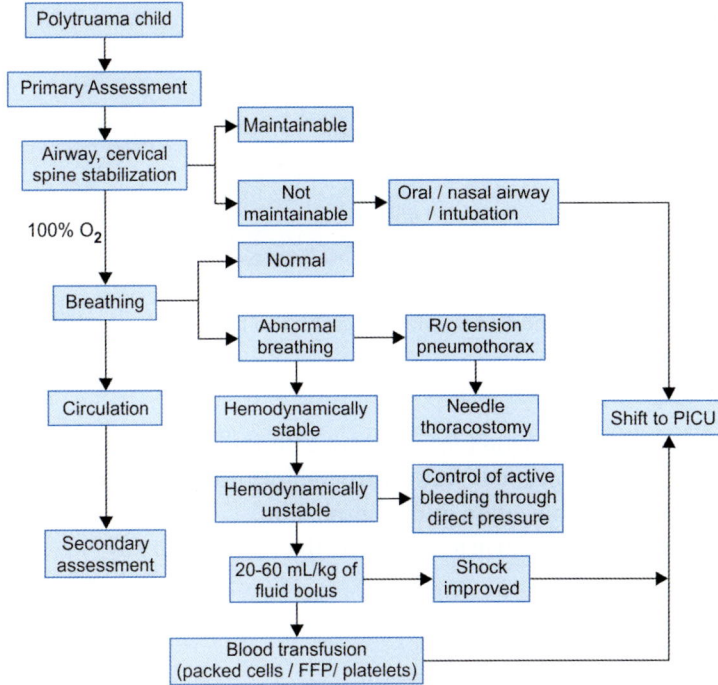

Fig. 1: Algorithm for initial assessment of a child with polytrauma.
(FFP: fresh frozen plasma; PICU: pediatric intensive care unit)

disability, and exposure (ABCDE) approach of Advance Trauma Life Support guidelines is a useful system for initial management of these children (Fig. 1).

Airway

First step is airway management with concomitant cervical spine stabilization (Fig. 2).

Inspect the mouth for:
- Secretions
- Foreign particles
- Broken teeth
- Facial lacerations

If any of the above is present, Yankauer-tip suction device is used to clear those. At the same time, the cervical spine is stabilized using inline immobilization (maintaining the cervical spine in a neutral position with bimanual cervical spine stabilization), followed by application of a semi-rigid cervical extrication collar. All victims of polytrauma should be given supplemental oxygen using FiO_2 while undergoing a primary survey. Artificial airway adjuncts should be used if the airway is not maintained even after manual positioning. An oral airway can be used in unconscious breathing patients as the gag reflex may be weak or absent, while a nasal airway is used for semiconscious patients who do not maintain the airway. Rapid

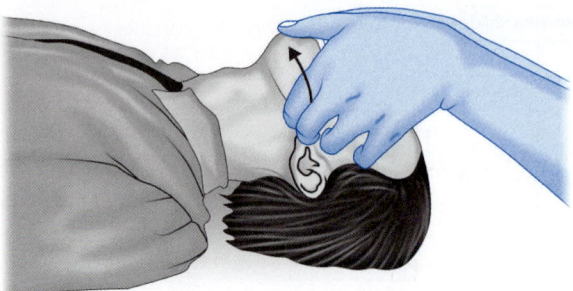

Fig. 2: Correct head position for intubation with cervical spine protection using the jaw thrust.

sequence intubation may be needed for children with rapidly deteriorating **Glasgow Coma Scale** (GCS) or GCS < 8 to prevent airway obstruction. However, the cervical spine should be stabilized using inline immobilization during intubation.

Before intubation, it is imperative to anticipate the "difficult airway."

Findings suggestive of difficult intubation:
- Small mouth
- Inability to open the mouth
- Temporomandibular joint abnormalities
- Narrow receding mandible
- Protuberant maxilla (overbite)
- Large tongue
- Inability to place in the "sniffing position" (such as with suspected cervical spine injury)
- Short, full, or bull neck
- Neck mass such as a large hematoma.

If the airway seemed to be difficult, bag–valve–mask ventilation may be preferred until a definitive airway can be established more safely. In patients with significant facial trauma, oral intubation is difficult. Under such circumstances, videoscope intubation or a needle cricothyrotomy may be required to maintain the airway.

Airway patency alone does not ensure adequate ventilation. Adequate ventilation is possible only when the function of the respiratory center, lungs, chest wall, and diaphragm is intact. These functions are assessed during examination of breathing and ventilation. The chest should be exposed and looked for respiratory pattern, breathing movement, external trauma, flail chest, splinting of chest wall during breathing, air entry, and diaphragmatic movement.

If the breathing pattern is shallow and irregular, then it should be assisted by a bag-mask ventilation followed by intubation and positive pressure ventilation. The end-tidal carbon dioxide ($EtCO_2$) can be monitored for adequate ventilation. Signs like decreased air entry on one side with tracheal deviation and unstable hemodynamics should give clues to a tension pneumothorax which should be relieved by a needle thoracostomy [insertion of a 14-gauge needle in the second intercostal space (ICS) in midclavicular line] followed by tube thoracostomy.

Circulation and Control of Hemorrhage

The third step in the primary assessment is the evaluation of circulation. Adequacy of circulation is quickly assessed by capillary refilling time, temperature, pulse volume, and color of the extremities. Active external hemorrhage can be best controlled by applying direct pressure on it either manually or using pneumatic splints. Use of tourniquets proximal to the bleeding site on the extremity is not a common practice to stop the hemorrhage.

Disability or Quick Neurological Survey

A rapid neurological evaluation is done in terms of responsiveness [using alert, voice, pain, unresponsive (AVPU) scale or GCS scoring system], papillary reaction, lateralizing signs. A depressed mental status indicates either cerebral injury or decreased cerebral perfusion or oxygenation which needs immediate attention.

Exposure

All children with injuries should be completely undressed and exposed to reveal all possible injuries. A head-to-toe survey is performed to look for all external injuries. While exposing the child, body temperature should be maintained using warm blankets and coverings to avoid hypothermia. Assessment and management protocols should go hand in hand to take care of any life-threatening situation.

Resuscitation

Resuscitation of a trauma victim should begin as soon as possible along with primary assessment. Class 1 and Class 2 categories of hemorrhagic shock (Table 3) usually require continuous monitoring whereas Class 3 and Class 4 require fluid resuscitation and monitoring. Two large bore intravenous (IV) cannulae are required for initial resuscitation. The fluid flow

Table 3: Classification of hemorrhagic shock in pediatric patients.

Clinical parameters	Class 1	Class 2	Class 3	Class 4
Blood volume loss	Up to 15%	15–30%	30–40%	≥40%
Pulse rate	Normal	Mild tachycardia	Moderate tachycardia	Severe tachycardia
Blood pressure	Normal/increased	Normal/decreased	Decreased	Decreased
Capillary blanch test	Normal	Positive	Positive	Positive
Respiratory rate	Normal	Mild tachypnea	Moderate tachypnea	Severe tachypnea
Urine output	1–2 mL/kg/h	0.5–1.0 mL/kg/h	0.25–0.5 mL/kg/h	Negligible
Mental status	Slightly anxious	Mildly anxious	Anxious/confused	Confused/lethargic

rate is directly proportional to the internal diameter and inversely proportional to the length of the cannula. Three successive attempts of failed cannulation are an indication for getting intraosseous (IO) access. All the medications and fluid which can be given by IV route can also be administered through IO line. IV cannulation can be tried again after initial resuscitation and restoration of intravascular volume.

Necessary baseline investigations can be done once IV or IO access is established. The stomach should be deflated to prevent aspiration of its contents. An orogastric tube is preferred over nasogastric tube for children with head and midfacial injury. A urinary catheter should be placed to monitor urine output in all children with multiple injuries unless urethral injury is suspected (blood at urethral meatus, perineal injuries and pelvic instability).

Pain management is one of the most ignored aspects in a child with polytrauma. Polytrauma victims have severe pain which causes persistent sympathetic stimulation and increased metabolic demand. This may lead to persistent shock and future psychological effects. So pain should be properly managed using opioid and non-opioid analgesics.

Fluid Therapy in Hemorrhagic Shock

Initial resuscitation for hemorrhagic shock should be performed with crystalloid-like normal saline (NS) or Ringer lactate (RL). Crystalloids are easily available, less reactogenic, more physiological, and cheap. Crystalloids are considered to be as efficacious as colloids for expanding the intravascular volume. Colloids are not found to be superior to crystalloids while comparing the outcome of patients with hemorrhagic shock. Colloids like starch and dextran are associated with coagulopathy, which can further increase the bleeding process and shock. If a patient with hemorrhagic shock remains hypotensive even after 40 mL/kg of crystalloids bolus, immediate blood transfusion should be given. Cross-matched blood products are always preferable; however, O-negative packed red blood cells (RBCs) can be transfused till cross-matched blood products become available. *Polytrauma is associated with coagulopathy and excessive use of fluid boluses and blood which can further dilute the available coagulant factors leading to increased risk of bleeding.* To prevent this dilution, one unit of fresh frozen plasma (FFP) and one unit of platelets should be transfused for every two units of packed cells used. Trauma exsanguination protocol has shown better outcome if packed RBCs, FFP, and platelets are used in the ratio of 1:1:1. On the other hand, if blood products are not available and shock continues despite 40–60 mL/kg of fluid boluses, albumin or other colloids can be considered to restore intravascular volume for longer duration. Fluid resuscitation target should be used to maintain systolic blood pressure just above the low normal as targeting high systolic blood pressure can increase the hemorrhage from the traumatic sites. This philosophy is known as damage control resuscitation. If shock persists despite volume expansion, other causes like persistent internal hemorrhages, neurogenic shock, cardiac tamponade, or myocardial contusion should be rule out. Under these extreme circumstances, inotropes like dopamine, dobutamine, norepinephrine, and epinephrine may be considered.

Monitoring of Resuscitation

Continuous monitoring of the clinical parameters is essential in any sick child. The important parameters to be monitored are heart rate, capillary refill time, blood pressure, core-peripheral temperature difference, urine output, GCS, pupillary reaction, partial pressure of oxygen (PaO_2), partial pressure of carbon dioxide ($PaCO_2$), and lactate.

Control of bleeding: Active hemorrhage can be life-threatening for polytrauma patients. It should be identified and controlled promptly. Unrecognized continuous hemorrhage can occur in body spaces like the thorax, retroperitoneum, pelvis, and thighs. External hemorrhage can be stopped by direct pressure in most of the patients. Application of tourniquets above the bleeding area is no longer advised. Continuous internal hemorrhages need emergency surgical intervention.

Secondary Survey

After completion of the primary ABCDE survey and initial resuscitation, a rapid secondary survey is performed. The secondary survey includes important history taking and a quick examination from head to toe. A pertinent history includes *SAMPLE* (see stabilization).

A head-to-toe examination should include the head and neck (altered sensorium, blunt head injury, bleeding from the ear and nose, midfacial injury, focal deficit), cervical spine, thorax (rib injuries, pneumothorax, hemothorax, flail chest), abdomen (external bruise or abrasions, abdominal distension, blood-stained vomiting or stool, altered bowel sounds), renal system (hematuria, anuria), and skeletal system (special consideration for pelvic stability and long bone fractures). Cervical spine injury should be given special attention. Measures for cervical spine stabilization should be taken care in such patients. Any child with one or more of the following signs and symptoms should be considered to have probable cervical spine injury.

- Altered mental status
- Neck pain and midline cervical tenderness
- Intoxication
- Focal neurological deficits or complaints
- Polytrauma
- Significant mechanism of injury (high-speed vehicle collision, fall from a significant height)
- Distracting painful injury.

Tertiary Survey

Ancillary Laboratory Studies

Laboratory investigations are an integral part of management and help in the continuous monitoring. A few basic laboratory parameters can provide information about the underlying injury and organ damage.

Important useful investigations include:
- Complete blood counts (CBC) and packed cell volume (PCV)
- Blood group and cross-match
- Baseline liver and kidney function tests
- Coagulation profile
- Serum amylase and lipase (liver and pancreatic injuries)
- Urine routine examination (hematuria and hemoglobinuria)
- Arterial blood gas analysis for PaO_2, $PaCO_2$, and lactate.

Table 4: Computerized tomography scans.

Without contrast for the head	With IV and oral contrasts for abdomen
Suspected blunt head injury	Blood-stained vomitus
Altered sensorium	Abdominal tenderness
Seizures	Bruising
Focal deficits	Lap-belt injury
Loss of consciousness	Persistent abdomen distension
Significant mechanism of injury	Hematuria

(IV: intravenous)

Radiological Survey

Radiological survey for blunt trauma patients should include cervical spine imaging (antero-posterior, lateral and odontoid view), chest, and pelvic X-ray. Other long bone imaging is done as required by secondary survey. A retrograde urethrogram is essential if urethral injury is suspected (Table 4).

A patient should be stabilized before being transported for radiological investigations. In an unstable patient, bedside investigations like ultrasonography (USG) are always preferable.

Ultrasonography Abdomen: Focused Abdominal Ultrasound in Trauma

Focused abdominal sonography has become the standard of care in adults and pediatric emergency medicine. Focused abdominal ultrasound in trauma (FAST) can be used during primary survey to detect any intraperitoneal fluid collections. In experienced hands, it is a very good tool for screening trauma patients for intra-abdominal injuries. It has several advantages of being at bedside with rapid repeatability and good sensitivity.

MANAGEMENT OF NON-NEUROLOGICAL INJURIES

Abdominal Trauma

Blunt abdominal injuries are more common compared to penetrating injuries in children. The most frequent injured organs during blunt trauma include the liver, spleen, and kidney whereas penetrating trauma is more likely to injure the intestine and liver. Abdominal trauma may present with abdominal pain, tenderness, rebound tenderness, decreased bowel sounds, abdominal wall contusion, or hematoma. A hemodynamically stable child with blunt trauma is conservatively managed with continuous monitoring to detect any deterioration. Penetrating injuries usually need operative management. Dropping hematocrit, repeated transfusion requirements, persistent signs of under-perfusion, and unstable hemodynamics should be alerts for surgical intervention.

Thoracic Trauma

Eight percent of children with polytrauma sustain chest injuries. Thoracic trauma is an indication of serious injury as two-thirds of these patients have other associated injuries. Blunt trauma to the chest can result in tension pneumothorax, pneumothorax, hemothorax, lung contusion, mediastinal injury, rib fractures, flail chest, or diaphragmatic injury. Penetrating injuries are more likely to cause open pneumothorax, tracheobronchial injury, aortic rupture, injury to major vessels, and esophageal tears. A plain chest X-ray is good enough for initial screening of these injuries. If lung parenchymal or mediastinal injuries are suspected, thoracic computerized tomography (CT) scan can be done. Most of the thoracic traumas are managed with tube thoracostomy and supportive treatment. However, open thoracotomy may be rarely required in some cases.

Genitourinary Trauma

Children are vulnerable for kidney and urinary tract injury following blunt trauma. Direct injury to the genitalia and injury to the pelvic region is associated with damage to the lower urinary tract. A gross hematuria is a reliable indicator for renal injury. Microscopic hematuria also indicates some amount of trauma sustained by the renal and urinary system. In case of direct injury to the genitalia, pelvic instability, or blood at the urethral meatus, urinary catheterization should be done only after retrograde urethrogram has been made to rule out urethral injury. Patients with suspected renal injury should have a contrast CT scan to assess the extent of injury. A pediatric surgeon and/or urologist should be involved early for further definitive management.

SUMMARY

Pediatric polytrauma is a multidisciplinary task; the management starts right from the field triage and immediate transport to a trauma center. A careful primary assessment with an ABCDE approach with aggressive resuscitation definitely improves the outcome of the child.

KEY MESSAGES

- Trauma is the leading cause of morbidity and mortality in the developed world.
- Blunt trauma is a most common mechanism of injury in children.
- ABCDE sequence of initial assessment should be followed in every child with multiple traumas.
- Continuous monitoring following initial resuscitation is mandatory to detect further deterioration.
- In a child with polytrauma, the cervical spine should always be taken care.
- Patients with persistent shock despite initial resuscitation may have neurogenic shock, cardiac contusion, or cardiac tamponade.

SUGGESTED READING

1. Advanced Trauma Life Support, 8th edition. Chicago: American College of Surgeons, 2008.
2. Barkin RM (Ed). Pediatric emergency medicine, 2nd edition. St. Louis, MO: BC Decker Mosby–Year Book; 1997.
3. Fleisher GR, Ludwig S (Eds). Textbook of pediatric emergency medicine, 6th edition. Philadelphia: Lippincott Williams & Wilkins; 2010.

4. Kay RM, Skaggs DL. Pediatric polytrauma management. J Pediatr Orthop. 2006;26(2):268-77.
5. Nichols DG (Ed). Roger's textbook of pediatric intensive care, 4th edition. Philadelphia: Lippincott Williams & Wilkins; 2008.
6. O'Neill JA. Advances in the management of pediatric trauma. Am J Surg. 2000;180(5):365-9.
7. Trunkey DD, Lewis FR (Eds). Current therapy of trauma, 3rd edition. St Louis, MO: BC Decker Mosby—Year Book; 1991.
8. Tuggle DW, Krug SE; American Academy of Pediatrics, Section on Orthopedics, Committee on Pediatric Emergency Medicine, Section on Critical Care, Section on Surgery, and Section on Transport Medicine. Management of pediatric trauma. Pediatrics. 2008;121(4):849-54.

Drowning 29

Kundan Mittal, Vinayak Patki

LEARNING OBJECTIVES

- Understanding the concepts of drowning
- Understanding the pathophysiological changes that accompany drowning
- Management of drowning

INTRODUCTION

Drowning is a leading cause of death, morbidity, and poor quality of life for survivors in children. "Drowning is the process of experiencing respiratory impairment from submersion/immersion in liquid. Drowning outcomes are classified as death, morbidity (moderately disabled, severely disabled, vegetative state/coma, and brain death), and no morbidity". Submersion is to plunge under the surface of the water and immersion is described as to plunge or dip being visible or exposed, especially into a fluid. If the victim dies it is known as "fatal drowning"; and if process is interrupted it is called as "nonfatal drowning". Drowning has two different physiological events:
- *Immersion*: Where the upper airway is above water. With immersion in thermoneutral water there is an increase in:
  - Venous return
  - Cardiac output
  - Work of breathing
  - Right to left shunt and diuresis
  - Natriuresis
  - Kaliuresis.

  Immersion in cold water causes:
  - Vasoconstriction
  - Increased right atrial pressure, heart rate, cardiac output, and venous return
  - Depressed respiratory drive after some time.
- *Submersion*: When the upper airway is below water, leads to:
  - Laryngospasm

- Hypoxia
- Hypercarbia
- Muscle relaxation
- Aspiration of water into lung.

It can be fresh water or salt water and also on the basis of temperature (cold water < 20°C and thermoneutral). Fresh water drowning or submersion injury is most common (47%). Epilepsy, cardiac rhythm disorders, male sex, intentional, inadequate supervision, child abuse, inadequate swimming skills, accidents, unexplained etiology, and hyperventilation (hypocapnia leading to less respiratory derive) before swimming are most common risk factors associated with drowning. Drug abuse and alcohol intoxication are risk factors commonly seen in older children. Children struggle for 20–30 seconds before final submersion.

Cold water submersion may lead to a "cold shock" response (gasp, hyperventilation, tachycardia, hypertension, vasoconstriction, increased myocardial oxygen requirement, and failure of motor coordination) and a "diving response" (apnea, bradycardia, and vasoconstriction in response to cold water touching eyes stimulating trigeminal nerve). Submersion in water leads to hypothermia because of large body surface to body mass ratio and even swallowing of cold water may induce brain cooling. All body organs are affected. Moderate hypothermia (32–35°C) is associated with increased sympathetic tone and shivering. Below 32°C shivering stops and heart rate and blood pressure fall and below 28°C extreme bradycardia occurs. Hypothermia can also lead to platelet dysfunction and coagulopathy. Difference in plasma and water osmolality leads to some electrolyte abnormalities, change in hematocrit, acute kidney injury, hypovolemia, and metabolic acidosis. Salt versus fresh water has no difference in pathology. Also, water contaminants, especially gram-negative bacteria, anaerobes, fungi, algae, and protozoa are common cause of severe pneumonia. Other respiratory changes are pulmonary edema, decreased compliance, increased intrapulmonary shunting, and acute lung injury/acute respiratory distress syndrome (ALI/ARDS). Chemicals in water can also lead to severe pulmonary abnormalities. Submersion may induce systemic inflammatory response syndrome (SIRS) leading to sepsis and disseminated intravascular coagulation. Hypoxia, acidosis, and hypothermia lead to cardiac disturbances, i.e., rhythm disturbances, bradycardia, tachycardia, pulseless electric activity, and asystole. Severity of neurological damage depends on the duration of submersion and effective resuscitation (<3 minutes). A child presenting with coma or resuscitation started after 5 minutes of the event often has a poor outcome.

MANAGEMENT

Prehospital Care

- Outcomes of submersion injury are better if immediate help is provided as soon as possible.
- Target is a secure airway, effective breathing, and circulation. Hypoxia, hypothermia, and vasoconstriction make the assessment of peripheral pulses difficult and, hence, the carotid artery may be palpated.
- Mouth-to-mouth breathing may be initiated even if the child is in water. Begin chest compression if there is no pulse. Basic life support (BLS) should be instituted immediately (sequence will be airway, breathing and circulation as hypoxia is major cause of physiological abnormalities) and call for advanced life support.
- There is no role of Heimlich maneuver.

- Defibrillation is not recommended below 28°C and rewarming should be avoided if temperature is less than 23°C.
- Spinal immobilization is indicated if the history and examination is consistent with a severe injury like diving.
- Immediate transfer to hospital should be planned and monitoring of vital parameters should be continued.

Hospital Management

- *Obtain a detailed history*: Type of water (fresh or salt), dry or wet submersion, temperature, time and length of submersion, any comorbid condition, any risk factor like seizure and cardiac rhythm disorder and event leading to drowning.
- Priority is to maintain airway, breathing, and circulation (ABC) with cervical spine immobilization and temperature monitoring and rewarming if needed.
- Rewarming with blankets should be started immediately if child is hypothermic.
- SAMPLE history and initial examination includes assessment of airway, breathing, circulation, consciousness level, evidence of trauma, and temperature measurement. Ancillary studies include blood glucose, arterial blood gas for knowing oxygenation, and ventilation status serum electrolytes, creatine phosphokinase (CPK), serum osmolality, hemoglobin, myoglobin, tracheal aspirate for culture, chest X-ray, and trauma-related imaging [computed tomography (CT) head and spine), toxicological screening, coagulation profile, and platelet count.
- Endotracheal intubation is indicated if there is hypoxemia, apnea, cardiopulmonary arrest, and poor response to high-flow oxygen. In a spontaneously breathing child, maintain blood oxygen saturation (SpO_2) more than 90% in room air using high-flow oxygen. Ventilatory management depends on pulmonary pathophysiology (ALI/ARDS and pneumonia), neuronal injury, and cardiac status.
- Intravenous access may be difficult due to hypoxia and vasoconstriction and, hence, the intraosseous route may come in handy.
- Shock should be treated and continued cardiovascular monitoring is needed.
- Vasoactive agents may be used as needed to improve perfusion or in suspected cardiac dysfunction.
- *Hypothermia*: Passive rewarming is sufficient if the core temperature is 32–35°C and in moderate to severe hypothermia, active external and internal rewarming is required. Goal is to increase temperature 1–2°C per hour to the target of 33–36°C.
    - Remove all wet clothes
    - Put warm blankets
    - Hot packs (40°C) and heat lamps or heat blowers.

  Active internal rewarming (core temperature is ≤30°C) include:
    - Warmed intravenous fluid (40–42°C)
    - Warmed and humidified oxygen (42–46°C)
    - Gastric, peritoneal, thoracic, and bladder lavage.
- No role of prophylactic corticosteroids and they may even harm the child.
- No role of sodium bicarbonate to correct acidosis.

- Antibiotics selection depends on type and contamination of water and laboratory results.
- Symptomatic support to be continued.

PREDICTORS OF DEATH

- Immersion duration more than 5 minutes
- Delayed cardiopulmonary resuscitation (CPR)/BLS
- Fixed dilated pupil
- Glasgow Coma Scale (GCS)–3
- pH less than 7.0
- Abnormal CT head.

SUGGESTED READING

1. Bierens JLMJ. Drowning: Prevention, Rescue, Treatment. 2nd edition. London: Springer; 2014.
2. Edibam C, Bowles T. Submersion. In: Bersten AD, Soni N (Eds). OH's Intensive Care Manual. 7th edition. China: Elsevier; 2014. pp. 817-20.
3. Fuhrman BP, Zimmerman JJ. Pediatric Critical Care. 5th edition. Philadelphia: Elsevier; 2017.
4. Irwin RS, Lilly CM, Mayo PH, et al. Intensive Care Medicine. 8th edition. Hong Kong: Wolter Kluwer; 2018.
5. Layon AJ, Modell JH. Drowning: update 2009. Anesthesiology. 2009;110(6);1390-401.
6. Semple-Hess J, Campwala R. Pediatric submersion injuries: emergency care and resuscitation. Pediatr Emerg Med Pract. 2014;11(6):1-21.
7. Wheeler DS, Wong HR, Shanley T. Pediatric Critical Care Medicine. USA: Springer; 2014.

Pediatric Emergency Care: Poisoning and Toxidromes

30

S Thangavelu, Nayani Sridevi

LEARNING OBJECTIVES

- To understand briefly, the pattern of poisoning in India
- Recognition and management of poisoning using toxidromes
- To understand the management of some common poisonings.

INTRODUCTION

Poisoning in children is a worldwide problem leading to morbidity and mortality and is one of the most common emergencies encountered in pediatric practice. Most poisoning in children is accidental and unintentional and preventable. Intentional poisoning is most likely in adolescents.

The factors that predict the severity and outcome of poisoning include nature, dose, formulation, route of exposure, co-exposure with other poisons, malnutrition, age, and pre-existing health conditions.

Accidental poisoning in children is due to ingestion of poisonous substances like household products like kerosene, pesticides, drugs as some of these toxic substances are removed from their original containers and stored in drinking water bottles or food containers, which are often mistaken by children for water or food and ingested.

EPIDEMIOLOGY OF POISONING

The profile and outcome of poisoned patients vary from place to place and is influenced by demography, socioeconomic status, education, local practices, and by the available medical care.

Childhood poisoning incidence in various studies ranges from 0.33% to 7.6%. Poisoning is most common in 1–5 years of age and constitutes 80% of all poisoning cases. In the first year of life, the common causes of poisoning are inadvertently erroneous dosing of medications by parents. There is a difference in poisoning patterns in children and adults (Table 1).

Table 1: Differences between poisoning in children and adults.	
Adult and adolescent	Child
• Mostly intentional with a suicidal attempt • Usually history of consumption of toxin will be available • Early diagnosis is possible • Prognosis influenced by underlying chronic disease	• Mostly accidental • They present as respiratory distress, convulsion or coma. Onus is on the pediatrician to identify • Diagnosis is delayed • Overall prognosis may be good

Household cleaning products cause most cases of poisoning at 2–3 years. The products are kept at low height or left open such that the toddler has access to them. During adolescence, intentional overdose of available medication is the main cause of poisoning. The mortality rate due to poisoning is 3–5%.

The profile of poisoning shows a variable trend and in India the epidemiological profile has local differences.

Household products predominated in studies done in Delhi and Chennai with an incidence of 53% and 61%, respectively. Neem, Eucalyptus, and Turpentine oils predominated in the South. Kerosene was common to all regions. Pesticides were found in about 16% and medication in about 20%. Unknown substances constituted 1–10%.

The pattern of poisoning in different regions might vary according to age group, type of exposure, nature of poisons, and social, cultural and demographic factors. Fatal poisoning rates in developing countries are four times that of developed countries. Africa, low- and middle-income countries in Europe and the Western Pacific Regions have the highest rates.

Categorization of Poisons

Classification of poisons can be done as:
- Household substances, e.g., kerosene, detergents (Table 2).
- Poisons that happens outside the house, e.g., pesticides, etc.
- Plant poisoning, e.g., *Dhatura*
- Medicines, e.g., Paracetamol, isoniazid
- Envenomation, e.g., Scorpion, snake.

GENERAL MANAGEMENT

When to suspect poisoning in a child presenting to an emergency without any history?

Any child with sudden change in the level of consciousness or change in behavior, without any clue from the history—consider the following: Table 3 shows the clinical features that help to suspect poisoning as the etiology of symptoms.
- *Unidentified trauma*: An unattended child with or without external injuries in area of danger
- *Seizures*: A child with a known seizure disorder may be in a postictal period. Will recover after 30–60 minutes unless he develops nonconvulsive status epilepticus
- *Intracranial bleed*: Child will be in deep and prolonged coma, with signs of increased intracranial pressure, focal signs, pupillary changes, and retinal bleeds

Table 2: Common household substances poisoning.

Substance	Manifestation	Treatment
Camphor	Delirium, seizures, rarely hepatic and renal damage	Gastric lavage, AC, lorazepam, no antidote
Naphthalene bathroom deodorant disc, preservative for wood, books or clothes, moth balls, air freshener	Acute hemolysis. Children with G6PD deficiency more susceptible. Pallor, jaundice, high colored urine, abdominal pain, dysuria due to irritation of the bladder. Headache. Methemoglobinemia jaundice and deranged liver function. Hemoglobinuria, and acute renal failure	Screening for G6PD. Symptomatic management for methemoglobinemia, renal replacement therapy
Vasambu (dried rhizome of the plant *Acorus calamus* commonly used in native medicine	Calamus oil causes hypothermia. CNS depression, sedation, hypothermia, hypotension, depression of respiration	Supportive management
Matchstick potassium chlorate, sulphur, gum, glass and red phosphorus	Methemoglobinemia and renal failure. Hypoxic brain injury can occur. MRI shows symmetric hyperintense signals within deep gray matter and medial temporal lobes consistent with hypoxia caused by potassium chlorate	Gastric lavage, activated charcoal. Methylene blue is used. Exchange transfusion or hemodialysis are done when needed. Hyperbaric oxygen may help. Symptomatic treatment
Eucalyptus oil	GI: abdominal pain, vomiting, diarrhea. CNS: loss of consciousness, hypoventilation, convulsions, Muscle weakness. Miosis or mydriasis, and ataxia; RS: bronchospasm, aspiration pneumonia CVS: Tachycardia, weak irregular pulse and irritation to skin and eyes	Avoid GI decontamination. Lavage and AC administration. Symptomatic and supportive management.
Neem oil	Recurrent seizures, toxic Encephalopathy, in the form of Reye like illness, metabolic acidosis, mitochondrial injury	Avoid GI decontamination. Lavage and AC administration. Symptomatic and supportive management

(AC: activated charcoal; CNS: central nervous system; CVS: cardiovascular system; GI: gastrointestinal; G6PD: glucose 6-phosphate dehydrogenase)

- *Unrecognized poisoning*: Suspect this when the child is found unconscious at home, seen amidst open bottles or opened strips. Mere availability of medicines may be an important clue. Examine the child looking for features of a toxidrome
- *Envenomation*: In a closed room, scorpion sting is likely and outside in fields or forests snake envenomation is more probable. A sudden crying spell in the night waking up a child,

Table 3: Differential diagnosis and analysis.

Differential diagnosis	For	Against
• Unidentified injury	Sudden onset of altered consciousness	Found in the bed, no external injuries, CT normal
• Unrecognized poisoning	Sudden onset of seizures, coma, she was alone	No evidence on arrival from the history
• Nonconvulsive status epilepticus	Recurrent seizures, may be underlying cause	Hyperglycemia, and acidosis
• Envenomation	Sudden onset of symptoms.	Both snake as well as scorpion usually does not lead to seizures or reddish vomiting within 3 hours
• Cerebrovascular accidents	Sudden onset of seizures, coma.	CT brain Normal

profuse sweating, cold extremities, priapism, bradycardia, or tachycardia may suggest scorpion sting. Bite marks, bleeding, local cellulitis, or neuroparalytic manifestation are more in favor of snake bite.

The stepwise management of a child with suspected poisoning is given in the Box 1.

> **Box 1:** Steps in the management a child with toxin ingestion.
>
> - Initial Stabilization—airway, breathing, circulation, mental status
> - Focused History of ingestion
> - Problem oriented examination
> - Laboratory investigations
> - Decontamination/removal of absorbed toxin, specific antidote
> - Monitoring and supportive care

Initial Assessment, Stabilization, and Management

The ABC management is vital and will not differ in poisoning. Shock is treated with fluid bolus and often needs a vasopressor.

If shock is caused by specific toxins such as beta-blockers, the specific antidote should also be given, for example, glucagon for hypoglycemia. Arrhythmias associated with poisoning are best treated by correcting precipitating factors (hypoxia, hypokalemia, hypomagnesemia, and acidosis) and by administering the antidote rather than resorting to antiarrhythmic agents. Antiarrhythmics may make situation worse due to negative inotropy.

Assess neurological function:
- *Level of consciousness*: AVPU (alert, voice, pain, unresponsive)/Glasgow coma scale
- *Pupillary size and reaction*: The pupillary reaction and size is a window for the recognition of the toxin (Table 4)
- *Blood glucose by glucometer*: Hypoglycemia can be corrected by 5 mL/kg of 10% dextrose, 2 mL/kg of 25% dextrose followed by serial monitoring of glucose level and maintain optimal glucose infusion rate (GIR)

Table 4: Pupillary size and clue for diagnosis.

Constricted pupil	Dilated pupil
• Organophosphates • Opiate compounds • Phenobarbitone • Clonidine	• *Dhatura* poisoning • Tricyclic antidepressants

- Seizures can be managed by treating the underlying factors, e.g., hypoglycemia, hypocalcemia and controlled by benzodiazepine, phenobarbitone, levetiracetam. Phenytoin should be avoided in seizures associated with poisoning which can aggravate cardiotoxicity.

Focused History

- It is important to get this from a reliable witness.
- Availability of drugs or toxins at home. Ask for all such medications and substances to be brought and count or measure the remaining amount.
- Was it accidental, intentional, time of ingestion, prior illness, time of onset, and worsening of symptoms, any other family members involved. Consider more than one medication consumed and more than one person involved.

Problem-oriented examination: In a child with critical presentation in an emergency situation, less time is spent on history and examination as assessment of the physiological status and resuscitation takes priority.

PHYSICAL EXAMINATION

Examine from head to toe, sting or snake bite marks, needle mark, odor, powder particles in the mouth, muscle twitching, and any stain on the clothing. The diagnosis may be assisted by the following descriptions.

Bradycardia: Organophosphorus compounds, anticholinesterases, beta-blockers, clonidine, calcium channel blocker, antiarrhythmics, alcohol, opioids, oleander.

Tachycardia: Anticholinergic, antihistamines, antipsychotic, sympathomimetics (cocaine, caffeine, amphetamine), theophylline, thyroid hormone, tricyclic antidepressant (TCA).

Hypothermia: Alcohol, sedatives and hypnotics, oral hypoglycemic agents, opioids, carbon monoxide (CO).

Hyperthermia: Anticholinergics, antidepressants, antipsychotic, antihistamines, salicylate, alcohol withdrawal.

Hypotension: Antihypertensive, rodenticide, antidepressants, sedatives, opiates, heroin.

Hypertension: Thyroid hormone, cocaine, sympathomimetics, caffeine, anticholinergic, nicotine.

Tachypnea: Organophosphate (OPC), chemical pneumonitis, salicylate toxin-induced metabolic acidosis and nerve agents, paraquat.

Bradypnea: Sedatives, alcohol, opioids, marijuana.

Coma: OPC, alcohol, ethylene glycol, tricyclic antidepressant, anticonvulsant agents, antipsychotics, antidepressants, antihistaminics, hypoglycemic agents, isoniazid, heavy metals, hepatic encephalopathy.

Agents causing seizure: Camphor, neem oil, gamma benzene hexachloride, organophosphorus poisoning, oral hypoglycemic agent, isoniazid, salicylate, tricyclic antidepressant.

Diaphoresis: OP poisoning, salicylates, sympathomimetics.

Dry skin: Antihistamines, anticholinergic.

Cyanosis: Dapsone, aniline dyes, naphthalene, nitrate, ergotamine, methemoglobinemia.

Hypoglycemia: Oral hypoglycemic agents; beta-blockers, alcohol.

Hyperglycemia: Theophylline; tricyclic antidepressants or isoniazid, salicylates.

Odor: Garlic – organophosphates, arsenic, phosphorus, thallium.
    Gasoline – petroleum products,
    Alcohol smell
    Bitter almond – cyanide, oil of winter green – salicylate.

Clinical features of many poisons resemble that of common disease processes. Table 5 helps to differentiate these mimics.

Toxidromes (Table 6)

A constellation of clinical features associated with certain classes or poisoning is known as a toxidrome and helps in making a diagnosis. This is not a theoretical description, but is of great practical importance as it helps in a child with an unknown ingestion. Currently biochemical toxicology assessment is not easy because we have to name a toxin and request for the assay, which is practically difficult, e.g., serum benzodiazepine or phenytoin or carbamazepine level.

Laboratory Investigations

- Rapid determination of blood glucose by glucometer strip
- Acid–Base status
- Electrolytes
- Blood urea nitrogen (BUN) and creatinine

Table 5: Poisons which mimic common diseases.

Symptoms and signs	Possible toxin	Differential diagnosis
Nonketotic hypoglycemia, collapse	Ethanol	Glycogen storage disease, fatty acid oxidation disorders.
Acute liver failure	Paracetamol	Idiopathic liver failure
Hyperthermia, tachypnea	Salicylate	Pneumonia
CNS depression, seizure, pyrexia	Ecstasy, LSD	Febrile seizure
Hyperglycemia, ketosis, CNS depression	Salicylate, Theophylline	Diabetic ketoacidosis

(CNS: central nervous system; LSD: lysergic acid diethylamide)

Table 6: Toxidromes.

Syndrome	Symptoms	Common causes
Cholinergic (Nicotinic)	Abdominal pain, fasciculation, hypertension, paresis, tachycardia, seizure	Organophosphorus compound, nicotine
Anticholinergic	Delirium, mydriasis, tachycardia, hyperthermia, dry skin, urinary retention	Antihistaminics, atropine, tricyclic antidepressants, psychoactive drugs
DUMBELS	Diarrhea, Urination, miosis/muscle weakness, bronchorrhea, bradycardia, emesis, lacrimation, salivation/sweating	Organophosphates
Sympathomimetics	Mydriasis, tachycardia, hypertension, seizure	Cocaine, amphetamine, ephedrine, theophylline
Sedative	Drowsiness, stupor, coma, bradycardia, bradypnea, hypotension, constricted pupil	Phenobarbitone
Myocardial depressant	Bradycardia, hypotension, tachyarrhythmia, acute cardiac failure, cardiogenic shock	Beta-blockers, calcium channel blocker, oleander, digoxin, tricyclic antidepressants
Hepatotoxicity	Raised transaminases, jaundice, bleeding tendency	Paracetamol, rat killers
Corrosive	Drooling of saliva, change in voice, lips and tongue appearing white and necrotic	Acids, detergents, bathroom cleaners, button battery

- Serum osmolality (suspected ingestion of toxic alcohols or presence of anion gap acidosis)
- Aspartate aminotransferase (AST) and alanine aminotransferase (ALT) (if acetaminophen or rat killer ingestion suspected)
- Quantitative acetaminophen serum concentration (if suicidal intent or if suspected based on history)
- Quantitative salicylate serum concentration (in patients with respiratory alkalosis and/or metabolic acidosis)
- Urine dipstick test
- Electrocardiogram
- *X-ray abdomen*: In addition, certain radiopaque toxins, including packets of illicit drugs smuggled internally by body packers, may be visualized by plain film radiograph. Very few toxins have specific antidotes as shown in Table 7. Supportive care is the mainstay of management.

Decontamination, Elimination of Absorbed Toxin

- *Gastric lavage*: Useful only when done within the first hour of toxin ingestion or later when there is ingestion of a sustained release preparation or when exact time of ingestion is not clear. The largest bore tube as appropriate for age is used and checked child is kept in left lateral decubitus (Fig. 1). This position increases the yield of gastric aspirate and also minimizes passage of toxins beyond the pylorus. Normal saline 10 mL/kg is infused into stomach by gravity and then drained by gravity assisted aspiration by syringe. The

Table 7: Toxins and specific antidote.

Poison indicated	Antidote
• Organophosphorus	• PAM
• Calcium channel blocker	• Calcium
• Acetaminophen	• N-acetyl cysteine
• Oral hypoglycemic agents	• Dextrose, glucagon, octreotide
• Benzodiazepines	• Flumazenil
• Opioid	• Naloxone
• Anticholinergic	• Physostigmine
• Methanol/ethylene glycol	• Ethanol/fomepizole
• TCA	• Sodium bicarbonate
• Digoxin	• Fab fragment
• Cyanide	• Nitrite
• Carbon monoxide	• Hyperbaric oxygen

(PAM: pralidoxime; TCA: tricyclic antidepressant)

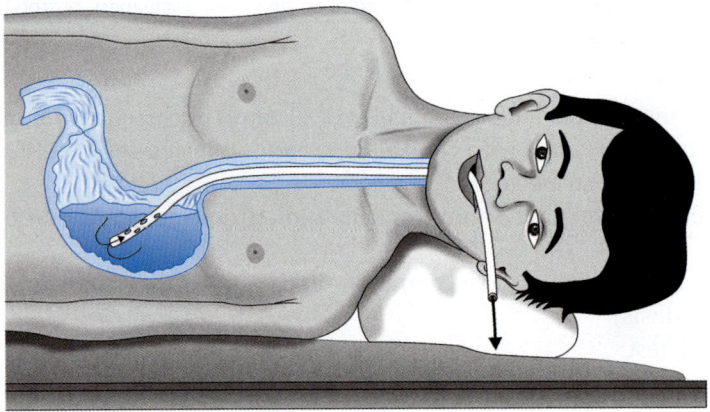

Fig. 1: Importance of left lateral position.
Source: www.obgynkey.com

first aspirate can be preserved for toxicological assay. Two or three lavages can be done till the returns are clear. In children, it should be done very gently to avoid aspiration and ulceration. During this procedure heart rate, respiratory rate, and saturation are to be monitored. Expected complications are aspiration, laryngospasm, mechanical injury, and bradycardia – due to vagal stimulation. Contraindications are remembered by the mnemonic – three Cs – carbons (hydrocarbon like kerosene), corrosives, and comatose child. In a comatose child with altered consciousness or respiratory distress, lavage can be done after airway protection.

- *Activated charcoal:* Activated charcoal is a special form of carbon that binds other substances on its surface. It is a bland, tasteless chemical substance with large surface area to absorb the toxin. One teaspoonful of activated charcoal has about the same total surface area of a football ground. It acts like enteral dialysate in poisoning caused by chemicals that undergo enterohepatic or enteroenteric circulation, e.g., salicylates, phenobarbital, carbamazepine, digoxin, theophylline, etc. Dose: 1 g/kg to be administered mixed with fruit juice in older kids and through nasogastric tube in younger children. It should be mixed with gradual addition of water with constant stirring to get a slurry. Approximate weight is calculated by small measuring cups. 5 mL is considered equivalent to 5 g. Side effects are nausea, vomiting, and a rare risk of aspiration in a child with reduced level of consciousness. It may not be useful in pesticides, hydrocarbons, alcohol, iron, lithium, and solvents (mnemonic PHAILS). Complications include bowel obstruction and perforation. But generally activated charcoal is well tolerated.

    Multiple-dose activated charcoal (MDAC): It should be considered in a patient who has ingested a life-threatening amount of carbamazepine, dapsone, phenobarbital, quinine, theophylline salicylates, slow release preparations, digoxin, phenytoin, sotalol, and piroxicam. Following the initial dose, 0.5 g/Kg every 6th hourly for 48 hours is used. Repeated doses of activated charcoal to remove toxins undergoing enterohepatic circulation is the simplest active elimination technique.

- *Whole bowel irrigation (WBI):* WBI is used to physically eliminate highly toxic substances that are not absorbed by activated charcoal and which have a long gastrointestinal (GI) transit time. WBI should not be used routinely in the management of a poisoned patient. WBI should be considered for potentially toxic ingestions of sustained-release or enteric-coated drugs particularly for those patients presenting more than 2 hours after drug ingestion and when there is a lack of other options for GI decontamination (e.g. substantial amounts of iron/ingestion of illicit packets of drugs).

    Treatment is based on the enteral administration of 10 mL/kg/h of osmotically balanced PEGylated polyethylene glycol electrolyte solution. Treatment is continued until the rectal effluent clears. WBI is contraindicated in patients with hemodynamic instability or compromised unprotected airway, bowel obstruction, perforation, and ileus.

    Urinary alkalinization is used to enhance the excretion of weakly acidic drugs. It increases the proportion of ionized drug in the tubule preventing its reabsorption. Examples include salicylate, isoniazid, phenobarbitone, methotrexate, etc. Administer 1–2 mL/kg 8.4% $NaHCO_3$ mixed with 5% dextrose solution in a separate IV line over 30–60 minutes followed by an infusion of bicarbonate. Check urine pH every 30 minutes. Titrate $NaHCO_3$ infusion rate to achieve urine pH more than 7.5, simultaneously avoiding serum hypernatremia or hypokalemia. Urinary pH manipulation is contraindicated in patients with established or incipient renal failure, pulmonary edema, and cerebral edema.

- *Extracorporeal treatment (ECT):* Removal of toxins by extracorporeal techniques is justified if there is an indication of severe toxicity and if the total body elimination of the toxin can be increased by 30% or more. Extracorporeal removal depends on characteristics of the toxin itself and of the elimination technique used as shown in Flowchart 1.

    Techniques available for extracorporeal removal of toxins are—(i) Hemodialysis; (ii) Continuous hemofiltration techniques; and (iii) Molecular adsorbent recirculating system (MARS).

    Toxins where ECTs are useful are given in Box 2.

Flowchart 1: Graphical abstract and algorithm for extracorporeal treatment.

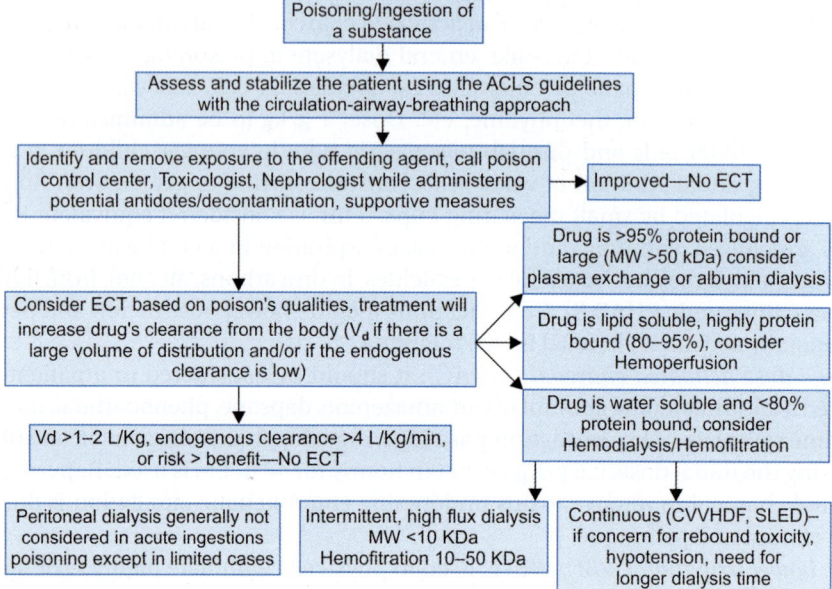

(ACLS: advanced cardiac life support; CVVHDF: continuous venovenous hemodiafiltration; ECT: extracorporeal treatment; SLED: sustained low-efficiency dialysis)

Situations where ECT are useful are given in Box 3.

Hemodialysis

Toxins and other substances must be water soluble and have a low molecular weight, low protein binding and a low volume of distribution in order to be removed by hemodialysis.

Molecular Adsorbent Recirculating System

It is a blood purification system, aimed at removing albumin-bound toxic molecules.

Although the efficacy of MARS in the removal of protein-bound drugs such as lithium, diltiazem, phenytoin, and theophylline has been demonstrated in case reports. Its use is limited by its availability, technical applicability, and high costs.

Box 2: Substances known to cause mortality in children at low doses.

- Calcium antagonists
- Camphor
- Clonidine and other imidazolines
- Opiates
- Salicylates
- Sulfonylureas
- Toxic alcohols
- Tricyclic antidepressants
- Lithium
  – Methanol, ethylene glycol
  – Sodium valproate, carbamazepine

Box 3: Situations that warrants extracorporeal treatment.

- Ingested quantity associated with severe toxicity
- Ingestion of a toxin with serious delayed effects
- Natural removal mechanism impaired
- Clinical evidence of severe toxicity and child is deteriorating: hypotension, coma, metabolic acidosis, respiratory depression, dysrhythmia/cardiac decompensation.

General Guidelines in the Management of Poisoning

- Consider poisoning when history is not clearly available
- Always try to identify the toxin ingested, at the same time resuscitate the child as per pediatric advanced life support (PALS) guidelines
- Focused history, problem-oriented examination and looking for features of toxidrome contacting poison information centers are very useful steps
- Always see whether any antidotes are available and useful. Ensure the availability of all antidotes. They are like fire extinguishers and not having an opportunity to use them is welcome event
- Making medicolegal entry in accident register and informing police is always a safe option for the medical team
- While treating a child with poisoning always look for more than one toxin ingested and more than one person who could have consumed the poison, e.g., siblings or other family members
- Always educate the parents and other family members about the safety precautions they have to follow
- In intentional poisoning always refer the child for pediatric psychiatry counseling.

INDIVIDUAL POISONS

Salicylate Poisoning

Methyl salicylate, a topical agent, also known as oil of wintergreen, is the most concentrated and toxic formulation of salicylate, containing 98% salicylate in its pure form.

Source

Usage of salicylate as medicine has reduced now, but nonaspirin salicylates available as topical agents, massage oils containing methyl salicylate or oil of wintergreen, teething gels and herbal products can be accidentally consumed. Oil of wintergreen 1 mL is equivalent to 7,000 mg or 21 (325 mg) aspirin tablets.

Mechanism of Toxicity

At therapeutic doses, salicylic acid is metabolized by the liver and eliminated in the urine within 2–3 hours after ingestion. In poisoning it interferes with multiple physiological processes which include direct stimulation of the respiratory center, uncoupling of oxidative phosphorylation, and hyperglycemia due to stimulation of glycolysis and gluconeogenesis and interference with TCA cycle. Renal function should be normal since up to 30% of free salicylate can be excreted in urine. Salicylate urinary excretion is markedly decreased in the presence of renal insufficiency, dehydration, low urine pH (< 6.5), or acidemia.

Toxic Dose

A toxic dose of acetylsalicylic acid (ASA) is 150 mg/kg. The lethal dose of 100% methyl salicylate in children is 4 mL. A 5-mL dose (1 teaspoon) of methyl salicylate is equivalent to 7,000 mg of salicylate. Degree of severity based on dose consumed (Box 4).

Although there is no absolute correlation between the plasma salicylate and toxic symptoms, most patients show signs of intoxication when the plasma concentration exceeds 30–50 mg/dL; the usual therapeutic range is 10–20 mg/dL.

> **Box 4:** Severity of acetyl salicylic acid toxicity.
> - <150 mg/kg ingested: No toxicity to mild toxicity
> - 150–300 mg/kg ingested: Mild-to-moderate toxicity
> - 301–500 mg/kg ingested: Serious toxicity
> - >500 mg/kg ingested: Potentially lethal toxicity

Salicylate dose and the patient's age, renal function, and hydration status are all factors in determining the degree of salicylate toxicity.

Clinical Manifestation

The classic triad of symptoms—hyperventilation, tinnitus, and GI irritation.
- *GI irritation*: Nausea, vomiting
- *Central nervous system (CNS) symptoms*: Cerebral edema, altered consciousness, seizures, and coma
- *Respiratory*: Initially hyperpnea, respiratory alkalosis, and later acute lung injury (ALI)
- *General symptoms*: Tachycardia, arrhythmia, diaphoresis leading to dehydration, hyperthermia, but fever may be absent in the first 12 hours., dehydration, bleeding tendency
- *Respiratory alkalosis*: Salicylate directly stimulates the respiratory center in the medulla oblongata; hyperventilation
- *Metabolic acidosis*: Uncoupling of oxidative phosphorylation in mitochondria leading to increased metabolic rate, increased oxygen consumption, increased carbon dioxide formation, increased heat production, increased glucose utilization, and lactic acidosis.

Differential Diagnosis

Diabetic ketoacidosis and sepsis are close differential diagnosis. Other poisons mimicking salicylate are iron, ethylene glycol, and ethanol.

Chronic salicylism can present with a confusing diagnostic picture, delaying an accurate diagnosis. Presenting signs and symptoms may suggest diagnoses such as congestive heart failure, hyperthyroidism, delirium, and psychosis.

Laboratory abnormalities:
- Initially hyperglycemia and later hypoglycemia
- ABG:
  - *Phase 1*: Respiratory alkalosis with alkaluria
  - *Phase 2*: Respiratory alkalosis and paradoxical aciduria (pH < 6.0)
  - *Phase 3*: Metabolic acidosis with or without respiratory alkalosis and hypokalemia
- Electrolytes
- *Serum salicylate level*: On arrival and every 4–6 hourly in deteriorating patients and in stable patients once in 24 hours. It is repeatedly done till two consecutive levels are declining or levels goes less than 30 mg/dL with clinical improvement. To some extent serum levels are useful. One should remember the fact that high levels are always dangerous irrespective of

clinical status. Decreasing plasma concentration, but deteriorating child can be seen due to rising CNS concentration or in chronic toxicity
- Complete blood count (CBC), coagulation studies, liver function tests: Leukocytosis and coagulopathy and raised transaminases
- Serum calcium
- Chest X-ray, electrocardiogram (ECG) to identify complications
- Urine analysis with serial monitoring of urine pH.

Therapeutic Approach

- *Resuscitation*: Assess and support the ABCs. If apnea or respiratory efforts are not adequate, intubation and ventilatory support is needed. But intubation also carries a risk of worsening of acidosis and cardiac arrest. Preloading with sodium bicarbonate, backed up by an experienced team can avoid this issue. While ventilating preventilation respiratory rate should be the initial setting and should aim to maintain pH at 7.45–7.50. Alkalemia will prevent redistribution of salicylate into brain
- Correction of metabolic acidosis by alkalinization with sodium bicarbonate helps in the management by two ways—(i) Alkalinizing the urine to enhance excretion of salicylate as salicylate levels cannot be reduced by metabolism. (ii) In severe poisoning respiratory compensation cannot manage the metabolic acidosis. (iii) Correction of metabolic acidosis is important to prevent CNS damage. Ideal maintenance fluid is 5% dextrose, 20–40 mEq/L of potassium, 1–2 mEq/kg of sodium bicarbonate titrating with blood pH. This fluid is given as 1.5–2.0 times maintenance rate, carefully watching for fluid overload. (iv) Urinary alkalinization: *Loading:* Sodium bicarbonate infusion 2 mEq/kg over 1 hour followed by maintenance infusion. Titration is done by serial monitoring of urine pH targeting a pH of 7.5. This is possible only when catheterization is done. In this situation, hypokalemia can occur due to increased loss and transcellular shift; hence, maintenance dose of potassium has to be increased to 20–40 mEq/L and serum level has to be monitored closely. *Caution—* Check urine pH hourly and serum electrolytes 4th hourly. Serum pH should not exceed 7.5
- *Supportive management*: Correct dehydration, shock, hypoglycemia and dyselectrolytemia. Aggressive rehydration and urinary alkalinization are the mainstay of therapy
- *Goals of therapy*: Maintaining the following targets are important.
  - Serum pH of 7.45–7.55
  - Urine output of 2 mL/kg/hr
  - Urine pH of 7.5–8.0. If urine pH is less than 7.5 bicarbonate concentration in the infusion has to be increased.
  - Serum potassium 4.0–4.5, because alkalinization cannot be achieved in the presence of hypokalemia
  - Treatment continued till plasma salicylate concentration reaches less than 30 mg/dL. Two situations make urine alkalinization impossible pulmonary edema and renal failure:
1. *GI decontamination*: Activated charcoal preferably within 2 hours and an upper limit of 4 hours in the presence of a coingestant that delays gastric motility or extended-release preparation. Multiple activated charcoal doses may be useful.

2. *Indication of hemodialysis*: (i) Moderate and severe toxicity as alkalinization is difficult to achieve in patients with significant neurotoxicity (e.g., focal neurologic signs, seizures, cerebral edema, coma); (ii) Renal insufficiency and pulmonary edema; (iii) A plasma salicylate level greater than 100 mg/dL in acute overdose or rising to 60 mg/dL despite treatment; (iv) Intractable acidosis, severe electrolyte disturbances, and/or progressive clinical deterioration; (v) Patients who require mechanical ventilation, unless that indication for mechanical ventilation is respiratory depression secondary to another coingestant.

Paracetamol Poisoning

This is the most common cause of hepatic failure requiring transplantation in Great Britain and in United States.

Source and Common Errors

Inadvertent overdose from confusing preparations, unintentional prescription of combination drugs, administration by different routes; iatrogenic overdose, intentional overdose in adolescent.

Acute single dose poisoning: 150 mg/kg or (>7.5 g in adolescence and 4 g in adult) within 24 hours both in pediatric and adults.

Repeated supratherapeutic ingestion (>24 hours staggered dose):
- In children (<6 years): 4 g or more than 100 mg/kg/day (whichever is less)
- In children (>6 years old) or adults: 6 g or 150 mg/kg/day (whichever is less).

Paracetamol kinetics: Paracetamol is rapidly absorbed from the small intestine. Its peak serum concentrations occur within 1–2 hours. 20% of the ingested dose undergoes first-pass metabolism in the gut wall (sulphation), while the rest undergoes hepatic biotransformation.

Mechanism of Paracetamol-induced Hepatotoxicity

- Normally 95% of the paracetamol ingested is metabolized into nontoxic compounds glucuronides and sulphates. And only 5% of the ingested paracetamol is converted to toxic compound called N-Acetyl-p-benzoquinone imine (NAPQI)
- In therapeutic doses, NAPQI is conjugated with glutathione and its byproducts, mercapturic acid and cysteine are excreted in urine
- In cases of a paracetamol overdose, the excess amount of the reactive metabolite NAPQI accumulates while the glutathione stores diminish to 30% of normal.

Excessively formed NAPQI, which is not metabolized by glutathione, covalently binds to hepatocellular proteins leading to formation of NAPQI protein adducts. This leads to mitochondrial dysfunction and oxidative damage, hepatocellular necrosis primarily in the centrilobular region (zone III), because of the excessive production of NAPQI by the cells in this region.

Stages of clinical features: Clinical features due to end organ toxicity does not manifest till 24–48 hours postingestion. They are arbitrarily divided into four stages with varying manifestations (Box 5).

The pathophysiology of hepatic necrosis following an overdose of acetaminophen has been hypothesized by molecular mechanisms
- Oxidative stress
- Kupffer cell activation

> **Box 5:** Various stages of paracetamol toxicity.
> - *Stage 1 (0.5–24 hours)*: Nonspecific – malaise, nausea, vomiting, pallor, diaphoresis
> - *Stage 2 (24–48 hours)*: Upper right quadrant pain and tenderness, oliguria, increasing liver enzymes. This may resemble viral hepatitis or tropical infection with hepatic impairment
> - *Stage 3*: Hepatic phase (72–96 hours) peak liver function abnormalities such as hypoglycemia, jaundice, hepatic encephalopathy, liver failure, renal failure, multiorgan failure
> - *Stage 4 (4 days–2 weeks) resolution of liver injury.*

- Nitration of the acetaminophen adducts with peroxynitrite formation.

In the presence of medications that induce cytochrome P450 (CYP) enzyme such as isonicotinic acid hydrazide (INH), rifampicin, carbamazepine, barbiturates, sulpha, zidovudine and alcohol, NAPQI production and hepatic damage is aggravated.

Risk Assessment

The key factors to consider for paracetamol poisoning are:
- The dose and concentration (early)
- The clinical and laboratory features which suggest liver damage (late)
- Children at high risk include those who are malnourished (anorexia, failure to thrive) or on CYP enzyme inducing drugs.

Management of Paracetamol Poisoning

- Where history of ingestion is suspected or the dose of ingested cannot be confirmed, blood paracetamol concentration should be measured at least 4 hours following ingestion, as the clinical features develop late. This can be repeated 4 hours later and if both levels are below the nomogram line N-acetylcysteine (NAC) is discontinued. This should be plotted in the Rumack-Matthew nomogram to predict the risk of hepatotoxicity. Patients who have taken an overdose or who present more than 8 hours postingestion should be started on treatment
- Baseline investigations include electrolytes, creatinine, liver enzymes, coagulation profile, urinalysis for renal tubular damage. Serum ammonia and arterial blood gas (ABG) are done in sick patients.

If the baseline results are within the normal range, the same investigations should be repeated daily for a minimum of 48 hours postingestion. Normal results at 48 hours exclude hepatic damage.

Alanine transaminase activity exceeding 1,000 IU/L is a marker of significant liver injury, but not prognosis. Serial measurements of prothrombin time (PT) and international normalized ratio (INR) are also important.

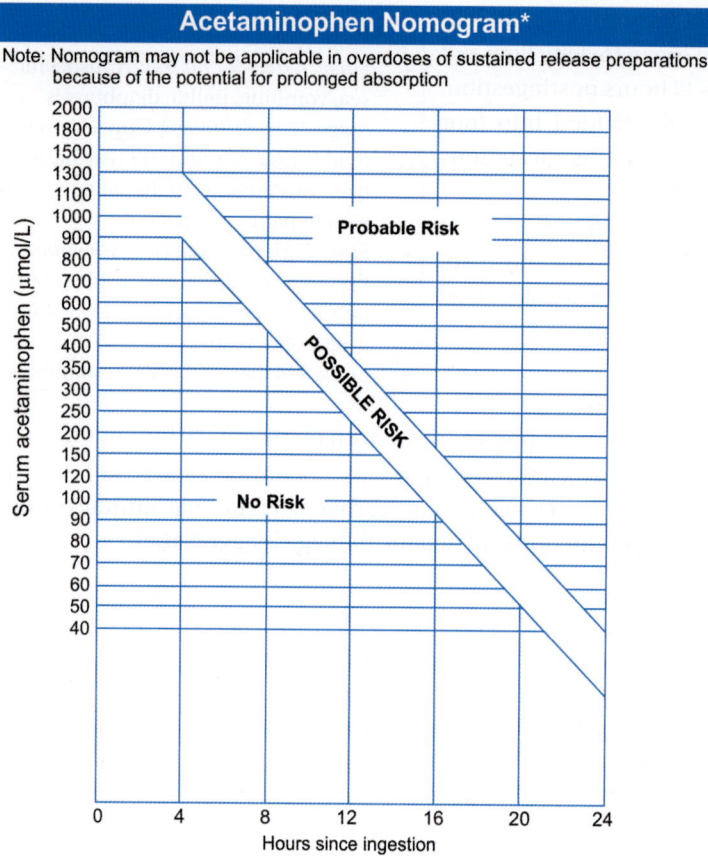

Fig. 2: Rumack-Matthew nomogram.

Rumack-Matthew Nomogram

Useful only in single, acute ingestion, and not useful for multiple dose ingestion or when levels are taken after 20 hours. Here paracetamol level is tracked between 4 hours and 24 hours of ingestion. Hepatotoxicity is expected in 60% of those levels seen above the probable line (Fig. 2).

N-acetylcysteine may be discontinued if both levels fall below the nomogram line.

Gastric lavage: If the child comes to the hospital within 1 hour, lavage is done.

Activated charcoal: Activated charcoal is given if patient reaches hospital within 1 hour and the time limit is extended if sustained release preparation is consumed or there is coingestion of drugs which delay gut motility.

N-acetylcysteine Infusion

N-acetylcysteine replenishes glutathione stores by converting to cysteine. In a single acute ingestion, if more than 150 mg/kg has been ingested, NAC should be started immediately. NAC is maximally useful when given within 8–10 hours of postingestion, and can be beneficial when give after 24 hours postingestion. NAC can be given both by oral route or intravenous route.

Oral route: The Food and Drug Administration (FDA)-approved regimen is as follows:
- Loading dose of 140 mg/kg
- 17 doses of 70 mg/kg given every 4 hours
- Total treatment duration of 72 hours.

Intravenous regimen:
- *Initial infusion*: An initial dose of 150 mg/kg of NAC diluted in 200 mL of 5% glucose and infused over 15–60 minutes
- *Second infusion*: Initial infusion is followed by a continuous infusion of 50 mg/kg of NAC in 500 mL of 5% glucose over the next 4 hours
- *Third infusion*: Second infusion is followed by a continuous infusion of 100 mg/kg of NAC in 1,000 mL of 5% glucose over the next 16 hours.

Side effects: Anaphylactoid reactions occur in 5–30% of patients during the first two NAC infusions.

Methionine can be considered as an alternative antidote for paracetamol poisoning, especially in the setting of known allergy to NAC. Charcoal hemoperfusion to be considered in severe paracetamol poisoning.

Indication of liver transplant: King's College criteria consist of the following laboratory abnormalities; any serological or clinical finding should prompt urgent transplantation consultation:
- Arterial pH less than 7.30 after fluid resuscitation
- Creatinine level greater than 3.4 mg/dL
- PT greater than 1.8 times control or greater than 100 seconds, or INR greater than 6.5
- Grade III or IV encephalopathy.

Prognosis

With aggressive, timely care the mortality rate is less than 2%.

Blood lactate levels more than 3.5 mmol/L before fluid resuscitation or more than 3 mmol/L after fluid resuscitation were found to be sensitive and specific indicators of survival.

Another early predictor is serum phosphate levels, which indirectly represent the balance between the development of renal failure and hepatic regeneration. Serum phosphate more than 1.2 mmol/L measured at 48–96 hours postingestion were sensitive and specific for increased mortality.

Other Antipyretics

Ibuprofen accounts for 65% of childhood NSAID ingestions, mefenamic acid for 10%, and diclofenac 6%. When consumed in toxic quantity they produce GI upset, headache, dizziness, tinnitus, and visual disturbance, hypotension, tachycardia and hypothermia, prolongation of the PT, electrolyte disturbances, metabolic acidosis, CNS depression, and respiratory failure can occur.

Ibuprofen may cause bradycardia or hepatic dysfunction. Mefenamic acid is associated with convulsions. Phenylbutazone can cause hepatic failure, arrhythmias, and bone marrow suppression.

Children who have consumed more than 100 mg/kg of ibuprofen and 25 mg/kg of mefenamic acid should receive activated charcoal. If sustained release preparations are consumed, a 12-hour period of observation is advised; managed by supportive treatment.

Antihistamines

It is one of the most commonly consumed medicines in both prescription as well over the counter sales. Because of these reasons this forms a major cause of poisoning.

Source

Commonly used medications in cough cold preparations are antihistamine (first and second generation) decongestants (phenylephrine, pseudoephedrine) cough suppressants (codeine, dextromethorphan), and expectorants (guaifenesin) and sometimes antipyretics like paracetamol is also included.

Mechanisms of Toxicity

Most of the antihistamines have diverse effects including CNS stimulation, depression, anticholinergic, and sympathomimetic effect.

Clinical Manifestations

- *CNS effects*: Commonly lead to sedation, altered consciousness, and respiratory failure. Paradoxically it can cause excitation, delirium, tremors, ataxia, and convulsions.
- *Anticholinergic effects*: Dryness of mouth, dilated pupils, and fever
- *Cardiovascular effects*: Majority of antihistamines this effect is mediated by myocardial sodium channel blockade. Two of the nonsedating antihistamines—terfenadine and astemizole, cause delayed cardiac repolarization by potassium channel blockade associated with prolongation of the QT interval and may predispose to the development of ventricular tachyarrhythmias and hence not used now. Severe cases are associated with hypertension, reflex bradycardia, arrhythmias, convulsions, and coma.

Management

- *Resuscitation*: If the child comes with seizures, altered level of consciousness, ABCs have to be assessed and stabilized
- *Decontamination*: Gastric lavage and activated charcoal administration are useful if the children are brought earlier. Multiple activated charcoal administration and WBI are needed in ingestion of sustained release preparations. Activated charcoal should be considered up to 4 hours postingestion as gut motility is impaired
- *Monitoring*: Vital signs, oxygen saturation, and ECG should be monitored in high dependency units. Cardiac monitoring and ECG: For detection of QTc interval prolongation or frank arrhythmias
- *Supportive and symptomatic management*: For convulsions, arrhythmias, and shock

- *Urinanalysis/microscopy and serum creatinine kinase*: Rhabdomyolysis in anticholinergic toxicity can occur secondary to prolonged seizures
- Sodium bicarbonate is the first drug of choice for QT prolongation with sodium channel blocking antihistamines. Class Ia and III antiarrhythmic drugs should be avoided in this situation. Magnesium sulphate to be considered for arrhythmia caused by terfenadine or astemizole.

Bronchodilator Medications

Salbutamol can be accidentally ingested by children and overdose can induce tremor, tachycardia, agitation, metabolic acidosis, hyperglycemia and hypokalemia. Symptoms are associated with ingestion of large doses (1 mg/kg).

Theophylline is more toxic but is encountered infrequently.

Symptoms include vomiting, tachycardia, tachypnea, tremors, agitation, convulsions, hyperglycemia, hypokalemia, hypophosphatemia, metabolic acidosis, and respiratory alkalosis.

Activated charcoal should be administered for children who have consumed more than 15 mg/kg of theophylline. Use of multiple doses of activated charcoal 0.5 g/kg administered on a 4 hourly can enhance theophylline elimination.

Propranolol can be used to prevent the metabolic disturbances caused by theophylline overdose. Hypokalemia implicated in cardiac arrhythmias and convulsions should be corrected with intravenous supplementation.

Theophylline can produce both supraventricular and ventricular arrhythmias by increasing cardiac conduction velocity, catecholamine liberation, reduced coronary blood flow and decreased ventricular fibrillation threshold. Arrhythmias are exacerbated by hypoxia, hypercapnia and acidosis and propranolol is the first line treatment, esmolol is an alternative in asthmatic patients.

Benzodiazepines

Sedatives or anxiolytics prescribed for adults are a common source. In overdose they produce drowsiness, ataxia, hallucinations, confusion, agitation, respiratory depression, bradycardia, and hypotension.

Activated charcoal should be administered if child presents within 1 hour of ingestion and conscious level is not impaired. Asymptomatic children should be observed for 4 hours.

Symptomatic children require hospital admission. Treatment is largely supportive.

The use of flumazenil, a competitive antagonist to benzodiazepines, is not generally indicated.

Iron Preparations

Iron compound is one of the serious poisons because of its potential to cause mitochondrial toxicity. Amount of elemental iron consumed should be calculated according to the iron formulation consumed (Fig. 3).

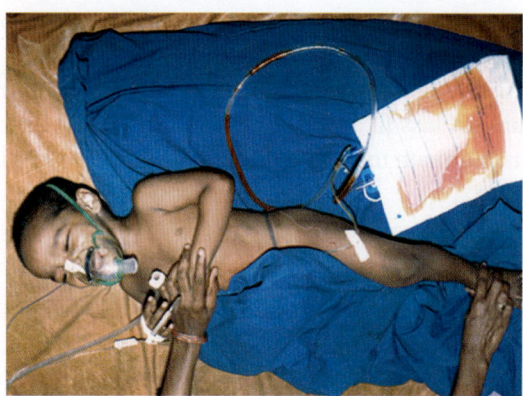

Fig. 3: Child receiving desferrioxamine.

Table 8: Various stages of intoxication.

Stage	Hours after ingestion	Clinical features
• Hemorrhagic enteritis	Starts 30–60 minutes after ingestion and lasts for 4–6 hours	Passage of black stools, shock, acidosis, coagulopathy, altered consciousness
• Apparent improvement	2–12 hours	Apparently child looks well
• Delayed shock	12–48 hours after ingestion	Fever, high anion gap metabolic acidosis, coma, leukocytosis
• Acute liver failure		
• Residual pyloric stenosis	4 weeks after ingestion	

Pathophysiology

High concentrations of intracellular iron disrupt mitochondrial function and result in cell death. Signs of multiorgan failure present at 12–48 hours postingestion. The liver is particularly prone to damage and symptoms of fulminant hepatic failure predominate.

Clinical Features

It depends on various phases that happen after ingestion (Table 8).

Diagnosis

History and examination:
- Ask about quality consumed and the formulation, time of consumption
- Black stools, reddish urine, change in level of consciousness
- Look for features of shock, metabolic acidosis and liver failure
- Most of the affected children developed symptoms between 30 minutes and 2 hours. The common presenting symptoms were vomiting, diarrhea, abdominal pain, hematemesis and black stools. Critical features are shock, jaundice, and encephalopathy

- Those with severe toxicity and presenting late may come with hepatic failure and respiratory failure
- Bacterial sepsis can also be observed as a complication
- Pyloric stricture is a late complication.

Laboratory investigation:
- Serum iron level at 4 hours after ingestion and 8 hours if delayed release preparations are consumed
- CBC, as leukocytosis is an evidence of toxicity
- *Liver function tests*: Raised transaminases and bilirubin
- Renal function tests
- Abdominal X-ray; presence of radiopaque shadows are associated with serious toxicity
- ABG: High anion gap metabolic acidosis
- *Coagulation studies*: Prolonged PT and INR are expected
- Blood grouping and cross matching.

Grading of poisoning based on serum levels:
Serum iron should be checked between 2 hours and 6 hours. Levels taken after 6 hours is misleading. And when iron sustained release preparations are consumed, it can be estimated in 8 hours. Toxic reference range for serum iron:
- More than 350 μg/dL: Mild toxicity
- More than 500 μg/dL: Moderate toxicity
- More than 1,000 μg/dL: Severe toxicity.

Management

- *Initial resuscitation:* Correction of shock with normal saline boluses and blood transfusion if warranted. Assessment and support of ABCs may be required if the child comes in shock, altered consciousness and liver failure.
- *Decontamination procedures*: Gastric lavage with normal saline ideally within 2 hours, but can be performed later if sustained release preparations are consumed or gut motility inhibiting drugs are co ingested. Activated charcoal will not be useful. WBI is very useful. Peglec solution is used and is administered through the feeding tube into the stomach continuously at the rate of 5–10 mL/kg/h. Usually done for 6 hours or till the rectal effluents are clear. Child should be monitored for electrolyte disturbances even though it is a balanced solution. Extracorporeal elimination techniques like hemodialysis is useful in the presence of ingestion of toxic levels and those presenting with serious toxicity.
- *Chelation therapy*: Desferrioxamine: This is indicated in the following circumstances (Box 6).

Box 6: Indications for chelation in iron poisoning.

Indications
- Serum iron level >350 μg/dL
- When serum iron levels are not available following factors will help
- Consumption of >60 mg/kg of elemental iron
- Presence of features of serious toxicity – shock, metabolic acidosis, coagulopathy, gastrointestinal (GI) bleeding, features of hepatic failure
- Presence of radiopaque shadows in the abdominal X-ray. Vitamin tablets containing iron may not be demonstrable radiologically.
- Blood glucose >150 mg/dL
- White blood cells (WBC) count >15,000/mm^3

Desferrioxamine should be given as infusion at the dose of 15 mg/kg/hr while carefully watching for features of toxicity like shock. In the presence of renal failure, dialysis has to be done to excrete iron desferrioxamine complex. Duration of desferrioxamine is decided by resolution of shock, metabolic acidosis, and glucose disturbances both hypo- and hyperglycemia and disappearance of Vin Rose color in the urine. As desferrioxamine can lead to acute respiratory distress syndrome (ARDS), it should not be continued beyond 24 hours.

- *Monitoring*: Close monitoring of vital signs 1–2 hourly and laboratory investigation 6–12 hourly will help in early identification and management of complications and reduce mortality.

A follow-up of the child after 4–6 weeks is essential to watch for the development of strictures and upper GI endoscopy is needed.

Poor prognostic factors: Irreversible shock, persistent metabolic acidosis, coagulopathy, hepatic failure, and GI bleeding are considered as poor prognostic factors.

Asymptomatic children, with a definite history of consuming less than 30 mg/kg of elemental iron, need to be closely monitored.

Beta-Blockers

These drugs have the potential to cause life-threatening toxicity in children even with 1–2 tablets of adult strength medication.

Source

Commonly used medication in adults for hypertension and in children for portal hypertension, migraine, and arrhythmia.

Mechanism of Toxicity

They competitively antagonize the binding of catecholamines to beta receptors. The effect of specific agents in overdose depends on their receptor specificity, lipid solubility, partial agonist activity, and dose. It reduces both the heart rate and decreases myocardial contractility and can also cause some peripheral vasodilatation. Other signs of cardiovascular toxicity include varying degrees of heart block, shock, and pulmonary edema.

Clinical features: Common presentations are bradyarrhythmia with wide QRS, hypotension, altered sensorium, seizures, hypoglycemia, bronchospasm especially in asthmatics and cardiogenic pulmonary edema.

Management

- All children with suspected beta-blocker overdose should be admitted and observed for at least 12 hours even if asymptomatic. For sustained preparation 24 hours observation may be needed. Heart rate, blood pressure, ECG, blood sugar, mental status, and urine output need to be observed
- Gastric lavage and administration of activated charcoal. Repeated dose of activated charcoal and WBI may be needed when sustained released preparations are consumed.

- Assess and support the ABC. Fluid used is 0.9% normal saline (NS) or Ringer's solution (RL) bolus in the presence of shock. Avoid repeated boluses due to risk of cardiogenic shock and pulmonary edema
- Symptomatic children require intensive monitoring. Hypotension may respond to intravenous fluids
- Goal in the management includes maintaining heart rate above 60/min and maintaining normal tissue perfusion (normal urine output and mental status). Bradycardia is initially treated with atropine though the success rate with atropine alone is poor
- In resistant cases, intravenous glucagon (50–150 mg/kg in 5% dextrose) is the treatment of choice. High-dose glucagon stimulates myocardial adenylate cyclase directly, bypassing beta receptors
- Sodium bicarbonate is used in the presence of severe metabolic acidosis, arrhythmia with QRS interval more than 120 ms. Beta-blockers with the so-called "membrane stabilizing effect" include acebutolol, betaxolol, carvedilol, metoprolol, oxprenolol, and propranolol. Thus, toxicity from these drugs may include widened QRS in addition to bradycardia
- Hemodialysis is useful only in toxicity due to certain drugs, e.g., atenolol, nadolol, and sotalol
- Cardiac pacing is indicated when pharmacological methods fail
- Intravenous fat emulsion rescue therapy is tried in severe beta-blocker poisoning. Beta-blockers with high lipid solubility (e.g., propranolol) rapidly cross the blood brain barrier into the CNS, predisposing to neurologic sequelae such as seizure and delirium. Beta-blockers with this characteristic are more amenable to treatment with lipid emulsions therapy. Intravenous lipid emulsions (20% solution) 1.5 mL/kg over 2 minutes, followed by 1.5 mL/kg as infusion over 60 minutes
- *Caution*: Always consider coingestions especially when it is intentional overdose. Toxicity is higher in the presence of other cardiotoxic drug coingestion, such as calcium channel blocker, cyclic antidepressant, and neuroleptics.

Calcium Channel Blocker Poisoning

Calcium channel blocker ingestion in infants and children has to be taken seriously, because even one tablet can be fatal.

Source

Commonly used medications are nifedipine, nicardipine, amlodipine, diltiazem, and verapamil.
Mechanism of toxicity: They block the L-type calcium channels in the myocardium and vascular smooth muscles resulting myocardial depression, hypotension, bradyarrhythmias, and delayed GIT motility.

Clinical Manifestations

Even though calcium channel blockers are well tolerated at therapeutic doses, in overdose it leads to serious complications such as hypotension and bradycardia. Toxicity depends on the type of tablet or sustained release preparation. Serious manifestations are bradycardia, hypotension, pulmonary edema, seizures, and altered mental status. Sometimes they present with nonspecific symptoms like nausea, vomiting, ileus, and constipation, headache, dizziness, syncope, lethargy, confusion, chest pain, palpitation, edema, cough and dyspnea, seizures, and altered mental status.

Management

- All children with calcium channel blockers ingestion need to be hospitalized for observation even if they appear asymptomatic and close monitoring for 24–36 hours is needed in high dependency unit (HDU)
- Continuous hemodynamic (ECG, HR, BP and perfusion) monitoring and serial estimation of blood sugar serum bicarbonate and calcium are essential. Assessment and stabilization of ABCs. IV fluid boluses to correct shock. Dobutamine is preferred over dopamine or vasopressors for correction of cardiogenic shock. Atropine is useful for bradycardia
- Intravenous calcium gluconate
- Hyperglycemia correlates with severity of toxicity and can occur before hemodynamic instability. Insulin is important first line therapy in calcium channel blockers overdose
- In refractory shock, pacemaker insertion for bradycardia, intralipid emulsion therapy, IV methylene blue and extracorporeal therapy for removal of toxins and extracorporeal membrane oxygenation (ECMO) are considered
- *Decontamination*: Gastric lavage and activated charcoal in view of delayed gastric emptying. Repeated doses of activated charcoal may be needed in case of sustained release preparation. WBI is useful.

Oral Hypoglycemic Agents

Source

(i) Sulfonylurea compounds. First generation compounds (e.g., chlorpropamide, others are tolazamide, tolbutamide) have longer half-life. Second generation is glipizide, glyburide, and glimepiride, which are more potent and have shorter half-lives. (ii) Biguanides, e.g., Metformin. Other agents: Alpha glucosidase inhibitors never cause hypoglycemia and glitazones very rarely cause hypoglycemia.

Mechanism of Toxicity

Sulfonylurea type drugs produce hypoglycemia by increasing insulin release. Ingestion of a single tablet can produce symptomatic hypoglycemia in children.

Clinical Features

Usually symptoms develop within 2 hours and may be delayed if food is taken. Most of the symptoms are due to hypoglycemia.

Management

- Asymptomatic children should be observed as effects can be delayed for up to 16 hours
- Decontamination: Activated charcoal should be administered. Multiple doses of activated charcoal may be useful in glipizide ingestion
- Level of consciousness, respiratory effort and saturation should be monitored capillary blood glucose and arterial or venous blood gas for metabolic acidosis should be monitored. In addition serum electrolytes and lactate estimation are needed. In adolescents with intentional overdose associated poisons such as alcohol, aspirin, and paracetamol should be checked.
- Started on intravenous dextrose infusion as intravenous glucose is faster and better than oral. Resistant hypoglycemia may respond to subcutaneous injection of octreotide, which inhibits pancreatic insulin release. *Dose*: 1 µg/kg SC or IV
- Advantage of glucagon that IM or SC when IV access is unavailable. Glucagon 0.02–0.03 mg/kg, octreotide 1 µg/kg/day SC/IV every 6th hourly
- Metformin does not cause hypoglycemia, but leads to lactic acidosis and significant GI disturbances
- As the effects of sulfonylurea may be prolonged upto 16 hours, 24 hours observation in hospital is necessary
- Hemodialysis may be useful in the presence of refractory acidosis or renal failure
- Other drugs which cause hypoglycemia, quinine, beta blockers, angiotensin-converting enzyme agents, and quinolones should be considered (Table 3).

Isoniazid

Isoniazid is widely used drug in the treatment of tuberculosis.

Source

Substance ingested may be a tablet or liquid or a compound along with rifampicin and here reddish color can give clue.

Mechanism of Toxicity

Pyridoxine is necessary for the production of the inhibitory neurotransmitter gamma aminobutyric acid (GABA). In overdose, isoniazid reacts with pyridoxine to form a compound which is rapidly excreted in the urine.

In overdose, INH metabolism yields a group of toxic compounds known as hydrazones which are significantly enhanced in acute overdose. Hydrazones adversely impact the metabolism of pyridoxine to its activated form, pyridoxal-5'-phosphate and reduced availability of pyridoxal-5'-phosphate. This leads to depletion of GABA (inhibitory neurotransmitter), along with an acutely elevated glutamic acid (powerful excitatory neurotransmitter), forces the brain into a state of hyperexcitation. Generalized tonic-clonic seizures are the end result. Replenishment of pyridoxine promptly restores production of GABA.

Cause of metabolic acidosis is seizures, leading to lactic acidemia.

Table 9: Toxins and medicines that lead to seizures.

Household substances	Medicines
• Gammexane, • OPC • Camphor • Neem oil • Mosquito repellents, eucalyptus oil, Insecticides	TCA Theophylline Oral antidiabetic hypoglycemia INH

(INH: isonicotinic acid hydrazide; OPC: organophosphate; TCA: tricyclic antidepressant)

Clinical Manifestations

Toxic symptoms following INH ingestion can develop over 30 minutes to 3 hours. Seizures are brief but multiple recurrent episodes will be noticed. Any child presenting with afebrile seizures without any clear etiology and associated with hyperglycemia and metabolic acidosis, isoniazid poisoning should be strongly considered. The toxicity appears within 2 hours of ingestion. Neurological symptoms predominate and seizures are likely if more than 70 mg/kg has been ingested. Secondary complications are rhabdomyolysis, renal failure, and cardiovascular collapse.

Differential diagnosis: Causes of seizures in a child with poisoning are given here (Table 9).
Following combinations, in addition to seizures further narrow down the possibilities:
- Hypoglycemia—oral hypoglycemic agents
- Hypoglycemia, bradycardia—beta-blockers
- Ventricular tachycardia, dilated pupil—tricyclic antidepressants
- Hyperglycemia, metabolic acidosis—isoniazid.

Laboratory findings: Lactic acidosis, hyperglycemia, hypokalemia, and ketonuria are common. Serum level of INH can be measured if facilities are available.

Management

- ABCs and full hemodynamic and respiratory support as required
- Symptomatic patients (seizures) should receive intravenous pyridoxine—at a dose equivalent to the amount of isoniazid ingested in milligrams. If the child's weight is 20 kg, 70 × 20 = 1,400 mg of pyridoxine is needed. Practical issue here is nonavailability of IV preparation and IM pyridoxine is 40 mg/mL. In addition, rest of the dose can be given as tablets crushed and administered through nasogastric tube. If expected response is not seen, repeat doses can be given after 30 minutes
- Hyperglycemia needs only monitoring and metabolic acidosis can be corrected bicarbonate IV infusion
- In refractory seizures, drug removal like extracorporeal support should be employed
- After INH poisoning, the metabolic pathways that leads to hepatic damage are saturated and hence it is rarely necessary to serially monitor serum transaminases.

Tricyclic Antidepressants

Source

These include imipramine and amitriptyline, which are commonly used in psychiatric disorders, nocturnal enuresis, and many other illnesses. Amitriptyline, clomipramine, doxepin, imipramine, trimipramine, amoxapine, desipramine, maprotiline, nortriptyline, and protriptyline are other compounds.

Mechanism of Toxicity

(i) Noradrenaline reuptake inhibitor, (ii) Central and peripheral anticholinergic effect, (iii) Fast sodium channel blockade in the myocardium, and (iv) Peripheral alpha-1 receptor blockade.

Clinical Manifestations

Remembered as three Cs and one A (tricyclic antidepressants), which are coma, convulsions, cardiac arrhythmias, and acidosis. In addition anticholinergic symptoms, dilated pupils, dry mouth, ileus, drowsiness, ataxia, agitation, initially hypertension and later hypotension.

Cardiac arrhythmias occur frequently and are the most common cause of death. Prolonged QRS, ventricular tachycardia (VT), ventricular fibrillation (VF), heart block, and cardiogenic shock are common. TCA poisoning should be considered in any child with unexplained encephalopathy, seizure, cardiac arrhythmia, or shock.

Laboratory monitoring: ECG, ABG/venous blood gas (VBG), electrolytes and renal function tests.

Serial monitoring of ECG changes is the single most important investigation that guides management. Prolongation of the QRS and QT intervals is indicative of toxin-induced sodium channel blockade.

Management

- *Assess and stabilize ABCs*: Hypertension need not be treated as it is transient. Seizures are managed with benzodiazepines and phenytoin is to be avoided. Shock correction should include small volume boluses and preferred vasoactive agents are dopamine and norepinephrine. Adrenaline may induce arrhythmias
- *Decontamination*: Gastric lavage and activated charcoal are useful
- Asymptomatic children, with a normal ECG, should be observed for a minimum of 6–8 hours. Symptoms of TCA toxicity generally present within 2 hours of ingestion
- Patients with any ECG abnormality should be monitored until resolution of the abnormality In all children with QRS more than 100 ms and those with arrhythmias, alkalinization is the mainstay of management. Treatment should be started with an initial bolus of 1 mL/kg of sodium bicarbonate followed by an infusion. Arterial pH should subsequently be maintained between 7.45 and 7.55
- Ventricular arrhythmias refractory to sodium bicarbonate may require treatment with lidocaine, magnesium sulphate or both.
- Hemodialysis and hemoperfusion may be considered in patients with very severe TCA poisoning.

Antipsychotic Drugs

These drugs are commonly used for psychiatric conditions and also for nonpsychiatric indications such as for vomiting, hiccup, vertigo, migraine headache, postherpetic neuralgia and Tourette's syndrome like tricyclic antidepressant poisoning the main system involved are the nervous and cardiovascular systems.

Source or Spectrum of Antipsychotics

They are classified into typical or first generation (butyrophenones and phenothiazines) and atypical or second generation antipsychotics (benzapines and indoles). (i) Butyrophenones (Haloperidol, droperidol) (ii) Phenothiazines (promethazine, chlorpromazine, thioridazine) (iii) Benzapines (clozapine, olanzapine, quetiapine) (iv) Indoles (risperidone, ziprasidone).

Mechanism of Toxicity

- All these drugs block dopamine D2 receptors but the second generation antipsychotics bind less avidly to the D2 receptor, and so less extrapyramidal effects.
- Second generation drugs antagonize serotonin receptors, mainly the 5HT2A receptor. A 1-adrenergic blockade cause orthostatic hypotension, muscarinic receptor antagonism leads to sedation, sinus tachycardia, and urinary retention. Adverse motor side effects are less in second generation drugs when compared with first-generation antipsychotics.

Clinical Manifestations

Symptoms begin mostly by 6 hours.
- *CNS*: (i) Extrapyramidal crisis manifests as episodes of torticollis, stiffening of the body, catatonia and inability to communicate lasting for few seconds to minutes. These are more common in typical antipsychotics. They are aggravated by dehydration. (ii) CNS depression, lethargy, and prolonged coma are the common manifestations, but rarely results in paradoxical hyperactivity. Seizures are not commonly seen.
- *Cardiovascular side effects*: Hypotension, tachycardia, QTc prolongation (common with thioridazine and ziprasidone). Sudden death can occur possibly due to torsades-de-pointes. QTc prolongation is most commonly reported and is dose related. Rarely, QRS prolongation can occur, resulting from sodium channel blockade, and is most frequently associated with quetiapine.
- *Neuroleptic malignant syndrome (NMS)*: This is a rare, idiosyncratic, and potentially fatal complication. This syndrome develops 1–2 weeks after initiation of therapy and characterized by confusion, coma, lead pipe rigidity, clonus, tachycardia, and hyperpyrexia. This can happen even at therapeutic doses.

Management

- Decontamination is done by gastric lavage and activated charcoal if they arrive within an hour

- Treatment is mainly supportive
- Extrapyramidal symptoms resolved within minutes by slow IV administration of diphenhydramine or diazepam. Agitations may need benzodiazepines
- ECG monitoring is essential to identify abnormalities and to treat them. Hypotension is treated by normal saline boluses
- NMS is treated with IV fluids, sedation, and control of hyperthermia.

Selective Serotonin Reuptake Inhibitors

These are commonly used as antidepressants.

Source

Frequently used compounds are citalopram, escitalopram, fluoxetine, fluvoxamine, paroxetine, and sertraline.

Mechanism of Toxicity

SSRI prevent the neuronal reuptake of serotonin at preganglionic sites, which leads to increased activity of serotonin.

Clinical Manifestations

Children and adolescent generally follow benign course, but rarely leads to serious life-threatening complications like delayed seizures, hypotension, and cardiac dysrhythmias. If there is coingestion of other serotonergic agents such as monoamine oxidase inhibitors, tramadol or serotonin and noradrenaline reuptake inhibitors (SNRIs), they are at significantly greater risk of serotonin syndrome. Citalopram or escitalopram poisoning can lead to arrhythmias like wide complex bradycardia, long QTc and torsade-de-pointes. Serotonin syndrome will occur when SSRI are given along with MAO inhibitors. This is characterized by hyperthermia, myoclonus, rhabdomyolysis, confusion, and tremors. Other features are extrapyramidal syndrome, prolonged bleeding time due to blocking of platelet serotonin activity. Hyponatremia can occur due to SIADH.

Laboratory Monitoring

ECG monitoring, electrolytes, renal function test, coagulation parameters, and creatine phosphokinase (CPK).

Management

Gastric lavage and activated charcoal are useful. There is no specific antidote. These children need to be monitored in pediatric intensive care unit (PICU) with ECG. Electrolyte disturbance is managed by supportive therapy. Benzodiazepines and cooling are used for hyperthermia. Hypotension may be treated by fluids and norepinephrine. Cyproheptadine may be useful serotonin syndrome. Bromocriptine and dantrolene are not recommended. Hemodialysis and charcoal hemoperfusion are not found to be beneficial.

Table 10: World Health Organization (WHO) color code for organophosphate compounds.

Red label	Extremely toxic	Monocrotophos, zinc phosphide, ethyl mercury acetate and others
Yellow label	Highly toxic	Endosulfan, carbaryl, quinalphos and others
Blue label	Moderately toxic	Malathion, thiram, glyphosate and others
Green label	Slightly toxic	Mancozeb, oxyfluorfen, mosquito repellant oils and liquids, and other household insecticides.

Organophosphate Compounds

It is a common poisoning in developing countries.

Sources

Organophosphates are used as pesticides (chlorpyrifos, dimethoate, malathion, parathion), nerve agents (e.g., tabun, sarin), and antilice medications. Most OPC compounds are divided into two types: (i) Diethyl (e.g., chlorpyrifos, diazinon, parathion, phorate, and dichlofenthion) and (ii) dimethyl (e.g., dimethoate, dichlorvos, fenitrothion, malathion, and fenthion).

Based on the severity of toxicity, these are classified low toxicity, moderate toxicity, and high toxicity compounds (Table 10).

Mechanism of Toxicity

Poisoning occurs after dermal, respiratory, or oral exposure to either organophosphate pesticides or nerve agents (e.g., tabun, sarin), causing inhibition of acetylcholinesterase at nerve synapses.

They produce irreversible acetylcholinesterase inhibition. Accumulation of acetylcholine stimulates muscarinic receptors at parasympathetic postganglionic synapses. Symptoms can be delayed for up to 24 hours postexposure.

In large doses, organophosphates produce muscle stimulation followed by paralysis because of a depolarizing block.

Pathophysiology

Organophosphates and carbamates bind to acetylcholinesterase and inhibits it, preventing degradation of acetylcholine and its accumulation at synapses.

Clinical Features

Symptoms develop usually at 8–12 hours. Spectrum of clinical manifestations are: (i) acute toxicity; (ii) intermediate syndrome; and (iii) delayed polyneuropathy.
Based on the effects they are grouped into following.
- *Acute toxicity*
  - *Muscarinic effects*: These are easily explained by the mnemonics. SLUDGE: salivation, lacrimation, urination, diarrhea, GI upset, emesis) or DUMBELS: diaphoresis, diarrhea, urination, miosis, bradycardia, bronchospasm, emesis, excess lacrimation, and salivation

- Nicotinic effects – these are life-threatening and involves CNS. Muscle fasciculation, hyper-reflexia, flaccid weakness, and reduced tendon reflexes
  - Autonomic nicotinic effects – hypertension, tachycardia, mydriasis, and pallor
  - CNS effects: Headache, dizziness, confusion, drowsiness, respiratory depression
  - Hyperglycemia and glycosuria also can occur.
- *Intermediate syndrome*
  - Begins 48 hours after poisoning in 20% of patients but may be delayed to 72–96 hours. It is a second stage of weakness with or without symptom free interval, if left unrecognised can lead to fatal respiratory depression
  - It reflects prolong action of Ach on nicotinic receptors. Manifestations are muscular weakness, dystonic posturing, cranial nerve palsies, respiratory depression, and sensory functions.
- *Organophosphate-induced delayed polyneuropathy*
  - Develops after 1–3 weeks of exposure due to ingestion of large amounts of OPC due to degeneration of long myelinated fibers. Common manifestations are cramping pain, numbness, paresthesia, foot and wrist drop, reflexes are lost
  - Aging means irreversible binding of OPC compounds to AChE for 24–72 hours. De novo synthesis Ach E is required to replenish the supply once the aging has occurred. Aging cannot occur in carbamates.

Diagnosis

- History of exposure, presence of garlic odor and characteristic manifestations will be indicative of OPC poisoning
- Estimation of plasma pseudocholinesterase (PChE) is a sensitive indicator of poisoning. But it is not specific as RBC acetylcholinesterase (AChE) activity. Latter is not freely available
- Every attempt is made to identify the product and chemical.

Management

All children with suspected OPC compounds must be hospitalized in HDU. Airway, breathing, and circulation.

Resuscitation

They may come with convulsions, unconsciousness, irritability, shallow breathing, and respiratory distress or failure. These children need to intubated and supported with mechanical ventilation. Succinylcholine should not be used. Vecuronium is an alternative (Table 11).

Decontamination is aggressively practiced, because of the potential of OPC to get absorbed through skin, inhalation, and ingestion.

Skin exposure would require irrigation of the skin with copious amounts of water and liberal use of soap. It is important for health care workers to wear appropriate protective gear before removing contaminated clothing and items from patients.
- Eye exposure should be irrigated with copious amount of normal saline
- Gastric lavage is useful, use of activated charcoal is controversial.

Table 11: Quick severity assessment.

	Severe	Moderate	Mild
Level of consciousness	Unconscious, no pupillary reflex. convulsions present	Conscious, anxious, restless, but cannot walk, miosis	Comes walking, headache, abdominal pain, vomiting
Respiration	Flaccid paralysis present, respiratory failure	Soft voice	–
Serum AChE	0.8 U/L	0.8–2.0 U/L	1.6–4.0 U/L

Specific antidotes: Atropine, Pralidoxime (P2AM).

Muscarinic antagonist:
- *Atropine*: Atropine reverses the cholinergic effects. Aim to dry bronchial secretions and reverse bronchospasm and to facilitate ventilation and oxygenation.

  Atropine acts as an antidote—blocking muscarinic receptors and preventing the excessive activity of acetylcholine.

Dose: 0.05 mg/kg IV every 5-10 min and it is targeted on drying of secretions including disappearance of crepitations. Once the desired target is achieved, it can be given in increasing intervals. Presence of fever, tachycardia, and delirium are features of atropine toxicity and warrant stopping of atropine for a short period. It will be always difficult to differentiate the delirium related to atropine toxicity from CNS effect of OPC. In this situation, atropine can be stopped and glycopyrrolate can be given for shorter periods.

Atropine test: If there is doubt regarding ingestion of OPC a single dose of atropine is given and if the heart rate does not go beyond 20 above the base line and pupils are dilated, it indicates mild toxicity or OPC not ingested.
- *Pralidoxime*: It is most effective as an antidote when given within the first 24 hours post-ingestion. Initially given as infusion 30 mg/kg in NS over 30 minutes followed by maintenance infusion of 8 mg/kg/hr for 8 hours or till signs of recovery is noticed. But P2AM is generally not given beyond 24 hours. Rapid push can lead to hypertension, arrhythmia, and cardiac arrest

  It is not used in carbamate poisoning as it is reversible.
- *Glycopyrrolate*: 1-2 mg IV in adolescents

    0.025 mg/kg IV in children
- Benzodiazepines are used to control seizures
- Intubation and ventilation is indicated in any child having increasing respiratory distress, shallow respiration, apnea, bradypnea, or coma
- Certain drugs are contraindicated – phenytoin, morphine, aminophylline
- *Controversies regarding P2AM*: Even though the World Health Organization (WHO) recommends usage of P2AM, there are many studies which do not favor P2AM. Use of P2AM is left to the discretion of treating physician and many prefer to use only in moderate to severe poisoning.

Organocarbamate poisoning: Toxic effects are less severe compared to organophosphate compounds. P2AM is not indicated here.

A prefix or postfix of carb is suggestive.

Propoxur (Baygon), aldicarb (Temik), bendiocarb (Ficam), Bufencarb, carbaryl (Sevin), carbofuran (Furadan), formetanate (Carzol), methiocarb (Mesurol), methomyl (Lannate, Nudrin), oxamyl (Vydate), and Pirimicarb (Pirimor).

Alcohol Poisoning

In adolescent and adults, this is a common cause of intoxication, uncommon cause in children. As increasing number of household products contain good quantity of ethanol this is considered as an important differential diagnosis. It may be intentional or accidental and unintentional.

Source: (Ethanol and other toxic alcohols – isopropyl alcohol, ethylene glycol and methanol). Large share of sources is available outside the bar. Except the first, other sources are available in plenty at every Indian home. Alcoholic beverages, cosmetics, mouth washes, alcohol rubs or sanitizers (60–70% alcohol) and tinctures. In some regions alcohol (brandy) is administered as cough, cold remedy even for young kids.

Mechanism of Toxicity

Complete absorption requires 30 minutes to 6 hours. Rate of metabolic degradation is 20 mg/hr in an adult. Main effects: CNS stimulation followed by depression, respiratory depression, hypoglycemia, acidosis, and risk of subarachnoid hemorrhage.

Clinical Features

- In any child, adolescent or adult who are euphoric, disoriented, or comatose without any reason, drug abuse including alcohol intoxication has to be suspected. Smell of alcohol may give clue
- It produces euphoria, talkativeness, increased pain threshold, unsteadiness, slurred speech, and impaired short-term memory
- Suspicion should be confirmed by estimation of serum levels. If the level of obtundation is disproportionately excessive to the serum level, suspect comorbidities like head trauma, hypoglycemia or other coingestions. At high serum levels, coma and respiratory depression occur.
- Infants and young children are prone to develop profound hypoglycemia, coma and hypothermia despite ingesting relatively small amounts of ethanol. Deaths have been reported
- Abdominal pain and vomiting may be due to gastritis or sometimes secondary to pancreatitis
- Licking a drop of hand sanitizers may not cause death but even one or two pumps 2.5 or 5.0 ml can lead to significant toxicity. Accuracy of quantity by history is unreliable, hence decision should be taken with caution
- Ethanol-induced hypoglycemia may be easily overlooked as adrenergic symptoms are frequently absent.

Toxic Levels (Adults)

- 50–100 mg/dL considered as intoxication; Up to 200 mg/dL is considered as moderate. Above 300 mg/dL is indicative of severe toxicity and more than 500 mg/dL is usually associated with fatal outcome
- No comparable values available for children. Absolute ethanol 1.0 to 1.5 mL/kg will result in a peak level of 100 mg/dL in 1 hour after ingestion
- Fatal hypoglycemia has occurred in young children with blood ethanol concentration below 100 mg/dL a serum level associated with minimum inebriation in adolescents and adults
- The minimum toxic dose in infants and young children is 0.4 mL/kg of 100% ethanol and would be expected to result in peak serum ethanol level of 50 mg/dL (11 mmol/L). The life-threatening dose expected to cause deep coma with respiratory depression is estimated at 4 mL/kg of 100% ethanol with an expected peak level of 500 mg/dL.

Differential Diagnosis

- Medical conditions, trauma, and other narcotic poisons leading to impaired level of consciousness
- But all these can coexist with alcoholic intoxication.

Laboratory Investigations

- Estimation of serum alcohol level is mandatory
- In addition, frequent capillary glucose estimation, amylase, lipase, electrolytes, renal and liver function tests are needed, wherever appropriate
- Neuroimaging when subarachnoid hemorrhage or head trauma is suspected.

Management

- Supportive care is the mainstay of managing ethanol intoxication in children. Treatment of respiratory depression, hypoglycemia, hypovolemia, and hypothermia are the key intervention to ensure good outcome
- Assessment and stabilization of ABCs, if the child is critically ill
- Gastric lavage will be useful if done early. Activated charcoal is not useful
- Cause of death is usually respiratory depression, cerebral edema, and hypoglycemia. So diagnosis and correction of hypoglycemia and ventilatory support are the two important strategies. Child should receive IV maintenance fluid containing D5 or D10 with serial monitoring of glucose. Correct hypoglycemia with 2 mL/kg of 25% dextrose or 4 mL/kg of 10% dextrose followed by dextrose containing IV fluids with frequent monitoring
- If metabolic acidosis develops correct with sodium bicarbonate
- Involve neurosurgical help if associated head trauma is suspected
- Many other sedative hypnotic and psychoactive agents may also produce somnolence and respiratory depression and are often coingested with ethanol recreationally or with suicidal intent especially in adolescents. Thus, even when is confirmed by serum or breathe

levels, the possibility of sedative hypnotic or opioid intoxication coingestion should be considered. In such cases presence of coingestants should be investigated and managed accordingly.

Ethylene Glycol

Ethylene glycol is found in certain types of antifreeze, brake fluid, and windscreen wash. Ethylene glycol is rapidly absorbed from the stomach, symptoms can occur within 30 minutes of ingestion.

Ethylene glycol is metabolized by alcohol dehydrogenase to form toxic metabolites including glycolic and oxalic acid.

Toxic effects include convulsions, coma, metabolic acidosis, hypocalcemia, and renal failure.

Blood gases, serum calcium, electrolytes, and renal function should be assessed.

Ethanol competes with ethylene glycol binding at the catalytic site of alcohol dehydrogenase.

Symptomatic children or those with a plasma ethylene glycol level of more than 200 mg/L, should receive intravenous fomepizole (15 mg/kg over 30 minutes). Fomepizole is a competitive alcohol dehydrogenase antagonist.

Its use replaces intravenous ethanol therapy, the disadvantages of which include CNS depression and hypoglycemia.

Where fomepizole is not available, ethanol remains an alternative treatment (7.5 mL/kg 10% ethanol in 5% dextrose over 30 minutes, then 1.65 mL/kg/h of 5% ethanol to keep blood level at 1–1.5 g/L).

Fomepizole should be given every 12 hours (10 mg/kg for four doses, then 15 mg/kg) until the plasma ethylene glycol level falls below 200 mg/L.

Patients require regular measurements of blood gases, renal function, and plasma calcium.

Patients with renal failure or resistant metabolic acidosis will require hemodialysis.

Kerosene and other Hydrocarbon Ingestion

The most common poison consumed by children across all states in India. More common in public sector hospital both in rural and urban areas. Less common in private sectors.

Source

Petrol, kerosene, lighter fluid, paraffin oil, diesel fuel, thinner oil, lubricating oil, furniture polishes, and mineral turpentine.

Mechanism of Toxicity

In the initial stages, kerosene vapor fills the lung and replaces the air which leads to hypoxia. Later after 1–8 hours it leads to the development of chemical pneumonia followed by bacterial pneumonia, sometimes ending up as necrotizing pneumonia. Hypoxia leads to CNS, respiratory, and cardiac complications.

Clinical Features

In the initial few hours, child may come with severe distressing cough, breathlessness, and with smell of kerosene. Child may have drowsiness or irritability, coughing, gagging, tachypnea, and desaturation. Some children may be asymptomatic. Usually symptoms develop as early as 1 hour or may be delayed up to 8 hours. Rarely, they may come with respiratory failure if the aspiration is massive leading to ARDS and hypoxia requiring early ventilatory support.

Respiratory: Wheeze, tachypnea, and pulmonary edema may indicate evolving chemical pneumonitis. Necrotizing pneumonia leads to pneumatocele, lung abscess, and empyema.

Cardiovascular: Rarely arrhythmias can occur which may be related to hypoxia

CNS: Altered consciousness, coma and seizures may occur with large acute exposures. It is only due to hypoxia in kerosene ingestion. But direct toxicity can occur in other hydrocarbons such as glue and tetrachloroethylene ingestion. Onset is usually within 2 hours.

GIT: Nausea, vomiting, and diarrhea also can occur (Figs. 4A and B).

Investigations: Monitoring saturation, chest X-ray if the child is symptomatic. If they are asymptomatic it is postponed to 8 hours later, ECG, electrolyte, and RFT.

Management

- All children with history or suspicion of kerosene ingestion needs hospitalization
- Oxygen administration, monitoring with pulse oximeter, and ECG are the initial steps
- Inducing emesis, gastric lavage, and activated charcoal administration are contraindicated. Child should be kept nil oral and started on IV fluid maintenance
- Indication of intubation: Increasing respiratory distress, desaturation, persisting depressed level of consciousness, recurrent seizures
- As air leak is common when ventilating a child with kerosene ingestion. High positive end-expiratory pressure (PEEP) and low tidal volume strategy should be used
- Antibiotics are not the initial choice, but can be given if fever and respiratory distress recurs or persists beyond 48 hours or with worsening radiological findings
- Steroids are not indicated and will be harmful

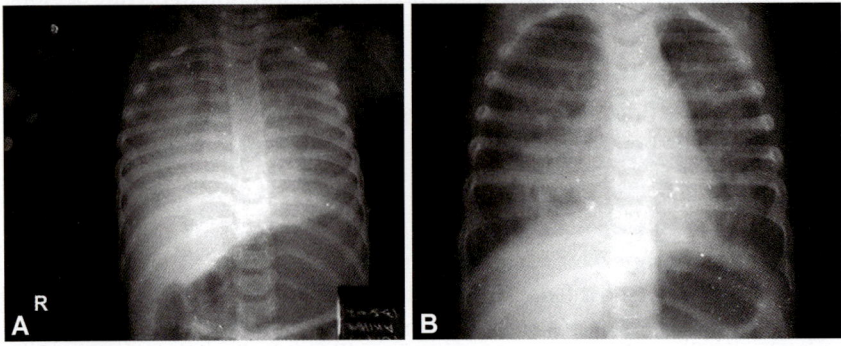

Figs. 4A and B: (A) Kerosene. Chest X-ray (CXR) showing acute respiratory distress syndrome (ARDS) like picture; (B) CXR showing bronchopneumonia.

- Patients with mild to moderate respiratory symptoms on presentation are at risk for the development of significant chemical pneumonitis with progression to respiratory failure over the next 24–48 hours
- *Outcome and prognosis*: Most of the children with kerosene ingestion recover with O2 and other supportive management. Risk factors of mortality are severe tachypnea, need for ventilator support, seizures, persistent shock, and altered consciousness.

Rat Killer Poisoning

One of the common household poisons available both in rural and urban environment, easy to procure.

Source

It is a heterogeneous product available as—(i) powders; (ii) pellets; (iii) pastes; and (iv) cakes. Following are the various chemicals present in the rodenticide. Highly toxic compounds are aluminum phosphide, sodium monofluoroacetate, and strychnine. Zinc phosphide, yellow phosphorus, arsenic, and thallium. In the study done by Suneetha et al., the most common poisoning agent was zinc phosphide (32.14%) followed by aluminum phosphide (21.4%), and yellow phosphorus (14.2%) and unidentified chemical in (28.5%) (Table 12).

Clinical Manifestations

- *Bleeding tendency (warfarin compounds)*: Usually develop 24–48 hours after ingestion. Epistaxis, flank pain with or without frank hematuria, excess bruising, hemoptysis, intracranial bleed, retroperitoneal bleed are all have been reported. They may present with shock following bleeding.
- Respiratory failure due to hemorrhagic pulmonary edema, acute respiratory distress syndrome

Table 12: Mechanism of toxicity of various chemicals.

Product	Chemical present	Mechanism of toxicity
Paste	Yellow phosphorus Yellow, waxy solid compound	Corrosive and highly cellular toxin Acute liver failure, Vomiting, diarrhea fluid loss It affects heart and vascular tone and leads to cardiovascular collapse. Multiorgan failure.
Powder	Zinc phosphide, (Gray or black powder; gray, green, or turquoise pellets or tablets radiopaque), thallium	Hemolysis, cardiogenic shock
Pellet	Aluminum, calcium, or magnesium phosphide used for fumigation/gassing	Arrhythmia, cardiogenic shock
Cake	Warfarin (short acting), super warfarin (long-acting warfarin derivatives) bromadiolone, brodifacoum, difenacoum, diphacinone	Oral anticoagulants. Inhibit the enzyme vitamin k1 2,3 reductase inhibiting synthesis of vitamin k dependent clotting factors

- *Corrosive effects (yellow phosphorus)*: Perioral, mucosal, and skin burns, vomiting, diarrhea, garlic odor on breath, acute liver failure, and acute kidney injury
- GI irritation marked by nausea, vomiting, hematemesis, and retrosternal chest and abdominal pain because of corrosive effect
- Cardiac arrhythmias, cardiogenic shock, hemorrhagic pulmonary edema – cardiovascular toxicity happens with following rodenticides: Zinc or aluminum phosphide, white (yellow) phosphorus, or barium carbonate. Arsenic, thallium, sodium monofluoroacetate (SMFA), or fluoroacetamide.

Laboratory Investigations

All symptomatic children need:
- PT, INR, and partial thromboplastin time (PTT) at 24, 48, and 72 hours.
- 12-lead ECG and continuous monitoring
- Plain radiographs of the chest and abdomen
- CBC
- VBG or ABG, serum calcium, and phosphorus,
- Blood glucose, serum electrolytes, BUN, and serum creatinine
- Liver enzymes (ALT and AST) and bilirubin (Table 13).

Management:
- *Decontamination procedures*: Gastric lavage, activated charcoal, if the child is brought within 1–2 hours of ingestion.
- *General support*: Oxygen and if needed ventilatory support, fluid management to correct shock, vasoactive medications for cardiogenic shock, in arrhythmia, IV magnesium sulphate is of greatest benefit. Cardiologist consultation is essential. Hypokalemia needs to be corrected

Table 13: Laboratory clues for the chemical consumed.

Finding	Chemical substance
QTc prolongation on ECG	Arsenic, white (yellow) phosphorus, sodium monofluoroacetate (SMFA), or fluoroacetamide
Hypocalcemia	White (yellow) phosphorus, SMFA, or fluoroacetamide
Lactic acidosis	SMFA or fluoroacetamide
Hyperphosphatemia	White (yellow) phosphorus
Hypokalemia	Zinc or aluminum phosphide or barium carbonate
Radiopaque substance on abdominal radiograph	Arsenic, thallium, or barium carbonate
Elevated liver enzymes, BUN, or creatinine	Thallium, white (yellow) phosphorus, arsenic, or zinc or aluminum phosphide
Elevated PT and INR	Anticoagulant

(BUN: blood urea nitrogen; ECG: electrocardiogram; INR: international normalized ratio; PT: prothrombin time)

- NAC infusion
- Vitamin K and fresh frozen plasma (FFP) in the presence of coagulopathy. Dosing of reversal agents for pediatric patients is as follows:
  - *PCC (3- or 4-factor) prothrombin complex concentrate*: 25–50 IU/kg (maximum dose 2000 IU)
  - *FFP*: 15–30 mL/kg (maximum single dose 2 units)
  - *Factor VIIa*: 20 µg/kg without maximum dose (as for congenital factor VII deficiency)
  - *Vitamin K_1*: 0.3 mg/kg intravenously (maximum single dose 10 mg).
- In asymptomatic children with an INR more than 4 and no bleeding, oral vitamin K_1 is preferred than intravenous vitamin K_1 to avoid the risk of anaphylaxis associated with intravenous administration
- Supportive management of acute liver failure
- Extracorporeal removal (hemodialysis, charcoal hemoperfusion, and continuous renal replacement therapy) also may be useful in the clearance of poison.

Prognosis

Fluoroacetate and zinc phosphide ingestion can lead to fatal outcome. Phosphorus intoxication produces serious corrosive injuries and may need reconstructive surgery.

Prevention

Government agencies and manufacturers should work together to bring out a strategy to produce a substance which is less toxic to humans and should make the availability difficult.

Caustics, Soaps, and Detergents

Detergents are powerful cleaning products that are made up of strong acids, alkalis, or phosphates. Cationic detergents are often used as antiseptics in hospitals. Anionic detergents are sometimes used to clean carpeting. Detergent poisoning occurs mostly due to ingestion of cationic or anionic detergents.

Soaps are natural products made from animal or vegetable fat.

Detergents are nonsoap synthetic chemicals used for cleaning because of their surfactant properties.

Sources

There are four types of detergents.
1. Cationic detergents (Acelepryn, diaparene, phemerol, zephiran, benzalkonium chloride, cetrimide, cetylpyridinium, dequalinium) are used as cleansing agents and antiseptics in dairy industries and hospitals. They are harmful to humans
2. Anionic detergents are present in most of the household products used for hand washing dishes, clothes, vessels, furniture, carpets, floor or hair. Among them automatic dish washer detergents can cause serious burns

3. *Nonionic detergents*: Lauryl, stearyl, oleyl alcohols and octyl phenol, e.g., alkyl ethoxylate-polyethylene glycol stearate
4. Recently introduced laundry detergent packets, which are colorful and attractive to children. They are marketed in the western countries in the names Tide Pods, All Mighty Pacs, and Gain Flings. Ethoxylated alcohols and propylene glycol are predominate compounds.

Detergents may also contain other chemicals such as phosphates, carbonates and silicates, bleaches to improve the cleaning, and also perfumes, and stain removers.

Nonionic detergents are usually nontoxic.

Laundry detergent packets: Stridor drooling, retractions, and respiratory distress are seen. Additional serious reactions included gastric burns, seizures, hematemesis, pulmonary edema, bradycardia, and respiratory arrest.

Clinical Manifestations and Treatment

Cationic detergents in dilute solutions cause mucosal irritation and in strong solutions (10–15%) may cause caustic burns. Can cause circulatory collapse, renal insufficiency, CNS effects are coma and convulsions which need anticonvulsants.

Cationic detergents and automatic dishwasher detergents cause corrosive effect.

Eye: Even one drop of a 2% solution has the potential to cause corrosive injury and severe corneal damage, irritation, tearing, erythema, and burning.

Clinical Features

Assessment is mainly based on clinical examination and X-ray neck, chest, and abdomen.

Immediate life-threatening problems: Injury can affect upper airway, lungs, oropharynx, esophagus, and stomach. All airway-related symptoms or signs are life-threatening which are dysphonia/aphonia, drooling, hoarseness, stridor, subcutaneous emphysema, chest pain, or respiratory distress. Lips and tongue may appear swollen with drooling of saliva. If there are no external signs like swollen lips, tongue and voice change, it is very unlikely that upper airway or esophagus is affected (Fig. 5).

- GI-related problems are bleeding, or signs of perforation like abdominal distension and rigidity. Some may present with shock due to vomiting, hemorrhage or third spacing
- *Eye*: Conjunctival bleed, blepharospasm, edema, or rarely loss of vision
- *Complications*: Respiratory – airway injury, mucosal edema, laryngeal edema, airway obstruction or ALI/ARDS; gastroesophageal: Perforation, hemorrhage and stricture on 2nd or 3rd day mediastinitis occur.

Laboratory Investigations

- Chest and abdominal X-ray showing pneumomediastinum, air under diaphragm are suggestive of life-threatening complications
- *Other laboratory investigations*: CBC, osmolar gap calculation, electrolytes, calcium, urea, creatinine, blood gases and anion gap, liver function tests, and disseminated intravascular coagulation (DIC) panel may also be helpful. If abnormal, it indicates severe injury follow-

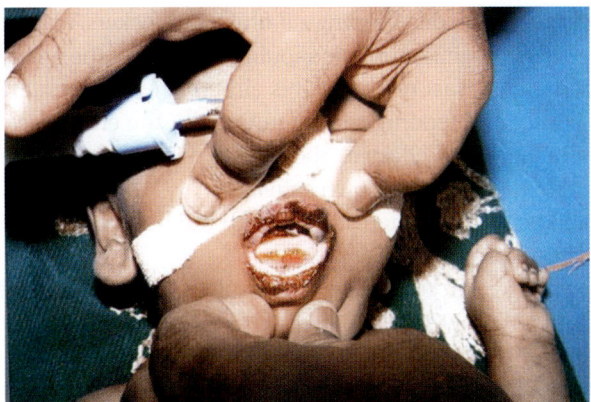

Fig. 5: Corrosive poisoning following inadvertent administration of corrosive.

ing acid ingestions. Blood grouping, typing and cross matching in the presence GI bleeding or when surgical intervention is planned
- Ask, examine and order other lab tests keeping the possibility of coingestions
- Hydrofluoric acid available in rust removers ingestion, can cause precipitous falls in calcium leading to sudden cardiac arrest. Because of long turnaround time, even before changes occur in ionized calcium cardiac arrest can occur.

Role of upper GI endoscopy: Early upper GI endoscopy between 6 and 24 or 48 hours will be useful to degree of severity and extent and will be helpful in planning the long-term nutritional support like gastrostomy. But the procedure should be done meticulously by an experienced person to avoid complications. Upper GI endoscopy is not indicated in mild ingestions (where there is no voice change, normal oral or upper airway or asymptomatic child. Indicated in children showing oropharyngeal changes, drooling of saliva, and dysphagia. Upper GI endoscopy is contraindicated in the presence of esophageal or GI perforation, significant airway edema, or necrosis and in those who are hemodynamically unstable.

Management

- Assessment and management of ABCs are the priority such as the need for intubation, need for fluid boluses to correct shock.
- Decontamination procedures like NG tube insertion and gastric lavage, activated charcoal, WBI are absolutely contraindicated. Dilution and neutralization should not be attempted. Burnt areas of skin, mucous membranes, and eye are irrigated with clean tap water or normal saline
- *Airway management*: Nebulized adrenaline is not useful and might delay intubation. Presence of voice change, stridor, and respiratory distress warrants intubation. Safer to visualize and intubate under the guidance of flexible fiberoptic bronchoscopy. Using IV propofol may be a safer option than using muscle relaxants and anesthetists help will be of immense benefit.

- Supportive management includes keeping nil oral, H2 blockers, or proton pump inhibitors. Opiates may be needed for pain. Antibiotic should be started in the presence of complication.
- Early nutrition is crucial for fast recovery. It is either by total parenteral nutrition (TPN) or through ostomy. Direct oral feeding can be initiated if the child does not have oral cavity involvement, dysphagia, voice change, abdominal distension or absent bowel sounds or when the child is able to swallow his own saliva.
- Surgical help should be sought if there is a need for tracheostomy or gastrostomy and in the presence of perforation or peritonitis.
- Repeat endoscopy and gastroenterologist consultation will be needed after 3-4 weeks anticipating strictures.

Button (Disc) Battery Ingestion

It is becoming more common because of wide availability of batteries in the toys. These are small lithium batteries. Majority of the victims are younger than 6 years which account for 66%, and the peak incidence is between 1 and 2 years of age..

The Centers for Disease Control (CDC) data from United States between 1997 and 2010: Estimated 40,400 children less than 13 years were treated for button battery ingestion. Approximately 75% were less than or equal to 4 years; 10% were hospitalized and 14 fatalities were reported ranging in age from 7 months to 3 years during 1995-2010.

Source

It is available in toys, watch and other household products, such as remote control devices, watches, calculators, pen, computer game, hearing aid, cameras, toys, games, flashing jewelery, some baby books, singing greeting cards as well as hearing aids. Button batteries vary in diameter from 7.9 to 23 mm. In 97% of cases diameter is less than 15 mm. Most frequently ingested sizes are 11.6 mm (63%) and 7.9 mm (30%).

Mechanism of Toxicity

Usually small batteries pass through GI tract and are expelled in the stools uneventfully (Table 14). Battery lodged in esophagus can cause burns in 2 hours. The negative pole has a slightly smaller diameter and anticipates complications based on battery position and orientation. Damage will be severe in tissue adjacent to the negative pole. But battery size more than

Table 14: Approximate duration of time through the gastrointestinal (GI) tract.

Time duration	Percentage in total
Within 24 h	23%
Within 48 h	61%
Within 72 h	78%
Within 96 h	86%
Takes >2 weeks	1%

15 mm are more likely to get lodged in esophagus and intestine. Child can ingest this without the knowledge of parents or insert into nose or ear. It acts in multiple ways: (i) Mechanical pressure effect leading to ischemic necrosis, (ii) corrosive effect of caustic alkaline electrolyte because they are strong alkalis, and (iii) electrical discharge.

Clinical Manifestation

Known history: Child may be brought with a history of battery ingestion and X-ray be ordered and will be followed for complications, so that they are identified early.

Unknown history: When the child has swallowed a battery and it was not known to any caretakers, child will be brought to the health care facilities with complications such as respiratory distress or GI bleeding or perforation.

GI issues: Drooling of saliva, vomiting, hematemesis, melena, abdominal pain, distension due to perforation of stomach or intestine. If ingestion is not recognized by parents or health care providers, serious complications can develop which are esophageal perforation, trachea esophageal fistula, exsanguination after eroding a major blood vessel, esophageal strictures, and vocal cord paralysis.

Airway and respiratory issues: Noisy breathing, stridor, breathlessness secondary to esophageal perforation, mediastinitis, and aspiration pneumonia.

Lodging in esophagus depends on the age of the child and size of the battery.

Investigations

X-ray: If the child comes with a history of foreign body or button battery ingestion, X-ray film should cover neck, chest and abdomen, first to ascertain the site where it is lodged. Next question is whether it is a coin or button battery? In addition, subcutaneous, emphysema, pneumomediastinum, or pneumothorax may be observed (Figs. 6 and 7).

Upper gastrointestinal endoscopy will be useful to confirm the location, directly visualize the ulcers or erosions and also the bleeding source.

Differential diagnosis: Difference between a coin and button battery: It is always prudent to assume any coin shadow as button battery to plan early removal and to avoid complications. But still two features favor button battery than coin. (i) Lateral view will show a plano-convex pattern and (ii) double halo will indicate button battery.

Management

- Assess the ABCs and stabilize the child as appropriate
- Child should be hospitalized when there is history or features suggestive a foreign body ingestion with a corrosive potential. Even X-ray is taken few hours prior, better to repeat as position of the battery might have changed
- X-ray and endoscopy are essential and immediate removal is planned. Even if the child is asymptomatic, immediate removal without any delay is mandatory when the battery is lodged in four places: (i) ear, (ii) nose, (iii) cricopharynx, and (iv) esophagus. If it is lodged in the stomach, it should be removed by endoscopy. Beyond pylorus, it is unlikely to get

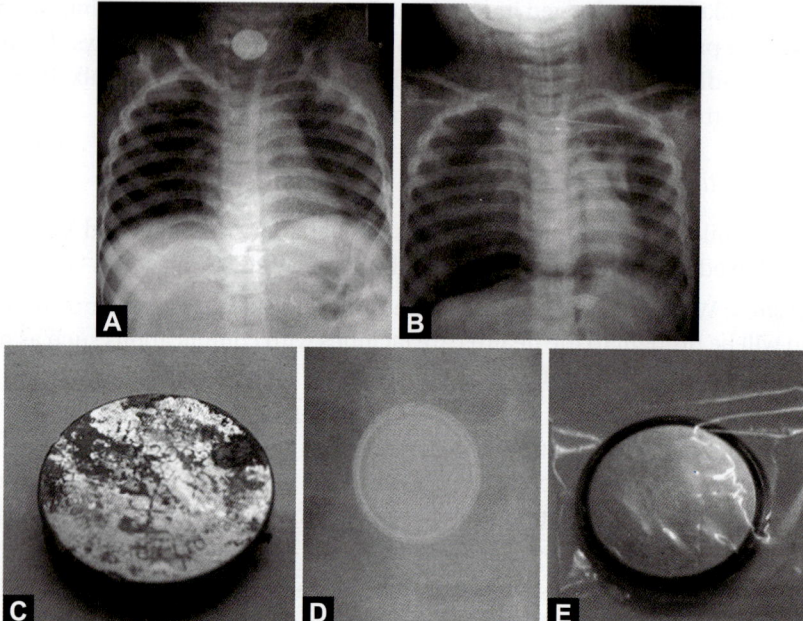

Figs. 6A to D: (A) Chest X-ray (CXR) with a coin shadow (button battery); (B) After removal—pneumothorax right, pneumomediastinum and subcutaneous emphysema; (C) Button battery after removal; (D) Radiological appearance of double line; (E) Photograph showing double lines.

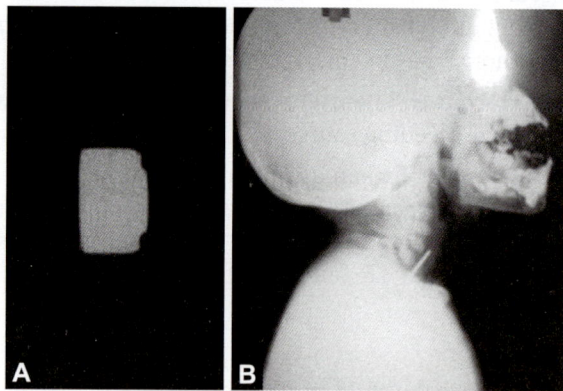

Figs. 7A and B: (A) Lateral view showing the differences between battery and coin. (A) Lateral view of button battery—planoconvex; (B) Lateral view of coin—thin symmetrical.

lodged in any place, hence observation is the only mode of management, unless the child develops bleeding, abdominal pain, or distension of abdomen
- In places where an endoscopy facility is not available Foley balloon catheter-enabled technique is followed

- Inducing vomiting and lavage are contraindicated. WBI is practiced by some, efficacy of which is not known
- Lateral view will differentiate as anterior location favors stomach and posterior location lodging in colon
- In western countries, National Button Battery Ingestion Hotline is available for guidance.

Complications

Nasal septum perforation, perforation of tympanic membrane, skin necrosis in external auditory canal, facial nerve paralysis, esophageal perforation, pneumothorax, and mediastinitis have been reported. Fatalities have occurred when ingestion is not witnessed or diagnosis is delayed. Death is most frequently associated with 3-volt lithium, coin-size batteries more than or equal to 20 mm in diameter, particularly lodged in esophagus.

Prevention

Both manufacturers and parents play a great role in prevention of battery-related injuries. (i) Battery size should be reduced; (ii) battery holding compartments should be tightly closed with screw type. Easily detachable compartment is a potential threat for disc battery ingestion (Figs. 6 and 7).

Mosquito Repellent Poisoning

One of the commonly encountered problems in children.

Source

Pyrethroids are the main chemicals dispensed in kerosene as a solvent in all vaporized liquids. Less commonly available are coils and mat. Transfluthrin, prallethrin (AllOut) and cypermethrin, permethrin, and allethrin are the common chemicals and others are tetramethrin, tralomethrin, and resmethrin.

Mechanism of Toxicity

These chemicals act on the voltage-dependent sodium channels, and GABA-gated chloride channels, leading to hyperexcitation of the nervous system. Cardiac dysfunction has also been described; lung injury is also less commonly reported, probably related to the hydrocarbon kerosene which is used as solvent in the liquid vaporizer. Fortunately these pyrethroids are 2,000 times more toxic to insects than humans.

Toxic dose: 100–1,000 mg/kg is toxic to humans. A refill of "All-Out" contains 45 mL is equivalent to 720 mg.

Clinical Manifestations

Systemic effects are seen within 4–48 hours after ingestion.

General: Sore throat, nausea, vomiting, and abdominal pain which develop within minutes. Others are mouth ulceration, increased secretions, and/or dysphagia, dizziness, headache, and fatigue.

CNS: Blurred vision, coma, and convulsions are the main life-threatening features.

CVS: Rarely causes arrhythmia

Rare complications: One case report from New Delhi reported intravascular hemolysis in a child with glucose 6-phosphate dehydrogenase (G6PD) deficiency and also methemoglobinemia. Both needed supportive management in the form of blood transfusion, plasma exchange and oxygen.

Respiratory: Because of the presence of hydrocarbon it can cause aspiration pneumonia or ARDS. This may need invasive or noninvasive ventilatory support.

Laboratory investigations: These are based on the symptoms. Afebrile seizure may require glucose, electrolytes, calcium, magnesium, neuroimaging, and EEG. In the presence of respiratory distress, arrhythmia chest X-ray, and ECG are required.

Management

- Management is mainly supportive
- Gastric lavage and activated charcoal are contraindicated as the solvent is kerosene
- Asymptomatic children may be kept in emergency room for 6–12 hours. Symptomatic children should be hospitalized. Child can be kept nil oral and should be started on Intravenous fluid maintenance
- In addition to monitoring clinical signs, pulse oximeter saturation and ECG monitoring are necessary to identify seizures, arrhythmia, and seizures
- Convulsions may be managed with IV lorazepam and as in any toxin mediated seizures, phenytoin is to be avoided
- There are no specific antidotes for pyrethroids poisoning.

Carbon Monoxide Poisoning

In India, only very few cases reported, despite the presence of conducive environment.

Probably most of them die on the spot with alternative wrong diagnosis. Simultaneous development of symptoms occurs among several persons from the same room or house one should consider the possibility of CO exposure.

Sources

- Usual setting for CO poisoning is smoke production (from a carbon source) and the victim staying inside an enclosed space where there is less oxygen.

Common sources are one of the following:
- Wooden or coal furnaces for warmth (bukhari or wood burning stove) commonly practiced in hill towns as an alternative for electric heaters, automobile exhaust in a car set, generator in a closed space, after explosive bursts or fire accidents with release of smoke in a closed environment

- Faulty heating systems, poorly maintained generators in enclosed spaces or in poorly ventilated rooms
- Gasoline-powered backup generators being run outside but near the air conditioner, through which CO was drawn into the home
- Kerosene camping stove used inside a closed tent or house even for 2 hours
- Gas geysers running on LPG can lead to CO poisoning in bathroom.

Chemical compound: It is a colorless, odorless, nonirritating, and tasteless gas but highly toxic, produced by partial oxidation (incomplete combustion) of carbon containing compounds in an enclosed space with less oxygen.

Mechanism of Toxicity

- Asphyxia and activation of inflammatory processes by CO leads to toxicity. There is high affinity between CO and hemoglobin (200 times higher affinity than oxygen). It combines with hemoglobin to produce carboxyhemoglobin (COHb), which seizes the space in hemoglobin and also leads to ineffective oxygen delivery to tissues. This shifts the oxyhemoglobin dissociation curve to the left, thereby decreasing the amount of oxygen available to cells
- CO also binds to cytochromes and guanylyl cyclase, and has increased affinity with myoglobin. This leads to its cardiovascular effects such as hypotension, ischemia, dysrhythmias, and myocardial impairment
- More recent research has shown that nitric oxide levels are increased in CO poisoning, resulting in vasodilation, which further causes hypotension, syncope, and cerebral lesions.

Clinical Features

Mild: Nonspecific symptoms like headache, dizziness, nausea, vomiting, and blurring of vision.

Moderate: In addition tachycardia, tachypnea, weakness, syncope.

Severe:
- *CNS*: Seizures, coma, cerebral edema, muscle necrosis
- *Cardiac*: Myocardial ischemia, arrhythmia
- *Respiratory*: ARDS, respiratory failure
- *Others*: Renal failure, rhabdomyolysis, permanent ocular toxicity
- Those with severe poisoning die in a short period or found unconscious
- Cherry red skin and retinal hemorrhage are seen only in severe cases or as postmortem findings
- Pulse oximetry is deceptive; may show normal SpO_2 despite cyanosis.

Toxic level: COHb concentration: In normal individuals up to 5% and up to 10% in smokers. Symptomatic 15%; Toxicity more than 20%; severe toxicity more than 25%; irreversible CNS damage at more than 50%.

Differential Diagnosis

Because of protean manifestations, CO poisoning is never suspected, instead other common conditions mistakenly suspected are viral fever, migraine, meningitis, alcohol intoxication, anxiety, arrhythmia, cyanide toxicity, and acute abdomen.

Laboratory Tests

- In suspected CO poisoning, O_2 saturation monitors are unreliable and it may show saturations of 100% occurring in the presence of significant hypoxia. Conventional blood gas analyzers can also be misleading
- COHb concentration is measured by means of CO-oximetry in ABG. Arterial sample is not needed, venous sample is enough
- As PaO_2 is normal and many ABG analyzers calculate SaO_2 from PaO_2, SaO_2 may be normal. ABG machines which measure these abnormal hemoglobins are available in hospitals (CO-oxymetry). CO-Hb levels may vary with time and treatment and may not reflect the true severity of the exposure
- *Chest X-ray (CXR)*: Noncardiogenic pulmonary edema
- *ECG*: Tachycardia, myocardial ischemia, arrhythmias
- *CT brain*: Bilateral globus pallidus lesions and white matter changes can occur within hours
- Serum lactate, cardiac enzymes, CPK and creatinine are also done. Persistent CNS impairment can occur in those with CT changes.

Management

- Promptly remove from source of CO
- *Mild*: O_2 using non-rebreathing mask
- *Moderate to severe*: Ventilation and 100% O_2
- In severe poisoning hyperbaric oxygen is used when available. Seizures and cardiac complications should be treated urgently
- *Monitoring*: All patients should have close cardiopulmonary and neurological monitoring throughout treatment. Monitor ABG and serum lactate to estimate metabolic acidosis, blood glucose to eliminate hypoglycemia (as a cause for altered mental status) and hyperglycemia and creatine kinase to monitor for rhabdomyolysis. ECG and cardiac enzymes may be monitored to detect evidence of end-organ damage. COHb can also be monitored, although levels may be low in patients receiving oxygen
- Oxygen should be given through a nonrebreather mask to all patients with CO poisoning regardless of pulse oximetry readings or SaO_2 (PaO_2 is not helpful in detecting CO poisoning since it does not distinguish COHb from oxyhemoglobin). An increase in the PaO_2 decreases the half-life of COHb, thereby facilitating the elimination of CO
- *Hyperbaric oxygen*: Hyperbaric oxygen is 100% oxygen in a pressurized chamber. It is used to eliminate hypoxic states and CO from the body. High concentrations of O_2 enhances the dissociation of COHb. It is indicated in severe poisoning as evident by patients with altered mental status, coma, focal neurological deficits, or seizures, cardiovascular dysfunction, or severe acidosis

- *Insulin*: As neurological outcomes following CO poisoning are worse in patients with hyperglycemia, insulin should be given as infusion to control hyperglycemia and avoiding hypoglycemia.

Some case scenarios from news: An adult was found dead in his car at Chennai suburb with the air-conditioner on, which happened on June 2012. Inhalation of poisonous gases, CO was suspected.

Newspaper report: A 35-year-old driver sitting inside his car with the air conditioner running was found dead in the sitting position in the afternoon in Coimbatore. The postmortem report indicated that the victim died of asphyxiation due to inhaling carbon monoxide that accumulated inside the vehicle.

Case report: One child from Kerala who fell asleep in a covered tractor, close to a working generator developed severe CO poisoning and died despite treatment.

Prevention

- Do not keep the generators close to air conditioner or the door of an enclosed space
- CO detectors with audible alarms should be installed in all homes
- Periodical servicing of automobile exhausts, heating devices
- When heating devices are used windows or doors are slightly opened to allow ventilation of the space
- Gas geysers should be fixed outside the bathroom, or should not be switched on when bathroom is closed.

Oleander Poisoning

This is a common cause of poisoning in rural areas by women, which contains multiple cardiac glycosides similar to digitalis. In young children even one flower or leaf and serious toxicity is less common.

Source

Two common sources are: (i) *Nerium oleander* (common oleander) and (ii) *Thevetia peruviana* (yellow oleander)

Mechanism of Toxicity

Reversible inhibition of the Na^+/K^+-ATPase pump leads to hyperkalemia leading to bradycardia with atrioventricular (AV) block, atrial tachycardias, ventricular tachycardia including bidirectional ventricular tachycardia and ventricular fibrillation (Table 15).

Clinical Features

Various clinical features can be grouped as GI, cardiac, and neurological.
- *GI*: Nausea, vomiting and abdominal colic
- *Cardiac*: Bradyarrhythmia and conduction block. Blood pressure will be preserved until late in the course. Often ends in ventricular fibrillation which is resistant to cardioversion.

Table 15: Plant toxidrome.

Constellation of clinical features	Cause of the toxins
Mucosal irritation and swelling	*Philodendron, Dieffenbachia* (dumbcane), *Spathiphyllum* species (peace lily), *Arisaema triphyllum* (Jack-in-the-pulpit), Rhubarb (leaf only), *Colocasia esculenta* (elephant ear), and *Symplocarpus foetidus* (skunk cabbage) contain calcium oxalate in the form of intracellular sharp projections, called raphides.
Gastroenteritis with systemic toxicity	Castor bean *(Ricinus communis)*, Jequirity beans *(Abrus precatorius)* Solanaceous steroidal glycoalkaloids (e.g., solanine, chaconine) which are present in cultivated and wild plants including unripe potatoes
Cardiac arrhythmias	*Nerium oleander* (common oleander), *Thevetia peruviana* (yellow oleander)
Cardiotoxicity and vomiting, diarrhea, paresthesias, numbness, weakness, diaphoresis, and altered mental status.	*Aconitum napellus (monkshood)* and other *Aconitum* species
Cholinergic symptoms: Tachycardia, Hot, flushed, dry skin, Dilated pupils and blurry vision, Disorientation, bizarre behavior, visual hallucinations, seizures, urinary retention	(Datura stramonium), angel trumpet (*Brugmansia* species), deadly nightshade (*Atropa belladonna*), and henbane (*Hyoscyamus niger*)
Status epilepticus, rhabdomyolysis, myoglobinuria, severe lactic acidosis, cerebral edema, and death.	*Cicuta* species (water hemlock) and Oenanthe crocata (hemlock water dropwort). The primary toxin is cicutoxin, a gamma-aminobutyric acid antagonist
Cyanide poisoning	Many fruit pits and seeds (e.g., cherry, apricot, peach, plum, pear, almond, apple) contain cyanogenic glycosides such as amygdalin that are converted to hydrogen cyanide by gut bacteria after ingestion of crushed or masticated seeds or pits of masticated seeds cause toxic side effects
Lychee fruit consumption followed by fasting	Edible when ripe and properly prepared, but the unripe fruit contains high concentration of the toxin, hypoglycin A, which, when metabolized, inhibits long chain fatty acid breakdown and transport into the mitochondria. Metabolites of hypoglycin A and methylene cyclopropylglycine were found in two-thirds of urine specimens from the victims. Toxicity manifests as a Reye-like syndrome. (Muzzafarpur, India, 2014)

Common ECG changes are sinus bradycardia, all types of AV block, sinus arrest and premature ventricular complexes
- *CNS*: Altered consciousness, seizure, and coma
- Hyperkalemia.

Differential Diagnosis

Bradyarrhythmia are commonly caused by beta-blockers, calcium channel blocker, digoxin, and oleander poisoning. CNS depressants poisoning like phenobarbitone also may present with bradycardia, but here child will be drowsy or comatose and bradypnea also may be a feature. Hypoglycemia in addition to bradyarrhythmia will be a feature of beta-blocker ingestion and hyperglycemia will favor calcium channel blocker poisoning. In OPC poisoning constricted pupil, excessive secretions, muscle twitching and convulsions will be the pointers.

Management

- *Decontamination*: Gastric lavage, multiple dose activated charcoal, and WBIs are useful
- All children should be admitted in HDU and closely monitored and all management is carried out with specialist advice from a pediatric cardiologist.

Laboratory Investigations

- 12-lead ECG and continuous monitoring, glucose, electrolytes, renal function tests are essential
- Bradyarrhythmia and AV blocks are managed by atropine
- Persistent tachycardia are managed by external or transvenous pacing
- Ventricular tachycardia is managed by lidocaine and magnesium sulphate (polymorphic VT). Defibrillation is found to be generally ineffective for patients with malignant ventricular dysrhythmias caused by yellow oleander poisoning.
- Cardiogenic shock is managed by small volume boluses and mechanical ventilation
- Digoxin-specific antibody fragments (DSFab) is expensive and not freely available in India, hence studies are limited. Western experience claims it is a safe and effective antidote in acute as well as chronic poisoning. The time taken for reversal of toxicity is found to be 30–45 min. Indications are (i) life-threatening tachy-brady arrhythmias, (ii) hyperkalemia (>6 mmol/L), and (iii) hemodynamic instability with an elevated digoxin concentration (>2 µg/L or 2.6 nmol/L). A randomized controlled trial (RCT) showed an early improvement in cardiac rhythm and hyperkalemia from antidigoxin Fab and no deaths were reported
- Fructose-1, 6-diphosphate (FDP) is a new antidote under experimental trials for the treatment of oleander poisoning, which will be a cost-effective alternative for digibind. It is a phosphorylated sugar, normal physiological intermediate in glycolysis
- Hyperkalemia management is similar except one difference. IV Calcium is better to be avoided as its effects are not clear and conflicting as intracellular calcium concentration is higher in digoxin poisoning. Hypokalemia can also occur because of vomiting and diarrhea and it has to be corrected with careful monitoring
- Bad prognostic factors are intake of more than 3 crushed seeds, delay in arrival of more than 120 minutes, persistent shock, ECG changes showing absent p wave, irregular rhythm
- According to one study from a rural Medical College in Tamil Nadu, India, there were 18 deaths, among a total of 101 patients and most of the death occurred within 24 hours of intake (Table 2).

Following are the clinical manifestations of antiepileptic drugs (Table 16).

Methemoglobinemia

Methemoglobin is a form of hemoglobin that contains ferric iron instead of ferrous form. Methemoglobinemia is a disorder characterized by the presence of a higher than normal level

Table 16: Clinical manifestation of anticonvulsant overdose.

Antiepileptic	Mechanism of action	Dose/half-life	Clinical features	Treatment
Carbamazepine	Voltage-gated sodium channel	Toxic dose 9 μg/mL	Cardiac–tachycardia, arrhythmia, hypotension CNS–nystagmus, mydriasis, seizures, respiratory depression, cerebellar and extrapyramidal signs GI – nausea, vomiting, hepatitis, cholestasis, hepatocellular necrosis Bone marrow suppression	Airway, breathing, circulation, gastric lavage, activated charcoal, WBI IV benzodiazepine
Phenytoin	Blocking voltage gated sodium channel	Toxic – half-life – 7–42 h	Ataxia, nystagmus, choreoathetoid movements, nausea, vomiting, seizures, opisthotonic posturing	Airway, breathing, circulation, gastric lavage, activated charcoal, hemodialysis
Phenobarbitone	GABA inhibition, opening of chloride channel	Toxic dose >60 mg/dL Half-life – 30–75 h	Respiratory depression, areflexia, coma, bradycardia, hypotension, ileus	Airway, breathing, circulation, activated charcoal, hemodialysis
Sodium valproate	Sodium channel inactivation GABA inhibition Attenuation of calcium channel	Toxic dose >200–400 mg/dL Half-life – 15 h	CNS depression – drowsiness, coma, ataxia, multiorgan involvement, severe hyperammonemic encephalopathy, cerebral edema, hepatotoxicity, pancreatitis, marrow failure, circulatory collapse	Airway, breathing, circulation Decontamination Symptomatic and supportive management for CNS, respiratory depression Hemodialysis – cardiovascular and neurotoxicity L-carnitine – 50 mg/kg 8th hourly

(CNS: central nervous system; GABA: gamma aminobutyric acid; GI: gastrointestinal; WBI: whole bowel irrigation)

of methemoglobin. Methemoglobinemia reduces the ability of the red blood cell to release oxygen to tissues causing tissue hypoxia.

One should suspect methemoglobinemia in the following situations.

- Any child who presents with clinical cyanosis or whose SpO_2 is less than or around 85% with no cardiac or pulmonary cause for cyanosis
- SpO_2 does not increase beyond 85% even with 100% FiO_2
- Presence of saturation gap, i.e., discrepancy between oxygen saturation in ABG and SpO_2 on pulse oximetry

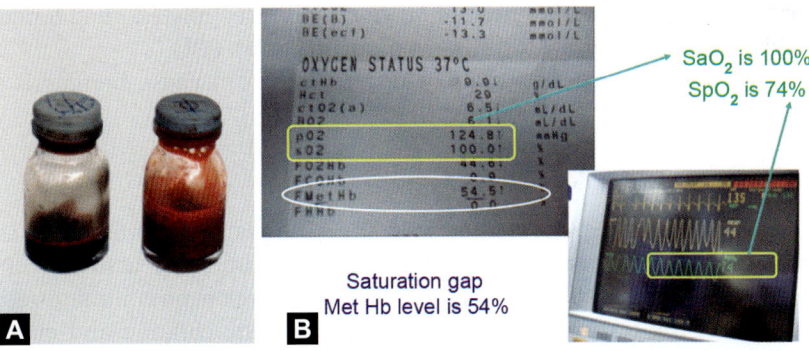

Figs. 8A and B: (A) Chocolate brown color of the blood with control; (B) Co-oximetry report and pulse oximeter reading.

- Presence of chocolate brown-colored arterial blood (color does not change with addition of O_2). This is a useful bedside test. Done on a blotting paper. If cyanosis was secondary to cardiac or pulmonary disease the chocolate brown color will change to red on exposure to air which contains oxygen, in methemoglobinemia the color continues to be brown (Figs. 8A and B).

Causes

Congenital or acquired.

Acquired causes include:
- *Drugs*: Dapsone, chloroquine, benzocaine, EMLA which contains lidocaine and prilocaine, flutamide, metoclopramide, nitrates, nitric oxide, nitroglycerine, nitroprusside, phenazopyridine, lidocaine, prilocaine, primaquine, amyl nitrate, silver nitrate, sodium nitrate, and sulfonamides
- *Others*: Aniline dyes, naphthalene, fume inhalation, herbicides, certain industrial chemicals, and pesticides, etc.

Clinical Features

Symptoms depend on the percentage of methemoglobin in the blood. Normally it should be less than 1%. Cyanosis occurs if more than 10% of hemoglobin is methemoglobin. As the percentage of methemoglobin increases the symptoms of tissue hypoxia develop.
- Irritability, altered mental status, tachypnea, tachycardia, abnormal cardiac rhythm, and seizures
- Older children can complain of headache, dyspnea, chest pain, palpitation, and confusion.

Investigations

- Perform co-oximetry analysis of the blood to confirm and know the degree of methemoglobinemia.

- *Other laboratory parameters that need to be monitored*: Electrolytes, renal function, ABG (varying degree of metabolic acidosis due to tissue hypoxia), CBC
- G6PD level before administering methylene blue as it can cause hemolysis in G6PD deficient individuals.

Management

- *General*: Give 100% oxygen (pulse oximeter reading is unreliable). Hydration and correction of acidosis. Remove the offending agent if possible, administer activated charcoal if methemoglobinemia secondary to drug ingestion and there are no contraindications
- *Methylene blue* is the treatment of choice in symptomatic children and children with methemoglobin level more than 30% (some treat >20%). Lower threshold is needed for treating children with chronic anemia, severe cardiopulmonary disease. It is contraindicated in patients with G6PD deficiency. Methylene blue 1–2 mg/kg IV as a 1% solution (max. 50 mg) over 10 minutes. Total dose should not exceed 7 mg/kg (in infants 4 mg/kg) – high dose can cause dyspnea, chest pain, hemolysis, and methemoglobinemia. The response to methylene blue is rapid and improvement in SpO_2 is seen during the infusion itself. The dose may be repeated in 2–4 hours if the level of MetHb is still high 1 hour after the initial infusion
- Rebound methemoglobinemia may occur up to 18 hours after methylene blue administration, due to prolonged absorption of lipophilic agents from adipose tissue
- It is reasonable to perform serial measurements of MetHb levels following treatment with methylene blue
- In G6PD deficiency, blood transfusion or exchange transfusion, hyperbaric oxygen, or ascorbic acid (2 mg/kg) may be tried
- Blood transfusion or exchange transfusion may be helpful in patients with shock.
- Cimetidine can be used in dapsone-induced methemoglobinemia.

SUGGESTED READING

1. Dargan PI, Wallace CI, Joneslate AL. An evidence-based management of acute salicylate (aspirin) overdose. Emerg Med J. 2002;19:206-9.
2. DeBaun MR, Frei-Jones M, Vichinsty E. Methemoglobinemia. In: Kliegman RM, Geme JS, Schor NF, et al. (Eds). Nelson Textbook of Pediatrics, 19th ed. Philadelphia, USA: Elsevier; 2011. pp. 1672-3.
3. Kohli U, Kuttiat VS, Lodha R, et al. Profile of childhood poisoning at a tertiary care centre in North India. Indian J Pediatr. 2008;75:791-4.
4. Menon J, Mathew L. A case of carbon monoxide poisoning. Indian Pediatr. 2004;41:291-2.
5. Patel NK, Bayliss GP. Current and forthcoming approaches for systemic detoxification. In: Leroux JC, Zhang L (Eds). Advanced Drug Delivery Reviews, Vol. 90. USA: Science Direct, Elsevier; 2015. pp. 3-11.
6. Riordan M, Rylance G, Berry K. Poisoning in children 1: General management. Arch Dis Child. 2002;87(5):392-6.
7. Vasanthan M, James S, Shuba S, et al. Clinical profile and outcome of poisoning in children admitted to a tertiary referral center in South India. Indian J Child Health. 2015;2(4).

Envenomation (Snake Envenomation and Scorpion Sting)

31

Mahesh A Mohite

LEARNING OBJECTIVES

- Approach to a child with snake and scorpion envenomation
- Identify clinical syndromes and initiate appropriate first aid measures
- Remember Do's and Dont's of snake and scorpion envenomation
- Appropriate indications for ASV and scorpion antivenin

SNAKE ENVENOMATION

INTRODUCTION

Snake envenomation is a common medical problem in Asia, Africa, and South America. In India, cases are more often seen in rural setup. Every year about 45,000 deaths are reported (it may not be actual figure). There are about 3,500 species of snake worldwide of which 200 are poisonous. In India about 216 species of snakes are seen of which 52 species are poisonous. The species are divided into Elapidae, Viperidae, and Hydrophidae (Box 1). Common poisonous snakes seen in India are common cobra, king cobra, krait, Russell's viper, and saw-scaled viper.

EPIDEMIOLOGY

Most bites occur during day time, except certain nocturnal habitat snakes

Box 1: Important species of venomous snakes found in India.

Elapids
- *Cobras*:
  - Spectacled cobra (Naja naja)
  - Monocled cobra (Naja kaouthia)
  - King cobra (Ophiophagus hannah)
- *Kraits*:
  - Common krait (Bungarus caeruleus)
  - Banded krait (Bungarus fasciatus)

Viperidae
- Russell viper (Vipera russelli/Daboia russelii)
- Saw scaled viper (Echis carinatus)
- Bamboo pit viper, Himalayan pit viper, and Levantine viper

Hydrophidae
- Sea snakes (Enhydrina schistosa)

like krait where bites occur at night time or early morning. Physically active males in the age group of 11–50 years, especially those working in farms or construction sites are at maximum risk. Majority of bites occur on hands and legs, and about 40% on feet. Envenomation are usually seen from May to August (early and peak rainy season). Around 30–40% of all bites are poisonous, out of which about 40% are dry bites (poisonous snake bite without injection of venom).

Toxicity depends on size of victim, dose of venom, penetration of fangs, condition of fangs and venom glands, bites on face and trunk (being more vascular area) and direct injection into blood vessel, exertion following bite, size of snake, previous bite by snake (decreases severity), and time elapsed between bite and start of treatment. Clinical manifestations vary according to the type of snake. In Western India, Krait bites leading to severe neurotoxicity predominates (60–70%). Early antivenom administration before signs of envenomation appear, decreases mortality from 40% to less than 10%.

The Snake Venom

Snake venom is a complex mixture of various enzymes, nonenzymatic proteins, and polypeptides. The clinical features vary depending upon predominance of a particular component.
- *Enzymes*: Multiple enzymes like hydrolases, hyaluronidase, and proteases present in the snake venom are responsible for the local damage at the site of bite
- *Nonenzyme proteins*:
  - *Nerve growth factors:* These are mainly present in elapid and viperid venom. Recently its role is being evaluated for transverse myelitis and few other neurological diseases.
  - *Hemorrhagins:* Seen in viper venom
  - *Neurotoxin and cardiotoxins:* Seen in elapids and hydropids.
- *Nonezyme polypeptides*: These are lethal components of snake venom and are of mainly four types, i.e., neurotoxins, vasculotoxins, hemorrhagins, and cardiotoxins.
  - *Neurotoxins*: These are lethal neurotoxin seen in the venom of cobra (cobratoxin), krait (alpha, beta, and gamma-bungarotoxin), and sea snakes (erabutoxins).

  Cobra toxin, alpha-bungarotoxin, and erabutoxin cause reversible blockade of postsynaptic receptors. Cobratoxin and erabutoxin effect is rapidly reversible, but alpha-bungarotoxin is slow or nonreversible. Because of this property, in neuroparalytic snake envenomation, antivenom, and a cholinesterase inhibitor like neostigmine increases the synaptic levels of acetylcholine which competitively removes the venom from receptor site, thus reverting paralysis. Beta-bungarotoxin (krait) damages the cholinergic synaptic vesicles (presynaptic blockade) and the paralysis persists till natural recovery and regrowth of presynaptic plate which may take 4–6 weeks
  - *Vasculotoxins*: These causes endothelial and basement membrane injury (mainly exhibited by vipers) and leading to capillary leak, edema, and sometimes shock
  - *Hemorrhagins*: These are mainly exhibited by vipers. They work at various level of coagulation cascade. The Russell's viper toxin works as activated factor X and with calcium and factor V converts prothrombin to thrombin and further coagulation and fibrinolysis is accentuated. Certain viper venom acts as active thrombin and activate the cascade, also may cause fibrinolysis directly and leading to disseminated intravascular coagulation (DIC)-like picture

- *Cardiotoxin*: Cardiotoxins have direct effect on cell membranes of cardiac, smooth muscles, and skeletal muscles. They may lead to membrane depolarization and cardiac arrest.

CLINICAL FEATURES (OPHITOXEMIA)

Often patients present late to hospital due to reliance on local first aid measures and traditional healers. By the time, they present to a healthcare facility the signs of toxicity are full blown. Clinical symptoms are divided into:
- Initial symptoms of fright
- Local signs of envenomation
- Systemic toxicity.

Local Signs of Envenomation

These appear within 10–30 minutes of a bite. Local signs in cobra bites appear rapidly and characterised by local swelling, pain, and bleeding. Krait bites exhibit only local mark (may be imperceptible) and no other local signs. Local findings are severe in case of viperine bites including edema, pain, redness, bleeding, gangrenous patch, and bullae. Compartment syndrome may be seen in severe cases. Sea snakes have minimal local swelling and pain. Nonpoisonous snakes cause local symptoms that are usually nonprogressive.

Systemic Toxicity

Systemic manifestations usually start within 15 minutes to 1 hour, but may appear as late as 12 hours in elapids and up to 48 hours in vipers. Therefore in confirmed elapid bite, patient should be observed for at least 24 hours and in viper bite for at least 72 hours.

Elapids

Abdominal pain may start within 1 hour, due to submucosal bleeds and splanchnic vasoconstriction and ischemia. Selective neuromuscular blockade may gradually cause ptosis, difficulty in swallowing, neck flop, weakness of limbs, and ultimately respiratory failure and death. Cardiotoxicity and hemolysis can be observed in cobra bites. Krait bites have typical story in which an asymptomatic child who went to sleep normally, gets up at midnight with abdominal pain and is found dead or in respiratory failure early in the morning. This is described as "early morning syndrome" and is due to the nocturnal habitat of krait. Due to this course, in Konkan region where it is commonly seen, krait is also called as "Surya Kandar" means "dead by sunrise".

Vipers

They exhibit mainly vasculotoxicity, hemolysis, and coagulopathy. Bleeding from local sites, progressive swelling with hemorrhagic bulle, and clotting abnormalities [prolonged bleeding time (BT), clotting time (CT), prothrombin time (PT), partial thromboplastin time (PTT)] are seen. In resource limited settings, a simple bedside test to detect viper envenomation is the 20 minutes whole blood clotting test (20-WBCT). For this test, 3–5 cc of blood is collected in a

Table 1: Clinical manifestations of different species.

Signs and symptoms	Viper	Krait	Cobra
Pain	+	–	+
Swelling	++ (minutes)	–	++ (hours)
Vomiting	+	+	+
Painful regional lymphadenopathy	+	+	+/–
Bleeding fang marks	+	–	–
Nonclotting blood	+	–	–
Hypotension/shock	+	+	+
Neuroparalysis	–	++	+
Musculoskeletal	+	–	–
Cardiotoxicity	+	–	+
Renal failure	++	–	–

clean and dry test tube and tube kept straight without disturbing for 20 minutes after which it is turned upside down. If blood is not clotted by then, the coagulopathy is confirmed. Progressive bleeding may lead to shock and multiorgan dysfunction leading to death. Kidneys are affected by shock, ischemia, myoglobinuria, and direct venom nephropathy.

Sea Snakes

Systemic manifestations start within 1–12 hours and leads to neurotoxicity similar to elapids. Additionally it is associated with severe myalgia, myoglobinuria, hyperkalemia, and renal failure. The comparison of clinical manifestations of different species is shown in Table 1.

TREATMENT

As in case of any emergency, first priority is to stabilize the victim. Ensure patent airway, proper breathing, and hemodynamic stability [airway, breathing, and circulation (ABC)] with necessary interventions. In case of impending neuroparalysis, if patient is to be transported to distant center, anticipate respiratory failure and pre-emptively intubate the patient to ensure adequate ventilation during referral.

First Aid

Reassurance

The fear of impending death causes fright reaction in victims. An older child should be counseled immediately while arranging other support systems. Parents also require counseling.

Immobilization

The affected (bite) area should be immobilized and splinted, if required. Any movement enhances proximal spread of the venom. Also the paralytic effect of elapid venom is aggravated by repeated movements and depolarization of presynaptic plate.

Tourniquet

Role of tourniquet is controversial and present evidence does not support it. Elapid venom being a very small molecule, quickly passes into circulation so tourniquet may not help. Similarly in vasculotoxic venom, its large molecule takes long to reach central circulation. Applying tourniquet may lead to local collection of venom causing more local damage.

Local Dressing (Pressure Immobilization)

Present recommendation is for local elastic bandage from distal to proximal limb, i.e., loose enough to allow two fingers slipping underneath it. The limb has to be monitored for vascular compromising effect, which may appear later due to progressive edema. If dressing is applied, it should be removed only after administration of antivenom.

Position of the Limb

The affected limb should be kept below the level of the heart until the antivenom is given. When there is severe local tissue damage (viper bite), the antivenom is given, by keeping the limbs at the level of the heart. In neurotoxic bite, limb should be below the level of the heart to reduce venom reaching central circulation.

Incision and suction is harmful and not recommended. Tetanus toxoid should be given to every victim as snake bite wounds are tetanus prone. Antibiotic prophylaxis may be needed in cases with contaminated wounds.

Treatment Inside Hospital

If the snake is killed, it should be identified so that type of toxicity can be anticipated and future catastrophe can be avoided. Be careful while examining dead snake as reflex bite may occur for a few hours after death of the snake. Treatment components include:
- Antivenin therapy
- Management of shock
- Neurological management
- Hematological management
- Supportive management.

Antivenom (Antisnake Venom)

Antisnake venom (ASV) is the mainstay of treatment. In India, a polyvalent antivenin, active against the four common poisonous snakes (cobra, krait, Russell's viper, and saw-scaled viper) is available in a lyophilized form. Each vial is reconstituted with 10 mL of distilled water. On average potency, 1 mL antiserum neutralizes 0.6 mg cobra, 0.45 mg krait, 0.6 mg Russell's viper, and 0.45 mg saw-scaled viper venom. A new Fab fragment antivenom (CroFab) for the treatment of crotaline envenomation, the predominant venomous snakebite in the United States is available commercially. It is not effective against king cobra, banded krait, and sea snake.

Antisnake venom is produced both in liquid and lyophilized forms. There is no evidence to suggest which form is more effective. Liquid ASV requires a reliable cold chain and has 2-year shelf life. Lyophilized ASV, in powder form, has 5-year shelf life and requires only to be

Table 2: Indication for administration of antisnake venom (ASV).

Local indications	Systemic indications
• Local swelling involving more than 50% of the affected limb within 48 hours • Swelling after bite on digits • Rapid extension of swelling • Enlargement of drainage lymph nodes	• Hemostatic abnormalities • Neurotoxicity • Cardiovascular abnormality • Actual renal failure • Hemoglobinuria or myoglobinuria

Table 3: Severity of snake envenomation and number of vials needed.

Severity	Features	Dose (number of vials)
Mild	Only local signs with or without lymphadenopathy	5–10
Moderate	Mild systemic signs, bleeding tendency, and hypotension	10–20
Severe	Severe local signs, disseminated intravascular coagulation (DIC), shock, and paralysis	20–30

kept cool. It is manufactured by Haffkine Institute, Mumbai and Center Research Institute, Kasauli. Haffkine Institute provides ASV as dry powder which is to be reconstituted and has longer shelf life.

Indications: It is indicated in all patients with signs and symptoms of local or systemic (i.e., coagulopathy or neurotoxicity) envenomation and asymptomatic bites occurring indoors and at night as it is highly indicative of krait envenomation. Essentially systemic envenomation will be evident from the 20-WBCT, signs of spontaneous bleeding or by visual recognition of neurological impairment such as ptosis. The various indications for administration of ASV are shown in Table 2. Only unbound, free flowing venom in bloodstream or tissue fluid can be neutralized by it. It carries the risk of anaphylactic reaction and doctors should be prepared to handle such reactions.

A common problem in our country is delayed presentation with renal failure (several days after the bite). The decision to give ASV depends on presence of unbound venom. Perform a 20-WBCT to determine if any coagulopathy is present. If it is present, administer ASV, otherwise treat renal failure. In the case of neurotoxic envenomation, with symptoms such as ptosis, respiratory failure, etc., it is wiser to administer one dose of 8–10 vials of ASV to ensure that no unbound venom is present. However, at this stage it is likely that most of the venom is bound and respiratory support will be required.

Dose and administration: Symptomatology is not of much help in determining the severity of envenomation as it is too dynamic and constantly evolving. ASV therapy should be individualized. The guidelines for ASV administration is given in Table 3.

The dose for children is same as for adults. The initial dose is 10 vials (10 mL each) for both adults and children; it is calculated to neutralize the average dose of venom injected. This ensures that the majority of victims would be covered by the initial dose. A maximum ASV dose of around 25 vials may be used. However, the available data do not suggest any advantage in following a high-dose regime.

Mode of administration: The total dose should be diluted with 10 mL/kg of distilled water or isotonic saline and infused intravenously at a rate of 2–4 mL/min. ASV should be administered over 1 hour at constant speed and patient should be closely monitored for 2 hours. Adrenaline infusion, antihistamines, and corticosteroids should be kept handy for hypersensitivity reaction. Local administration of ASV near or at the bite site should not be done. It is ineffective, painful and can raise the intra-compartmental pressure.

Adverse reactions, either anaphylactic or pyrogenic, have often been cited as reasons for not administering ASV in smaller local hospitals. The fear of these potentially life-threatening reactions has caused reluctance amongst some doctors to treat snakebite. However, if handled early, these reactions are easily surmountable and should not restrict doctors from treating snakebite.

At the first sign of any of the following—urticaria, itching, fever, shaking chills, nausea, vomiting, diarrhea, abdominal cramps, tachycardia, hypotension, bronchospasm, and angioedema, ASV should be discontinued and 0.01 mg/kg body weight of 1:1,000 adrenaline should be given intramuscular (IM). In addition, to provide protection against anaphylactic reactions, 0.2 mg/kg of antihistamine and 2 mg/kg of hydrocortisone should be administered intravenously. If after 10–15 minutes the patient's condition has not improved or is worsening, a second dose of adrenaline is given IM. This can be repeated for a third and final dose, but in the vast majority of reactions, two doses of adrenaline will be sufficient. Once the patient has recovered, the ASV can be restarted slowly for 10–15 minutes, keeping the patient under close observation. Then the normal drip rate should be resumed. Late serum sickness can be treated with oral prednisolone and/or antihistaminics.

Antisnake venom test doses have been abandoned. They have no predictive value in anaphylactic or late serum reactions and may sensitize the patient to the protein. There are no systematic trials of sufficient power to show that any prophylactic regimes are effective in preventing ASV reactions.

Repeat doses of antisnake venom: In antihemostatic bites, once the initial dose has been administered over 1 hour, no further ASV is given for 6 hours. This is due to the inability of the liver to replace clotting factors in less than 6 hours. The 20-WBCT test needs to be repeated every 6 hourly, which will determine if additional ASV is required. If repeat WBCT is more than 20 minutes repeat dose of 5–10 vials of ASV should continue 6 hourly till coagulation is restored. In the case of neurotoxic bites, once the first dose has been administered, and a neostigmine test given, the victim is closely monitored. If after 1–2 hours the victim has not improved or has worsened, then a second and final dose (10 vials) should be given. Once the patient develops respiratory failure, and has received 20 vials, ASV therapy should be discontinued assuming that all the circulating venom is neutralized.

Support Management

Shock management of snake bite is just the same as distributive and hypovolemic shock with crystalloids, colloids, vasopressor drugs, and noninvasive and invasive monitoring.

Neurological Support

Mechanical ventilation is needed for neuromuscular paralysis and respiratory failure. Neostigmine is an anticholinesterase, which is particularly effective in postsynaptic neurotoxins such as those of cobra and is not useful against presynaptic neurotoxin, i.e., common krait and the Russell's viper. Neostigmine should be started at the earliest evidence of neuroparalysis. Five intravenous (IV) doses of 0.05 mg/kg are administered every 30 minutes initially. The interval between doses is then gradually increased till neurological recovery occurs. Each dose of neostigmine is preceded by IV dose of atropine (0.02 mg/kg). Respiratory muscle paralysis may require mechanical ventilatory support.

Renal Failure

It is a poor prognostic sign and continuous monitoring of intravascular volume and urine output can prevent it. If acute kidney injury is established, fluid restriction, correction of electrolyte abnormalities, and renal replacement therapy may be needed.

Surgical Management

Severe local edema, tissue necrosis, and compartment syndrome may require surgical decompression. Compartment syndrome in a limb can be diagnosed from pain, paresis, pressure, paresthesia, tingling numbness, absent pulses, and pain on passive stretch. Decompression is rarely required and usually not done within first 3–4 days of bite.

Advances

The cost of antivenin is exorbitant and prohibitive in developing world. A polypeptide molecule is under research, which will bind the venom molecule before it binds the target tissue and this will prevent the further catastrophe. Being a polypeptide molecule manufactured commercially it will be much economical.

Prognosis

A lower body weight increases children's susceptibility to the lethality of the venom. The degree of provocation, number of bites, state of the fangs, number of bites by the snakes in preceding few hours as well as the quantitative and qualitative characteristics of venom are the major determinants of outcome. The location of the bite is of extreme clinical importance. Incidental injection of venom into an artery or vein greatly enhances the potential for systemic envenomation, commonly resulting in the victim's death. Bites to the head and faces are much more serious than bites sustained on an extremity. Bites on an upper extremity tend to have a worse prognosis than bites on a lower extremity. In hospitalized children, death occurs in 3–5% patients. The death in viper envenomation occurs because of severe DIC and hemorrhage (internal or from local site), hypotension or pulmonary edema, and in Elapidae bites is due respiratory paralysis.

KEY POINTS

- *Do it right*: Reassure, immobilize the limb, get to hospital, and tell doctor about snake bite and symptoms.
- Avoid incision and suctioning, tourniquet, tight bandage, killing the snake, and wasting time with traditional healers.

- Provide first aid and shift the patient to a center with all backup facility after giving antivenin immediately.
- Give ASV dose as soon as possible.
- Supportive care is cornerstone in management of snake envenomation.

SCORPION ENVENOMATION

INTRODUCTION

Scorpion sting envenomation (SSE) is common medical emergency predominantly seen in rural India. SSE is associated with substantial morbidity and mortality in children. It is commonly seen in Konkan region of Maharashtra, northern Karnataka, Andhra Pradesh, Tamil Nadu, and Puducherry. Recent improvement in understanding of basic pathophysiology, clinical profile, use of prazosin (an α-blocker), and use of scorpion antivenom has resulted in significant decrease in mortality.

INCIDENCE

The SSE is more common in rural areas. Scorpions are found in dry paddy farms, house roofs, and soil burrows. The sting happens accidentally in young males while working in farms and is common on hands and feet. Small children may get stings at home from scorpions, which drops from roofs or while playing near house. SSE commonly occur in early monsoon when rain water enters burrows of scorpion thus displacing them out. Stings are common from March to June and October to December.

The Scorpion

There are about 1,500 species of scorpion world over of which 50 are poisonous. In India, about 86 species are found of which *Mesobuthus tamulus* is the most poisonous and common. *M. tamulus* commonly known as the red scorpion is the most poisonous and found in Konkan, Karnataka, and Pondicherry. Its venom predominantly leads to cardiotoxicity. Poisonous scorpions are also found in West Asia, South America, and Mexico.

The Venom

The venom contains enzymes and nonenzymatic proteins. The venom of *M. tamulus* causes autonomic storm and leads to predominant cardiotoxicity. Few American scorpions cause neurotoxicity leading to neuromuscular paralysis. Few West Indian scorpions cause pancreatitis and severe metabolic derangements. The Indian red scorpion causes three major derangements either serially or simultaneously.
- Parasympathetic stimulation
- Sympathetic storm
- Metabolic derangements.

Flowchart 1: Pathogenesis of scorpion venom.

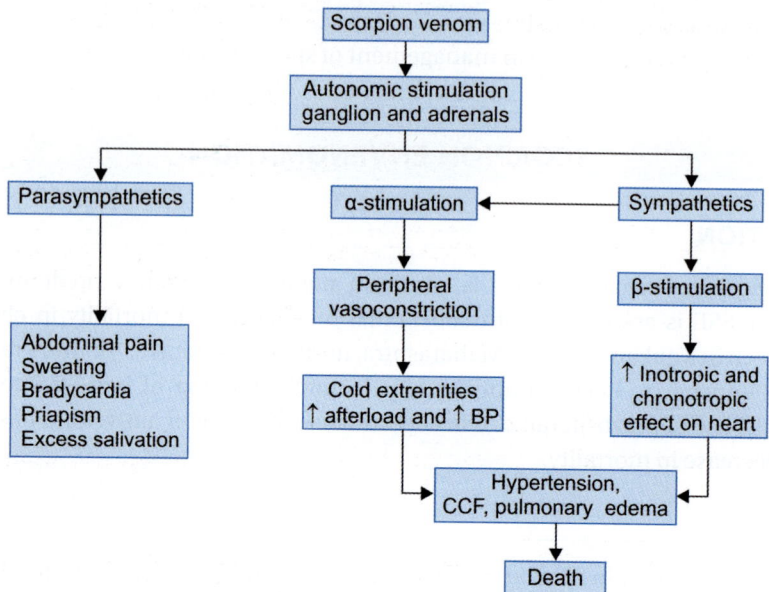

(CCF: congestive cardiac failure; BP: blood pressure)

PATHOGENESIS

The pathogenesis in red scorpion is the characteristic "autonomic storm". There is intense stimulation of autonomic system initially parasympathetic followed by sympathetic (Flowchart 1). The former manifests as bradycardia, hyperperistalsis, abdominal pain, excess sweating, salivation, and priapism. The latter due to strong α-receptor stimulation leads to vasoconstriction and severely increased cardiac afterload. The β-receptor stimulation increases cardiac contraction and heart rate. Combined effect of the two leads to extreme hypertension, cardiac failure, pulmonary edema, and if not treated appropriately, to death.

Certain metabolic derangements also appear with SSE (Flowchart 2). The venom stimulates α-receptors in pancreas inhibiting insulin secretion and causing hyperglycemia and diabetic ketoacidosis like states. Stress hormones come into play leading to breakdown of fats that leads to increase plasma lipids and free fatty acid levels. This can induce severe arrhythmias and DIC.

CLINICAL FEATURES

Clinical features reflect the underlying pathological process. Many times the sting is nonpoisonous leading to only local symptoms; pain and tingling. The poisonous stings are usually minimally painful or painless and pain may appear after vasodilator treatment is started.

In case of poisonous sting, the symptoms evolve through the following phases (Flowchart 3):

Flowchart 2: Metabolic derangements of scorpion sting envenomation.

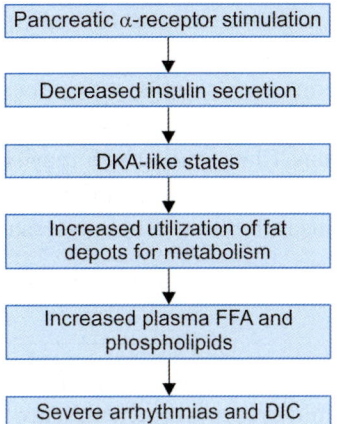

(DIC: disseminated intravascular coagulation; DKA: diabetic ketoacidosis; FFA: free fatty acid)

Flowchart 3: Phases of poisonous and nonpoisonous sting.

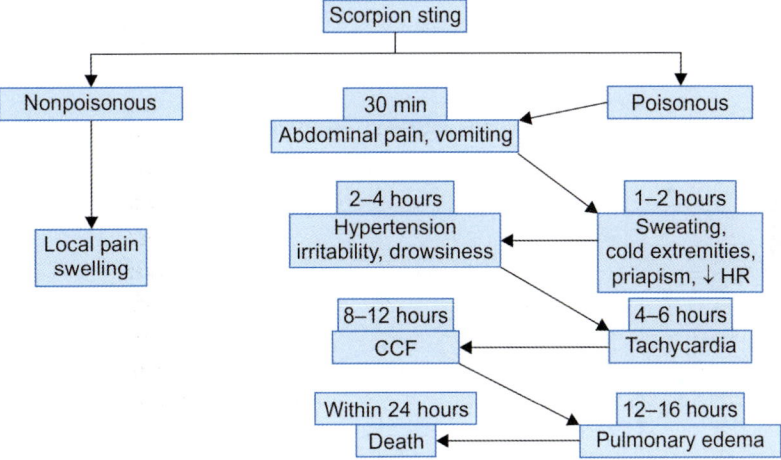

(CCF: congestive cardiac failure)

- *Parasympathetic phase*: It is characterized by intense sweating, abdominal pain, vomiting, borborygmi, bradycardia, and priapism (the pathognomonic sign in male victims). Usually this stage lasts for 2–4 hours, but at times this phase can be very short
- *Sympathetic phase*: The rapid onset of sympathetic phase indicates severe envenomation. In sympathetic phase child will have tachycardia, cold extremity, poor pulses, narrow pulse pressure, and hypertension. This phase usually lasts for 4–6 hours. If not treated appropriately, this phase culminates into cardiac failure and pulmonary edema. With no treatment death may ensue after 6–12 hours of sting.

DIAGNOSIS

Diagnosis is clinical and there is no laboratory test to confirm the diagnosis. Mostly patient is brought with history of sting and scorpion seen at site. The rural population brings killed scorpion for recognition. Seldom definitive history is not available and the clinical toxidrome of autonomic storm helps diagnose the case. In late stages, electrocardiogram (ECG) may show ischemic changes and arrhythmias. Chest radiograph may show signs of pulmonary edema. Cardiac enzymes may be abnormal; propeptide of brain natriuretic peptide (proBNP) levels may be raised; however, the trends rather than single assessment are more helpful for assessing cardiac function.

TREATMENT

Scorpion sting envenomation is a medical emergency and treatment depends upon the phase of envenomation in which the child presents to a healthcare facility. For nonpoisonous sting, usually pain relief, proper hydration, and reassurance is sufficient. If in doubt, the child may be observed for evolution of symptoms.

Local treatment has no role. In case of poisonous stings, the venom molecule is very small and quickly slips into central circulation, hence negating the role of tourniquet or local suction. When patient presents with signs of envenomation, following graph (Fig. 4) of management can be followed.

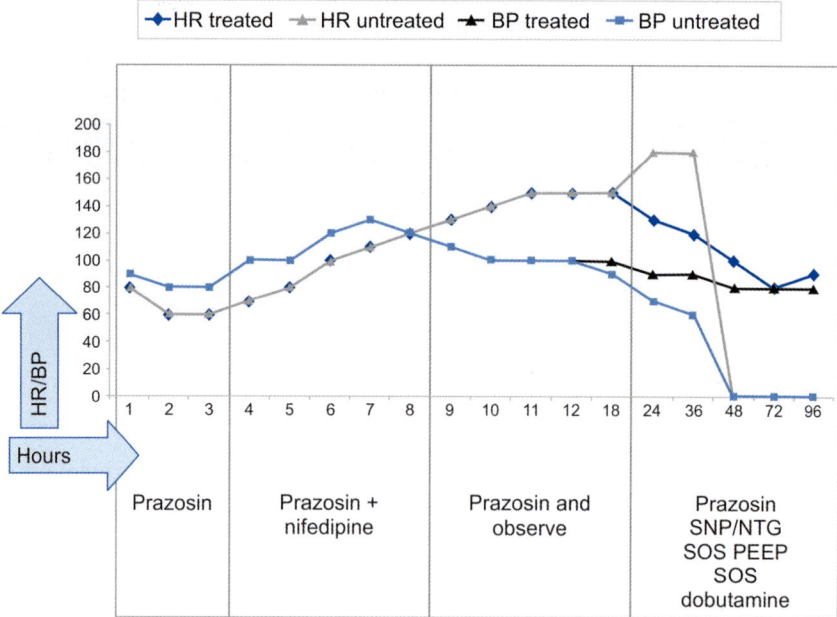

Fig. 4: Time correlation of clinical features of scorpion sting (based on pathophysiology) and appropriate treatment.
(BP: blood pressure; HR: heart rate; NTG: nitroglycerine; PEEP: positive end-expiratory pressure; SNP: sodium nitroprusside)

Treatment is guided by the stage of envenomation:
- *Early parasympathetic phase*: Hydrate well administer prazosin 30–40 µg/kg stat orally. If patient can not take orally given by nasogastric (NG) tube. Monitor patient for further progress. Repeat two doses of prazosin in the dose of 20 µg/kg each at 4 hourly intervals. Monitor hemodynamics, repeat same dose after next 6 hours twice. After 24 hours usually no more doses are needed.
- *Sympathetic phase*: Prazosin 40 µg/kg stat and subsequent doses as mentioned above. If patient has hypertension without congestive cardiac failure (CCF), sublingual nifedipine 0.5 mg/kg single dose is given (maximum 5 mg) and blood pressure (BP) is monitored. Repeat dose can be given 4–6 hourly. If signs of CCF are present, nifedipine (calcium channel blocker) or any other negative inotropic drug should be avoided. Sometimes vasodilators may be useful to counter the α-receptor stimulation induced vasoconstriction and hypertension; however, stringent monitoring is required.
- *Cardiac failure and pulmonary edema*: Prazosin along with supportive management for CCF is to be done. Intubation and positive pressure ventilation [positive end-expiratory pressure (PEEP)] will help tide over the crisis. Sometimes children present in pulmonary edema and severe vasoconstriction. In such situations, inotropic support with adrenaline (if hypotensive pulseless) or dobutamine [normotensive of at third percentile of Measures of Academic Progress (MAP)], along with a small dose of vasodilator (sodium nitroprusside or nitroglycerine) can be used under invasive monitoring.

The critical phase lasts for 3–4 days. On recovery most patients have severe bradycardia probably due to adrenaline exhaustion. If patient is hemodynamically stable, no treatment is required. The bradycardia may last for 1 week. In the intensive phase, dysglycemias and electrolyte derangements should be managed as per standard protocols.

Recently some trials are showing promising results with respect to scorpion antivenom. The antivenom should be derived from local species of poisonous scorpion. It has to be given in early stages of envenomation. Antivenom along with prazosin protocol has shown better results. Exact dose of antivenom is not standardized but initially two vials are given IV and are repeated after 6 hours if clinical features of envenomation persist.

PROGNOSIS

Following factors determine severity of envenomation and prognosis:
- Size of the victim
- Posthibernation sting has severe envenomation
- Number of victims in one stage sting; first victim getting maximum dose
- Stage of presentation; later sympathetic stage has grave prognosis
- Intensity of management received.

SUGGESTED READINGS

Snake Envenomation

1. Simpson ID. The pediatric management of snakebite the national protocol. Indian Pediatr. 2007;44(3):173-6.
2. Mahadevan S, Ingrid Jacobsen. National snakebite management protocol (India), 2008. l. Indian J Emerg Pediatr. 2009;1(2):63-84.

3. Simpson ID. A study of current knowledge base in treating snake bite among doctors in high risk countries of India and Pakistan: Does snake bite treatment training reflect local requirements? Trans R Soc Trop Med Hyg. 2008;102:1108-14.
4. Kasturiratne A, Wickramsinghe AR, DeSilva N, et al. The global burden of snakebite: A literature analysis and modelling based on regional estimates of envenoming and deaths. PLOS Med. 2008;5:e218.
5. Bawaskar HS, Bawaskar PH. Profile of envenoming in western Maharashtra in India. Royal Soc Trop Med Hua. 2002;96:79-84.
6. Warrel DA. Venom, toxins and plant poisons. In: Weatneral DS (Ed). Oxford textbook of medicine. NY, Oxford University Press; 1996. pp. 1124-39.
7. Dayal S, Lall SB. Management of common Indian snake and insect bites. New Delhi: Noble Vision; 1997. pp. 17-23.
8. Alirol E, Sharma SK, Bawaskar HS, et al. Snake bite in South Asia: a review. PLoS Negl Trop Dis. 2010;4:e603.
9. Simpson ID, Tanwar PD, Andrade C, et al. The Ebbinghaus retention curve: training does not increase the ability to apply pressure immobilisation in simulated snake bite—implications for snake bite first aid in the developing world. Trans R Soc Trop Med Hyg. 2008;102:451-9.
10. Anil A, Singh S, Bhalla A, et al. Role of neostigmine and polyvalent antivenin in Indian common krait (Bungarus caeruleus) bite. J Infection Public Health. 2010;3(2):83-7.
11. Simpson ID. Snakebite management in India, the first few hours: A guide for primary care physicians. J Indian Med Assoc. 2007;105:324-35.
12. Schmidt JM. Antivenom therapy for snakebites in children: is there evidence? Curr Opin Pediatr. 2005;17(2):234-8.

Scorpion Envenomation

1. Bawaskar HS, Bawaskar PH. Scorpion sting: update. J Assoc Physicians India. 2012;60:46-55.
2. Bawaskar HS, Bawaskar PH. Quarterly Medical Review: Management of Snake Bite and Scorpion Sting. Mumbai: Raptakos, Breet & Co. Ltd., 2009. pp. 4-26.
3. Sagindar. Handbook on treatment guidelines for snake bite and scorpion sting. Chennai: Tamil Nadu health systems project health and family welfare Department; 2008. pp. 45-64.
4. Bawaskar HS. Scorpion sting. Trans R Soc Trop Med Hyg. 1984;78(3):414-15.
5. Bawaskar HS, Bawaskar PH. Efficacy and safety of scorpion antivenom plus prazosin compared with prazosin alone for venomous scorpion (*Mesobuthus tamulus*) sting: randomised open label clinical trial. BMJ. 2011;342:c7136.
6. Mahadevan S. Scorpion sting. Indian pediatr. 2000;27:504-14.
7. Santhanakrishnan BR, Ranganathan G, Ananthasubramanium P. Cardiovascular manifestations of scorpion stings in children. Indian Pediatr. 1977;14:353-6.
8. Bawaskar HS, Bawaskar PH. Management of scorpion sting. Heart. 1999;82:253-4.
9. Bawaskar HS, Bawaskar PH. Prazosin in the management of cardiovascular manifestations of scorpion sting. Lancet. 1986;1:510-1.
10. Bawaskar HS. Diagnostic cardiac premonitory signs and symptoms of red scorpion sting. Lancet. 1982;2:552-4.
11. Prasad R, Misra OP, Pandey N, et al. Scorpion sting envenomation in children: factors affecting the outcome. Indian J Pediatr. 2011;78(5):544-8.
12. Natu VS, Murthy RK, Deodhar KP. Efficacy of species specific anti-scorpion venom serum (AScVS) against severe, serious scorpion stings (Mesobuthus tamulus concanesis Pocock)—an experience from rural hospital in western Maharashtra. J Assoc Physicians India. 2006;54:283-7.
13. Bawaskar HS, Bawaskar PH. Management of the cardiovascular manifestations of poisoning by the Indian red scorpion (Mesobuthus tamulus). Br Heart J. 1992;68:478-80.

32. Oncological Emergencies

Lalitha AV, Mounika Reddy, Vinay Munikoty

LEARNING OBJECTIVES

- Core concepts: Brief physiology and the altered pathophysiology in oncological emergencies
- Early recognition and assessment
- Structured approach and management.

INTRODUCTION

Oncological emergencies in children may be the first presentation of an underlying malignancy or may occur later in the course of disease or treatment. They often develop acutely and progress rapidly, therefore, anticipation, a high index of suspicion and astute clinical assessment are vital to the prevention, early recognition, and management of these emergencies. The common pediatric oncological emergencies are presented in Table 1.

Table 1: Common pediatric oncologic emergencies.

At the time of the diagnosis:	Metabolic:
• Tumor bulk causing metabolic disturbances • Tumor bulk causing obstructive problems **After intensive chemotherapy:** • Metabolic complications • Infectious complications	• Tumor lysis syndrome (TLS) • Syndrome of inappropriate antidiuretic hormone (SIADH) • Hypercalcemia **Hematological:** • Hyperleukocytosis • Disseminated intravascular coagulation (DIC) **Cardiovascular:** • Superior mediastinal syndrome (SMS)/superior vena caval syndrome (SVCS) • Malignant pericardial/pleural effusion **Infections:** Febrile neutropenia (FN) **Neurological:** • Spinal cord compression • Brain metastasis and raised intracranial pressure

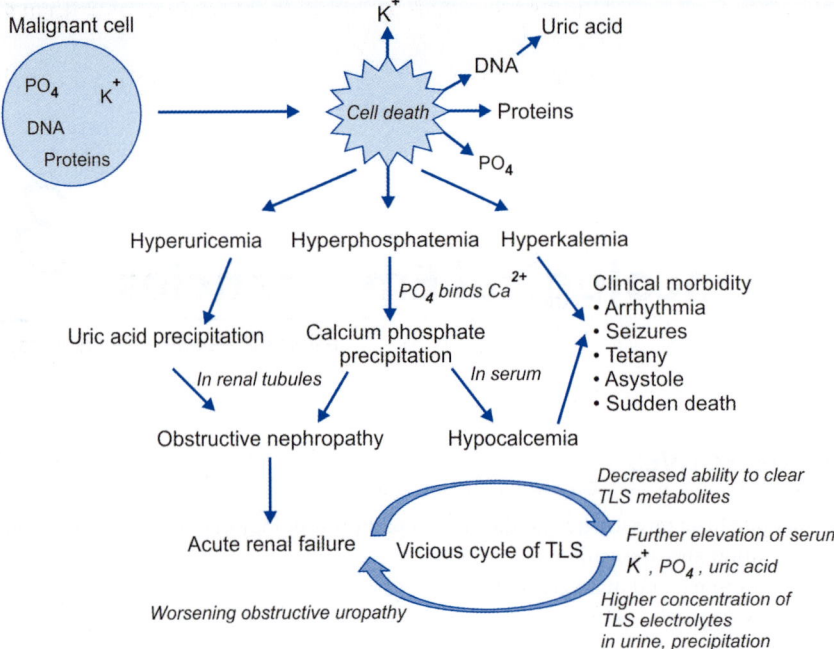

Fig. 1: Pathophysiology of TLS.
(TLS: tumor lysis syndrome)

TUMOR LYSIS SYNDROME

Core Concepts: Pathophysiology

Tumor lysis syndrome (TLS) is a constellation of metabolic derangements with or without systemic manifestations secondary to release of intracellular contents from rapid breakdown of tumor cells. It may result from spontaneous lysis of tumor cells or in response to therapy. The released intracellular contents—potassium, phosphate, and uric acid (product of nucleic acid metabolism) overwhelm the body's homeostatic mechanisms and renal excretion capacity. This results in acute kidney injury by their precipitation in renal tubules, secondary hypocalcemia, and inflammatory cytokine mediated multiorgan failure (Fig. 1).

Definition

The Cairo and Bishop Classification for TLS defines and classifies TLS as described in the text.

Biochemical or Laboratory (Asymptomatic) TLS

More than or equal to 2 of following metabolic abnormalities occurring simultaneously within 3 days before or up to 7 days after initiation of therapy.
- *Hyperuricemia*: Uric acid more than 8.0 mg/dL or above the upper limit of normal range for age in children
- *Hyperkalemia*: Potassium more than 6.0 mmol/L

- *Hyperphosphatemia*: Phosphorus more than 6.5 mg/dL in children or more than 4.5 mg/dL in adults
- *Hypocalcemia*: Corrected calcium less than 7.0 mg/dL or ionized calcium less than 1.12 mg/dL.

Clinical (Symptomatic) TLS

Laboratory TLS accompanied by any end-organ dysfunction.
- Acute kidney injury
- Cardiac arrhythmias, sudden death
- Seizures, neuromuscular irritability (tetany, paresthesias, laryngospasm, etc.).

Risk Factors and Risk Stratification

Though any malignancy can result in TLS, some tumor types and their specific characteristics predispose to high risk of TLS. The risk factors for TLS include:

Tumor Characteristics

- *Large tumor burden*: Hyperleukocytosis, massive intra-abdominal or mediastinal mass, massive hepatosplenomegaly
- *Rapid turnover*: For example, acute lymphoblastic leukemia (ALL), non-Hodgkin's lymphoma (NHL)
- *Highly chemosensitive*: Rapid lysis
- *Highly effective targeted therapies*: For example, rituximab in NHL.

Host Characteristics

- Small children
- *Volume-depleted state*: Poor oral intake, gastrointestinal losses such as vomiting, diarrhea
- Compromised baseline renal function
- Acidosis.

Others

- Coadministration of nephrotoxic drugs or contrast
- Tumor infiltrating kidneys or obstructing ureters.

Risk Stratification by Tumor Type

- *High risk*:
  - Burkitt's lymphoma or leukemia
  - ALL or leukemia [total leukocyte count (TLC) >50,000/mm^3]
  - Acute myeloid leukemia (TLC >20,000/mm^3)
  - Diffuse large B-cell lymphoma.

- *Low risk*: (Solid tumors)
  - Hepatoblastoma
  - Neuroblastoma
  - Nephroblastoma
  - Germ cell tumor.

Clinical Evaluation

The clinician should attempt to discern the rate of progression of malignancy by history and physical examination. Relevant history includes time of onset of symptoms referable to the malignancy, pace of growth of any palpable mass, symptoms of dehydration including decreased urine output, thirst, dizziness, vomiting, bleeding, and diarrhea. Other pertinent historical components that will help guide clinical decision making include presence of cramps, spasms, tetany, seizures, and altered consciousness suggestive of hypocalcemia. On examination, special attention should be given to blood pressure, heart rate and rhythm, abnormal masses, lymphadenopathy, hepatosplenomegaly, and presence of pleural or pericardial effusions or ascites.

Laboratory Evaluation

- Complete blood counts
- *Serum electrolytes*: Sodium, potassium, chloride, phosphate, calcium (total and ionized if indicated), bicarbonate
- Blood urea nitrogen, serum creatinine, uric acid, lactate dehydrogenase
- *Urinalysis*: pH, crystals, hematuria
- Electrocardiogram
- *Imaging studies*: Chest radiography is useful to determine the presence any mediastinal mass or effusions. Ultrasonography or computed tomography (CT) scanning of the abdomen and retroperitoneum is indicated if abdomen mass is present; intravenous contrast may be contraindicated in a patient with renal insufficiency.

Management

Early anticipation and prevention rather than treating established TLS is the key to management. Timely recognition and management of the metabolic derangements prevents the severe, life-threatening complications associated with TLS. The onset of oligoanuria is an ominous late sign. The principles of prevention and management of TLS are:
- *Aggressive intravenous hydration* is the cornerstone to both prevention and treatment. Potassium and calcium-free saline dextrose fluids up to 3 L/m^2/day (2–4 times maintenance fluids) are given to rapidly improve renal perfusion and glomerular filtration, targeting urine output of at least 2–4 mL/kg/h. High urine output is renoprotective. Hydration is started 48 hours prior and continued at least till 72 hours of initiation of chemotherapy.
- *Diuretics* (e.g., furosemide) should be tried in patients whose urine output remains low (<2 mL/kg/h) even after volume repletion with optimal hydration.
- *Management of hyperuricemia*: *Allopurinol* inhibits xanthine oxidase and prevents conversion of hypoxanthine and xanthine into uric acid. However, it does not remove

Flowchart 1: Pathway of nucleic acid metabolism and drugs acting on it.

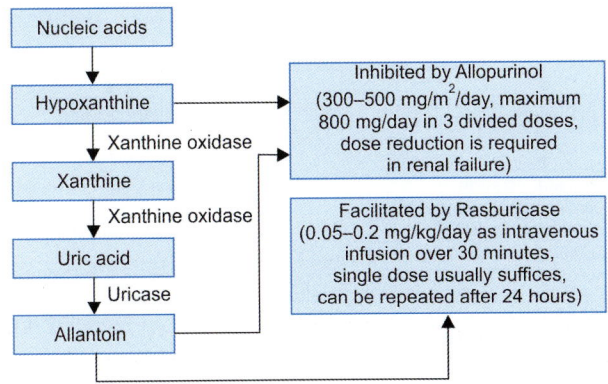

existing uric acid and can result in xanthine accumulation and nephropathy. In contrast, rasburicase (recombinant urate oxidase) removes uric acid by enzymatically degrading it into water-soluble allantoin, without accumulation of precursors like xanthine. Thus, rasburicase is more effective than allopurinol for prevention and treatment of TLS and reducing need for dialysis. When using rasburicase, blood samples for uric acid measurement must be transported in ice, to prevent breakdown and spuriously low level. It is contraindicated in glucose-6-phosphate dehydrogenase deficiency due to risk of methemoglobinemia and hemolytic anemia. The pathway of nucleic acid metabolism and the sites of action of allopurinol and rasburicase are depicted in Flowchart 1.

- *Management of individual metabolic abnormalities*:
  - *Hyperkalemia:* Avoid oral potassium and give calcium gluconate for membrane stabilization. Treat with insulin-dextrose infusion or beta-agonists for intracellular shift of potassium, and oral or per-rectal sodium polystyrene sulfonate to promote gastrointestinal excretion of potassium. Diuretics can be used for urinary excretion of potassium, if renal function is preserved. Renal replacement therapy is indicated, if hyperkalemia is refractory to medical management.
  - *Hyperphosphatemia:* Avoid oral phosphate. Oral phosphate binders like aluminum hydroxide, sevelamer may be considered.
  - *Hypocalcemia:* Treat only if symptomatic. Treat with the lowest dose of calcium required to relieve symptoms. Excess calcium increases calcium-phosphate product (>60 mg/dL^2) and promotes precipitation as calcium phosphate (ectopic calcification). Treating hyperphosphatemia in turn prevents hypocalcemia.
- *Urinary alkalinisation* was used previously as it increases uric acid solubility. However, it reduces calcium phosphate solubility, resulting in hyperphosphatemia and symptomatic hypocalcemia. It also aggravates obstructive uropathy due to precipitation of calcium, phosphate, and xanthine. As it is more difficult to correct hyperphosphatemia than hyperuricemia, urinary alkalinisation should be avoided, especially when rasburicase is available.

Flowchart 2: Algorithmic approach to the prevention and management of TLS.

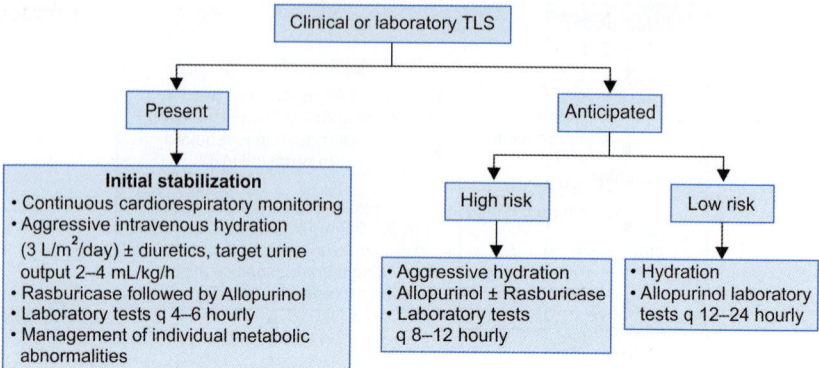

- *Treatment prophase in patients at high risk for TLS:* Low-intensity initial therapy with slower cancer cell lysis is preferred to allow better renal clearance. For example, a week of prednisone monotherapy in ALL, low-dose cyclophosphamide, vincristine, and prednisone for a week before intensive chemotherapy in advanced B-cell NHL or Burkitt's leukemia.
- *Indications of renal replacement therapy in TLS:* Should be considered if one or more of the following exists:
  - Hyperkalemia, hyperphosphatemia, hyperuricemia, hypocalcemia or metabolic acidosis refractory to medical management
  - Refractory volume overloads (pulmonary edema, etc.)
  - Uncontrolled hypertension
  - Severe uremia with neurological toxicity or bleeding diathesis

The algorithmic approach to the prevention and management of TLS is presented in Flowchart 2.

FEBRILE NEUTROPENIA

Core Concepts

Febrile neutropenia (FN) is suspected in any patient with malignancy on chemotherapy presenting with fever. Fever may be the only manifestation of serious infection in neutropenic children as other signs of systemic inflammation may be attenuated.

Definitions

- *Fever*: Single oral temperature more than or equal to 38.3°C (101°F) (or) oral temperature more than or equal to 38.0°C (100.4°F) for more than or equal to 1 hour
- *Neutropenia*: Absolute neutrophil count (ANC) less than 500/mm³ or expected to fall less than 500/mm³ in next 48 hours
- *Profound neutropenia*: ANC less than 100/mm³
- *Prolonged neutropenia*: Lasting more than 7 days.

Clinical Evaluation

Detailed history regarding the symptoms, possible focus of infection and the underlying risk factors must be elicited. The salient points in history include:
- Symptoms onset, duration, severity, localizing symptoms
- Phase of chemotherapy (intensive vs. nonintensive)
- Duration since last chemotherapy
- Recent hospitalization and antibiotics received
- Prior episodes of FN, organisms isolated, and course.

A thorough physical examination is warranted to not miss any clues to the diagnosis. Head to toe examination including ear, nose, throat, sinuses, oral cavity, eyes, skin, and nails along with respiratory, gastrointestinal, cardiovascular, neurological, genitourinary, and musculoskeletal system examination will be helpful. Do not forget to look at the perineum, intravascular catheter insertion site, and bone marrow aspiration site.

Laboratory Evaluation

- Complete blood counts including differential count
- Serum electrolytes, urea, creatinine
- Blood culture: Two sets from different venipuncture sites (one from central venous catheter, if present)
- Cultures from other sites, as clinically indicated: urine, stool, respiratory secretions, pus, cerebrospinal fluid (CSF), etc.
- *Chest radiograph*: if respiratory symptoms and signs are present
- Additional investigations may be indicated, if fever persists, for e.g., CT chest or paranasal sinuses, bronchoalveolar lavage, galactomannan, fungal cultures.

Risk Stratification

Risk stratification of FN patients is important in determining the appropriate choice of antimicrobials, route of administration (oral vs. intravenous), setting (outpatient vs. inpatient), and duration of therapy. The characteristics of low-risk and high-risk FN patients are as follows:

Low-risk Febrile Neutropenia Patients

- Clinically stable
- Nonintensive phase of chemotherapy, e.g., maintenance phase
- ANC is more than or equal to $100/mm^3$ and anticipated neutropenia is less than 7 days
- Absolute monocyte count is more than or equal to $100/mm^3$
- No focus of infection
- No comorbidities
- Assured follow-up and compliance with good oral intake.

High-risk Febrile Neutropenia Patients

- *Clinically unstable*: Respiratory distress, hypotension, encephalopathy, etc.
- Intensive phase of chemotherapy, e.g. induction, consolidation, intensification phases

- Profound or anticipated prolonged neutropenia
- Focus of infection presents, e.g. pneumonia, diarrhea, cellulitis, etc.
- Comorbidities present
- Mucositis causing poor oral intake and diarrhea
- Concerns regarding compliance and follow-up.

Management

Febrile neutropenia patients have a high probability of serious bacterial infection and must be attended to promptly. Any fever in a child on chemotherapy warrants immediate attention. Rapid triaging and administration of first-dose of empirical, broad-spectrum intravenous antibiotics within 30 minutes of presentation, after collecting appropriate cultures, improves outcomes. The choice of initial antimicrobials depends on local bacterial epidemiology and susceptibility patterns. Initially, two antibiotics with broad-spectrum gram-negative cover (e.g., Fluoroquinolone or cefoperazone-sulbactam or piperacillin-tazobactam ± aminoglycoside) are usually initiated. Additional gram-positive cover with vancomycin is indicated in the presence of hemodynamic instability, suspected catheter-related infection, pneumonia, skin and soft tissue infection, severe mucositis, or in case of known colonization with gram-positive organisms. The patient must be admitted and continuously monitored as there is high risk of rapid deterioration. Organ dysfunctions like respiratory failure and hemodynamic instability should be managed with appropriate supports.

Further management depends on the clinical course, response to treatment, and recovery of neutrophil counts. Once positive cultures are available, the antimicrobials are modified according to the susceptibility pattern. If fever is persistent or recurrent after 48–72 hours, send repeat cultures, and upgrade antibiotics. Risk of fungal infections increases with profound or persistent neutropenia and requires consideration of appropriate work-up and addition of an antifungal agent.

Rarely, a low risk FN patient may be managed on an outpatient basis with oral antibiotics provided follow-up and compliance to treatment is ensured. If fever persists for 48 hours, admission and intravenous antibiotics are warranted. The algorithmic approach to management of febrile neutropenia is presented in Flowchart 3.

SUPERIOR MEDIASTINAL SYNDROME

Core Concepts: Pathophysiology

Superior mediastinal syndrome (SMS) is a constellation of signs and symptoms caused by compression of the mediastinal structures (airway, great vessels) by mediastinal pathology. Superior vena caval syndrome (SVCS) is due to superior vena cava (SVC) obstruction secondary to external compression or internal thrombosis, thus impeding venous return. SMS includes SVCS and tracheobronchial obstruction. In children, it is most commonly due to a malignant mediastinal mass, usually lymphoma.

Flowchart 3: Algorithmic management of febrile neutropenia.

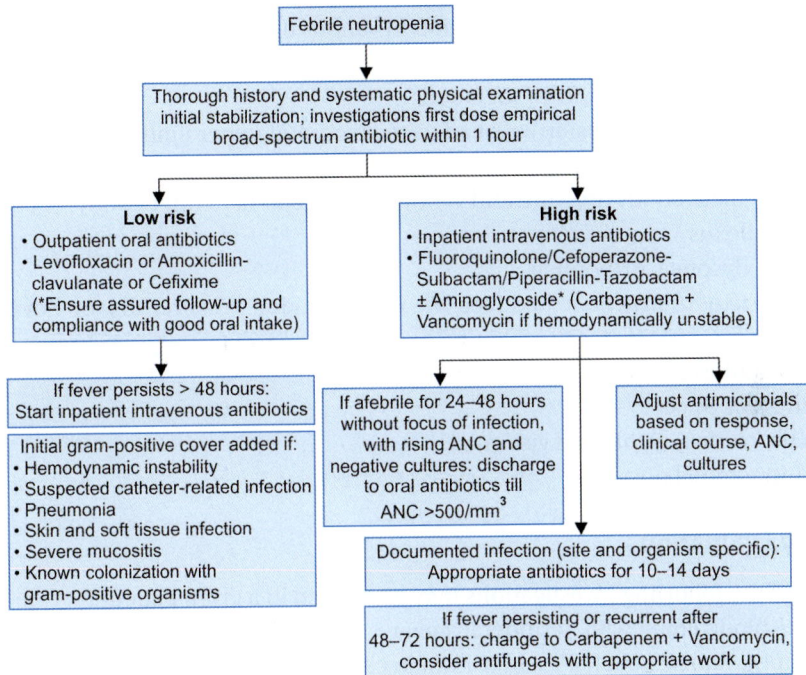

(ANC: absolute neutrophil count)

Etiology

Malignant masses are most common and include:
- *Anterior mediastinal masses*: (more likely to cause compression)
    - Non-Hodgkin lymphoma
    - ALL, usually T-cell ALL
    - Hodgkin lymphoma
    - Germ-cell tumor, teratoma
    - Thymic tumor
    - Acute myeloid leukemia (AML).
- *Posterior mediastinal masses*:
    - Neuroblastoma
    - Sarcoma
    - Rhabdomyosarcoma.

Nonmalignant causes include:
- *Infections*: Tuberculosis, fungal infections
- Mediastinal cysts
- Venous thrombosis (e.g. due to a central line).

Clinical Features

The clinical features are due to the obstruction to venous drainage of upper body and tracheobronchial obstruction. However, the severity of symptoms and signs does not always correlate with the degree of obstruction. They include:
- Edema and plethora (suffusion) of head, face, neck, and upper limbs
- Conjunctival edema or suffusion
- Elevated jugular venous pressure and venous engorgement in upper body
- Pulses paradoxus
- Tachypnea, dyspnea, orthopnea
- *Signs of airway obstruction*: Reduced air entry, stridor, wheeze, dry or bovine cough, cyanosis
- Chest discomfort
- Hoarseness of voice
- Headache, confusion, blurred vision
- Raised intracranial pressure.

Laboratory Evaluation

All or some of the following investigations may be needed in a given patient:
- Complete blood count with peripheral smear
- Serum alpha-feto protein (AFP), beta human chorionic gonadotropin (β-HCG)
- TLS work-up
- Chest imaging: X-ray or contrast CT or ultrasound—to look for mass location, size, airway compression, associated pleural or pericardial effusions (Fig. 2)
- Pleural or pericardial fluid for malignant cytology
- Fine needle aspiration cytology (FNAC) from an affected peripheral node
- Bone marrow aspiration and biopsy.

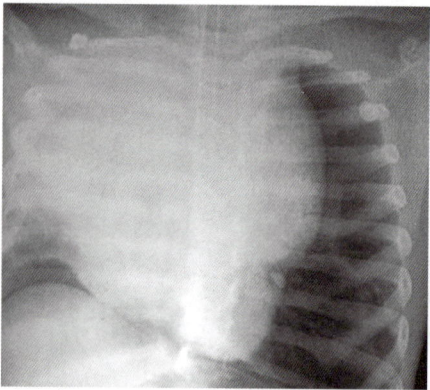

Fig. 2: Chest X-ray showing mediastinal mass.

Flowchart 4: Algorithmic management of superior mediastinal syndrome.

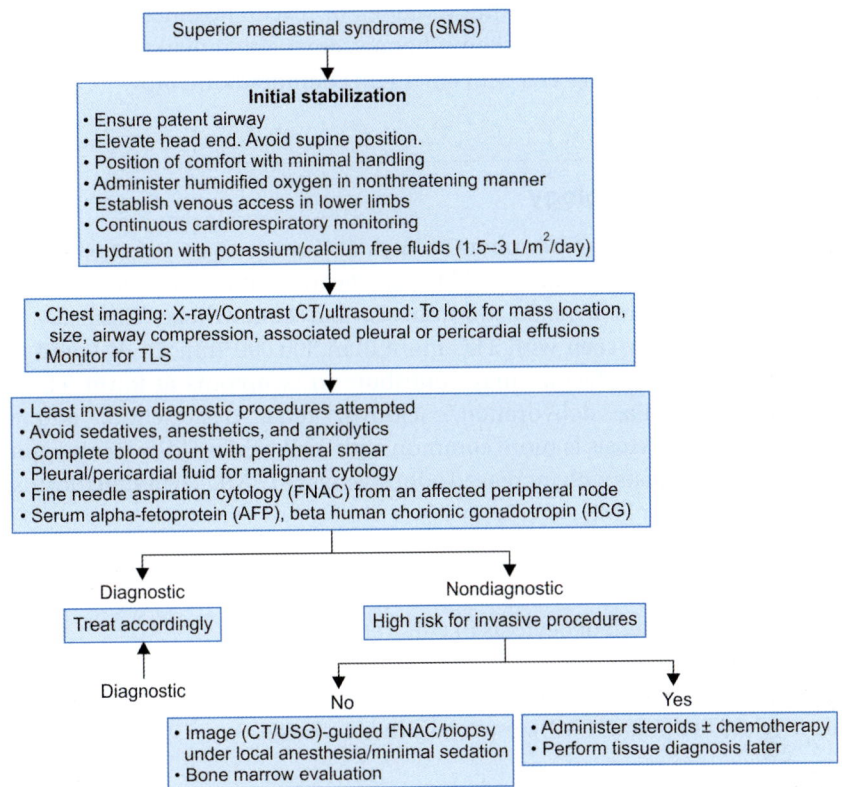

(CT: computed tomography; USG: ultrasonography)

Management

These children are at high risk of sudden adverse cardiorespiratory events and should be on continuous cardiorespiratory monitoring. Keep the head end elevated to 30–45° and ensure a parent airway. Avoid upper limb venous access for fluids and infusions as the increased hydrostatic pressure in the upper body venous system can worsen edema.

Tissue diagnosis and staging is desirable but not mandatory before initiating emergency management in SMS. The least invasive investigations or procedures enabling most rapid diagnosis are preferred and should be performed under local anesthesia avoiding the use of sedation or general anesthesia. The algorithmic approach to the management of SMS is presented in Flowchart 4.

In addition to stabilization and supportive measures, emergent chemotherapy may be required in life-threatening SMS to rapidly reduce tumor mass. Systemic steroids are usually the first line therapy as the most common cause of SMS in children is lymphoma or leukemia. Dexamethasone 4–6 mg/m²/day or hydrocortisone 5 mg/kg/dose 6 hourly intravenous can be given. A single dose of steroids usually suffices to stabilize the patient to allow diagnostic procedures and prolonged steroids (>24–48 hours) may impair subsequent tissue diagnosis. Additional agents like vincristine, anthracycline, or cyclophosphamide are sometimes required. If the tumor is insensitive to chemotherapy, emergent radiation may be considered. One must beware of precipitating TLS with emergent chemoradiotherapy.

HYPERLEUKOCYTOSIS

Core Concepts: Pathophysiology

Hyperleukocytosis is defined as peripheral blood TLC more than 100,000/mm³. It results in increased blood viscosity, leukemic blast aggregation and stasis in microcirculation causing organ damage from hypoxia, thrombosis, and hemorrhage. Clinically significant hyperleukocytosis is usually seen with TLC more than 300,000/mm³ in ALL and more than 200,000/mm³ in AML. Other factors may contribute to symptoms at lower TLC including anemia, thrombocytopenia, dehydration, acidosis, renal dysfunction, and infection. Symptomatic hyperleukocytosis is more common with AML while TLS is more common with ALL, likely due to larger blasts with increased adhesiveness in AML. Hyperleukocytosis is often associated with TLS and/or SMS.

Etiology

The common causes of hyperleukocytosis in children include:
- Acute myeloid leukemia
- Acute lymphoblastic leukemia (ALL), especially T-cell ALL, infant ALL, hypodiploid ALL
- Chronic myeloid leukemia (CML), especially in blast crisis.

Clinical Features

The various clinical presentations include:
- *Neurological*: Headache, vomiting, irritability, altered sensorium, seizures, focal neurological deficits, raised intracranial pressure
- Visual disturbance, papilledema
- *Respiratory*: Respiratory distress, hypoxia, diffuse lung infiltrates
- *Gastrointestinal*: Pain abdomen, hematemesis, melena
- *Others*: Priapism, clitoral enlargement, dactylitis
- Metabolic derangements and TLS due to increased tumor burden.

Differential Diagnosis

- *Leukemoid reaction*: High TLC (mostly mature cells), usually 50,000–1,00,000/mm³ in non-malignant conditions, especially infections like pertussis, and inflammatory disorders. They are usually mature leukocytes
- High nucleated red cell count may be erroneously interpreted as elevated TLC in counter, e.g., in neonates and in thalassemia major patients
- In these conditions, the count is usually less than 1,00,000/mm³, and are easily differentiated by history, examination, and peripheral smear examination.

Flowchart 5: Algorithmic management of hyperleukocytosis.

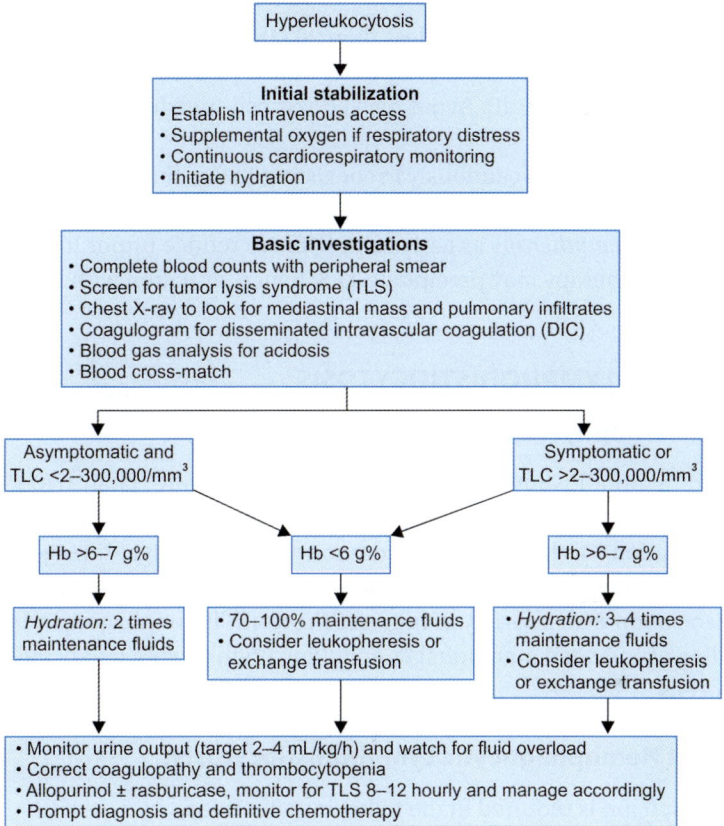

Management

Aggressive supportive care with prompt diagnosis and initiation of cytoreductive chemotherapy is the key to management of hyperleukocytosis. The algorithmic approach to the management of hyperleukocytosis in children is elaborated in Flowchart 5.

- *Aggressive hydration* with 2-4 times maintenance fluids (potassium and calcium-free saline dextrose fluids). The fluid rate depends on tumor burden and hemoglobin level. Target urine output of 2-4 mL/kg/hour and monitor for fluid overload
- Start allopurinol (250-500 mg/m^2/day) to *prevent TLS*. Monitor for and correct metabolic abnormalities. Rasburicase may be considered
- In symptomatic hyperleukocytosis or with very high counts, consider *leukopheresis or exchange transfusion*. Nonavailability, need for technical expertise, difficult venous access in young children and risks of anticoagulation are the limitations of leukopheresis. Exchange transfusion is preferred in hyperleukocytosis with severe anemia as it reduces risk of volume overload and hyperviscosity with hydration and blood transfusion respectively. Leukopheresis or exchange transfusions are temporary measures to stabilize the patient

while establishing diagnosis. The procedure may be repeated around 24 hours later for successful leukoreduction
- *Blood products*: Transfuse platelets if less than 20,000/mm³ or if active bleeds are present. Correct coagulopathy with 10–15 mL/kg fresh frozen plasma (FFP). Give cryoprecipitate if fibrinogen is less than 1 g/dL. Avoid packed red cell transfusion as it further increases viscosity
- Diuretics may be considered cautiously in coexisting TLS or fluid overload as it can worsen dehydration and hyperviscosity
- Initiate *definitive chemotherapy* as early as possible to reduce tumor load. Regular dose of multi-agent chemotherapy may precipitate TLS; hence, initiation with low-dose steroids is preferred.

HEMOPHAGOCYTIC LYMPHOHISTIOCYTOSIS

Core Concepts: Pathophysiology

Hemophagocytic lymphohistiocytosis (HLH) is a potentially fatal hyper-inflammatory state due to hyper-stimulated but ineffective immune response. It is characterized by non-neoplastic proliferation of histiocytes of monocyte-macrophage lineage with extensive organ infiltration and hemophagocytosis. It may be a familial or a sporadic condition, often occurring in association with a variety of triggers. The term "hemophagocytosis" describes the pathologic finding of activated macrophages engulfing erythrocytes, leukocytes, platelets, and their precursor cells.

When to Suspect Hemophagocytic Lymphohistiocytosis?

A high index of suspicion is required in the following situations:
- Prolonged fever with pancytopenia and hepatosplenomegaly
- Prolonged fever of unknown origin, unresponsive to antibiotics
- Pancytopenia of unknown origin
- Unexplained liver dysfunction with elevated ferritin.
- Systemic inflammatory response syndrome (SIRS) with falling erythrocyte sedimentation rate (ESR).

Clinical Features

- Persistent and high grade hectic fever
- Pallor and bleeding manifestations
- Hepatosplenomegaly
- Lymphadenopathy
- *Rash*: Maculopapular erythematous rash, erythroderma, petechiae, and purpura
- Jaundice
- *Central nervous system (CNS) symptoms*: Irritability, seizures, encephalopathy.

Laboratory Abnormalities

- Anemia, neutropenia, and thrombocytopenia
- Coagulopathy, conjugated hyperbilirubinemia, and raised transaminases
- Hypertriglyceridemia and hypofibrinogemia
- *Elevated serum ferritin*: Although level more than 500 ng/mL is defined as the cut-off, it is often very high
- Hypoalbuminemia, hyponatremia, and elevated lactate dehydrogenase (LDH)
- CSF pleocytosis and elevated protein.

Diagnostic Criteria for Hemophagocytic Lymphohistiocytosis (2004)

The diagnosis of HLH can be established, if one of either 1 or 2 below is fulfilled:
1. A molecular diagnosis consistent with HLH is made.
2. *Diagnostic criteria for HLH are fulfilled (5 of the 8 criteria below)*:
   - Fever
   - Splenomegaly
   - *Cytopenias (Two or more cell line involvement)*:
     - Hemoglobin less than 9 g/dL (< 10 g/dL in infants < 4 weeks age)
     - Platelet count less than 1,00,000/mm^3
     - Absolute neutrophil count <1,000/mm^3.
   - *Hypertriglyceridemia and/or hypofibrinogenemia*:
     - Fasting triglycerides more than 3.0 mmol/L (>265 mg/dL)
     - Fibrinogen less than 1.5 g/L.
   - Hemophagocytosis in bone marrow, spleen, or lymph nodes
   - Low or absent NK-cell activity
   - Ferritin more than 500 g/L
   - Soluble CD25 more than 2400 U/mL.

   Familial forms often present early in life (<4 years) and should have no evidence of malignancy.
- Absence of hemophagocytosis does not exclude a diagnosis of HLH.
- Neurological and hepatic abnormalities often are supportive evidence.

Classification of Hemophagocytic Lymphohistiocytosis

Primary or Familial Hemophagocytic Lymphohistiocytosis

- *Familial HLH (FHL)*: FHL1, FHL2, FHL3, FHL4, FHL5
- *Overlap syndromes*:
  - *Associated with albinism and immunodeficiency*: Griscelli syndrome, Chédiak–Higashi syndrome, Heřmanský–Pudlák syndrome
  - *Associated with immunodeficiency*: X-linked lymphoproliferative disorder.

Flowchart 6: Algorithmic approach to hemophagocytic lymphohistiocytosis (HLH).

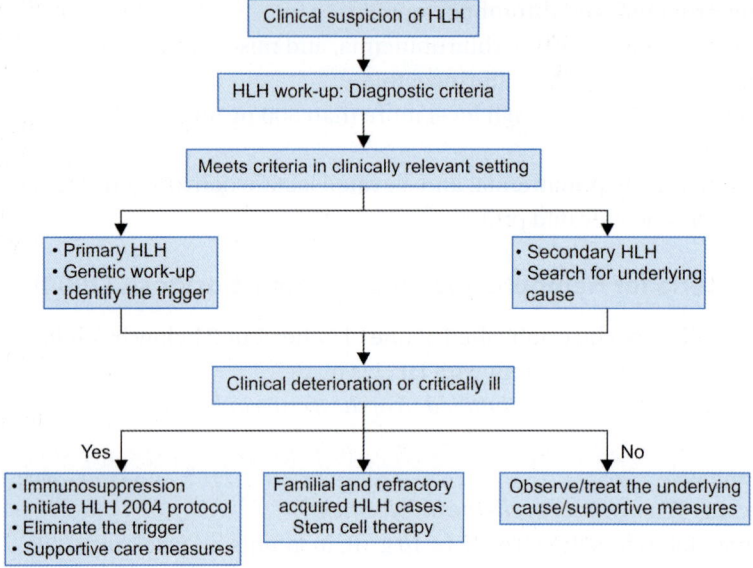

Secondary or Acquired Hemophagocytic Lymphohistiocytosis

- *Infections*:
  - *Virus*: Herpes simplex virus, Ebstein Barr virus, cytomegalovirus, Human immunodeficiency virus, dengue virus, parvovirus, influenza
  - *Bacteria*: Mycoplasma, brucella, staphylococcus, streptococcus, gram-negative organisms
  - *Parasites*: Leishmaniasis, malaria
  - Mycobacterial and fungal infections.
- *Malignancies*: Leukemia, lymphoma, and solid tumors
- *Autoimmune and rheumatological conditions*: Juvenile idiopathic arthritis, systemic lupus erythematosus, Kawasaki disease, Sjögren syndrome, mixed connective tissue disorder
- *Miscellaneous*: Stem cell transplant.

Management

The aim of treating the syndrome is to suppress the severe hyper-inflammation and to eliminate the triggering factors. HLH-2004 trial is an international prospective trial formulated for protocol-based management of these patients. The design includes initial intense therapy (dexamethasone, etoposide, and cyclosporine) for 8 weeks; followed by continuation therapy for 32 weeks. Familial forms and refractory secondary HLH cases would necessitate and benefit from an early allogeneic hematopoietic stem cell transplant. These trials have demonstrated a 5-year overall survival of 57–66%. The algorithmic management of HLH is presented in Flowchart 6.

SUGGESTED READING

1. Fisman DN. Hemophagocytic syndomes and infection. Emerg Infect Dis. 2000;6(6): 601-8.
2. Freifeld AG, Bow EJ, Sepkowitz KA, et al. Clinical Practice Guideline for the Use of Antimicrobial Agents in Neutropenic Patients with Cancer: 2010 Update by the Infectious Diseases Society of America. Clin Infect Dis. 2011;52(4):e56-93.
3. Henry M, Sung L. Supportive care in pediatric oncology. Pediatr Clin North Am. 2015;62(1):27-46.
4. Henter JI, Horne A, Aricó M, et al. HLH-2004: Diagnostic and therapeutic guidelines for hemophagocytic lymphohistiocytosis. Pediatr Blood Cancer. 2007;48(2):124-31.
5. Howard SC, Jones DP, Pui C-H. The tumor lysis syndrome. N Engl J Med. 2011;364(19):1844-54.
6. Jain R, Bansal D, Marwaha RK, et al. Superior Mediastinal Syndrome: Emergency Management. Indian J Pediatr. 2013;80(1):55-9.
7. Jain R, Bansal D, Marwaha RK. Hyperleukocytosis: Emergency management. Indian J Pediatr. 2013;80(2):144-8.
8. Klastersky J, de Naurois J, Rolston K, et al. Management of febrile neutropaenia: ESMO Clinical Practice Guidelines†. Ann Oncol. 2016;27(suppl_5):v111-8.
9. Lehmberg K, Ehl S. Diagnostic evaluation of patients with suspected haemophagocytic lymphohistiocytosis. Br J Hematol. 2012;160(3):275-87.
10. Lewis MA, Hendrickson AW, Moynihan TJ. Oncologic emergencies: Pathophysiology, presentation, diagnosis, and treatment. CA Cancer J Clin. 2011;61(5):287-314.
11. Oberoi S, Suthar R, Bansal D, et al. Febrile Neutropenia: Outline of management. Indian J Pediatr. 2013;80(2):138-43.
12. Prusakowski MK, Cannone D. Pediatric Oncologic Emergencies. Emerg Med Clin North Am. 2014;32(3):527-48.
13. Rajendran A, Bansal D, Marwaha RK, et al. Tumor lysis syndrome. Indian J Pediatr. 2013;80(1):50-4.
14. Seth R, Bhat AS. Management of common oncologic emergencies. Indian J Pediatr. 2011;78(6): 709-17.
15. Stephanos K, Picard L. Pediatric oncologic emergencies. Emerg Med Clin North Am. 2018;36(3): 527-35.
16. Taplitz RA, Kennedy EB, Bow EJ, et al. Outpatient management of fever and neutropenia in adults treated for malignancy: American society of clinical oncology and infectious diseases society of America clinical practice guideline update. J Clin Oncol. 2018;36(14):1443-53.
17. Usmani GN, Bruce A. Woda BA, Newburger PE. Advances in understanding the pathogenesis of HLH. Br J Hematol. 2013;161(5):609-22.
18. Wagner J, Arora S. Oncologic metabolic emergencies. Emerg Med Clin North Am. 2014;32(3): 509-25.
19. Weitzman S. Approach to hemophagocytic syndromes. Hematology Am Soc Hematol Educ Program. 2011;2011:178-83.

Blood Components in Intensive Care Practice

33

Nitin K Shah

LEARNING OBJECTIVES

- Component therapy in transfusion medicine
- Rational use of blood products.

INTRODUCTION

Availability of blood components has improved the outcome for many children. However, these are often misused in the pediatric intensive care unit (PICU) setting.

There are major differences between an adult and a child in the etiology of cytopenias and the effect of cytopenia on physiological responses. This is even more so for a newborn. Accordingly, the guidelines for the use of blood components differ in adults and children as well as in newborns. Various recent publications are available which define the guidelines for the use of blood components specific to children and newborns.

WHY NOT WHOLE BLOOD AND WHY COMPONENTS?

Each unit of whole blood has at least 4 basic components which include: (i) red blood cells (RBCs), (ii) white blood cells (WBCs), (iii) platelets, and (iv) plasma. Each of these components has specialized functions. All these functions are not deranged in all patients and hence all the components are not required all the time. Blood is always in short supply and making components from one unit of whole blood will satisfy the needs of more than one patient. Besides, giving whole blood can lead to harmful effects like plasma overload; lymphocyte mediated toxicities or allosensitization, etc. Some components can only be given effectively as component, e.g., platelets, which are otherwise, destroyed in refrigerated stored whole blood. Some components are better given as component, e.g., clotting factors as effective levels cannot be achieved by using fresh frozen plasma (FFP) alone. It is a social crime to use whole blood and waste this rare commodity!

WHICH COMPONENTS?

From one unit of unrefrigerated whole blood packed RBCs, platelet pack (random donor platelet), granulocytes pack, and fresh plasma can be made. Fresh plasma can be further frozen at −30°C and be used as FFP. Pooled-plasma can be converted into further components like cryoprecipitate, albumin, gamma globulins, anti-D globulins, plasma proteins, etc. These components can be modified and manipulated to obtain neocyte red cells, frozen red cells, washed red cells, platelets, filtered red cells, or platelets, ultraviolet (UV) light or gamma irradiated red cells or platelets. Cytomegalovirus (CMV) negative blood components, human leukocyte antigen (HLA) matched blood components or blood products from specific minor blood group compatible donors can be obtained from selected donors. Lastly, stem cells from the umbilical cord blood of a newborn or peripheral blood of an older child for autologous or allogeneic bone marrow transplant or rescue can be collected.

STORAGE AND SHELF LIFE

Whole blood is stored at 1–4°C. Shelf life will depend upon the type of anticoagulant and additive used. Acid citrate dextrose (ACD) is no longer used. Citrate-phosphate-dextrose (CPD) or CP-2D blood can be kept for 21 days. CPDA1-A2 blood can be kept for 35 days. With additives like Nutrisol or Adsol, the blood can be stored for 42 days. Packed RBC is stored at 1–4°C and should be used within 24 hours, if packed using open system. Platelets are stored at 20–22°C on a constant agitator as resting platelets tend to aggregate. The shelf life is 3–7 days. Granulocytes are kept at room temperature and should be used within 24 hours of collection. FFP and cryoprecipitate have shelf life of 1 year and are stored at -30°C. Frozen RBCs can be kept at −70°C and have shelf life of 5–7 years.

ABO AND Rh COMPATIBILITY

Tables 1 and 2 describe the choice of the ABO and Rh type of the donor blood component in various recipient ABO and Rh settings.

Table 1: Choice of ABO blood group of donor components in children.

Patient's ABO group	Donor ABO group		
	Red cells	Platelets	FFP[Δ]
O			
First choice	O	O	O
Second choice	–	A	A or B or AB
A			
First choice	A	A	A or AB
Second choice	O*	O*	
B			
First choice	B	B[#]	B or AB
Second choice	O*	A or O*	
AB			
First choice	AB	AB[#]	AB
Second choice	A or B	A	A
Third choice	O*		

*Group O component without high anti-A or anti-B titers should be selected.
[#]Platelet concentrates of B or AB group may not be easily available.
[Δ]Group O FFP should be given only to O group patients and no one else. AB group FFP may not be easily available.
(FFP: fresh frozen plasma)

Table 2: Choice of Rh blood group of donor components in children.

Patient's Rh group	Donor Rh group		
	Red Cells	Platelets	FFP^Δ
Rh positive			
First choice	Rh +ve	Rh +ve	Rh +ve
Second choice	Rh –ve	Rh –ve	Rh –ve
Rh negative			
First choice	Rh –ve	Rh –ve	Rh –ve
Second choice	–	Rh +ve*	Rh +ve

*If Rh +ve platelets are given to an Rh negative recipient, anti-D globulin in the dose of 250 µg should be given to the recipient, which will cover up to five platelet transfusion for up to next 6 weeks.
^ΔFFP usually are not labeled as Rh positive or negative.
(FFP: fresh frozen plasma)

WHOLE BLOOD

Whole blood has all the components, but, i.e. only in the first 6–8 hours only when stored at room temperature. The platelets are the first to disappear in the first 4–48 hours, the labile clotting factors V and VII are the next to disappear and the other clotting factors go down thereafter. On prolonged storage the potassium levels go up whereas the pH, the 2-3-DGP levels and the ATP levels fall. Hence, for exchange transfusions, the preference is to use less than 7-day-old blood. Whole blood is stored at 1–4°C and has a shelf life of 21–42 days as discussed before.

Indications

Whole blood is used only when massive transfusions are required like in exchange transfusion, massive blood loss with at least one volume blood transfused or during extracorporeal membrane oxygenation (ECMO). It is reconstituted and there is nothing like 'fresh' blood! 10 cc/kg body weight of whole blood will raise the hematocrit (HCT) by 5% and hemoglobin (Hb) by 1–1.5 g%.

PACKED RED BLOOD CELLS

Packed RBCs (PRBCs) are the backbone of any transfusion service as they help in improving both the oxygen carrying capacity as well as volume. Ideal HCT for PRBC is 70–75% and it should not be too tightly packed. For newborns, while doing exchange transfusion, HCT can be adjusted to 50–55% using additional FFP or albumin. The lower volume reduces the risk of circulatory overload. Reduced-plasma reduces citrate-related toxicity. It is mainly used in patients with hemorrhage or anemia needing transfusions. As it contains significant amount of plasma and leukocytes, it can lead to toxicities related to them like allergic reactions, febrile nonhemolytic transfusion reaction (FNHTR), allosensitization, graft-versus-host disease (GVHD), etc. Full cross-match for ABO and Rh and screening for abnormal antibody should be done before each transfusion. 10-cc/kg body weight of PRBC will raise the HCT by 10% and Hb by 3–4 g%.

> **Box 1:** Indications of using packed red blood cell in a greater than 4-month-old child.
>
> - Acute blood loss of > 15-20% blood volume with hypovolemia
> - Hb <8 g% with
>   - Symptomatic periopertaive anemia
>   - Chronic congenital/acquired transfusion dependent anemia
>   - Emergency surgery with anticipated blood loss
>   - Uncorrectable preoperative anemia
>   - Severe infections
>   - Associated severe pulmonary disease
> - Hb <7.0 g% with chronic transfusion dependent states, e.g.
>   - Hemoglobinopathies other than Thalassemia major
>   - Bone marrow failure syndrome including Fanconi's anemia
>   - Congenital dyserythropoietic anemia
>   - Sideroblastic anemia
>   - Chronic hemolytic anemia like congenital spherocytosis
>   - Chronic hemolytic anemia like hereditary nonspherocytic anemia
> - *Pediatric oncology*:
>   - Hb <8 g% with chemotherapy/radiotherapy
>   - Hb <10 g% if
>   i. Intensive chemotherapy planned
>   ii. Presence of febrile neutropenia
>   iii. Severe LRTI
>   iv. Thrombocytopenic bleeding
>   - Hyperleukocytosis (partial exchange preferred)
> - Patient on ventilatory support
>   - Hb <11 g% with significant ventilatory support
>   - Hb <10 g% with minimal ventilatory support
>
> (LRTI: lower respiratory tract infection)

Indications

The 'cut-offs' used in various indications are shown in Box 1. It is used for replacement of volume as well as oxygen carrying capacity. It is used in acute hemorrhage where more than 15-20% blood volume is lost, monitoring vitals, blood pressure, and central venous pressure (CVP). The commonest indication of PRBC is chronic transfusion dependent anemia as seen in thalassemia, sickle cell disease, congenital dyserythropoietic anemia, Diamond-Blackfan syndrome, Fanconi's anemia, aplastic anemia, chronic renal failure, cancer patients, sideroblastic anemia, etc. It is also useful in episodic transfusions for acute hemolysis like in G6PD deficiency, malaria, autoimmune hemolytic anemia, etc. It is rarely, if at all, used in nutritional anemia, if patient has severe anemia with impending cardiac failure or has associated cardio-respiratory disease. Lastly, it can be used before surgery, where patient is anemic with Hb less than 7 g% and where moderate blood loss is expected during surgery. In PICU, it is also useful to maintain hb in a patient who is on ventilator support as shown in Box 1.

It is most often misused as "top-up" in patients with nutritional anemia, or during surgery to keep Hb above "10 g%". In such cases, it is counterproductive as it can lead to immune suppression of the recipient and delay healing.

PLATELET TRANSFUSIONS

Whenever possible use ABO and Rh compatible platelets. Store the platelets at 22°C on a constant agitator. Use a designate donor repeatedly to obtain single donor platelet using an apheresis machine. Transport the platelets quickly and infuse the same in 20–30 minutes. Use plastic tubes and never use glassware as they will stick to the glass surface and get activated. Remember, platelets should never be stored in a refrigerator!

Types of Platelets

There are two types of platelets, random donor platelet (RDP) obtained by centrifugation of a unit of whole blood or single donor platelet (SDP) obtained by apheresis. One can use a HLA matched or CMV negative donor in specific situation. Use of WBC filters helps reduce allosensitization and febrile reactions.

Random Donor Platelet

Random donor platelet is obtained by centrifugation of a unit of whole blood within 68 hours of collection, and it contains $5–6 \times 10^{10}$ platelets in 50–60 mL of plasma per pack. One unit/10 kg body weight will raise the platelet count by 20,000–30,000/cumm. RDP is less costly and easily available from the blood bank shelf, however it is less efficacious than SDP as it contains 6–7 times less number of platelets. Hence, patients needing repeated platelet transfusions may benefit by using SDP which will reduce the exposure to a fewer donors.

Single Donor Platelet

It is obtained from a designate single donor using apheresis machine like COBE spectra cell separator. Compatible donor is selected and subjected to continuous or discontinuous apheresis and platelets are collected over 4–6 hours period. It contains $2–3 \times 10^{11}$ platelets in 50–70 cc of plasma. Thus, it has 6–7 times more platelets than RDP. The donor should be healthy, off medicines like aspirin and should have platelet count of more than 1.5 lakhs/cumm. The same donor can donate again after 2–3 weeks. Specific donor selection like CMV negative or HLA matched donor is possible. But SDP is extremely costly and needs sophisticated cell separator.

Criteria to Transfuse

Platelet transfusions are usually given to those with thrombocytopenia due to decreased production rather than to those with increased destruction. Platelet transfusions are given when they have significant mucosal bleeds. Only skin bleeds do not warrant platelet transfusion, but such patients should be closely monitored for any further mucosal bleeds.

It is controversial as to when to give prophylactic platelet transfusion. Children with thrombocytopenia usually do not bleed spontaneously unless the platelet count falls under 50,000/cumm. The chances of spontaneous bleeds increase when the count drops to less than 10–20,000/cumm. Hence, the decision when to transfuse platelets prophylactically is based on basic disease, type of thrombocytopenia, platelet count, and presence of associated coagulation abnormalities. A well-child is a given prophylactic transfusion when the platelet count is less than 5,000–10,000/cumm. In patients with massive hemorrhage, it should be

> **Box 2:** Indications of using platelets in a greater than 4-month-old child.

- Prophylactic platelets (without bleeding)
  - <5–10,000/cumm in a non-sick child
  - <20,000/cumm in a sick child with:
    i. Severe mucositis
    ii. DIC
    iii. Platelet likely to fall <10,000/cumm before next evaluation
    iv. Associated coagulopathy/anticoagulation
  - Before surgery
    i. Bone marrow aspiration/biopsy can be without platelet support
    ii. Lumbar puncture <30,000/cumm
    iii. Other surgeries <50,000/cumm
    iv. Surgery at critical sites like CNS, eyes <100,000/cumm
  - <50,000/cumm with acute bleeding, massive hemorrhage, head trauma, multiple trauma
- Chronic stable thrombocytopenia only in presence of significant mucosal bleeding
- Platelet dysfunction only in presence of significant mucosal bleeding
- Chronic stable DIC only in presence of significant mucosal bleeding

(CNS: central nervous system; DIC: disseminated intravascular coagulation)

given when the count is less than 50,000/cumm as most of the circulating platelets are likely to be non-functional platelets of the infused stored blood. The 'cut-off' used in various indication is shown in Box 2.

Indications

Platelet transfusions are given for thrombocytopenia or for platelet dysfunction.

Decreased Platelet Production

This is seen when bone marrow failure occurs like in aplastic anemia, Fanconi's anemia, thrombocytopenia with absent radius (TAR) syndrome, and other constitutional hypoplastic anemia. It is also seen when the bone marrow is infiltrated, e.g., in leukemia and other metastatic cancers or in presence of bone marrow suppression due to chemoradio therapy or fulminant infections. Platelet transfusions have revolutionized the treatment and the outcome of pediatric cancers. The cause of mortality has shifted from bleeding to infections with better platelet support available now.

Increased Consumption of Platelets

It is indicated in disseminated intravascular coagulation (DIC), necrotizing enterocolitis (NEC), and Kasabach-Merritt syndrome. In these cases, there is good platelet recovery at 1 hour after transfusion, but not at 24 hours suggesting consumption. However, it is contraindicated in thrombotic thrombocytopenic purpura (TTP) and hemolytic uremic syndrome (HUS).

Increased Platelet Destruction

Idiopathic thrombocytopenic purpura (ITP) is the most common scenario in this category. It can occur due to immune or nonimmune mechanisms. Immune destruction can occur in posttransfusion purpura, autoimmune diseases, ITP, and alloimmune disease of newborn. Platelet transfusions are generally not effective in this group of diseases, as they will be immediately destroyed after transfusion. However, in ITP with life-threatening bleeding like intracranial hemorrhage one may give platelet packs just to tide over crisis till splenectomy is done or intravenous immunoglobulin (IVIG) is administered. Nonimmune destruction can occur following drugs or infections.

Hypersplenism

Normally one-third of platelets are pooled in the spleen. This proportion will increase in patients with hypersplenism due to any reason. Again platelet transfusions may not be effective in such cases, as they will be immediately removed from the circulation into the enlarged spleen.

Dilutional

Dilutional thrombocytopenia can occur following massive transfusions in patients with massive hemorrhage or following exchange transfusions. Supplemental platelet transfusions may be required in such cases.

Platelet Dysfunction

Various congenital and acquired platelet functional disorders may present with significant bleeding. If local measures fail to control bleeding, platelet transfusions will be required. One should use platelets sparingly in such cases as allosensitization may prevent good recovery in future after a number of transfusions are given. One can use HLA matched platelets in such cases.

Platelet Transfusion Efficacy

One unit of RDP per 10 kg body weight increases platelet count by 20,000–30,000/cumm. SDP is 5–7 times more effective than RDP. The efficacy of platelet transfusion depends upon various factors. Platelet factors like source of platelets, type of platelets, storage, collection and administration will affect the efficacy. Similarly, factors in recipient that affect the efficacy include pretransfusion count, fever, sepsis, size of liver and spleen, presence of antibodies or consumption coagulopathy, and drugs taken by the recipient.

Clinically, one can judge the efficacy by seeing the cessation of bleeding. One can look for the expected increments by calculating Corrected Count Increment ($\times 10^9/L$) (CCI) as follows by doing platelet count at 1 hour and 24 hours after transfusion.

$$CCI = \frac{\text{Post-transfusion platelet count} - \text{Pretransfusion platelet count}}{\text{Platelets infused} \times 10^{11}} \times BSA\ (m)^2$$

Normal CCI is greater than $7.5 \times 10^9/L$ at 1 hour and greater than $4.5 \times 10^9/L$ at 20–24 hours. If CCI is normal at 1 hour, but less at 24 hours, it suggests consumption coagulopathy. If CCI is less at 1 hour itself, it suggests immune destruction.

GRANULOCYTES

Though, its use in infections may sound logical, granulocytes are rarely used in current clinical practice. People have tried giving granulocyte transfusion in patients with severe uncontrollable infection in presence of congenital or acquired neutropenia or neutrophil dysfunction. It is usually reserved for neutropenic patients with fulminant sepsis not controlled by antibiotics and antifungal with absolute neutrophil count (ANC) less than 300 in newborn, ANC less than 100 in infants and ANC less than 500 in immune compromised host. It should always be used along with antibiotics and antifungals. As colony stimulating factors are now easily available and affordable, use of granulocytes has fallen in to disrepute.

Buffy coat preparations are not very satisfactory as the cells tend to become nonfunctional. Packs obtained by apheresis are the best. They should be used within 24 hours of collection and stored at room temperature. Each pack has 10^{11} granulocytes in 200 cc of plasma. Dose recommended is 10^9 granulocytes/kg each time. It can be repeated every 12–24 hours for 4–6 days. It should be given obviously without using the WBC filter. It leads to all the side-effects related to plasma and lymphocytes. One should use ABO/Rh compatible donor.

LEUCODEPLETED BLOOD COMPONENTS

Why Leucodepletion?

Various side effects and toxicities are associated with the presence of significant number of donor lymphocytes in the unit of blood component transfused. These include nonhemolytic febrile transfusion reactions; allosensitization; increased chances of rejection of graft in candidates for future transplant; lymphocyte-mediated lung toxicity like acute respiratory distress syndrome (ARDS); transmission of viral infections like HIV, human T-cell lymphotropic virus (HTLV), Epstein–Barr virus (EBV), CMV, etc. which are intracellular pathogens; transfusion associated graft versus host disease (TA-GVHD) in immune compromised patients and in transfusion from first degree relatives; and immune suppression of the recipient especially in surgical patients. These donor lymphocytes ordinarily do not serve any beneficial effects and hence should be removed or depleted from the unit transfused to eliminate or reduce the chances of these side effects and toxicities.

Nonhemolytic febrile transfusion reactions (NHFTR) occur when more than 5×10^6 lymphocytes are present in the unit, whereas for TAGVHD it is more than 10^7 cells/kg body weight. One pack of PRBC has 10^9 WBC, RDP has $4\text{–}6 \times 10^7$ WBC, SDP has $2\text{–}4 \times 10^8$ WBC and granulocyte pack has 10^{11} WBC. Ideally all the transfusion should be leucodepleted, especially in patients needing recurrent transfusions and in immunocompromised hosts.

Methods of Leucodepletion

There are various ways of leucodepletion. Each method has its own merits and demerits and efficacy.

White Blood Cell Filter

Third generation WBC filters are 99.5 % efficient in removing the donor lymphocytes. Activated lymphocytes can release cytokines like interleukin-2 (IL-2), tumor necrosis factor (TNF-α) during storage and hence it is best to remove the lymphocytes while collecting blood from the donor using in-line WBC filter, rather than using the WBC filter at bedside while giving the transfusion to the recipient. The advantage of WBC filter is its high efficacy and simplicity to use. The disadvantages include its high cost and inability to prevent TA-GVHD. Each filter costs ₹ 400–500/– and is not reusable. Ideally, all transfusions should be given using filters especially if patient needs recurrent transfusions and develops NHFTR.

Washed Cells

Ninety percent of lymphocytes and 99% of plasma are removed by washing the PRBC with saline or blood processor. This will help reduce NHFTR, allosensitization, and other toxicities related to WBC as well as allergic reactions to plasma proteins. It is a simple technique and needs cold centrifuge but is not as effective as the WBC filter for leucodepletion. One can combine washing and use of WBC filter where the patient is prone to severe allergic reactions. Washing does not prevent TA-GVHD. Lastly, washed platelets from mother are given in a baby suffering from alloimmune thrombocytopenia.

Gamma Irradiation

The TA-GVHD can be only prevented by gamma irradiating the blood. Dosages of 2,500–3,500 cGy are used to irradiate the components. The only disadvantage is need for the sophisticated and expensive irradiator. There are chances of membrane leak from the irradiated cells which can result in to increased potassium levels. Hence, blood should be irradiated just before infusion or else supernatant plasma should be removed before transfusion.

Ideally, all blood should be irradiated where there is risk of TA-GVHD. This includes transfusion given to newborn especially preterms less than 1,200 g, intrauterine transfusions, patient with primary or secondary immunodeficiency, cancer patients, organ transplant recipients and transfusion given to normal person from a first degree relative donor.

Frozen Cells

This is routinely available in the west but is rarely available in India. RBC frozen at –70°C has shelf life of 5–7 years. While freezing, deglycerolization is done to prevent intracellular ice formation. It should be thawed gradually and once thawed should be used within 24 hours. The efficacy for leucodepletion is 90% and plasma depletion is 99%. Hence, it reduces toxicities related to both lymphocytes and plasma. Advantage of frozen cells is its availability in emergency where one can use O –ve frozen cells in AB negative plasma. One can collect blood from CMV negative donors; HLA matched donor or rare blood group donor and freeze it for future use. Lastly autologous blood collected for surgery can be frozen and used in future if surgery gets postponed for some reasons. Disadvantage of frozen cell is that it needs sophisticated instruments to prepare and store it and is extremely costly. It cannot prevent TA-GVHD.

FRESH FROZEN PLASMA

This is made by freezing the plasma obtained at the end of centrifugation of the whole blood unit and is stored at less than –30°C. The shelf life of FFP is one year when properly stored. It should be thawed at 37°C over 30 minutes in the water bath. Thawed FFP should be used within 4 hours, if used for hemophilia A or used within 24 hours if used for other conditions provided it is stored properly. FFP contains all the plasma proteins including albumin, gamma globulins, and most important clotting factors. As labile factor V and VIII tend to decrease on storage, freezing of the plasma should be done within 4–6 hours of collection to prevent loss of these factors. One unit of FFP has 200–250 mL of plasma and 1 mL of plasma contains approximately 1 unit of each clotting factor. As the maximum tolerated dose of FFP is 10–15 cc/kg every 12 hours, one cannot achieve very high plasma level of the missing clotting factors without volume overloading the patient.

Fresh frozen plasma is often misused as volume expander. As FFP can lead to allergic reactions, anaphylaxis in IgA deficient patient and can transmit all the plasma borne infections, albumin should be used as a volume expander which is much safer. Similarly, albumin and not FFP should be used to replace proteins or albumin. If patient needs both volume expansion as well as clotting factors like in DIC, sepsis, NEC, etc. one can use FFP. However, FFP should not be used in a case of DIC without clinical bleeding. FFP should also not be used prophylactically to prevent intracranial bleeding in neonate.

Box 3 summarizes the indications of using FFP in clinical practice. FFP is mainly used to replace clotting factors. It can be given when the patient presents with bleeding for the first time where the diagnosis is uncertain as to which factor is deficient. In known cases of hemophilia, it is better to use factor concentrates, as they are more efficient and safe. FFP is used for deficiencies of other factors like factor V, VII, etc. where factor concentrates are not available. It is also used where multiple factors need to be replaced as in case of hemorrhagic disease of newborn, liver disease, preterm with liver dysfunction, DIC, etc. FFP also contains antithrombin

---

Box 3: Indications of using FFP considered as appropriate.

- *Inherited factor deficiency*:
  - Patient with unknown clotting factor deficiency presenting for the first time
  - Single clotting factor where factor concentrate is not available like factor V or XI
  - Multiple clotting factor deficiency.
- DIC with clinical bleeding
- Hemorrhagic disease of newborn
- Liver disease with coagulopathy for prevention and control of bleeding
- Dilutional coagulopathy as seen after massive transfusion (surgical patients) to maintain PT, aPTT to <1.5 time the control
- Plasma exchange for TTP/HUS
- Sick newborn with coagulopathy and bleeding

(aPTT: activated partial thromboplastin time; DIC: disseminated intravascular coagulation; FFP: fresh frozen plasma; HUS: hemolytic uremic syndrome; PT: prothrombin time; TTP: thrombotic thrombocytopenic purpura)

III, protein C and protein S and hence is useful in the deficiency of these factors too like in the treatment of purpura fulminans; however in the west activated protein C concentrates are easily available. FFP is used for plasma exchange in patients with TTP or HUS. It can be used to reconstitute whole blood along with PRBC or to adjust HCT of PRBC for exchange transfusion in newborn. Lastly, FFP is useful to prevent and treat coagulopathy due to L-asparaginase in cancer patients.

The FFP leads to all the side effects related to plasma like allergic reactions like urticaria, anaphylaxis, especially in IgA deficient patient and transmission of plasma borne infections to the recipient. In small babies, it can lead to hemolysis if it contains high levels of antibodies against recipient's blood group antigens. FFP has also been associated with rare but significant toxicities like TRALI.

SUGGESTED READING

1. Beulter E. Platelet transfusion: the 20000/L trigger. Blood. 1993;81:1411-13.
2. Boulton F. Transfusion guidelines for neonates and older children. Brit J Hematol 2004;124:433-53.
3. Consensus Conference on Platelet Transfusion. Br J Cancer. 1998;78:290-91.
4. Ennio CR. Red cell Transfusion Therapy in Chronic anemia. Hemat Oncol Clin North Am. 1994;8:1045-52.
5. Estcourt LJ, Birchall J, Allard S, et al. Guidelines for the use of platelet transfusions. Brit J Hematol. 2003;122:10-23.
6. Green L, Cardigan R, Beattie C, et al. Guidelines for the use of fresh-frozen plasma, cryoprecipitate and cryosupernatant. Brit J Hematol. 2004;126:11-28.
7. Indian Academy of Pediatrics transfusion guidelines for neonates and older children (under publication).
8. Miller JP, Mintz PD. The use of leucocyte- reduced blood components. Hemat Oncol Clin North Am. 1995;9:69-90.
9. Rentels PB, Kenney RM, Crowley JP. Therapeutic support of the patient with Thrombocytopenia. Hemat Oncol Clin North Am. 1994;8:1131-51.
10. Roseff SD, Luban NL, Manno CS. Guidelines for assessing appropriateness of pediatric transfusion. Trans. 2002;42:1398-413.
11. Roseff SD. Pediatric Transfusion: A Physician's Handbook; 1st Edition. American Association of Blood Banks; 2003.
12. Rosen NR, Weidner JG, Boltd HD, et al. Prevention of transfusion associated graft-versus-host disease: selection of sufficient dose of gamma irradiation. Transf. 1993;33:125.
13. Shah N, Lokeshwar MR. Blood components in pediatric practice. Proc South Pedicon. 2000:55-68.
14. Strauss RG, Levy GJ, Sotelo-Avila C, et al. National survey of neonatal transfusion practices: ii. Blood component therapy. Pediatrics. 1993;91:530-36.
15. Voak D, Cann R, Finney RD, et al. Guidelines for administration of blood product transfusion of infants and neonates. British Committee for Standards in Hematology Blood Transfusion Task Force. Transf Med. 1994;4:1411-13.

Ventilator-associated Pneumonia and Hospital-acquired Pneumonia

34

VSV Prasad, Dilip Jain

LEARNING OBJECTIVES

- The reader should be able understand the etiopathogenesis of ventilator-associated pneumonia (VAP) and hospital-acquired pneumonia (HAP)
- The reader should be able to use the concept of prevention and treatment of VAP and HAP in day-to-day practice
- The reader should have evidence-based protocol for management of patient with VAP and HAP.

INTRODUCTION

Nosocomial infection is quite common in pediatric and neonatal intensive care units, and pneumonia is second most common nosocomial infection in this setting. Health-care-associated pneumonia (HCAP) comprises 6–36% of nosocomial infections and mechanical ventilation increases the risk of nosocomial pneumonia by 6–13 times and VAP is the most common nosocomial infection in mechanical ventilated patients. VAP rates in the pediatric intensive care unit (PICU) range from 6 per 1,000 ventilation days to 31 per 1,000 ventilation days.

Nosocomial pneumonia is associated with higher risk of mortality (25–40%), increased duration of ventilation by 5–11 days and prolonged hospital stay by 20–34 days. VAP comprises of highest risk of mortality among nosocomial infections.

There are different categories of nosocomial pneumonia and they have different terminologies such as HAP, VAP, and HCAP. HAP is generally considered less severe than VAP, but serious complications such as respiratory failure, pleural effusion, empyema, septic shock, renal failure occur in approximately 50% of the HAP patients.

DEFINITIONS

Healthcare-associated Pneumonia

Health care-associated pneumonia is defined as development of pneumonia in any patient who was hospitalized in an acute care hospital for 2 or more days within 90 days of the infection;

resided in a nursing home or long-term care facility; received recent intravenous antibiotics therapy, chemotherapy, or wound care with the past 30 days of the current infection; attended a hospital or hemodialysis clinic.

Hospital-acquired Pneumonia

Hospital-acquired pneumonia is defined as pneumonia not incubated at the time of hospital admission and occurring 48-hours or more after admission.

Ventilator-associated Pneumonia

Ventilator-associated pneumonia is defined as pneumonia occurring more than 48 hours after endotracheal intubation in mechanically ventilated patients.

PATHOGENESIS

An imbalance between host defense and microbial propensity for colonization and invasion is the process responsible for the pathogenesis of VAP. Colonization of the aerodigestive tract may occur endogenously or exogenously. Exogenous colonization may result in primary colonization of the oropharynx or may be the result of direct inoculation into the lower respiratory tract during manipulations of respiratory equipment, during using of respiratory devices, or from contaminated aerosols.

For causing VAP microorganisms first gain access to the normally sterile lower respiratory tract, where they can adhere to the mucosa and produce sustained infection. Microorganisms gain access by one of the four mechanisms (Fig. 1)—(i) by aspiration of microbe laden

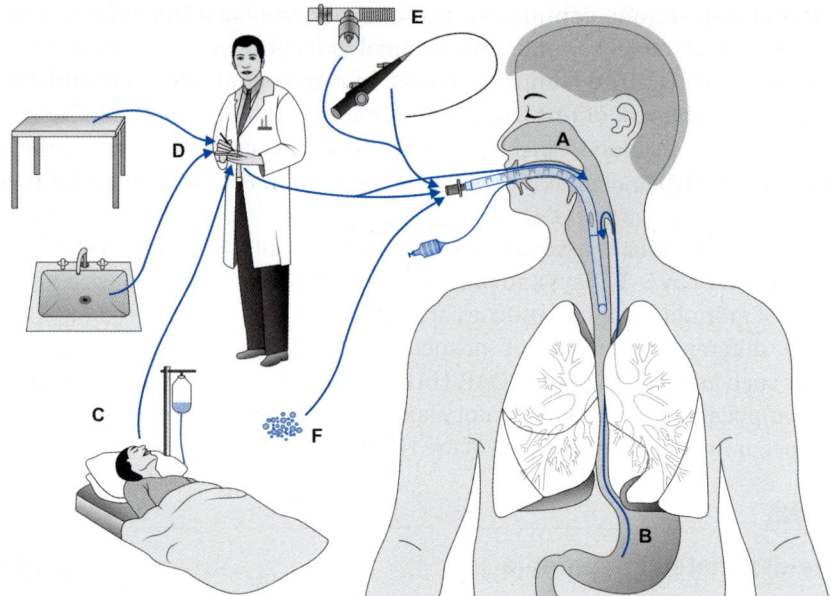

Fig. 1: Routes of colonization: (A and B): Endogenous colonization (oropharyngeal and gastric); (C to E): Exogenous colonization (contaminated devices, instruments, and aerosol).

secretions, either from the oropharynx directly or, secondarily by reflux from the stomach into the oropharynx, then into the lower respiratory tract; (ii) by direct extension of a contiguous infection, such as a pleural space infection; (iii) through inhalation of contaminated air or medical aerosols; or (iv) by hematogenous carriage of microorganisms to the lung from remote sites of local infection, such as vascular or urinary catheter-related bloodstream infection.

After colonization of microbes into respiratory tract they overwhelm the host's mechanical (ciliated epithelium and mucous), humoral (antibody and complement), and cellular (polymorphonuclear leukocytes, lymphocytes and their respective cytokines) defenses' to establish infection. This alteration in the host immune system causes abnormal cough reflex, compromised mucociliary clearance formation of the biofilm, damage to the tracheal mucosal epithelium, and a direct conduit for rapid access of bacteria from upper respiratory tract into lower respiratory tract.

Other suggested mechanisms for pathogenesis of VAP include:
- Sources of pathogens for VAP include health care devices, the environment (air, water, equipment, and fomites), and commonly the transfer of microorganisms between the patient and staff or other patients
- A number of host and treatment related colonization factors, such as the severity of the patient's underlying disease, prior surgery, exposure to antibiotics, other medications, and exposure to invasive respiratory devices and equipment, are important in the pathogenesis of HAP and VAP
- Aspiration of oropharyngeal pathogens or leakage of secretions containing bacteria around the endotracheal tube (ETT) cuff is the primary route of bacterial entry into the lower respiratory tract
- Inhalation or direct inoculation of pathogens into the lower airway, hematogenous spread from infected intravenous catheters, and bacterial translocation from the gastrointestinal tract lumen are uncommon pathogenic mechanisms
- Infected biofilm in the ETT, with subsequent embolization to the distal airways, may be important in the pathogenesis of VAP
- The stomach and sinuses may be potential reservoirs of nosocomial pathogens that contribute to bacterial colonization of the oropharynx, but their contribution is controversial, may vary by the population at risk, and may be decreasing with the changing natural history and management of HAP.

The risk of VAP is highest early in the course of hospital stay, and is estimated to be 3% per day during the first 5 days of ventilation, 2% per day during 5–10 days of ventilation, and 1% per day after this. Because most mechanical ventilation is short-term, approximately half of all episodes of VAP occur within the first 4 days of mechanical ventilation. The intubation process itself contributes to the risk of infection, and when patients with acute respiratory failure are managed with noninvasive ventilation, nosocomial pneumonia is less common (Table 1).

RISK FACTORS

Risk factors associated with VAP are mainly divided into modifiable and nonmodifiable as mentioned in Table 2.

Table 1: Reported outbreaks of ventilator-associated pneumonia traced to environmental source.

Source of outbreak	Organisms
Reusable electronic ventilator probes and sensors	• *Burkholderia cepacia* • *Stenotrophomonas maltophilia*
Nebulized medication	• *Burkholderia cepacia* • *Pseudomonas aeruginosa*
Ventilator circuits and equipment, humidifiers, and respirometers	• *Acinetobacter calcoaceticus* • *Burkholderia cereus* • *Pseudomonas aeruginosa*
Ice and water	• *Legionella pneumophila* • *Pseudomonas aeruginosa* • Nontuberculous mycobacteria
Bronchoscopes	• *Pseudomonas aeruginosa* • *Mycobacterium tuberculosis* • *Nontuberculous mycobacteria*
Fingernails and hands of healthcare workers:	• *Pseudomonas aeruginosa* • *Klebsiella pneumonia*
Miscellaneous: • Milk bank pasteurizer • Blood-gas analyzer • Mouthwash • Food coloring dye	• *Pseudomonas aeruginosa* • *Pseudomonas aeruginosa* • *Burkholderia cepacia* • *Pseudomonas aeruginosa* • *Burkholderia cepacia*
Infected patients or healthcare workers	• SARS human coronavirus • Influenza A, respiratory syncytial virus • *Mycobacterium tuberculosis* • Methicillin-resistant *Staphylococcus aureus*
Ambient air	*Aspergillus, zygomycetes*

(SARS: severe acute respiratory syndrome)

Table 2: Modifiable and nonmodifiable risk factors for development of ventilator associated pneumonia

Modifiable	Nonmodifiable
Effective infection control measures • Education • Hand hygiene • Isolation • Routine surveillance	Age
Intubation and reintubation	Sex
Use of NIV	Existing lung diseases
Orotracheal intubation and OG tube over nasotracheal intubation and NG tube	Immunodeficiency

Contd...

Contd...

Modifiable	Nonmodifiable
Aspiration of subglottic secretions	Underlying chronic diseases • Chronic kidney diseases • Chronic lung diseases • Chronic heart diseases
ET cuff pressure < 30 cm H_2O	Lung malformations
Care of condensate in ventilator tubing	Presence of high pulmonary blood flow lesions
Humidification and utilization of HME (heat and moisture exchanger)	Multi organ dysfunction syndrome
Duration of ventilation	Disease severity
Patient position and early feeding, nutrition	Genetic syndromes
VAP bundle and oral care	Neurological impairment
Sedation control and allowing spontaneous ventilation	
Stress ulcer prophylaxis	
Use of prolonged antibiotics	

(NG: nasogastric tube; NIV: noninvasive ventilation; OG: orogastric tube; VAP: ventilator associated pneumonia)

DIAGNOSIS

It should serve two purposes:
1. To define whether a patient has pneumonia as the explanation for a constellation of new signs and symptoms
2. To determine the etiologic pathogen when pneumonia is present.
   Diagnosis of VAP is based on clinical, radiological, laboratory and microbiological characteristics as mentioned below:
- Clinical diagnosis is established when the following criteria are met:
  - New onset fever or persistence of fever despite appropriate antibiotics
  - Increasing oxygen requirement (worsening oxygenation)
    - Increase in daily minimum fraction of inspired oxygen (FiO_2) of more than or equal to 0.20 above the baseline, sustained for more than or equal to 2 calendar days.
    - Increase in daily minimum positive end-expiratory pressure (PEEP) values of more than or equal to 3 cm H_2O above the baseline, sustained for more than or equal to 2 calendar days.
  - New clinical chest findings such as tachypnea, crepitations, etc.
  - Changes in tracheal secretions:
    - Frequent suctioning
    - Change in the color and consistency of secretions
    - Purulent secretions.

- *Laboratory*:
  - Blood white blood cells (WBC) count (>15,000/mm³ or <4,000/mm³)
  - Broncho–alveolar–lavage (BAL) suggestive of purulent sputum [>25 neutrophils and <10 squamous cells per low-power field (LPF)]
    - Cellularity
    - Microscopy.
- *Radiological*:
  - *Serial chest radiographs*:
    - More than or equal to 1 for patients without underlying disease
    - More than or equal to 2 for patient with underlying disease.
  - *With at least one of following*:
    - New or progressive and persistent infiltrate
    - Consolidation
    - Cavitations
    - Pneumatoceles in infants less than or equal to 1-year-old.
- *Microbiological diagnosis*: The following samples can be obtained through the ETT (all of these samples are assessed for adequacy and then processed for gram stain, quantitative and qualitative cultures). Qualitative cultures have high sensitivity (75%) but low specificity and are useful in excluding VAP particularly in patients who are not exposed to antibiotics. Quantitative cultures performed by serial dilutions and are reported as colony-forming unit (CFU).
  - Lung tissue (biopsy)
  - *Bronchoscopic*:
    - BAL
    - Protected specimen brush.
  - *Nonbronchoscopic*:
    - Tracheal aspirate or endobronchial secretions
    - Blinded protected sampling brush (BPSB)
    - Blinded bronchial sampling (BBS).

Characterization of Pneumonia (VAP) based on Clinical, Radiological, and Microbiological Criteria (Flowchart 1 and Box 1)

Ventilator associated pneumonia can be divided into three types depending upon the microbiological results:

1. *Definite ventilator-associated pneumonia*:
   - Pathogen from lung biopsy, or positive growth in culture of pleural fluid, or histopathologic examination
   - Positive culture of lung parenchyma, or fungal hyphae
   - Meets quantitative criteria definition.
2. *Probable ventilator-associated pneumonia*:
   - Below quantitative criteria
   - Quantitative culture (endotracheal aspirate) with a threshold of more than or equal to 10^6 CFU/mL

Flowchart 1: From centers for Disease Control and Prevention algorithm for clinically defined pneumonia.

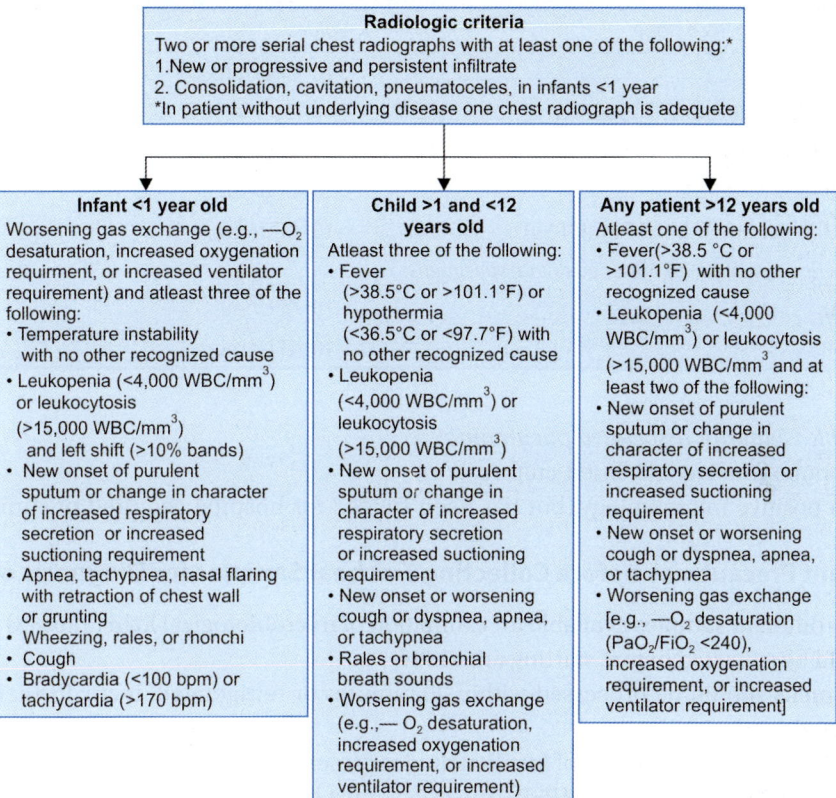

(FiO$_2$: fraction of inspired oxygen; PaO$_2$: partial pressure of arterial oxygen; WBC: white blood cells)

Box 1: Microbiological criteria for diagnosis of VAP.

Microbiological criteria:
- Positive growth in blood culture not related to another source of infection
- Positive growth in culture of pleural fluid
- Positive quantitative culture from minimally-contaminated LRT specimen (e.g., BAL or protected specimen brushing)
- ≥ 5% BAL-obtained cells contain intracellular bacteria on direct microscopic examination (e.g., Gram's stain)
- Positive quantitative culture of lung tissue
- Histopathologic exam shows at least one of the following evidences of pneumonia:
  – Abscess formation or foci of consolidation with intense PMN accumulation in bronchioles and alveoli
  – Evidence of lung parenchyma invasion by fungal hyphae or pseudohyphae.

(BAL: broncho-alveolar-lavage; LRT: lower respiratory tract; PMN: polymorphonuclear neutrophils; VAP: ventilator-associated pneumonia)

Table 3: Quantitative cultures of different sample collection methods and their significance.

Specimen collection/technique	Value
Lung tissue	>10^4 CFU/g tissue
Bronchoscopically (B) obtained specimens:	
• Bronchoalveolar lavage (B-BAL)	>10^4 CFU/ mL
• Protected BAL (B-PBAL)	>10^4 CFU/ mL
• Protected specimen brushing (B-PSB)	>10^3 CFU/ mL
Nonbronchoscopically (NB) obtained (blind) specimens:	
• NB-BAL	>10^4 CFU/ mL
• NB-PSB	>10^3 CFU/ mL

3. *Possible ventilator associated pneumonia*:
    - Nonquantitative specimen culture or
    - No positive microbiology, but has been treated for hospital acquired pneumonia.

Important Precautions before Collecting Tracheal Samples for Diagnosis of VAP

There are different samples available for estimation of microbiological load (Table 3)
- Should be collected before starting antibiotics
- Specimens should be processed within 30 minutes or refrigerated, if any further delay is expected
- In BAL, less than 10% return of instilled fluid represents inadequate sampling
- In protected specimen brush (PSB), the brush must be placed into exactly 1 mL of fluid
- If squamous to bronchial epithelial cells ratio is more than 1% or more than 10/LPF, then reject the sample.

COMMON ETIOLOGICAL ORGANISMS

Organisms differ from institution to institution, but the common organisms are mentioned below. Their overall and approximate prevalence in India is depicted in Figure 2. There are certain risk factors which make individuals prone for infection with multidrug resistant organism as mentioned in Box 2.

Prevalence of organisms causing VAP in the Indian scenario in decreasing order:
- *Acinetobacter* species
- *Pseudomonas aeruginosa*
- *Klebsiella* species
- *E.coli*
- Methicillin-resistant *Staphylococcus aureus*
- *Candida*
- *Enterobacter*
- *Citrobacter*
- Coagulase negative *Staphylococcus* (CONS).

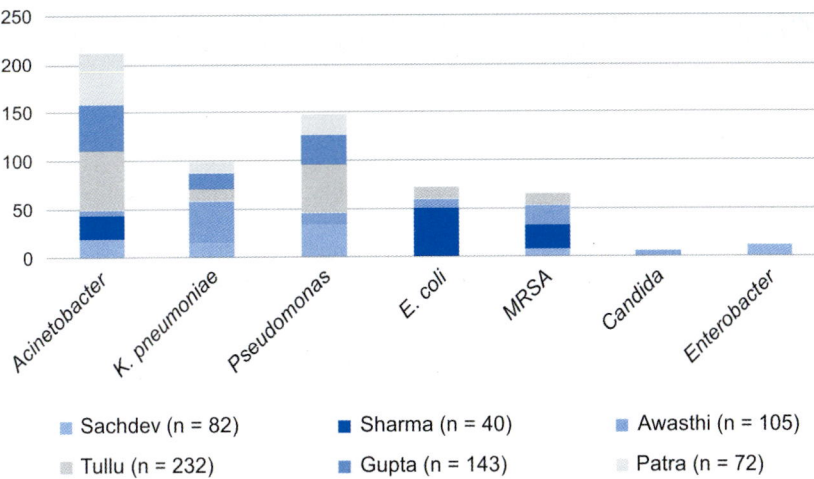

Fig. 2: Common etiological organisms in India.[10]
(MRSA: methicillin-resistant *Staphylococcus aureus*)
Source: Gupta D, Agarwal R, Aggarwal AN, et al. Guidelines for diagnosis and management of community- and hospital-acquired pneumonia in adults: Joint ICS/NCCP (I) recommendations. Lung India: Off Organ Indian Chest Soc. 2012;29(Suppl 2):S27.

> **Box 2:** Risk factors for multidrug-resistant pathogens causing hospital-acquired pneumonia, healthcare-associated pneumonia, and ventilator-associated pneumonia.
>
> - Antimicrobial therapy in preceding 90 days
> - Current hospitalization of 5 days or more
> - High frequency of antibiotic resistance in the community or in the specific hospital unit
> - Presence of risk factors for HCAP:
>   – Hospitalization for 2 days or more in the preceding 90 days
>   – Residence in a nursing home or extended care facility
>   – Home infusion therapy (including antibiotics)
>   – Chronic dialysis within 30 days
>   – Home wound care
>   – Family member with multidrug-resistant pathogen
> - Immunosuppressive disease and/or therapy

(HCAP: healthcare-associated pneumonia)

MANAGEMENT

Management consists of: (i) Prevention and (ii) Treatment.

Prevention

There are various preventive modalities postulated for VAP. Some of them have a strong evidenced base, while others have weak evidence. These are shown in Tables 4 and 5.

Table 4: Measures for prevention of ventilator-associated pneumonia based on our understanding of pathogenesis and epidemiology.

Source of VAP pathogen	Prevention goal	Specific measures
Aerodigestive colonization	Prevent colonization by exogenous routes	• Hand hygiene • Microbial surveillance and targeted barrier isolation • *Pre-emptive barriers*: 　– Routine gloving 　– Routine gowning 　– Dedicated equipment
	Suppress oropharyngeal mucosal colonization	• Oral decontamination with chlorhexidine • Selective digestive tract antimicrobial decontamination • Aerosolized antimicrobials • Sucralfate instead of H_2-blockers
	Prevent aspiration	• Noninvasive ventilation • Semirecumbent positioning • Novel endotracheal tubes permitting continuous subglottic suctioning
Contaminated respiratory therapy equipment and medical aerosols	Safe equipment and medical aerosols	• Procedures for reprocessing bronchoscopes and reused respiratory therapy equipment • Training and education of reprocessing staff and respiratory therapists • Procedures for use of aerosolized medications
	Reducing contamination of ventilator circuits	• Heat and moisture exchanger • Periodically draining of condensate from the circuit • Sterile water for bubble-through humidifiers • Aseptic procedures for suctioning of ventilated patients
Contaminated tap water (*Legionella* species, *Pseudomonas aeruginosa*)	Safe water	• *Sterile water for*: 　– Cleaning respiratory therapy equipment 　– Rinsing bronchoscopes 　– Aerosolized medications • Hospital surveillance for cases of nosocomial legionellosis • Microbial surveillance of hospital water for contamination by *Legionella* • *Engineering controls for contaminated water*: 　– Superheat and flush 　– Ultraviolet light 　– Hyperchlorination 　– Silver-copper ionization 　– Ozonation

Contd...

Contd...

Source of VAP pathogen	Prevention goal	Specific measures

Contaminated ambient air (filamentous fungi, *Mycobacterium tuberculosis*, SARS coronavirus)	Safe air	• Procedures for minimizing communicable airborne infections:
		  – Disease recognition
		  – Administrative controls
		  – Engineering controls
		• Procedures for minimizing risk to immunocompromised patients:
		• High-efficiency particulate arrester (HEPA)-filtered rooms
		• N95 masks for intrahospital transports policies and procedures for management during periods of construction and renovation.

(SARS: severe acute respiratory syndrome)
Source: Safdar N, Crnich CJ, Maki DG. The pathogenesis of ventilator-associated pneumonia: its relevance to developing effective strategies for prevention. Resp Care. 2005;50(6):725-41.

Table 5: Preventive modalities in ventilator-associated pneumonia.

Evidence based	Evidence is weak
Head end elevation 30–45°	Systematic use of closed tracheal suction system
Avoiding gastric over distention	Heat and moisture exchanger
Avoiding unplanned extubation and reintubation	Periodic change of ventilator circuits
Use of cuffed endotracheal tubes (where feasible) and maintaining safe cuff pressures	Regular oral care with chlorhexidine 0.12%
Change of circuits when visibly soiled or malfunctioning	Clearing of oral secretions followed by endotracheal tube secretions while suctioning
Implementation of protocols to reduce sedation and minimize the duration of mechanical ventilation	Use of subglottic suction catheters
Reduce the length of treatment for ventilator-associated pneumonia except for nonfermenting gram-negative bacilli	–

Source: Safdar N, Crnich CJ, Maki DG. The pathogenesis of ventilator-associated pneumonia: its relevance to developing effective strategies for prevention. Resp Care. 2005;50(6):725-41.

Treatment

Appropriate choice of antibiotics depends upon institutional antibiograms. Antibiotics should be individualized as per patient characteristics, sickness, and local antibiograms. General choice of antibiotics in different organisms is mentioned in Tables 6 and 7.

Table 6: Suggested empiric treatment options for clinically suspected ventilator-associated pneumonia in units where empiric methicillin-resistant *Staphylococcus aureus* coverage and double antipseudomonal/gram-negative coverage are appropriate.

A. Gram-positive antibiotics with MRSA activity	B. Gram-negative antibiotics with antipseudomonal activity: β-lactam-based agents	C. Gram-negative antibiotics with antipseudomonal activity: Non-β-lactam-based agents
Glycopeptides[a] Vancomycin Or Oxazolidinones Linezolid	Antipseudomonal penicillins[b] Piperacillin-tazobactam Or Cephalosporins[b] or Cefepime or Ceftazidime Or Carbapenems[b] or Imipenem or Meropenem Or Monobactams[d] Aztreonam	Fluoroquinolones- Ciprofloxacin or Levofloxacin Or Aminoglycosides[a,c] Amikacin or Gentamicin or Tobramycin Or Polymyxins[a,e] Colistin or Polymyxin B

Choose one gram-positive option from column A, one gram-negative option from column B, and one gram-negative option from column C.
[a] Drug levels and adjustment of doses and/or intervals required.
[b] Extended infusions may be appropriate.
[c] On meta-analysis, aminoglycoside regimens were associated with lower clinical response rates with no differences in mortality.
[d] Polymyxins should be reserved for settings where there is a high prevalence of multidrug resistance and local expertise in using this medication. Dosing is based on colistin-base activity (CBA); for example, one million IU of Colistin is equivalent to about 30 mg of CBA, which corresponds to about 80 mg of the prodrug colistimethate. Polymyxin B (1 mg = 10,000 units).
[e] In the absence of other options, it is acceptable to use aztreonam as an adjunctive agent with another β-lactam–based agent because it has different targets within the bacterial cell wall.
Source: Adapted from American Thoracic Society and Infectious Diseases Society of America guidelines. Feb 2005.

Table 7: Recommended initial empiric antibiotic therapy for hospital-acquired pneumonia (nonventilator-associated pneumonia).

Not at high risk of mortality[a] and no factors increasing the likelihood of MRSA[b,c]	Not at high risk of mortality[a] but with factors increasing the likelihood of MRSA[b,c]	High risk of mortality or receipt of Intravenous antibiotics during the prior 90 days[a,c]
One of the following:	One of the following:	Two of the following, avoid 2 β lactams:
Piperacillin-tazobactam[d] Or Cefepime[d] Or Levofloxacin Or Imipenem[d] or Meropenem[d]	Piperacillin-tazobactam[d] Or Cefepime[d] or ceftazidime[d] Or Levofloxacin or Ciprofloxacin Or Imipenem[d] or Meropenem[d] Or	Piperacillin-tazobactam[d] Or Cefepime[d] or ceftazidime[d] Or Levofloxacin or ciprofloxacin Or Imipenem[d] or Meropenem[d] Or

Contd...

Contd...

Not at high risk of mortality[a] and no factors increasing the likelihood of MRSA[b,c]	Not at high risk of mortality[a] but With factors increasing the likelihood of MRSA[b,c]	High risk of mortality or receipt of intravenous antibiotics during the prior 90 days[a,c]
	Aztreonam[e]	Amikacin or Gentamicin or Tobramycin Or Aztreonam[e]
	Plus: Vancomycin with goal to target 15–20 mg/mL trough level (consider a loading dose of 25–30 mg/kg × 1 for severe illness) Or Linezolid	Plus: Vancomycin with goal to target 15–20 mg/mL trough level (consider a loading dose of 25–30 mg/kg IV × 1 for severe illness) Or Linezolid If MRSA coverage is not going to be used, include coverage for MSSA. Options include: Piperacillin-tazobactam, cefepime, levofloxacin, imipenem, meropenem. Oxacillin, nafcillin, and cefazolin are preferred for the treatment of proven MSSA, but would ordinarily not be used in an empiric regimen for HAP.

If patient has severe penicillin allergy and aztreonam is going to be used instead of any β-lactam–based antibiotic, include coverage for MSSA.

[a] Risk factors for mortality include need for ventilatory support due to pneumonia and septic shock.

[b] Indications for MRSA coverage include intravenous antibiotic treatment during the prior 90 days, and treatment in a unit where the prevalence of MRSA among *S. aureus* isolates is not known or is > 20%. Prior detection of MRSA by culture or non-culture screening may also increase the risk of MRSA. The 20% threshold was chosen to balance the need for effective initial antibiotic therapy against the risks of excessive antibiotic use; hence, individual units can elect to adjust the threshold in accordance with local values and preferences. If MRSA coverage is omitted, the antibiotic regimen should include coverage for MSSA.

[c] If patient has factors increasing the likelihood of gram-negative infection, 2 antipseudomonal agents are recommended. If patient has structural lung disease increasing the risk of gram negative infection (i.e., bronchiectasis or cystic fibrosis), two antipseudomonal agents are recommended. A high-quality Gram stain from a respiratory specimen with numerous and predominant gram-negative bacilli provides further support for the diagnosis of a gram-negative pneumonia, including fermenting and non-glucose-fermenting microorganisms.

[d] Extended infusions may be appropriate.

[e] In the absence of other options, it is acceptable to use aztreonam as an adjunctive agent with another β-lactam–based agent because it has different targets within the bacterial cell wall.

(HAP: hospital-acquired pneumonia; IV: intravenous; MRSA: methicillin-resistant *Staphylococcus aureus*; MSSA: methicillin-sensitive *Staphylococcus aureus*)

Source: Adapted from American Thoracic Society and Infectious Diseases Society of America guidelines. Feb 2005.

Inhaled Antibiotics

Inhaled antibiotics have been tried in multiple case reports and series but with limited efficacy and so they are not the standard line of management in pediatric patients with VAP.
- High concentration of antibiotics in lung tissue, which leads to following advantages theoretically:
  - Improved bacterial elimination
  - Decrease in emergence of resistant strains
  - Decrease in systemic side effects of treatment
  - Decrease in complications like *Clostridium difficile* infection.
- Factors affecting delivery of aerosol into lung parenchyma while on inhaled antibiotics
  - Particle size (1–5 microns optimal)
  - *Nebulizers type*:
    - *Jet nebulizer (Venturi principle)*: least efficient, delivers less than or equal to 15% aerosol
    - *Ultrasonic nebulizers*: delivers 30–40% aerosol
    - *Vibrating mesh plate nebulizers*: Most efficient, delivers 40–60% aerosol.

ASSESSING RESPONSE TO THERAPY

- Assess response to therapy by clinical criteria and modification of therapy should mandate clinical and microbiological data
- Clinical improvement usually takes 48–72 hours, and thus therapy should not be changed during this time unless there is rapid clinical decline. No responsive to therapy is usually evident by day 3, using an assessment of clinical parameters
- The responding patient should have de-escalation of antibiotics, narrowing therapy to the most focused regimen possible on the basis of culture data
- The nonresponding patient should be evaluated for noninfectious mimics of pneumonia, unsuspected, or drug-resistant organisms, extra pulmonary sites of infection, and complications of pneumonia and its therapy. Diagnostic testing should be directed to whichever of these causes is likely.

RECENT ADVANCES IN THE MANAGEMENT OF VENTILATOR-ASSOCIATED PNEUMONIA

Modification of Endotracheal Tube

Recent studies suggest that use of silver-coated ETT prevent the formation of biofilm and micro aspiration by which it reduces the incidence of development of VAP. Further studies of ETT design are required to prove the safety, efficacy, and cost effectiveness for the use of silver coated ETTs.

Use of Endotracheal Tubes with Subglottic Secretion Drainage

In patients who required prolonged mechanical ventilation, the use of ETTs with subglottic secretion drainage (SSD) reduces the development of VAP. Using ETTs with SSD for all

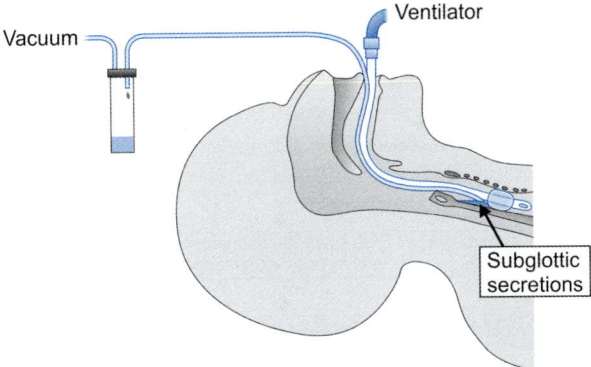

Fig. 3: Subglottic secretion drainage. The endotracheal tube has a dorsal lumen (black arrow) above the cuff, which is connected to suction to remove the secretions that pool above the cuff in the subglottic space.

mechanically ventilated patients would lead to significant unjustified incremental costs and is unadvisable. Replacing standard ETTs by ETTs with SSD at ICU admission would increase the risk of micro aspiration and is not advisable either. Identifying patients who are at risk to be mechanically ventilated for at least 72 hours at the time of intubation before ICU admission, or using convertible ETTs that feature a separate suction line allowing for subglottic secretion suctioning on demand are suggested solutions to reduce VAP (Fig. 3).

Role of Probiotics for Preventing VAP in Mechanically Ventilated Patients

In a recent meta-analysis it is found that use of probiotics in mechanically ventilated patients reduces the incidence of development of VAP. Probiotic also provide clinical benefits in mechanical ventilated patients. Further studies using large samples and high quality randomized controlled trials (RCTs) are needed to evaluate the effect of probiotics on preventing VAP in mechanically ventilated patients.

Diagnosis of VAP by Analysis of Volatile Organic Compounds in Exhaled Breath

A recent study has demonstrated that it is possible to diagnose VAP based on the profile of only 12 volatile organic compounds (VOCs) in exhaled breath analysis is a promising, safe, and noninvasive technique for rapid diagnosis of VAP. A larger study population is warranted to confirm this finding.

Diagnosis of VAP by using Lung Ultrasound

Recent published data shows that lung ultrasound (LUS) is an accurate bedside tool to detect and monitor VAP in critical care units. It reduces the overexposure of patients to radiation and therefore the use of LUS for diagnosis and monitoring of VAP should be encouraged, especially in ICUs. Further research is needed regarding LUS in VAP diagnosis.

Flowchart 2: Algorithm for the management of VAP.

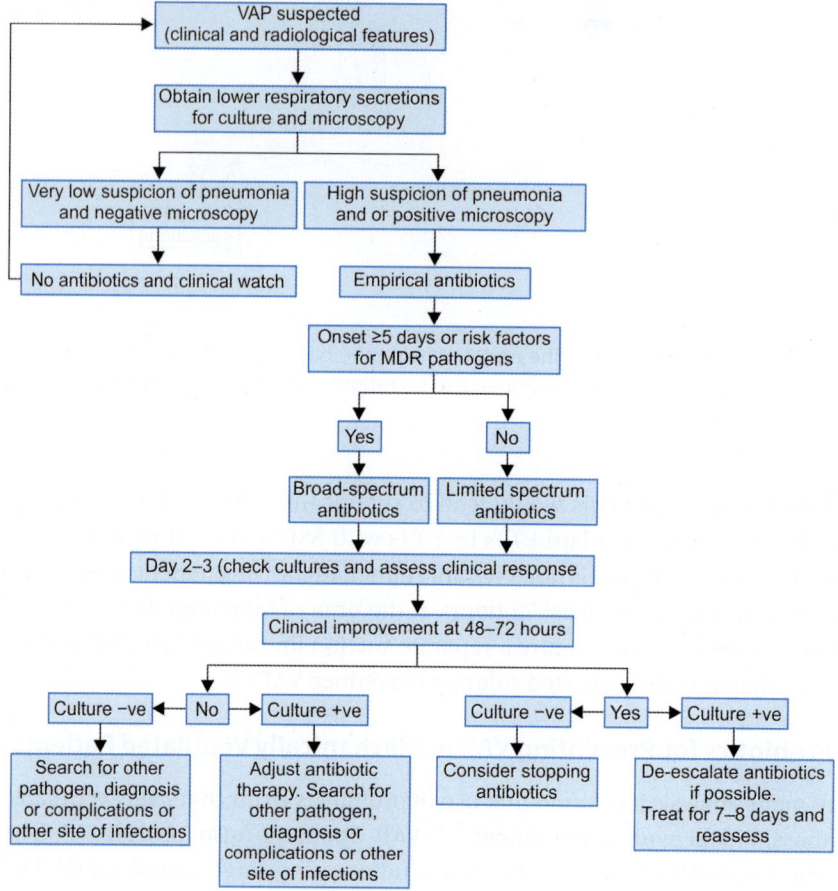

(MDR: multidrug-resistant; VAP: ventilator-associated pneumonia)

KEY MESSAGE

- Ventilator-associated pneumonia and HAP are preventable condition to a large extent by using infection control practices.
- A good understanding of etiopathogenesis helps in prevention and management of VAP and HAP.
- Diagnosis of VAP by using by using clinical, laboratory, radiological, and microbiological criteria and treatment by using antibiotic stewardship is important in the management.
- There are a lot of scopes for advances in the management of VAP by further RCTs (Flowchart 2).

SUGGESTED READING

1. Adair CG, Gorman SP, Feron BM, et al. Implications of endotracheal tube biofilm for ventilator-associated pneumonia. Intens Care Med. 1999;25(10):1072-6.
2. American Thoracic Society, Infectious Diseases Society of America. Guidelines for the management of adults with hospital-acquired, ventilator-associated, and healthcare-associated pneumonia. Am J Resp Crit Care Med. 2005;171(4):388.
3. Bergmans DC, Bonten MJ, van Tiel FH, et al. Cross-colonisation with Pseudomonas aeruginosa of patients in an intensive care unit. Thorax. 1998;53(12):1053-8.
4. Brochard L, Mancebo J, Wysocki M, et al. Noninvasive ventilation for acute exacerbations of chronic obstructive pulmonary disease. New Engl J Med. 1995;333(13):817-22.
5. CDC Statement (2017). Device-associated Module PNEU, Pneumonia (Ventilator-associated [VAP] and non-ventilator-associated Pneumonia [PNEU]) Event 2017 January [online] Available at https://www.cdc.gov/nhsn/pdfs/pscmanual/6pscvapcurrent.pdf. [Accessed November 2018].
6. Cook D, De Jonghe B, Brochard L, et al. Influence of airway management on ventilator-associated pneumonia: evidence from randomized trials. JAMA. 1998;279(10):781-7.
7. Craven DE, Steger KA. Nosocomial pneumonia in mechanically ventilated adult patients: epidemiology and prevention in 1996. Semin Respir Infect. 1996;11(1):32-53.
8. Craven DE. Ventilator-associated tracheobronchitis (VAT): questions, answers, and a new paradigm?. Crit Care. 2008;12(3):157.
9. Deem S, Treggiari MM. New endotracheal tubes designed to prevent ventilator-associated pneumonia: do they make a difference?. Resp Care. 2010;55(8):1046-55.
10. Gupta D, Agarwal R, Aggarwal AN, et al. Guidelines for diagnosis and management of community- and hospital-acquired pneumonia in adults: Joint ICS/NCCP (I) recommendations. Lung India: Off Organ Indian Chest Soc. 2012;29(Suppl 2):S27.
11. Kalil AC, Metersky ML, Klompas M, et al. Management of adults with hospital-acquired and ventilator-associated pneumonia: 2016 clinical practice guidelines by the Infectious Diseases Society of America and the American Thoracic Society. Clin Infect Dis. 2016;63(5):e61-111.
12. Kollef MH. Prevention of hospital-associated pneumonia and ventilator-associated pneumonia. Crit Care Med. 2004;32(6):1396-405.
13. Loupec T, Petitpas F, Kalfon P, et al. Subglottic secretion drainage in prevention of ventilator-associated pneumonia: mind the gap between studies and reality. Crit Care. 2013;17(6):R286.
14. Magill SS, Edwards JR, Bamberg W, et al. Multistate point-prevalence survey of health care-associated infections. New Engl J Med. 2014;370(13):1198-208.
15. Montravers P, Harpan A, Guivarch E. Current and future considerations for the treatment of hospital-acquired pneumonia. Adv Ther. 2016;33(2):151-66.
16. Pássaro L, Harbarth S, Landelle C. Prevention of hospital-acquired pneumonia in non-ventilated adult patients: a narrative review. Antimicro Resis Infect Cont. 2016;5(1):43.
17. Pittet D, Hugonnet S, Harbarth S, et al. Effectiveness of a hospital-wide programme to improve compliance with hand hygiene. The Lancet. 2000;356(9238):1307-12.
18. Quartin AA, Scerpella EG, Puttagunta S, et al. A comparison of microbiology and demographics among patients with healthcare-associated, hospital-acquired, and ventilator-associated pneumonia: a retrospective analysis of 1184 patients from a large, international study. BMC Infect Dis. 2013;13(1):561.
19. Ramirez P, Lopez-Ferraz C, Gordon M, et al. From starting mechanical ventilation to ventilator-associated pneumonia, choosing the right moment to start antibiotic treatment. Crit Care. 2016;20(1):169.
20. Rouby JJ, Laurent P, Gosnach M, et al. Risk factors and clinical relevance of nosocomial maxillary sinusitis in the critically ill. Am J Resp Crit Care Med. 1994;150(3):776-83.

21. Safdar N, Crnich CJ, Maki DG. The pathogenesis of ventilator-associated pneumonia: its relevance to developing effective strategies for prevention. Resp Care. 2005;50(6):725-41.
22. Schnabel R, Fijten R, Smolinska A, et al. Analysis of volatile organic compounds in exhaled breath to diagnose ventilator-associated pneumonia. Sci Rep. 2015;5:17179.
23. Sehulster L, Chinn RY, Arduino MJ, et al. Guidelines for environmental infection control in health-care facilities. Morbid Mortal Weekly Rep Recommend Rep RR. 2003;52(10).
24. Van Hueveln N. Ventilator-associated pneumonia and the effectiveness of endotracheal tubes coated with silver sulfadiazine. Master's Thesis, RIC. 2017.
25. Wang G, Ji X, Xu Y, et al. Lung ultrasound: a promising tool to monitor ventilator-associated pneumonia in critically ill patients. Crit Care. 2016;20(1):320.
26. Weng H, Li JG, Mao Z, et al. Probiotics for preventing ventilator-associated pneumonia in mechanically ventilated patients: A meta-analysis with trial sequential analysis. Front Pharmacol. 2017;8:717.

Catheter-related Bloodstream Infection   35

Azeem Khan

LEARNING OBJECTIVES

- To define and recognize central line-associated bloodstream infection (CLABSI)
- To correctly manage devices for prevention of CLABSIs by using a bundled approach.

INTRODUCTION

For every device inserted and for everyday, the device is in place, there is a real danger of a hospital-acquired infection (HAI), often by a multidrug resistant organism, afflicting the patient. While the desired rate would be zero, this is not possible and the best possible action would be to take measures for prevention, early detection, and best possible treatment and management for the patient and the unit. Every HAI is a threat to the patient as well as to other patients in the unit. There is increased morbidity, mortality, length of stay, and cost involved. Every unit needs a robust infection control and antibiotic stewardship program to help manage this threat.

DEFINITION

Bacteremia or fungemia in a patient who has an intravascular device, with at least one positive blood culture obtained from a peripheral vein, with clinical manifestation of infection and no other appropriate of source of bloodstream infection (BSI). The growth of an organism in the bloodstream must be documented by:
- Positive semi quantitative (>10 CFU) or quantitative (>10^3 CFU/catheter segment) culture of a catheter segment with an organism identical in species and antibiogram as isolated from peripheral blood culture OR
- Simultaneously drawn peripheral and line quantitative blood culture with more than 3:1 ratio in catheter blood versus peripheral blood colony counts or
- Differential time to culture positively of more than 2 hours between the catheter and peripheral blood culture, where the catheter culture is positive first.

Catheter-related bloodstream infection (CR BSI) is the terminology not typically used for surveillance purposes due to the clinical needs of the patient (the catheter is not always pulled out to investigate), limited availability of microbiologic methods (many laboratories do not use quantitative blood cultures or differential time to positivity), and procedural compliance by direct care personnel (labeling must be accurate).

A CLABSI is a primary BSI in a patient who had a central line within the 48-hour period before the development of the BSI and is not related to an infection at another site. It requires less strict criteria for its diagnosis and can be used for surveillance purposes.

RISK FACTORS

Critically ill children have many factors, which increase their risk for CR BSI. The risk factors for CR-BSI have been enlisted in Box 1.

Box 1: Risk factors for CRBSI.

- *Patient-related risk factors*:
    - Severity of underlying infection
    - Prolong duration of hospitalization before central line insertion
    - Prolong hospitalization
    - Immunosuppression
    - Prematurity
    - Parenteral nutrition
    - Loss of skin integrity
    - Prolonged antibiotic therapy
- *Catheter-related*:
    - *Catheter material*:
        - Highest infection risks with polyvinyl chloride and polyethylene catheter
        - Polyurethane and silicone elastomer (polytetrafluorethylene)—less thrombogenic and seem to have lesser infection complications
    - Length or size of the catheter
    - Catheter lumen—more the number of lumens more risk of infections
    - *Site of catheter*: The risk of colonization in the following ascending order—subclavian < femoral < internal jugular
    - Catheter inserted in the ICU/emergency room has higher incidence of infection.
    - Lack of maximal sterile barrier for central venous catheter insertion
    - Heavy microbial colonization at the insertion site
    - *Duration of placement*: Risk increases with duration
    - *Type of placement*: Risk is more with venous cut down than percutaneous line insertions. Tunneling reduces the risk of infection regardless of the site of insertion.
- *Pathogen–related*:
    - Some strains of coagulase negative *Staphylococcus* (CONS) produce an antiphagocytic exocalyx.
    - Host factor-binding protein such as fibrinogen receptor ClfA and fibronectin-binding protein (FbpA and FbpB) appear to be important in the adherence of *Staphylococcus aureus* to catheter surface.

ETIOLOGICAL AGENTS

A study by Singh et al. in 2009, from Gujarat, India, showed that the common organisms responsible for BSIs were—Coagulase negative *Staphylococcus* (CONS), enterococci, staphylococci, and *Candida* species. Others include extended spectrum beta-lactamase (ESBL)-producing organisms (*Pseudomonas, Klebsiella, E. coli, Serratia,* etc.). The *Candida* BSIs are caused by nonalbicans (*C. krusei* and *C. glabrata*), which are not susceptible to fluconazole.

Certain pathogens are associated with specific host, treatment, and catheter characteristics. *Staphylococcus aureus* infections are disproportionately represented in infections of hemodialysis catheters. Gram-negative bacilli have been associated with infections of patients with cancer, and they are typically the pathogens recovered in instances of infusate contaminations. Gram-negative bacilli and yeast have been affiliated with catheters placed in femoral veins, while *Candida* have been associated with infections of lines used for administration of parenteral nutrition.

DIAGNOSTIC CRITERIA

Catheter-related bloodstream infection should be suspected in a patient with an intravascular catheter who develops the clinical or laboratory criteria of the systemic inflammatory response syndrome (i.e., temperature <36°C or >38°C, heart rate >2 SD for age, respiratory rate > 2 SD for age, or peripheral white blood cell count <4,000/mL or >12,000/mL).

- A positive result of semiquantitative (>15 CFU/catheters/segment) or quantitative (>102 CFU/catheter segment) culture
- Same organism (specimen and antibiogram) is isolated from a catheter segment and peripheral blood
- Suggestive organisms (*CONS, S. aureus,* and *Candida species*) isolated from blood
- Lack of other sources of bacteria
- Differential time to positivity (DTP), best defines CRBSI. It is defined as growth from a catheter hub blood sample is seen at least 2 hours before growth is detected in a blood sample obtained from a peripheral vein.
- Three-fold greater bacterial count from the central venous catheter (CVC) site compared with the peripheral vein is predictive of CR BSI.

At least two blood cultures should be obtained when catheter infection is suspected. When the tip of a catheter is sent for culture, the two blood cultures may be obtained by peripheral venipuncture. Alternatively or when culture of the tip of the catheter is not performed, one blood culture should be obtained by peripheral venipuncture and at least one blood culture should be obtained from a lumen of the catheter.

As per few reports drawing multiple catheter blood cultures, one from each lumen of the catheter suspected of infection, in addition to one blood culture obtained by peripheral venipuncture will enhance detection of catheter infection.

For patients with multiple central venous and/or arterial catheters, a blood culture should be drawn through each catheter in addition to that obtained by peripheral venipuncture; in these circumstances drawing blood cultures from all lumens of all catheters is not endorsed. To reduce the incidence of blood culture contamination, the skin and the hub of the catheter must be cleansed with alcohol, tincture of iodine or alcohol chlorhexidine, and allowed to dry, before specimen collection.

MANAGEMENT (SHORT-TERM CENTRAL VENOUS LINE)

Management requires good clinical judgment and it can be challenging in the absence of specific pediatric data. The decision to remove the catheter should be based on many factors such as underlying illness, need for intravascular access, catheter type, pathogen type and the likelihood of successful replacement at another site. Catheter removal is strongly recommended for high virulence infections such as those caused by *Staphylococcus aureus, Candida species* and coliform bacteria because of their tendency to result in metastatic infection. It is also indicated for the patients who deteriorate on appropriately chosen antibiotics.

Following guidelines have been proposed by the IDSA in its 2009 guidelines:
- Empiric antibiotics against gram negative bacilli should be based on local susceptibility patterns and severity of illness
- Antibiotics active against *Pseudomonas aeruginosa*, based upon local susceptibility patterns, are to be used in the setting of neutropenia, severe illness, or known colonization
- Antimicrobials active against *Candida*, preferably an echinocandin, should be used in the setting of femoral catheterization, total parenteral nutrition, prolonged administration of broad-spectrum antibiotics, hematologic malignancy, or solid organ or hematopoietic stem cell transplantation
- Vancomycin is recommended in institutions where the prevalence of methicillin resistance in staphylococci is increased (otherwise use a first-generation cephalosporin such as cefazolin or an anti-staphylococcal penicillin such as nafcillin)
- Daptomycin in lieu of vancomycin in facilities where the prevalence of methicillin-resistant *S. aureus* with reduced vancomycin susceptibility (minimum inhibitory concentration >2 µg/mL) is increased.

For patients with short-term central venous or arterial CR BSI, the infected catheter, or the catheter placed over a guidewire in exchange for the infected catheter, should be removed expeditiously.

For uncomplicated BSI (i.e. no associated supportive thrombosis, endocarditis, or metastatic infection) that arises in the absence of factors that increase the risk of hematogenous spread of infection (e.g., no intravascular hardware, immunosuppression) and which resolves within 72 hours of catheter removal, systemic therapeutic, intravenous antibiotic treatment is recommended for:
- 5–7 days for coagulase-negative staphylococci
- 7–14 days for enterococci and gram-negative bacilli
- 14 days in the absence of evidence of fungal retinitis for Candida species
- 14 days in the absence of evidence of endocarditis clinically and by transesophageal echocardiography (TEE), for *S. aureus*.

For patients with susceptible pathogens and a functioning gastrointestinal tract, orally administered linezolid, fluoroquinolones, or fluconazole may be considered for treatment of methicillin-resistant staphylococci, gram-negative bacilli, and *Candida*, retrospectively.

For patients with short-term central venous or arterial CR BSI lasting over 72 hours, or with factors that increase the risk of metastatic infection, longer duration of antibiotic administration directed by patient, pathogen, and disease characteristics will be required. Expert opinion in the form of infectious diseases consultation should be considered to assist the evaluation and management of these more complicated infections.

Long-term Central Venous Line

Patients with long-term CR BSI associated with septic thrombosis, endocarditis, metastatic infection (e.g., osteomyelitis), subcutaneous catheter tunnel track or port infection, the catheter should be removed immediately. Catheter removal is also recommended for *S. aureus*, *Bacillus* species, micrococcus, *Propionibacterium*, *P. aeruginosa*, *Candida*, or mycobacterial infection.

About 4–6 weeks of therapy is often required for *S. aureus* infection, the specific duration depends on the patient, pathogen, and disease characteristics. Fourteen days of administration can be considered for non-neutropenic, non-immunosuppressed patients without septic thrombosis, endocarditis, metastatic infection, or prosthetic intravascular devices when *S. aureus* or other bacterial infection resolves within 72 hours of antibiotic initiation and catheter removal. For patients with *Candida* infection in whom there is no suspicion or evidence of metastatic infection (including candida retinitis) and for whom fungemia and evidence of infection resolve promptly upon catheter removal, antifungal therapy should be continued for 14 days after the first negative blood culture.

A new long-term CVC can be placed at a new anatomic site after 72 hours of effective antibiotic administration and lack of growth in repeat blood cultures.

Antibiotic lock therapy and systemic therapy can be tried for patients with highly needed catheter, when infection with CONS is documented and there are no systemic signs of sepsis.

For patients with long-term central venous CR BSI unassociated with septic thrombosis, endocarditis, metastatic infection, tunnel track, or port infection caused by coagulase-negative staphylococci, enterococci, or non-*Pseudomonas* gram-negative bacilli, treatment without catheter removal can be attempted. Systemic therapeutic antibiotics should be given for 10–14 days.

Bundle approach to prevent vascular catheter associated BSIs was one of the first to be reported in the literature. Pronovost et al. demonstrated that intervention using care bundles decreased infection rates by up to 66%. The individual elements included:
- Hand washing
- Using full barrier precautions during central line insertion
- Cleaning the skin with chlorhexidine
- Rapidly removing unnecessary catheters.

The CDC/IDSA guidelines for the prevention and management of catheter-related infections are evidence-based and a must-read for every health team member involved with prevention of CRBSI (Box 2).

Box 2: Methods to prevent catheter-related bloodstream infections.

- Limit insertion to trained personnel
- Avoid use of the femoral vein
- Use subclavian vein in lieu of the internal jugular or femoral vein depending upon risk of injury during insertion
- Use a central venous catheter with the minimum number of lumens required for patient care
- Complete hand hygiene prior to insertion or dressing change of catheter exit site
- Prepare insertion site with more than 0.5% chlorhexidine plus alcohol
- Do not administer systemic antimicrobial prophylaxis

Contd...

Contd...

- Use a chlorhexidine/silver sulfadiazine or a minocycline-/rifampin-impregnated central venous catheter when the local rate of central line-associated bloodstream infection is not declining despite:
  - Education of optimal insertion and maintenance practices
  - Use of maximum sterile barrier precautions during insertion
  - Use of more than 0.5% chlorhexidine plus alcohol for preparation of skin before insertion
- Use maximum sterile barrier precautions, including cap, mask, sterile gown, sterile gloves, and a sterile full-body drape for insertion and during guidewire exchange
- Place semipermeable transparent or gauze dressing over insertion site
- Gauze is favored when exit site is bloody or moist
- Restrict application of antimicrobial ointment to exit sites of hemodialysis catheters
- *Assess exit site daily*:
  - Visually for transparent dressings
  - By palpation for gauze dressings (remove for visual inspection, if tender)
- Exchange exit site dressing whenever damp, loosened, or soiled
- Replace gauze dressings every 2 days
- Replace semipermeable transparent dressings every 7 days
- When adherence to aseptic technique was compromised during insertion, replace the catheter as soon as possible
- Do not routinely replace central venous catheters to prevent infection
- Remove any intravascular catheter as soon as it is no longer required for patient care

What probably works	*What does not work*
• Antibiotic lock solution	• Cut down for arterial/central access
• Use of antibiotic/antiseptic impregnated catheter (adult studies show efficacy)	• Scheduled guidewire exchanges of central venous catheter
• Heparin bonded catheter	• Topical antibiotics at insertion site
	• Systemic antibiotic prophylaxis

SUGGESTED READING

1. Bell T, O'Grady NP. Prevention of central line-associated bloodstream infections. Infect Dis Clin North Am. 2017;31(3):551-9.
2. Mermel LA, Allon M, Bouza E, et al. Clinical practice guidelines for the diagnosis and management of intravascular catheter-related infection: 2009 update by the Infectious Disease Society of America. Clin Infectious Dis. 2009;49(1):1-45.
3. O'Grady NP, Alexander M, Burns LA. Guidelines for the prevention of intravascular catheter-related infections. Clin Infect Dis. 2011;52(9):162-93.
4. Rosenthal VD, Maki DG, Salomo R, et al. Device associated nosocomial infections in 55 intensive care units of 8 developing countries. Ann Intern Med. 2006;145:582-91.
5. Shah H, Bosch W, Thompson KM, Hellinger WC. Intravascular catheter-related bloodstream infection. Neurohospitalist. 2013;3(3):144-51.
6. Singh S, Pandya Y, Patel R, et al. Surveillance of device-associated infections at a teaching hospital in rural Gujarat-India. Indian J Med Microbiol. 2010;28:342-7.

Catheter-associated Urinary Tract Infection

36

Vishal Baldua, Deepali Wankhade

LEARNING OBJECTIVES

- Understanding the mechanisms leading to development of catheter-associated urinary tract infection (CAUTI)
- Understanding the signs, symptoms, and lab tests appropriate for diagnosing CAUTI
- Identify current best practices in the management of urinary catheters and CAUTI prevention.
- Rational management of bacteriuria and candiduria esp. differentiating infections from colonization.

INTRODUCTION

Urinary tract infection (UTI) accounts for almost 25% of hospital-acquired infections and is mostly attributable to an indwelling urethral catheter. It adds significantly to morbidity and intensive care unit (ICU) cost-of-care, though very rarely causing mortality.

DEFINITION

The Infectious Diseases Society of America (IDSA) guidelines define catheter-associated bacteriuria as follows:
- *Symptomatic bacteriuria UTI*—culture growth of $\geq 10^3$ colony forming units (CFU)/mL of uropathogenic bacteria in the presence of symptoms or signs compatible with UTI without other identifiable source in a patient with indwelling urethral, indwelling suprapubic, or intermittent catheterization
- *Asymptomatic bacteriuria*—culture growth of $\geq 10^5$ CFU/mL of uropathogenic bacteria in the absence of symptoms compatible with UTI in a patient with indwelling urethral, indwelling suprapubic, or intermittent catheterization.

Patients who are no longer catheterized but had urethral, suprapubic, or condom catheters within the past 48 hours are also considered to have CAUTI or asymptomatic bacteriuria if they meet these definitions.

Epidemiology and Risk Factors

The daily risk of acquisition of bacteriuria varies from 3 to 7% with an indwelling urethral catheter of which 10–25% develop symptoms of UTI. The burden of CAUTI in pediatric patients is not well defined.

Examples of appropriate indications for indwelling urethral catheter use are limited and include the following:
- Perioperative use for selected surgical procedures
- Hourly assessment of urine output in critically sick patients in an ICU
- Management of acute urinary retention and urinary obstruction

Some risk factors for the development of CAUTI:
- The duration of catheterization
- Not maintaining a closed drainage system
- Neutropenia, renal disease, and female sex
- Diarrhea, diabetes, absence of antibiotics
- Renal insufficiency and immunocompromised or debilitated states.

Etiopathogenesis

Source of microorganisms in CAUTI may be endogenous (meatal, rectal, or vaginal colonization) or exogenous (contaminated hands of healthcare professionals). The biofilm that forms around the catheter helps extra-luminal bacteria to proliferate into the bladder. Such extraluminal bacteria may be difficult to eradicate without catheter removal. Common culprits of CAUTI include *Escherichia coli, Pseudomonas species, Enterococcus species, Staphylococcus aureus,* coagulase-negative staphylococci, *Enterobacter species,* and yeast. Proteus and *Pseudomonas species* are often associated with biofilm growth on catheters.

CLINICAL PRESENTATION

New onset fever or septic shock in the appropriate clinical background may be the first hint of urosepsis due to an in situ urinary catheter. Fever, irritability, poor feeding, nonspecific gastrointestinal (GI) symptoms, and abdominal pain may be the presenting features. Most patients are asymptomatic. The use of clinical signs such as fever, leukocytosis, and decreased renal function cannot reliably distinguish between asymptomatic fungiuria and actual infection.

LABORATORY FINDINGS

Specimen collection—Correct technique is vital to correct diagnosis and treatment.
- Ideally remove the catheter and obtain a midstream specimen
- If ongoing catheterization is needed, the catheter should be replaced prior to collecting a urine sample for culture, to avoid culturing bacteria present in the biofilm of the catheter but not in the bladder
- Many systems have a "needleless" site that can be cleansed prior to specimen collection. If a sample is being collected without catheter removal, urine should be obtained from the port in the drainage system.

For circumstances in which the above approaches are not possible, the culture should be obtained by separating the catheter from the drainage system.

Pyuria is a common finding in catheterized patients with bacteriuria, whether they are symptomatic (implying an actual infection) or not. Quantitative urine white blood cells (WBCs) >10 cells/μL had low sensitivity for predicting growth of >10^5 CFU/mL. By definition, all patients with CAUTI have bacteriuria or funguria on culture specimen as described above.

Odorous or cloudy urine has not been demonstrated to be indicative of either bacteriuria or UTI.

CANDIDURIA: "INFECTION VERSUS COLONIZATION"

Most patients with candiduria are asymptomatic and the yeasts merely represent colonization. It is found that neither the presence of pseudohyphae in the urine nor the number of colonies growing in culture, unlike bacterial urine cultures, help to distinguish colonization from infection.

Persistent candiduria should prompt blood cultures and radiologic imaging—computed tomography (CT) scans or sonography—that may show hydronephrosis, fungus balls, or perinephric abscesses associated with ascending infection.

TREATMENT

- *Antibiotics*: Antimicrobial selection should be based on the culture results when available. In select cases, empiric antimicrobial choice should be tailored to results of past cultures, use of ongoing antibiotics and community prevalence of antimicrobial resistance. Urine Gram stain, if available, can also guide empiric antimicrobial choice. Treatment of incidentally discovered asymptomatic bacteriuria is not indicated as per current guidelines.
- *Catheter management*: Patients who no longer require catheterization should have the catheter removed and receive antibiotics as per locally prevalent microbial growth. If long-term catheterization is needed and intermittent catheterization is not feasible, the catheter should be replaced at the initiation of antimicrobial therapy. Catheter replacement is associated with fewer and later relapses than retaining the original catheter, as biofilm penetration of most antimicrobials is poor.
- *Candiduria:* Elimination of predisposing factors, such as indwelling bladder catheters, is recommended whenever feasible. Treatment for asymptomatic candiduria is recommended only for neutropenic patients, very-low-birth-weight infants (<1,500 g) and patients who will undergo urologic manipulation as these groups risk dissemination.

Symptomatic candiduria should be treated with appropriate antifungal. Fluconazole achieves high urinary concentrations and is effective in most cases. Nonalbicans candiduria is an emerging threat and may need the usage of amphotericin or flucytosine.

PREVENTION

Recommendations for prevention of infections associated with short-term indwelling urethral catheters are based on the 2009 Centers for Disease Control and Prevention (CDC) and IDSA guidelines:
- Documentation of catheter insertion
- Trained personnel

- Hand hygiene—during and after insertion
- Evaluation of necessity and alternative methods
- Regular review of ongoing need
- Choice of catheter and use of smallest gauge catheter
- Aseptic technique/sterile equipment
- Barrier precautions for insertion
- Antiseptic cleaning of meatus
- Secure catheter and use closed drainage system (using preconnected systems)
- Obtain urine samples aseptically
- Replace system if there is a break in asepsis
- No routine change in catheter
- Routine hygiene for meatal care
- Avoid irrigation for purpose of preventing infection
- Utilize bladder scanners to measure urine volume and promote catheter removal when feasible.

Approaches that should not be considered as a routine part of CAUTI prevention:
- Do not routinely use antimicrobial/antiseptic-impregnated catheters
- Do not screen for asymptomatic bacteriuria in catheterized patients
- Do not treat asymptomatic bacteriuria in catheterized patients except before invasive urologic procedures
- Avoid catheter irrigation
- Do not use systemic antimicrobials routinely.

Nurses can be educated and trained to implement CAUTI prevention bundles:
- Provide daily reminders to physicians to remove unnecessary catheters
- Standardize indications for urinary catheter placement
- Utilize bladder bundle
- Develop a nurse-driven protocol to discontinue catheter if no longer meeting criteria
- Mandatory order to remove catheter after 5 days
- Standardize products, increase availability of bedside commodes
- Create educational materials, e.g., posters in units—pocket cards.

Some Interesting Studies

- A prospective randomized trial of thoracic surgery patients managed with epidural analgesia compared morning-after-surgery catheter removal with the catheter remaining in place as long as the thoracic epidural analgesia was functioning. There was a longer time to reach post void residuals of less than 200 mL with early removal and increased need for recatheterization

    (*Ref.*: Annals of Thoracic surgery, 2016 September)
- Suganya et al. demonstrated that a workable initiative focusing on removal of unnecessary central line (CL) and urinary catheter (UC) can be easily implemented requiring minimal time and resources. A rebound increase in urinary catheter device utilization ratios

(UC-DURs) to preintervention levels after intervention end indicates that continued vigilance is required to maintain performance (*Ref.*: Open Forum Infectious Diseases volume 5, issue 7, July 2018)
- Implementation of the CAUTI prevention bundle was associated with a 50% reduction in the mean monthly CAUTI rate (95% confidence interval: -1.28 to -0.12; $P = 0.02$) from 5.41 to 2.49 per 1,000 catheter days (*Ref.*: Pediatrics, volume 134, number 3, September 2014)
- The implementation of CAUTI bundle care successfully reduced CAUTI in Taiwanese high-risk units (*Ref.*: Journal of Microbiology, Immunology and Infection (2017) 50, 464e470).

KEY MESSAGES

- Catheter-associated UTI is a serious problem even in tertiary ICUs. The most important risk factor is the duration of catheterization followed by errors in catheter care
- The diagnosis of a CAUTI is made by the finding of bacteriuria in a catheterized patient who had signs and symptoms that are consistent with UTI or systemic infection and are otherwise unexplained
- Methods of urine collection for cultures should be strictly followed as described above to avoid unnecessary treatment and increase in drug resistance in the unit. Antimicrobial selection should be based on the culture results when available
- Treatment of incidentally discovered asymptomatic bacteriuria is not indicated. Avoidance of unnecessary catheterization, use of sterile technique for insertion, and removal as soon as possible are essential to the prevention of CAUTI
- Implementation of bundle approach and nurses' training and involvement in catheter usage may help decrease the incidence of CAUTI.

SUGGESTED READING

1. Bardossy AC, Jayaprakash R, Alangaden AC, et al. Impact and Limitations of the 2015 National Health and Safety Network Case Definition on Catheter-Associated Urinary Tract Infection Rates. Infect Control Hosp Epidemiol. 2017;38:239.
2. CDC. (2018). Urinary Tract Infection (Catheter-Associated Urinary Tract Infection [CAUTI] and Non-Catheter-Associated Urinary Tract Infection [UTI]) and Other Urinary System Infection [USI]) Events. Available from: http://www.cdc.gov/nhsn/PDFs/pscManual/7pscCAUTIcurrent.pdf
3. Goyal RK, Sami H, Mishra V, et al. Nonalbicans candiduria: An emerging threat. J App Pharm Sci. 2016;6(3):48-50.
4. Hooton TM, Bradley SF, Cardenas DD, et al. Diagnosis, prevention, and treatment of catheter-associated urinary tract infection in adults: 2009 International Clinical Practice guidelines from the Infectious Diseases Society of America. Clin Infect Dis. 2010;50:625.
5. Kauffman CA. Diagnosis and management of fungal urinary tract infection. Infect Dis Clin North Am. 2014;28(1):61.
7. Neelakanta A, Sharma S, Kesani VP, et al. Impact of changes in the NHSN catheter-associated urinary tract infection (CAUTI) surveillance criteria on the frequency and epidemiology of CAUTI in intensive care units (ICUs). Infect Control Hosp Epidemiol. 2015;36:346.
6. Leuck AM, Wright D, Ellingson L, et al. Complications of Foley catheters--is infection the greatest risk? J Urol. 2012;187:1662.

8. Pappas PG, Kauffman CA, Andes DR, et al. Clinical Practice Guideline for the Management of Candidiasis: 2016 Update by the Infectious Diseases Society of America. Clin Infect Dis. 2016;62(4):e1-50.
9. Richards MJ, Edwards JR, Culver DH, et al. Nosocomial infections in medical intensive care units in the United States. National Nosocomial Infections Surveillance System. Crit Care Med. 1999;27(5):887.
10. Tambyah PA, Maki DG. Catheter-associated urinary tract infection is rarely symptomatic: A prospective study of 1,497 catheterized patients. Arch Intern Med. 2000;160:678.

Antimicrobial Stewardship in PICU

37

Rachna Sharma

LEARNING OBJECTIVES

- To describe the evidence-based approach to antimicrobial stewardship program.
- To describe the components of an ideal antimicrobial stewardship program.

INTRODUCTION

Antimicrobial resistance (AMR) is a looming threat to the current medical practice. Irrational antibiotic combinations and lower thresholds for starting antibiotics in fragile pediatric patients in the pediatric intensive care unit (PICU) lead to the emergence of multi-drug resistant (MDR) microorganisms and failure of our "faithful antibiotics". Drug toxicity and drug interactions complicate it further. In India, the infectious disease burden is among the highest in the world and a recent WHO report showed the inappropriate and irrational use of antimicrobial agents has led to the increase in development of antimicrobial resistance.

Pediatric intensive care unit children are at a higher risk of acquiring infections because of the use of different invasive procedures, invasive devices, and extended length of stay. Hospital-acquired infections (HAIs) are a serious concern in them and have been reported to occur in 16–23% of patients admitted to PICUs.

Antimicrobial stewardship program (ASP) is one approach to optimize drug use and improve patient outcomes. Infectious Disease Society of America (IDSA) defines ASP as "a set of coordinated interventions, designed to improve and measure the appropriate use of antimicrobials by promoting the selection of the optimal antimicrobial drug regimen (including the appropriate agent, dose, route of administration, and duration of therapy)". ASP as a strategy was introduced in IDSA in 2007. The 2006 Centres For Disease Control (CDC) guideline "Management of Multi-drug-Resistant Organisms in Healthcare Settings" stated that control of multi-drug resistant organisms in healthcare "must include attention to judicious antimicrobial use". In 2009, CDC launched the "Get Smart for Healthcare Campaign" to promote improved use of antibiotics in acute care hospitals and in 2013 the CDC highlighted the need to improve antibiotic use as one of four key strategies required to address the problem of growing antibiotic resistance in the US. In recognition of the urgent need to improve antibiotic use in hospitals and the benefits of antibiotic stewardship programs, in 2014 CDC recommended that all acute care hospitals implement Antibiotic Stewardship Programs (ASP's).

While there are guidelines and evidence for ASPs in adult ICUs, there is limited evidence for the same in PICUs. Data evaluating the impact of ASPs on HAIs and AMR in PICUs are lacking. In addition, there is also limited information on effective components of a successful ASP in PICU. In 2010, the Pediatric Infectious Diseases Society (PIDS) formed the Paediatric Committee on Antimicrobial Stewardship with the mission of advancing pediatric AS in various clinical settings, promoting research in pediatric AS, and developing AS educational programs. The American Academy of Paediatrics also recommends implementation of AS programs for healthcare organizations that provide inpatient and outpatient pediatric care.

PRINCIPLES AND STRATEGIES OF ANTIBIOTIC STEWARDSHIP PROGRAMS

Antimicrobial stewardship strategies and protocols incorporate core principles as laid down by the CDC. Understanding these core principles can help identify opportunities to develop ASP (Table 1).

Table 1: Principles and strategies for AS programs.

Timely antibiotic therapy management	• Ensuring prompt initiation of antibiotic therapy when indicated as in critical illness such as sepsis and high-risk patients with serious bacterial infections • Avoiding use of antibiotics when not indicated as in viral upper or lower respiratory tract infections, asthma exacerbations and viral pharyngitis • Use of clinical guidelines and algorithms that facilitate provider recognition of clinical syndromes that do and do not require antibiotics
Appropriate selection of antibiotics	• Ensuring that proper antibiotic regimens are selected for specific clinical syndromes and infections • Minimizing redundant antibiotic regimens for gram negative or anaerobic bacterial infections • Use of antibiograms and clinical guidelines to optimize antibiotic selections
Appropriate administration and de-escalation of antibiotic therapy	• Ensuring proper dosing of antibiotics • Peer review of antibiotic use at 48–72 h after initiation to determine if therapy should be continued, changed, or discontinued • Monitoring for serum therapeutic levels of antibiotics • Proper administration of antibiotics for surgical prophylaxis
Use of expertise and resources at point of care	• Formation of multidisciplinary AS committees • Obtaining administrative and leadership support
Continuous and transparent monitoring of antibiotic use	• Auditing antibiotic use to identify opportunities for stewardship and education • Prospective monitoring to assess efficacy of AS program

Appropriate and Prompt Antimicrobial Therapy Initiation

Appropriate and timely antibiotics have been shown to reduce morality in septic shock patients when administered within the first hour of resuscitation. Barriers to antibiotic administration may be due to delayed order entry, pharmacy related issues, shortage of staff and lack of emergency medicines in the stock. AS Protocols and interventions have been shown to be effective in reducing the time to antibiotic administration by addressing these barriers. ASPs can facilitate prompt initiation of therapy by developing protocols and guidelines based on evidence and best practices. AS also prevents misuse and overuse of antibiotics. These programs incorporate educational material for physicians and patients and also conduct clinical audits and offer feedbacks to review the state of antibiotic use.

Appropriate Selection of Antibiotics

Empirical antibiotics have to be chosen wisely based on the knowledge of prevalent strains and resistance patterns. Antibiograms help in proper selection of antibiotics and limit inappropriate use of irrational combinations of antibiotics thus saving resources and preventing resistances.

Appropriate Administration and De-escalation of Antibiotic Therapy

Pediatric AS programs use involves protocols and standardized prescription orders along with periodic surveillance of antibiotic use. Appropriate dosing using therapeutic drug level monitoring for drugs like vancomycin is useful for better efficacy. De-escalation of antibiotics is one of the most widely adopted and advocated principles of AS. It involves reducing the number of antibiotics, selecting narrow over broad-spectrum antibiotics, or converting parenteral to oral therapy as soon as possible.

Use of Expertise and Resources at Point of Care

Infectious Disease Society of America guidelines on ASPs advocate development of local AS teams or committees composed of experts from multiple fields, including infectious diseases, pharmacy, microbiology, infection control, and information technology. Support from hospital administration and medical staff leadership in establishing appropriate authority and securing financial resources for an AS program is essential to its success.

Continuous and Transparent Monitoring of Antibiotic Use

Consistent and standardized surveillance is required to promote appropriate use of antibiotics and to judge the effectiveness of active AS programs with an aim to improve performance of the existing protocols.

IDSA ANTIBIOTIC STEWARDSHIP GUIDELINES (2016)

Infectious Disease Society of America (IDSA)/Society for Healthcare Epidemiology of America (SHEA) recommends that ASPs be multidisciplinary, including a pediatric infectious disease physician leader, a clinical pharmacist (preferably with infectious disease training), a clinical microbiologist, an information system specialist, an infection prevention specialist, and a hospital epidemiologist. The new guidelines focussed more on specific strategies to ensure the program will be more effective and sustainable. A summary of the guidelines and relevant points has been listed below:

- Preauthorized and prospective audits with feedback form part of a multi-combed approach for consistent implementation. These have been shown to reduce antibiotic use, reduce antibiotic resistance, and reduce *Clostridium difficile* infection (CDI) rates without a negative impact on patient outcomes like mortality. The focus is more on active teaching and develop curriculum to ingrain principles of AS in the clinician's mind. Effective implementation requires the support of hospital administration, allocation of necessary resources for a persistent effort by dedicated, well-trained personnel, and ongoing communication with clinicians
- Patients with specific disease syndromes such as community-acquired pneumonia, healthcare-associated infections due to organisms such as methicillin-resistant *Staphylococcus aureus* (MRSA) or MDR *Pseudomonas* will benefit from targeted and timely drug therapy. Early active alert by microbiologists after positive blood cultures of ASP team has shown benefits in terms of reduced mortality and reduced length of stay
- Antibiotic review by the prescriber can have an important stewardship impact if done with appropriate reminders and sustained efforts
- Antibiotic cycling (substitution with a different class of antibiotics but with the same spectrum over a designated period of time) and antibiotic mixing (in which consecutive patients with the same diagnosis receive an antibiotic from a different class in rotation) are not advised as yet in ASP
- Use of pharmacokinetics and pharmacodynamics for some antibiotics like vancomycin, aminoglycosides etc. has been found to be useful in reducing nephrotoxicity but definite guidelines advocating their use cannot be recommended
- ASPs should implement strategies to assess patients who can safely complete therapy with an oral regimen to reduce the need for IV catheters and to avoid outpatient parenteral therapy
- Antibiotics should be used for the shortest effective duration. Studies have shown that shorter courses of antibiotic therapy are associated with outcomes similar to those with longer courses in both adults and children
- Use of stratified antibiograms, e.g., based on location (ICU vs. non-ICU), population (medical and surgical; pediatrics vs. adults) are helpful to ASPs for the development of guidelines for empiric therapy
- Use of specialized tests like rapid molecular assays, PCR for viral testing, and specific fungal markers like galactomannan may be useful
- Outcome measures should study the effectiveness of ASP including antibiotic cost per patient-day and patient outcome analysis like mortality and length of hospital stay.

CORE ELEMENTS OF HOSPITAL ANTIBIOTIC STEWARDSHIP PROGRAMS

The centres for Disease Control have laid down the core elements (Table 2) of successful hospital ASPs. It complements existing guidelines on ASPs from organizations including the

Table 2: Core elements of hospital Antibiotic Stewardship Programs.

Leadership commitment	Dedicating necessary human financial and information technology resources
Accountability	Appointing a single leader responsible for program outcomes. Experience with successful programs show that a physician leader is effective
Drug expertise	Appointing a single pharmacist leader responsible for working to improve antibiotic use
Action	Implementing at least one recommended action, such as systemic evaluation of ongoing treatment need after a set period of initial treatment (i.e., "antibiotic time out" after 48 h)
Tracking	Monitoring antibiotic prescribing and resistance patterns
Reporting	Regular reporting information on antibiotic use and resistance to doctors, nurses, and relevant staff
Education	Educating clinicians about resistance and optimal prescribing

IDSA/SHEA. The success of any ASPs is dependent on defined leadership and a coordinated multidisciplinary approach

The following checklist (Table 3) is a companion to core elements of hospital antibiotic stewardship programs. This checklist should be used to systematically assess key elements and actions to ensure optimal antibiotic prescribing and limit overuse and misuse of antibiotics in hospitals. Facilities using this checklist should involve one or more knowledgeable staff to determine if the following principles and actions to improve antibiotic use are in place. The elements in this checklist have been shown in previous studies to be helpful in improving antibiotic use though not all of the elements might be feasible in all hospitals.

COMMON BARRIERS TO DEVELOPMENT AND IMPLEMENTATION OF ANTIBIOTIC STEWARDSHIP PROGRAMS (TABLE 4)

The most common barriers are lack of funding or time to support a program, lack of physician participation, lack of diagnostic facilities, awareness lack of hospital administration, awareness of the value of AS programs, and concerns about the effect of the stewardship program on physician autonomy, such as potential antagonism between physician groups. A potential strategy to overcome these barriers is to use a conceptual framework that identifies potential categories of barriers as knowledge, attitude, and practice barriers.

- *Knowledge barrier*: Physicians should be aware of the ASP and its role. Evidence-based guidelines and strategies for overcoming the reluctance of administrative leaders to invest in AS should be encouraged
- *Attitude barrier*: Multidisciplinary groups should review existing evidence and develop consensus guidelines and physician's fears and beliefs should be addressed. Recommendations should not cause antagonism because they challenge long-standing clinical practices. Senior consultants should bridge the gap between the AS team and their colleagues

Table 3: Checklist for core elements of hospital Antibiotic Stewardship Programs.

Leadership support	A. Does your facility have a formal, written statement of support from leadership that supports efforts to improve antibiotic use (antibiotic stewardship)? ☐ Yes ☐ No B. Does your facility receive any budgeted financial support for antibiotic stewardship activities (e.g., support for salary, training, or IT support)? ☐ Yes ☐ No
Accountability	A. Is there a physician leader responsible for program outcomes of stewardship activities at your facility? ☐ Yes ☐ No
Drug expertise	A. Is there a pharmacist leader responsible for working to improve antibiotic use at your facility? ☐ Yes ☐ No

Key support for the antibiotic stewardship program

Does any of the staff work with the stewardship leaders to improve antibiotic use?	B. Clinicians ☐ Yes ☐ No C. Infection Prevention and Healthcare Epidemiology ☐ Yes ☐ No D. Quality Improvement ☐ Yes ☐ No E. Microbiology (Laboratory) ☐ Yes ☐ No F. Information Technology (IT) ☐ Yes ☐ No G. Nursing ☐ Yes ☐ No

Actions to support optimal antibiotic use

Policies	A. Does your facility have a policy that requires prescribers to document in the medical record or during order entry a dose, duration, and indication for all antibiotic prescriptions? ☐ Yes ☐ No B. Does your facility have facility-specific treatment recommendations, based on national guidelines and local susceptibility, to assist with antibiotic selection for common clinical conditions? ☐ Yes ☐ No
• Specific interventions to improve antibiotic use – Are the following actions to improve antibiotic prescribing conducted in your facility? https://www.cdc.gov/antibiotic-use/healthcare/pdfs/checklist.pdf	C. Is there a formal procedure for all clinicians to review the appropriateness of all antibiotics 48 hours after the initial orders (e.g. antibiotic time out)? ☐ Yes ☐ No D. Do specified antibiotic agents need to be approved by a physician or pharmacist prior to dispensing (i.e., pre-authorization) at your facility? ☐ Yes ☐ No E. Does a physician or pharmacist review courses of therapy for specified antibiotic agents (i.e., prospective audit with feedback) at your facility? ☐ Yes ☐ No
• Pharmacy-driven interventions – Are the following actions implemented in your facility?	F. Automatic changes from intravenous to oral antibiotic therapy in appropriate situations? ☐ Yes ☐ No G. Dose adjustments in cases of organ dysfunction? ☐ Yes ☐ No H. Dose optimization (pharmacokinetics/pharmacodynamics) to optimize the treatment of organisms with reduced susceptibility? ☐ Yes ☐ No I. Automatic alerts in situations where therapy might be unnecessarily duplicative? ☐ Yes ☐ No J. Time-sensitive automatic stop orders for specified antibiotic prescriptions? ☐ Yes ☐ No

Contd...

Contd...

• Diagnosis and infections specific interventions – Does your facility have specific interventions in place to ensure optimal use of antibiotics to treat the following common infections?	K. Community-acquired pneumonia ☐ Yes ☐ No L. Urinary tract infection ☐ Yes ☐ No M. Skin and soft tissue infections ☐ Yes ☐ No N. Surgical prophylaxis ☐ Yes ☐ No O. Empiric treatment of Methicillin-resistant *Staphylococcus aureus* (MRSA) ☐ Yes ☐ No P. Non-C. *Difficile* infection (CDI) antibiotics in new cases of CDI ☐ Yes ☐ No Q. Culture-proven invasive ☐ Yes ☐ No (e.g., blood stream) infections
Tracking: Monitoring antibiotic prescribing, use, and resistance	
Process measures	A. Does your stewardship program monitor adherence to a documentation policy (dose, duration, and indication)? ☐ Yes ☐ No B. Does your stewardship program monitor adherence to facility-specific treatment recommendations? ☐ Yes ☐ No C. Does your stewardship program monitor compliance with one of more of the specific interventions in place? ☐ Yes ☐ No
Antibiotic use and outcome measures	D. Does your facility track rates of CDI? ☐ Yes ☐ No E. Does your facility produce an antibiogram (antibiotic susceptibility report?) ☐ Yes ☐ No
Does your facility monitor antibiotic use (consumption) at the unit and/or facility wide level by one of the following metrics:	F. By counts of antibiotic(s) administered to patients per day (days of therapy; DOT)? ☐ Yes ☐ No G. By number of grams of antibiotics used (defined daily dose, DDD)? ☐ Yes ☐ No H. By direct expenditure for antibiotics (purchasing costs)? ☐ Yes ☐ No
Reporting information to staff on improving antibiotic use and resistance	
	A. Does you stewardship program share facility-specific reports on antibiotic use with prescribers? ☐ Yes ☐ No B. Has a current antibiogram been distributed to prescribers at your facility? ☐ Yes ☐ No C. Do prescribers ever receive direct, personalized communication about how they can improve their antibiotic prescription? ☐ Yes ☐ No
Education	
	A. Does your stewardship program provide education to clinicians and other relevant staff on improving antibiotic prescribing? ☐ Yes ☐ No

- *Practice barriers*: Lack of funds and technical resources and time may limit the benefit of ASPs. Apart from short-term costs benefits, long-term economic benefits of improved patient outcomes secondary to AS, such as decreased lengths of stays in the ICUs and hospitals, HAIs, and antibiotic-associated adverse events will also pave the way for the success of a long-term program.

Table 4: Common barriers to development and implementation of antibiotic stewardship programs.

Category	Barriers	Examples
Knowledge	• Lack of awareness • Lack of familiarity	• No knowledge of AS guidelines • Unfamiliar with guidelines in general or with specific guideline(s) • Reluctance to invest in ASP
Attitude	• Lack of agreement • Lack of self-efficacy • Lack of outcome expectancy	• Disagreement with specific guidelines • Physicians lack of confidence or inacceptance of guidelines • Lack of belief that guideline will lead to an important health outcome
Practice	• External factors	• Lack of time, staff, administrative support, reimbursement, supplies, educational materials to support stewardship program

STATE OF ANTIBIOTIC STEWARDSHIP PROGRAMS IN INDIA

Antimicrobial resistance is a major public health problem in India. Except policies or guidelines for appropriate use of antimicrobials like Integrated Management of Neonatal and Childhood Illness (IMNCI) in diarrheal diseases and respiratory infections, there are no guidelines available for other diseases of public health importance like enteric fever and others. Another major issue is that there is no national data based on antimicrobial resistance in different pathogens except for those where there is a specific national health program like RNTCP. Increasing incidences of multidrug resistant extended-spectrum β-lactamase (ESBL) producing *Klebsiella pneumoniae*, vancomycin intermediate staphylococci, *Pseudomonas aeruginosa*, and *Acinetobacter baumannii* resistant to carbapenems is being encountered. Metallo-β-lactamases (MBL) are the enzymes that mediate resistance to carbapenems. MBL producing *P. aeruginosa* are emerging as important causes of nosocomial infection. Prevalence of MBL producing organisms ranges from 7% to 65% in India and is major health issue plaguing ICUs. According to survey conducted on antimicrobial programs in India by Sureshkumar et al., more than 50% hospitals in India did not have an ASP.

The first major step toward curtailing rising antibiotic resistance was taken in 2009 with the launch of the Global Antibiotic Resistance Partnership. It was started to create a platform for developing actionable policy proposals on antibiotic resistance in low and middle income countries. India, Kenya, South Africa and Vietnam in 2011, in a multidisciplinary approach,-made multiple recommendations so as to implement it at a priority stage and second-tier stage. Priority stage recommendations included surveillance on antibiotic resistance and use, increasing use of diagnostic tests, strengthening infection control committee, in-service training for physicians, continuing education for pharmacist, distributing Standard Treatment Guidelines (STGs) to the hospital staff, and regulate veterinary use. The second tier recommendations were to regulate over the counter sale, prioritize funding for research, issue guidelines and checklists, and study impact of seasonal influenza vaccine on pregnant females.

- The National Policy for Containment of Antimicrobial Resistance has created a task force to review the current situation regarding manufacture, use and misuse of antibiotics in the country; to recommend the design for creation of a national surveillance system for antibiotic resistance; to initiate studies documenting prescriptions patterns and establish a monitoring system for the same; to enforce and enhance regulatory provisions for use of antibiotics in human and veterinary and industrial use; to recommend specific intervention measures such as rational use of antibiotics and antibiotic policies in hospitals; and to review the diagnostic methods pertaining to antimicrobial resistance monitoring.

Chennai Declaration

A joint meeting of Medical Societies in India was held in 2012 at the 2nd Annual Conference of the Clinical Infectious Disease Society (CIDSCON) in Chennai to develop a road map to tackle the challenge of antimicrobial resistance. Chennai Declaration was a major step toward antibiotic stewardship policy in India. The aim was to initiate efforts to formulate a policy to control the rising trend of antimicrobial resistance with following objectives (Box 1):

- To regulate over-the-counter sale of antibiotics
- In-hospital antibiotic usage monitoring
- Audit and feedback
- Initiate measures to step up microbiology laboratory facilities
- National antimicrobial resistance surveillance system.

Box 1: Goals of the Chennai declaration.

1. *First year*
   - Formulation of a national policy to combat antimicrobial resistance
   - Efforts to implement major components of the policy
   - 60% compliance rates to major recommendations by stakeholders
2. *Second year*
   - Compliance rate 70%
   - Efforts to implement minor components of policy
   - India achieving the status of a country with a functioning antibiotic policy despite limitations
3. *Next 5 years*
   - >90% compliance to major components of the policy
   - India achieving the status of a country with a functioning antibiotic policy comparable to countries with high quality infection control and antibiotic policy compliance rates.

The Indian Council of Medical Research also recently (2012) carried out a survey in the Government and private corporate hospitals to understand the quality of infection control and antibiotic stewardship activities being practiced. The results from the survey indicated that while most of the hospitals have guidance document on infection control, the infrastructure required was often lacking in hospitals. Standard treatment guidelines even if present are not strictly followed. The monitoring and audit of antimicrobial usage is rarity. They advocated the need to have uniform infection control practices in the country and also standard treatment guidelines for all hospitals which can be customized based on the hospital requirement. A better coordination among the microbiologists and physicians was stressed along with sustained monitoring and auditing mechanisms to have feedbacks to strengthen ASP. The Indian Academy of Paediatrics (IAP) joined hands with ICMR in 2014 to discuss and deliberate over the magnitude of the problem, reasons and possible solutions to tackle the antimicrobial resistance among children in India. The meeting culminated in formulating a 4-point plan (Box 2).

OUTCOME MEASURES FOR A SUCCESSFUL ANTIBIOTIC STEWARDSHIP PROGRAMS

Evaluation of ASPs is based on their performance on antimicrobial consumption, as well as on clinical and microbiological outcomes and cost-effectiveness. Studies have shown that hospital ASPs result in significant decreases in antimicrobial consumption and cost. The benefit is higher in the critical care setting. In contrast, relatively fewer studies have examined patient-oriented clinical outcomes of AS programs, such as lengths of hospital or ICU stays, HAIs, readmissions, mortality, CDI, and adverse events associated with antibiotic therapy. Most studies reported unchanged mortality rates, HAI rates, and lengths of ICU and hospital stays after AS implementations. Variations of clinical outcomes reported from various studies highlight the need for further research and data to assess the impact of AS.

> **Box 2:** IAP-ICMR 4-point plan to tackle antimicrobial resistance.
>
> - Developing and disseminating National Antibiotic Guidelines for Children 2014—the IAP-ICMR document
> - Educating doctors—both pediatricians and other doctors, as well as public on rational antibiotic use
> - Developing infection control guidelines for small hospitals and nursing homes, training the owners of such establishments and ensuring compliance by the members
> - Collecting and collating data on antimicrobial resistance from the clinicians.

KEY MESSAGES

- Antibiotic stewardship is urgently required to counter the ever increasing problem of antimicrobial resistance.
- Any antibiotic stewardship program should be implemented in a structured manner and requires an interdisciplinary team, educational interventions, system innovations, process indicator evaluation, and feedback to healthcare workers.

SUGGESTED READING

1. Abbas Q, Haq A, Kumar R, et al. Evaluation of antibiotic use in pediatric intensive care unit of a developing country. Indian J Crit Care Med. 2016;20(5): 291-4.
2. Barlam TF, Cosgrove SE, Abbo LM. Implementing an Antibiotic Stewardship Program: Guidelines by the Infectious Diseases Society of America and the Society for Healthcare Epidemiology of America. Clin Infect Dis. 2016;62(10):e51-77.
3. CDC. 2014. Core Elements of Hospital Antibiotic Stewardship Programs. Atlanta, GA: US Department of Health and Human Services. CDC 2014. [online] Available from http://www.cdc.gov/getsmart/healthcare/ implementation/core-elements.html [Accessed December 2018].
4. Chennai Declaration Team. The Chennai Declaration: Recommendations of a roadmap to tackle the challenge of antimicrobial resistance. A Joint Meeting of Medical Societies of India. Indian J Cancer. 2012;49:84-94.
5. Directorate General of Health Services, Ministry of Health and Family Welfare. (2011). National Policy for Containment of Antimicrobial Resistance. [online] Available from http://www.mohfw.nic.in/showfile.php?lid=2727 [Accessed December 2018].

6. Global Antibiotic Resistance Partnership (GARP) - India Working Group. Rationalizing antibiotic use to limit antibiotic resistance in India. Indian J Med Res. 2011;134:281-94.
7. Hyun D, Hersh A, Namtu K, et al. Antimicrobial stewardship in pediatrics-how every pediatrician can be a steward. JAMA Pediatrics. 2013;167(9).
8. Karanika S, Paudel S, Grigoras C, et al. Systematic review and meta-analysis of clinical and economic outcomes from the implementation of hospital-based antimicrobial stewardship programs. Antimicrob Agents Chemother. 2016;60(8):4840-52.
9. Kumar G, Adithan C, Harish B, et al. Antimicrobial resistance in India: A review. J Nat Sci Biol Med. 2013;4(2):286-91.
10. Silva A, Dias D, Marques A, et al. Role of antimicrobial stewardship programmes in children: a systematic review. J Hosp Infect. 2018;99(2):117-12.
11. Sureshkumar D, Gopalakrishnan R, Ramasubramanian V. Survey of infection control programs in India. [online] Available from https://idsa.confex.com/idsa/2013/webprogram/Paper42762.html [Accessed December 2018].
12. Walia K, Ohri V. Antibiotic stewardship activities in India: Current scenario. International J Infect Dis. 2014;21:214.
13. Yewale VN. IAP-ICMR Call to Action to tackle the antimicrobial resistance. Indian Pediatr. 2014;51:437-9.

Pain and Sedation

38

Arun Bansal, Amish Vora

LEARNING OBJECTIVES

- To familiarize the reader with the drugs used in sedation and analgesia.
- To provide a framework on which to use these drugs.
- To use a weaning protocol for prevention of withdrawal.

INTRODUCTION

Pain is defined by the International Association for the Study of Pain (IASP) as "an unpleasant sensory and emotional experience associated with actual or potential tissue damage or described in terms of such damage." The important elements of this definition to be emphasized are—(1) pain encompasses both peripheral physiologic and central cognitive/emotional components and (2) pain may or may not be associated with real tissue damage—pain may exist in the absence of demonstrable somatic pathology.

One of the major objectives in the pediatric intensive care unit (PICU) is to treat children less invasively, thus avoiding physical and emotional suffering. Sedatives are necessary to reduce the anxiety and agitation that result from the admission to a hostile environment and from medical procedures. Analgesics are used to treat pain secondary to surgical interventions and/or invasive methods, besides the pain inflicted by the disease itself. Moreover, the combined use of analgesics and sedatives allows patients to adapt to mechanical ventilation through the hypnotic effects of these drugs, their potential to cause decreased cough reflex and respiratory drive. Regrettably, administration of sedative drugs in the PICU is often approached in a generic way and as an afterthought, with more attention paid to the primary disease, which can lead to avoidable morbidity.

However, under-sedation and over-sedation are both harmful. Inadequate sedation is unacceptable in a vulnerable child who may be unable to move or communicate distress as a result of the use of muscle relaxants, while the unparalyzed child may "fight" the ventilator leading to ineffective ventilation, accidental extubation, or the loss of invasive access or monitors. In intensive care, agitation and inadequate sedation has been correlated with adverse short- and long-term outcome. The use of protocols that facilitate the selection of appropriate drugs, their adequate administration and careful monitoring can improve the quality of sedation and analgesia and prevent their adverse effects. Over-sedation delays recovery, promotes tolerance to the drugs, and leads to distressing symptoms on their withdrawal (agitation, seizures, halluci-nations, psychosis, fever, and tachycardia). Maintaining ideal analgesia while at the same time promoting earlier extubation and PICU discharge can be difficult to achieve.

The ideal sedative regimen in ICU patients should—(1) provide adequate coverage for pain, sedation, and anxiety; (2) have evidence to support routine or extended use in various critical care populations; (3) have favorable kinetics and clinical effect (e.g., rapid onset of action, short half-life, minimal bioaccumulation or drug interactions); (4) be easily titrated and monitored; (5) have tolerable adverse effects; and (6) have a reasonable cost. Unfortunately, none of the commonly available agents satisfies all of these criteria. There are significant limitations associated with each drug, many fitting the definition of "high-risk medications"—those that have the highest risk of causing injury when misused.

There is a wide availability of sedative and analgesic drugs that can be used in critically ill children, and each one of them has advantages and disadvantages. Nevertheless, no analgesic or sedative meets all the criteria of an ideal drug—rapid onset action, short half-life, metabolization and elimination by organs that are less susceptible to failure (liver and kidney), minimum secondary effects without hemodynamic or respiratory involvement, no interaction with other drugs, and availability of a specific antidote. When choosing a medication, one should bear the following in mind—pharmacodynamics of the drug, its route of administration, secondary effects, patient's age, underlying disease, mechanical ventilation, nutritional status, kidney and liver functions, cost, etc.

Simply put analgesic drugs should be given for pain relief, sedative drugs for reduction in conscious level, and muscle relaxants for specific situations when paralysis is essential (e.g., low cardiac output states). However, there is some cross-over in these roles—morphine has sedative properties, ketamine provides analgesia and anesthesia, and even muscle relaxants may have an additive effect on reduction of conscious state through deafferentation.

NON-PHARMACOLOGICAL TREATMENT

Several non-pharmacological interventions can improve the routine of children in the PICU, reducing their anxiety, improving their sleep-wake cycles, and minimizing the necessity for sedative and analgesic drugs. Music therapy has proven efficient in overcoming anxiety and increasing relaxation of critically ill patients of any age, including preterm infants. Other effective measures include noise control in the PICU, control of lighting to maintain the day and night pattern and the sleep-wake cycle, massage, and communication, if patient's age and health status allow so.

SEDATION

Goals of Sedation

The effective management of pain, anxiety, and sleep (hypnosis) are the major aims of a sedation therapy regimen. The goals of effective sedation include:
- Unconsciousness (virtual anesthesia) or reduction in conscious level

- Reduced awareness
- Loss of explicit and implicit memory
- Compliance with the need to lie in a confined space, attached to monitors and invasive lines
- Prevention of distress during procedures such as physiotherapy, radiological scanning, or minor surgical intervention, which may require enhanced levels.

Different drugs fulfill these roles to varying extents. Benzodiazepines, for example, provide anterograde amnesia, with reduced or complete unconsciousness at different doses, while phenothiazines and butyrophenones (chlorpromazine and haloperidol), used as major tranquillizing drugs in schizophrenia, have psychotropic properties that render the patient disinterested in activity. Some analgesic drugs reduce both pain and consciousness—ketamine provides analgesia and a dissociative anesthesia/sedation, clonidine produces analgesia and a calmed, relaxed state, and morphine has additional sedative properties. Therefore, choice of a sedative regimen needs to be tailored to the individual rather than generic.

Sedative Drugs

Sedation inhibits the neuroendocrine effects caused by stress (hypertension, tachycardia, tachypnea, and hyperglycemia), which increases oxygen consumption and hinders synchronism with the ventilatory support equipment. In addition, it prevents anxiety, which is accountable for sleep deprivation and subsequent psychological disorders. Despite the fact that there are a wide variety of drugs with different indications, there is no sedative that suits all situations. Table 1 summarizes the basic characteristics of the most important drugs. The selection of the drug depends on several factors, such as age, disease, and organ dysfunction/failure.

Table 1: Recommended sedative agents.

Drug	Dosing	Notes

Midazolam	• Intravenous bolus
	  – <60 kg; 0.1–0.2 mg/kg/dose.
	  – >60 kg; 5 mg/dose
	• Intravenous infusion
	  – <60 kg; 2–10 µg/kg/min
	  – >60 kg; 5–15 mg/h
		• May be associated with tolerance and withdrawal syndrome
		• Prolonged sedation possible on discontinuation

Clonidine	• NG
	  – 1–5 µg/kg/dose 8 hourly.
	• Intravenous infusion
	  – 0.1–2 µg/kg/h
		• May be associated with withdrawal syndrome
		• Avoid sudden discontinuation

Chloral hydrate Triclofos	• NG; 20–50 mg/kg/dose 4–6 hourly • Maximum 2 g per dose • Maximum daily dose; 200 mg/kg/day	• May cause gastric irritation • Risk of accumulation
Promethazine	• NG; 1–2 mg/kg/dose 6 hourly • Maximum 50 mg per dose	• Use with caution in neonates
Alimemazine	• NG; 2–4 mg/kg/dose 6 hourly • Maximum 90 mg per dose	• Use with caution in renal and hepatic failure

Benzodiazepine

The most commonly used drugs are diazepam, midazolam, and lorazepam, which are given in continuous intravenous doses. Midazolam is the benzodiazepine of choice for continuous sedation of critically ill children. When given quickly, it may reduce systemic vascular resistance and cause hypotension in hypovolemic patients. However, its continuous intravenous infusion produces few hemodynamic effects. For sedation, it is necessary to administer a bolus dose prior to continuous infusion. Prolonged infusion produces tolerance, and hence the necessity to gradually increase the dose in order to achieve the same sedative effect. In this situation, midazolam should be combined with another sedative (opioid, propofol or other). High doses may lead to "midazolam infusion syndrome," which consists of delayed arousal hours to days after discontinuation, increasing the length of ventilatory support. In case of prolonged use for several days, it is necessary to gradually decrease midazolam infusion so as not to induce the withdrawal syndrome. Lorazepam has a similar effect to that of midazolam, but its use in critically ill children is less documented. The enteral route has been used for its administration in order to minimize the need of continuous midazolam infusion and to prevent subsequent withdrawal syndrome.

Propylene glycol is used as a diluent in many medications, but parenteral formulations of lorazepam contain a substantial amount that can accumulate and cause toxicity in patients receiving large lorazepam doses. Although initially thought to accumulate only with very high lorazepam doses in the 15 to 25 mg/h range, data suggest that total daily lorazepam doses (including infusion and bolus administration) as low as 1 mg/kg are associated with toxic propylene glycol concentrations and adverse effects such as acute kidney injury and metabolic acidosis. These clinical features of propylene glycol toxicity occur so frequently from other causes in critically ill patients that it is easy to overlook that lorazepam administration may cause these events. Because most hospitals do not have the ability to quickly measure propylene glycol concentrations, the serum osmol gap has been used as a reliable screening and surveillance tool. An osmol gap greater than 10 to 12 may help identify patients accumulating this toxic substance, and some physicians have recommended screening patients at least every other day when lorazepam doses approximate 1 mg/kg/d.

Propofol

The major characteristics of propofol are its rapid onset of action and its rapid elimination of adverse effects after withdrawal ("rapid arousal"). This can be particularly useful in patients who require frequent neurological assessment (e.g., traumatic brain injury or convulsive status epilepticus). Propofol has vasodilator properties and may cause reduced cardiac contractility and negative chronotropic effects, especially in patients with hypovolemia and/or abnormal myocardial contractility. For quick procedures (e.g., respiratory endoscopy), we use a loading dose of 1.5 mg/kg, with small bolus doses of 0.5 mg/kg, as necessary. The maximum dose of propofol recommended for children is 4 mg/kg/h. The least understood, least predictable, and most dangerous adverse effect is the propofol infusion syndrome (PRIS). Higher doses for prolonged periods are associated with the "PRIS," which consists of cardiogenic shock (reduced myocardial contractility and conduction disorders) in addition to metabolic disorders (lactic acidosis, hypertriglyceridemia) and/or rhabdomyolysis with high mortality.

Despite these concerns, and its contraindications for use by regulatory authorities in the USA and UK, it continues to be used short-term, at low dose (<4 mg/kg/h) for specific cases. Patients on a propofol infusion should be closely monitored for rising lactate, acidosis, reduced urine output or dysrhythmias.

There are numerous studies comparing both drugs. Midazolam allows maintaining adequate sedation and amnesia levels at a low cost, but its use is more complex, requiring more ventilatory support and showing a greater association with the withdrawal syndrome after its discontinuation. Propofol has a more rapid action and allows earlier weaning from the ventilator, but it causes more vascular depression during induction, it is also more expensive and should be given through an independent intravenous route. Midazolam is still the drug of choice in patients who need sedation with intravenous infusion.

Etomidate

Etomidate is one of the intravenous anesthesia-inducing agents that causes the fewest hemodynamic alterations. For some time, it was the drug of choice for rapid and emergency intubation in critically ill patients. However, recently, it has been contraindicated as it causes adrenal failure, even when it is used as a single dose for intubation. In addition, it may cause trismus during anesthetic induction, so it must be used with a neuromuscular blocking agent (NMBA). Therefore, its single and repeated administration or infusion is contraindicated in septic patients, since it may cause suprarenal failure.

Barbiturates

Other sedative drugs include barbiturates such as pentobarbital and thiopental. Among other indications, they are recommended in the treatment of refractory seizures and traumatic brain injury with severe intracranial hypertension. Currently, they are seldom used in critically ill patients, as they cause hemodynamic instability and accumulate in peripheral tissues after prolonged infusion, delaying the patient's arousal. Phenobarbital can also be used as supplementary treatment in patients submitted to prolonged ventilatory support in remarkable need for sedation. Chloral hydrate given orally or rectally can be used as sedative in rapid interventions (e.g., echocardiogram), but its onset and length of action vary considerably.

Techniques that can be used in PICU to limit the problems associated with long-term sedation include:
- *Drug cycling*: Changing pharmacological drug groups routinely to reduce the emergence of tolerance.
- *Sedation holidays*: Temporary cessation of sedative drugs to evaluate emergence.
- *Non-pharmacological techniques*: Oral sucrose, reducing environmental stress (noise, light, interruption of day–night cycle), swaddling, etc.
- Transfer to oral sedation where possible.

ANALGESIA

Children admitted to the PICU have pain caused either by the underlying disease or by the diagnostic or therapeutic procedures. More often than not, patients receive insufficient analgesic treatment, even for painful procedures. A recent study showed that 44% of children

Table 2: Recommended analgesic agents.

Morphine	Intravenous bolus • <60 kg; 100–200 µg/kg/dose. • >60 kg; 5–10 mg/dose Intravenous infusion • <60 kg; 10–60 µg/kg/h • >60 kg; 0.8–3 mg/h	• Potential histamine release • Consider reducing dose in renal and hepatic impairment
Fentanyl	Intravenous bolus • <60 kg; 1–2 µg/kg/dose. • >60 kg; 50–200 µg/dose Intravenous infusion • <60 kg; 4–10 µg/kg/h • >60 kg; 25–100 µg/h	• Rapid following prolonged use onset and relatively long elimination half-life, especially

Paracetamol	• <60 kg; 10–15 mg/kg/dose, 4 hourly
	• >60 kg; 650–1,000 mg/dose, 4 hourly
	• Maximum daily dose
	  – <3 months; 60 mg/kg/day
	  – 3 months–12 years; 90 mg/kg/day
	  – >12 years; 4 g/day
		• Rectal administration is associated with variable uptake
		• Intravenous preparation available

Ibuprofen	• <60 kg; 6–10 mg/kg/dose, 6 hourly
	• >60 kg; 200–600 mg/dose, 6 hourly
	• Maximum daily dose
	  – <60 kg; 30 mg/kg/day
	  – >60 kg; 2.4 g/day
		• Use with caution in renal failure
		• Potential for gastrointestinal bleeding and water retention

recalled the painful experiences they had been put through during their PICU stay. As occurs with sedation, there is not such a thing as an all-purpose analgesic, and the selection of drugs depends on numerous factors. Table 2 summarizes the characteristics of the most commonly used drugs.

Opioid derivatives and non-steroidal anti-inflammatory drugs (NSAIDs) are the most widely used analgesics in critically ill patients. Opioids are the drugs of choice for mechanically ventilated patients, especially if combined with benzodiazepines, since they have shown a synergistic effect that allows reducing the dose of both medications. Morphine and fentanyl are widely used in continuous infusion, but remifentanil, tramadol, and meperidine have been increasingly used as well (Table 2).

Morphine

Morphine has low solubility, which explains its delayed maximum effect on the central nervous system (CNS)—15 minutes and its longer effect—3-6 hours. It is metabolized by the liver, originating two active metabolites that accumulate in case of renal failure. When given intravenously, it may cause hypotension by producing venodilation and by releasing histamine. Usually, its elimination half-life is longer, but its elimination is smaller in newborn (NB) infants, compared to other children and to adults. The greater difference is mostly perceived in preterm NB infants. Nonetheless, less morphine binds to the protein in NB infants, leading to a higher amount of morphine, increasing the risk for respiratory depression. The elimination half-life and clearance similar to that of an adult is obtained at 2 months of life.

Fentanyl

Fentanyl is 60–100 times more potent than morphine. Its fat-solubility is higher, which explains its rapid action and short duration, due to its fast distribution. If given for a prolonged time, there is rapid tolerance and accumulation in the adipose tissue; therefore, its half-life is longer than that of morphine. It does not produce active metabolites. It does not release histamine, allowing for greater hemodynamic stability than morphine. An infrequent adverse effect is chest wall rigidity, which is related to the dose used, rate of infusion and age less than 6 months.

Remifentanil

Remifentanil is a fentanyl derivative with similar potency and rapid onset action. Its peak effect is achieved in less than 3 minutes and it is short-acting (its effect disappears within few minutes, being metabolized by nonspecific plasma esterases), regardless of the length of its infusion and of the presence of liver and/or renal dysfunction. This profile allows earlier extubation than other opioids and the use of higher doses, in which the analgesic effects combine with sedative effects without any risk of accumulation. Only approximately 30% of patients may need another sedative at low doses in order to achieve the goals of sedation and analgesia. Disadvantages include large economic cost, quick development of tolerance, and higher frequency of hypotension compared to fentanyl. Its use as continuous infusion has been more frequent, among NB and infants. Due to its potency, hemodynamic stability and short action at low doses, fentanyl is ideal for short painful procedures in children, especially in the PICU.

Non-steroidal Anti-inflammatory Drugs

Mild-to-moderate pain can be effectively managed with non-opioid analgesics, such as acetaminophen (paracetamol), or with NSAIDs. Acetaminophen has a very good therapeutic power, with few contraindications. It may be used in any age group, even in preterm infants, and it is possible to obtain synergistic effects with other NSAIDs or opioids, due to its analgesic effect on the central nervous system.

The NSAIDs have analgesic and anti-inflammatory properties, both of which are useful in the management of postoperative and chronic pain or of mild-to-moderate pain. An advantage is that they do not cause respiratory depression or sedation. The mechanism of action occurs through the inhibition of cyclooxygenase (COX), the enzyme in charge of arachidonic acid metabolization. In recent years, they have been increasingly used in combination with opioids in the postoperative period, as they produce a synergistic analgesic effect that allows better pain management with fewer secondary effects and lower doses.

Ibuprofen and naproxen are the most common NSAIDs in pediatrics. They are not indicated in the initial stages of septic shock, due to their secondary effects on the gastric mucosa, renal function, and platelets. Metamizole is one of the non-opioid analgesic drugs most widely used in European, South American, and African countries and can be used to treat moderate-to-severe pain, combined with opioids in order to enhance the analgesic effects and delay the

Neuromuscular Blocking Agents

In certain situations, in addition to sedative and analgesic drugs, the use of NMBAs is necessary. They are subdivided into depolarizing and non-depolarizing agents. Table 3 shows the most widely used NMBAs.

Succinylcholine is still the most widely used muscle relaxant for emergency intubations, due to its rapid action, whereas rocuronium is the most efficient alternative with fewer secondary effects.

Table 3: Characteristics of the neuromuscular blocking agents.

Drug	Action	Dose (mg/kg)	Onset (Minutes)	Length (Minutes)	Advantages	Comments
Succinylcholine	Depolarizing	1–2 Not recommended for infusion	Immediate	3–5	Short action (intubation)	Hyperkalemia Fasciculations
Vecuronium	Non-depolarizing	Initial bolus: 0.08–0.2 INF: 0.08–0.2 mg/kg/h	2–4	20	No cardiovascular effects	Muscle weakness
Pancuronium	Non-depolarizing	Initial bolus: 0.1 INF: 0.1 mg/kg/h	2–4	30–45	Longer action	Tachycardia, hypertension Increase in intracerebral hemorrhage
Atracurium	Non-depolarizing	Initial bolus: 0.3–0.6 INF: 0.3–0.6 mg/kg/h	2–3	25–30	Not metabolized by the liver and kidney	Bronchospasm Bradycardia
Rocuronium	Non-depolarizing	Initial bolus: 0.6–1.2 INF: 5–15 µg/kg/min	1–2	30–40	No cardiovascular effects	Tachycardia at high doses
Mivacurium	Non-depolarizing	Initial bolus: 0.1–0.2 INF: 10–14 µg/kg/min	2–4	12–18	Short action	Bronchospasm Coughing
Cisatracurium	Non-depolarizing	Initial bolus: 0.15 INF: 1.5 µg/kg/min	3–4	30	Not metabolized by the liver and kidney	No cardiovascular effects

Clinical scores are the most common tools for monitoring the levels of sedation. However, these scores are limited, since they are subjective, their assessment is intermittent, they sometimes interrupt patient's rest, and sometimes give more importance to pain sensitivity than to the sedation level. Moreover, their usefulness is quite limited in deep levels of sedation and in patients with muscle relaxation. The Ramsay and Comfort scores are the most widely used tools for determining the level of sedation in pediatrics.

Various scales that can be used are the:
- Ramsay's score
- Sedation-agitation scale—better on doctor
- COMFORT scale 8 part score
- OAA/S
- Visual analog scale (VAS)
- Facial expression scale.

Studies in assessment have shown that most scales consistently underestimate; even in awake patients 74% felt pain when staff thought control was adequate.

The Ramsay scale has 6 levels (Box 1). The ideal level would be level 2 (cooperative, oriented, tranquil patient) which is easier said than done when dealing with children. What we usually achieve is either too much or too little with a child who is asleep with little or no response, i.e., level 5-6.

The COMFORT scale, is an objective measure of distress in ventilated pediatric patients, validated in all age groups. It comprises eight variables, each rated 1-5: alertness, calmness/agitation, respiratory response, physical movement, heart rate, blood pressure, muscle tone, and facial tension, the scale ranging from 0 to 40, with a target range of 17-26. As with other scoring systems, it is limited by inter observer variability, provides only intermittent data, and cannot be used in the context of neuromuscular (NMJ) blockade. Cardiovascular responses are also difficult to assess in patients who are paced. A recent study has described a simplified Comfort score with the same value as the original score, in which physiological variables were eliminated.

Box 1: Ramsay sedation scale.
- Patient is anxious and agitated or restless, or both
- Patient is cooperative, oriented, and tranquil
- Patient responds to commands only
- Patient exhibits brisk response to light glabellar tap or loud auditory stimulus
- Patient exhibits a sluggish response to light glabellar tap or loud auditory stimulus
- Patient exhibits no response.

Neurophysiological methods and auditory evoked potentials have been evaluated in the research domain. Bispectral Index (BIS) monitoring utilizes data from electroencephalogram (EEG) to measure depth of anesthesia. This technique assumes changes in frequency are related and looks for phase coupling among frequency bands (biocoherence). In awake individuals, there is minimal synchronization because of multiple signal generators within the brain, whereas during sleep, there is less activity and the EEG reflects coupling between signal generators. A dimensionless value, "the BIS number", is calculated, which ranges from 0 to 100, 0 indicating an isoelectric state, with 100 correlating with a fully awake individual. Values of 40-60 are seen with general anesthesia. While it may provide an accurate assessment of depth of sedation for single agents such as midazolam, propofol, and volatile agents, this is not the case for opiates or ketamine.

an analgesic in intrathecal perfusion, and for the control of tolerance and of the deprivation syndrome of other sedatives.

Dexmedetomidine is a highly selective α2 adrenoceptor agonist that has been shown to have both sedative and analgesic effects. Compared with clonidine, which is an α2 agonist that has been used for the treatment of hypertension, dexmedetomidine has an α2:α1 adrenoceptor ratio of approximately 1,600:1 (seven to eight times higher than clonidine). This makes it primarily a sedative–anxiolytic. The elimination half-life of dexmedetomidine is 2 versus 8 hours for clonidine and the half-life of dexmedetomidine is 6 minutes. The short half-life of dexmedetomidine makes it an ideal drug for intravenous titration. Dexmedetomidine is only available as an intravenous infusion. The hypnotic effect of dexmedetomidine is mediated by the hyperpolarization of noradrenergic neurons in the locus coeruleus. When the α2 adrenergic receptor is activated, it inhibits adenylyl cyclase. This latter enzyme catalyzes the formation of cyclic adenosine monophosphate (cAMP), a crucial second messenger molecule that acts in many catabolic cell processes.

The use of dexmedetomidine was initially considered as a sedative to be used in mechanically ventilated adults, but now its use in children is also documented. Although dexmedetomidine has been primarily investigated for its sedative effect, it apparently has analgesic effects that are appropriate for cases where opioids are needed, therefore allowing for a lower opioid use.

The following protocol is useful but needs to be individualized for each patient (Flowchart 1).

ASSESSMENT OF PAIN AND SEDATION

Assessment of depth of sedation, with titration of analgesic and sedative drugs, is important to ensure comfort and avoid adverse outcomes, associated with under or over-sedation.

Flowchart 1: Protocol for sedation and analgesia.

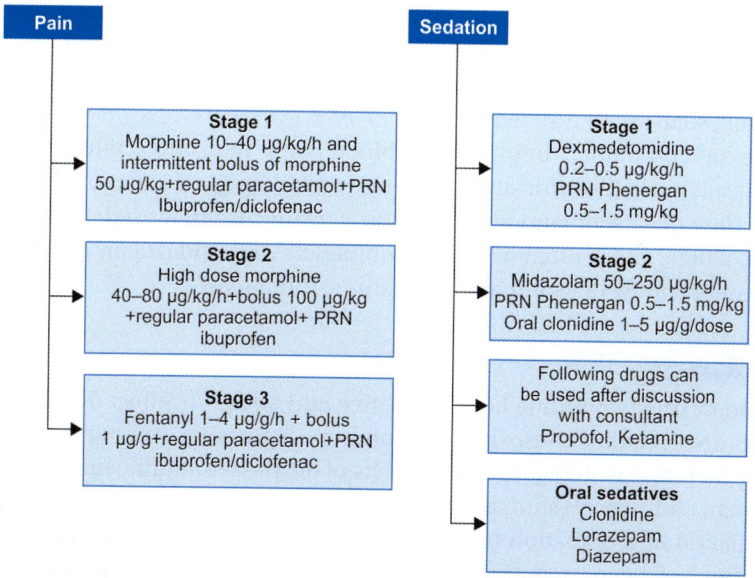

development of tolerance. It may cause hypotension as a result of vasodilation if administered as rapid intravenous infusion. The risk of agranulocytosis and bone marrow aplasia is very low. At some centers, they are frequently used in continuous infusion in the immediate postoperative period, including heart surgeries, with excellent results.

Tramadol is an atypical opioid structurally related to codeine. Its double mechanism of action includes central inhibition of norepinephrine as serotonin reuptake inhibitor and weak agonist action on the theta receptor, due to an active metabolite. Tramadol is 10 to 15 times less potent than morphine. It is known for producing fewer side effects than other opioids. The use of tramadol should be avoided in patients with seizures or traumatic brain injury or who are being treated with drugs that lower the seizure threshold. In general, tramadol is a safe and efficient analgesic in the management of mild-to-moderate pain in children.

Analgesic and Sedative Drugs

Ketamine

It is a phencyclidine derivative that produces dissociative anesthesia. It has analgesic effects, even at lower doses than the sedative dose. It is a potent analgesic at sub-anesthetic doses and regularly used in painful procedures in children in the emergency room (e.g., fracture reduction, burn dressings) and in the PICU. Its half-life ranges from 2 hours to 3 hours, and may be extended if continuous infusion is used or in case of liver failure. Unlike other sedative drugs, it activates the sympathetic nervous system (by releasing endogenous norepinephrine), with increase in heart rate, in vascular resistance, and with bronchodilation. Although it has a negative inotropic effect, sympathetic stimulation runs counter to this effect, except in cases of catecholamine refractory cardiogenic shock. The difference between intramuscular and intravenous administration lies only in the onset of action (1–2 min and 5–10 min). Intravenous doses provide around 10 minutes of sedation and analgesia for each mg/kg, i.e., 1 mg/kg of IV ketamine produces analgesia and sedation for 10 minutes, whereas 2 mg/kg produces approximately 20 minutes of analgesia and sedation. However, the residual effect may last for 2–3 hours. One IV dose of 1–2 mg/kg is usually well tolerated in procedures that involve a larger amount of pain, such as fracture reduction.

Ketamine in continuous infusion combined with benzodiazepines can be used in hemodynamically unstable critically ill patients, providing good sedation and analgesia and reducing the dose of catecholamines. Ketamine is mostly useful for sedation and analgesia in invasive procedures, and is often used in combination with midazolam and as an anesthesia inducing agent in emergency intubation in status asthmaticus.

Adrenergic Alpha-2-agonists

Clonidine and dexmedetomidine have a sedative and analgesic effect due to their action on alpha-2 receptors. Clonidine causes minor respiratory depression. There are some contradictory reports in the literature with regard to the effects of dexmedetomidine on ventilatory function in some (human and animal) studies, suggesting mild respiratory depression, reduction of the minute ventilation and reduction of CO_2 response, whereas other reports do not show this effect. Clonidine has been used as premedication before surgery, for peripheral blockade, as

Muscle relaxants are also useful in some patients in which sedation and analgesia are not enough to allow adaptation to mechanical ventilation. In certain situations, in addition to sedative and analgesic drugs, the use of NMBAs is necessary. They are subdivided into depolarizing and non-depolarizing agents. Box 1 shows the most widely used NMBAs.

Muscle relaxants are also useful in some patients in which sedation and analgesia are not enough to allow adaptation to mechanical ventilation. They increase the compliance of the respiratory system, reducing the pressure that is necessary to ventilate and minimize oxygen consumption. It has been suggested that their early use in mechanically ventilated patients with acute respiratory distress syndrome (ARDS) can prevent progression of inflammation and ventilator-induced lung injury.

Vecuronium is more widely used in critically ill patients, as it does not cause hemodynamic changes and does not release histamine. It has an intermediate half-life; it does not often bind to proteins, has a high distribution volume, and is metabolized by the liver into active metabolites that are eliminated by the kidneys. This explains why its effects last longer in patients with renal and/or liver dysfunction.

All patients on muscle relaxants must be previously sedated to avoid anxiety of involuntary immobilization in alert patients. Neuromuscular blocking agents must be given at the least effective dose and for the shortest time. Their main risk includes residual neuromuscular blockade and accumulation due to prolonged administration, which may lead to muscle weakness and neuromyopathy, being more frequent when combined with the use of corticosteroids in patients with sepsis, renal or liver failure.

Withdrawal Syndrome

The withdrawal syndrome results from sudden discontinuation of sedative and analgesic drugs in patients with physical tolerance due to prolonged administration of such drugs. The signs and symptoms vary substantially in terms of presentation and severity, depending on the drug and on the patient's status. Among these signs and symptoms are CNS activation (irritability, abnormal reflexes, tremors, clonus, hypertonicity, delirium, and seizures), gastrointestinal disorders, and activation of the sympathetic nervous system (tachycardia, hypertension and tachypnea). This is a less recognized but important problem in children who cannot express distress. Most children get symptomatic treatment as the diagnosis of withdrawal is often missed. Slow withdrawal of opioids in a protocolized stepwise fashion would prevent many of these symptoms.

Weaning guidelines adapted from those used commonly in UK PICUs are as follows:
- *Morphine*:
  - *Oral doses*: 0.05–0.1 mg/kg PO 4–6 hourly
  - *Side effects*: Respiratory depression, hypotension, histamine release, pruritus (not an issue if child is on steroid), miosis, constipation, and urinary retention (patients on morphine infusion do not always need in-dwelling urinary catheters), chest wall rigidity, and withdrawal syndrome.
  - *Weaning or stopping*:
    - On IV/oral opiates
    - *Less than 7 days*: Stop or intermittent/PRN dose for pain
    - *7–14 days*: Wean and stop over 3 days, if no withdrawal symptoms

- More than 14 days or withdrawal symptoms: Start clonidine and decrease morphine dose by 10% every 24 or 48 hours rounding dose to nearest 0.2 mg to enable more accurate dosing (Oramorph® is available as 2 mg/mL solution). Once dose is weaned to 0.2 mg every 4 hours, extend interval rather than reducing dose, i.e., 4 hourly to 6 hourly to 8 hourly. Stop after 48 hours at 200 μg 8 hourly for infants/children or 200 μg 12 hourly in neonates.
  - For IV to oral conversion of morphine: Conversion factor is 2, i.e., multiply the IV dose patient is receiving for 24 hours by 2 that's the total dose of oral morphine for 24 hours. Divide that by 6 and give that dose every 4 hourly. Then titrate it up and down according to patient's clinical condition. Hence write an extra oral dose on PRN.
- Clonidine:
  - Bolus dose: NG/PO 2–5 μg/kg/dose tds or qds
  - Infusion rates: 0.5–2 μg/kg/h IV infusion
  - Side effects: Hypotension, bradycardia, opiate potentiation, withdrawal usually manifest as hypertension
  - Weaning or stopping: Oral clonidine
    - Less than 7 days: Stop
    - 7–14 days: Reduce dose by 50% of original dose for 24 hours, then by a further 25% of original dose for 24 hours, then stop
    - Monitor blood pressure throughout the weaning period and for 24 hours after stopping. If mean blood pressure increases by more than 50% over 24 hours (and other causes are excluded), consider slowing the weaning of clonidine wean and stop over 3 days, if no withdrawal symptoms
    - More than 14 days or withdrawal symptoms: Reduce dose by 1 μg/kg/dose every 24 hours once benzodiazepine and Oramorph® have stopped. When dose reaches 1 μg/kg/dose, increase interval to 8 hourly if on 6 hourly, and stop after 24 hours at 1 μg/kg/dose 8 hourly.
- Fentanyl(s) bolus dose 1 μg/kg
  - Infusion rates: 1 to 4 μg/kg/h
  - Side effects: Glottis and chest wall rigidity following rapid infusions of more than or equal to 5 μg/kg and the development of bradycardia
  - Weaning or stopping: After 3 to 5 days of fentanyl infusion, convert the total daily dose of fentanyl to morphine. 1 μg of fentanyl = 100 μg of morphine.
- Dexmedetomidine bolus dose; 0.5 to 1 μg/kg over 10 min is often avoided
  - Infusion: 0.2 to 1 μg/kg/h
  - Side effects: Bradycardia, hypotension, and adrenal insufficiency with prolonged infusions
  - Weaning: Once on full feeds convert dexmedetomidine to oral clonidine.

SUGGESTED READING

1. Al-Samsam RH, Cullen P. Sleep and adverse environmental factors in sedated mechanically ventilated pediatric intensive care patients. Pediatr Crit Care Med. 2005;6:562-7.
2. Bartolomé SM, López-Herce CJ, Freddi N. Analgesia and sedation in children: practical approach for the most frequent situations. J Pediatr (Rio J). 2007;83:S71-82.

3. Bergendahl H, Lonnqvist PA, Eksborg S. Clonidine in paediatric anaesthesia: review of the literature and comparison with benzodiazepines for premedication. Acta Anaesthesiol Scand. 2006;50: 135-43.
4. Carollo DS, Nossaman BD, Ramadhayani U. Dexmedetomidine: a review of clinical applications. Curr Opin Anaesthesiol. 2008;21:457-61
5. Cornfield DN, Tegtmeyer K, Nelson MD, et al. Continuous propofol infusion in 142 critically ill children. Pediatrics. 2002;110:1177-81.
6. Fayaz MK, Abel RJ, Pugh SC, et al. Opioid-sparing effects of diclofenac and paracetamol lead to improved outcomes after cardiac surgery. J Cardiothorac Vasc Anesth. 2004;18:742-7.
7. Finkel JC, Rose JB, Schmitz ML. An evaluation of efficacy and tolerability of oral tramadol hydrochloride tablets for the treat¬ment of post-surgical pain in children. Anesth Analg. 2002;1994: 1469-73.
8. Gurbet A, Goren S, Sahin S, et al. Comparison of analgesic effects of morphine, fentanyl, and remifentanil with intravenous patient-controlled analgesia after cardiac surgery. J Cardiothorac Vasc Anesth. 2004;18:755-8.
9. Ista E, van Dijk M, Tibboel D, et al. Assessment of sedation levels in pediatric intensive care patients can be improved by using the COMFORT "behavior" scale. Assessment of sedation levels in pediatric intensive care patients can be improved by using the COMFORT "behavior" scale. Pediatr Crit Care Med. 2005;6:58-63.
10. Jackson WL Jr. Should we use etomidate as an induction agent for endotracheal intubation in patients with septic shock?: a critical appraisal. Chest. 2005;127:1031-8.
11. Jacobi J, Fraser GL, Coursin DB, et al. Clinical practice guidelines for the sustained use of sedatives and analgesics in the critically ill adult. Crit Care Med. 2002;30:119-41.
12. Joshi GP, Warner DS, Twersky RS, et al. A comparison of the remifentanil and fentanyl adverse effect profile in a multicenter phase IV study. J Clin Anesth. 2002;14:494-9.
13. Kart T, Christup LL, Rasmussen M. Recommended use of morphine in neonates, infants, and children based on a literature review: Part 1 Pharmacokinetics. Paediatr Anaesth. 1997;7;5-11.
14. Martin LD, Bratton SL, Quint P, et al. Prospective documentation of sedative, analgesic, and neuromuscular blocking agent use in infants and children in the intensive care unit: a multicenter perspective. Pediatr Crit Care Med. 2001;2:205-10.
15. Petrillo TM, Fortenberry JD, Linzer JF, et al. Emergency department use of ketamine in pediatric status asthmaticus. J Asthma. 2001;38:657-64.
16. Raimer PL, Shanley TP. Bispectral index monitoring in the PICU. In: Shanley TP, Zimmerman JJ (Eds). Current Concepts in Pediatric Critical Care. Illinois, IL: SCCM; 2008. pp. 89-93.
17. Richman PS, Baram D, Varela M, et al. Sedation during mechanical ventilation: a trial of benzodiazepine and opiate in combination. Crit Care Med. 2006;34:1395-401.
18. Tobias JD. Dexmedetomidine: applications in pediatric critical care and pediatric anesthesiology. Pediatr Crit Care Med. 2007;8:1-17.
19. Tonner P, Weiler N. Sedation and analgesia in the intensive care unit. Curr Opin Anaesthesiol. 2003;16:113-21.
20. Twite MD, Rashid A, Zuk J, et al. Sedation, analgesia, and neuromuscular blockade in the pediatric intensive care unit: survey of fellowship training programs. Pediatr Crit Care Med. 2004;5:521-32.
21. Welzing L, Roth B. Experience with remifentanil in neonates and infants. Drugs. 2006;66:1339-50.
22. Wolf AR, Jackman L. Analgesia and sedation after pediatric cardiac surgery. Pediatr Anes. 2011;21:567-76.
23. Yaster M, Kost-Beyerly S, Maxwell LG. Opiods agonists and antagonists. In: Schechter NL, Berde CB, Yaster M (Eds). Pain in infants, children, and adolescents, 2nd edition. Baltimore: Lippincott; 2003. pp. 181-224.

Nursing Issues in the PICU

39

Nirmal Chorari

LEARNING OBJECTIVES

- To have a comprehensive guide to nursing duties in critical care
- To understand the role of the nurse in holistic care
- To enable nurses and doctors to act as a team

INTRODUCTION

The word "nurse" stems from the Latin word for nurture; this origin provides us with the nurse's first obligation to the patient and is the source of one of the most persistent metaphors for the nurse, i.e., a mother substitute.

The Association of Critical Care nurses further defines critical care nursing as "the utilization of the nursing process (assessment, planning, implementation, and evaluation) in the prevention of or intervention in life-threatening situations". At its most fundamental level, then it can be said that all of nursing is care, rather than cure, orientation, a wellness (prevention of disease or crisis), in addition to illness and concerns a whole person—rather than one organ or subsystem.

PATIENT POPULATION

The pediatric critical care population traditionally consists of patients who range in age from full-term neonates to adolescents and their families. Unlike system-specific adult critical care units, a wide spectrum of illnesses are found in most pediatric intensive care units (PICUs). Extremes in age and illness require pediatric critical care nurses to function as generalists within a subspecialty area.

Levels of PICU Care

The guidelines recommend that level III PICUs provide multidisciplinary definitive care for a wide range of complex, progressive, rapidly changing, medical, surgical, and traumatic disorders, occurring in pediatric patients of all ages, excluding newborns. The guidelines also recommend that level II PICUs provide stabilization of critically ill children before transfer to another center or, to avoid long-distance transfers, provide care for disorders of less complexity or lower acuity.

DESCRIBING WHAT NURSES DO: THE SYNERGY MODEL

The synergy model describes nursing practice based on the needs and characteristics of patients. The fundamental premise of this model is that patient characteristics drive nurse competencies. When patient characteristics and nurse competencies match and synergize, optimal patient outcomes result.

The following presents the major tenets of the Synergy Model:
- Patient characteristics of concern to nurses
- Nurse competencies important to the patient
- Patient outcomes that result when patient characteristics and nurse competencies are mutually enhancing.

Patient Characteristics of Concern to Nurses

Contextually, each patient and family is unique with:
- Varying capacities for health
- Vulnerability to illness
- Genetic and biologic makeup
- Variable socioeconomic and environmental factors.

Each person brings a unique cluster of personal characteristics, to a healthcare situation, which are:
- *Stability* refers to the person's ability to maintain a steady-state equilibrium.
- *Complexity* is the intricate entanglement of two or more systems (e.g., body, family therapies).
- *Predictability* is a summative patient characteristic that allows the nurse to expect a certain trajectory of illness.
- *Resilience* is the patient's capacity to return to a restorative level of functioning using compensatory and coping mechanisms.
- *Vulnerability* refers to an individual's susceptibility to actual or potential stressors that may adversely affect outcomes.
- *Participation in decision making and in care* is the extent to which the patient and family engage in decision making and in aspects of care.
- *Resource availability* refers to resources the patient, family, or community brings to a healthcare situation which includes personal, psychological, social, technical, and fiscal resources.

These seven continua are applicable to patients in all practice settings, which are important for nurse-to-nurse communication of patient characteristics across traditional unit and system boundaries. For example, a healthy uninsured 4-year-old girl undergoing a preschool physical examination could be described as an individual who is (1) stable, (2) not complex, (3) very predictable, (4) resilient, (5) not vulnerable, (6) parent able to participate in decision making and care, but (7) has inadequate resource availability; whereas a critically ill infant in multisystem organ failure can be described on the other end of the continuum in some areas but very similar in others, e.g., as an individual who is (1) unstable, (2) complex, (3) unpredictable, (4) resilient, (5) vulnerable, (6) unable to become involved in decision making and care with (7) adequate resource availability.

Nurse Competencies Important to the Patient

Nursing competencies, derived from the needs of patients, are also described in terms of essential continua.

Clinical Judgment

It is clinical reasoning that includes clinical decision making, critical thinking, and a global grasp of the situation, coupled with nursing skills acquired through a process of integrating formal and experiential knowledge.

The expert nurse anticipates the needs of patients, predicts the patient's trajectory of illness, and envisions the patient's level of recovery.

Advocacy/Moral Agency

It is defined as working on another's behalf and representing the concerns of the patient, family, or community. In the PICU, it is especially challenging to balance technology with values that emphasize the quality of life, consumer choice, risk-benefit decisions, access, and integrity of human life.

This, almost never talked about, intimate aspect of care, which is learnt from role modeling is nursing's most profound contribution to human kind.

Caring Practices

Caring practices optimize and make clinical competence and expertise more visible. Caring practices include not only what nurses do but also how they do it. From the patient's perspective, caring practices are expressive activities that help the patients and families feel cared for. Important caring practices are:
- Demonstration of professional knowledge and skill
- Surveillance
- Reassuring presence
- Vigilance
- Nurturance.

Care is focused at supporting the entire family unit, having empathetic practices that value the family and provides close, attentive care to the patient. More than any other subspecialty, pediatric critical care nurses have made significant progress in role modeling family-centered care in critical care.

Few areas of patient care where vigilance is required are:
- Proper identity of patient before drug delivery
- Proper drug dosing, proper dilution and avoidance of incompatible drug mixing
- Avoidance of verbal orders except in emergency and mandatory notation of the same, later
- Proper management of the medication chart with appropriate notation of any change in dose or frequency made by the physician
- Notation of any adverse reaction with any drug and conveying that to the physician
- Adjustment of parameters on the ventilator exactly as advised by the physician and timely notation of change in any parameter

- Proper delivery of life-saving medication like inotropes infusion, insulin infusion etc. through properly working instruments
- Proper observation and notation of vital parameters of a patient and early notification when any sudden change, like in SpO_2, ABP, vent alarms, intake/output, etc., occurs
- Proper fixation and management of invasive lines and tubes like ET, CVC, HD catheter, arterial lines, etc
- Checking the prescribed drug for proper content, dosage, expiry date and dilution according to physician's orders
- Assisting in procedures
- Assisting and able to handle CPR.

Facilitator of Learning

Nurses facilitate patient learning so that patients can:
- Understand the healthcare system
- Provide the opportunity, accountability, and responsibility to make informed choices
- Allay anxiety.

A nurse takes on various roles with respect for values, beliefs, and rights of the patient:
- She becomes an important person medically as well as emotionally to the patient and the family because of her long presence, frequent contacts and delivery of continuous attention in the absence of family in the critical care unit
- She acts as a liaison between the patient, the patient's family and other healthcare professionals
- She intercedes for patients who cannot speak for themselves in situations that require immediate action
- She provides education and support to help the patient or the patient's designated surrogate to make informed decisions.

Collaboration

Jacques, an organization theorist who studied the structural dimensions of nurses' work, noted: "The nurse is the one person on the unit whose job is to care about anything that might happen in the universe of the patient and to connect any parties who need to be connected in order to assure a successful outcome for the patient." Optimal collaboration requires multidisciplinary socialization.

Hospitals with positive organizational climate, good collaboration, good communication, job satisfaction, and high morale amongst the staff lead to:
- Low mortality ratio
- Low complication rate
- High patient satisfaction.

Systems Thinking

Nurses are leaders in creating and managing systems. Today, as Angela McBride notes,

True nurses:
- Design, implement, and evaluate whole programs of caregiving

- Manage units in which care is provided
- Monitor whether the healthcare system as a whole is sensitive to patient needs
- Play a role in ethical decision making around caregiving.

A PICU nurse's responsibilities include:
- Documentation:
  - Admission/discharge criteria fulfillment
  - Indoor case sheet
  - Consents
  - Daily notes by consultants, registrars, fellows
  - Medicine dosage chart
  - Confirmation chart for drug delivery
  - Charts for vital parameters
  - Procedure notes
  - Sentinel events
  - Proper notation of procedures and consultations to facilitate proper billing.
- Inventory work:
  - To keep records of all the equipment in the unit with new additions
  - Inward/outward movement of equipment
  - Proper working and maintenance of equipment
  - Timely calibration of equipment
  - Maintenance of drug supply
  - Segregations of drugs like emergency drugs, look alike-sound alike drugs, narcotics etc. as per the institutional policy
  - Stationary.
- Legal issues:
  - Meticulous record keeping
  - Proper communication with legal authorities when required
  - Conform diligently to physician's advice in sensitive situations like end-of-life care, autopsy request, organ donation, etc.
  - Proper documentation and consent forms.

Response to Diversity

Response to diversity is the sensitivity to recognize, appreciate, and incorporate differences into the provision of care. Response to diversity is required because the individual differences that exist in everyday life. This approach requires:
- Effective communication with patients and families at their level of understanding
- Tailoring the healthcare culture to meet the diverse needs and strengths of families.

Clinical Inquiry

Clinical inquiry helps push the limits of current practice so that patients receive evidence-based care.

A PICU nurse's daily activities include:
- *General care (nursing aides or assistants can take on this role to unburden the nurse)*:
  - Care of patient's personal hygiene, eye care, mouth care
  - Bed making
  - Maintaining proper position of the patient as per the physician's advice
  - Frequent changing of posture to prevent bedsores
  - Physiotherapy
  - Biomedical waste disposal.
- *Infection control*: Most important aspects of critical care nursing include:
  - Strict adherence to institutional guidelines
  - Proper hand hygiene
  - Strict asepsis during procedures, CVC handling, IV drug administration, changing of tubing and peripheral cannulas
  - Proper dressing of CVC, arterial line, and surgical sites
  - Proper management of urinary catheters, surgical drains, ventilator tubing, ICDs, etc.
  - Endotracheal and oral suctioning when indicated
  - Maintenance of general cleanliness and proper disposal of waste
  - Strict surveillance of breech in asepsis.
- *Nutritional assistance*:
  - Providing oral and/or parenteral feeds as per the physician's and dietician's advice.

These competencies reflect a dynamic integration of knowledge, skills, experience, and attitudes necessary to meet patients' needs and optimize patient outcomes. For example, if the gestalt of a patient were stable but unpredictable, minimally resilient, and vulnerable, primary competencies of the nurse would be centered on clinical judgment and caring practices (which includes vigilance).

Optimal Patient Outcomes

"Optimal patient outcomes" are what patients (or the people of significance to the patient), themselves, define as important.

According to the Synergy Model, when patient characteristics and nurse competencies match and synergize, optimal patient outcomes result. Many outcome measures have been proposed including:

Physiological status	Psychological outcomes
Functional measures	Behavior
Knowledge	Symptom control
Quality of life	Home functioning
Family strain	Goal attainment
Utilization of services	Safety
Problem resolution	Patient satisfaction

Three levels of outcomes are delineated:
1. Patient level outcomes
2. Patient–nurse level outcomes
3. Patient–system level outcomes.

Patient Level Outcomes

Trust results from the nurse knowing the patient and patient knowing the nurse with great emphasis on the nurse's clinical competency and moral agency. Caring practices create a compassionate and therapeutic environment with the aim of promoting comfort, and preventing unnecessary suffering. Patient satisfaction measures involving nursing typically include:
- Technical–professional factors
- Trusting relationships
- Education experiences
- Patient-perceived functional change
- Quality of life.

Patient satisfaction, functional status, and quality of life are interrelated.

Patient–Nurse Level Outcomes

Patient–nurse level outcomes include:
- Physiologic changes
- The presence or absence of complications
- Attainment of care or treatment objectives.

Nurses carry out these activities by:
- Monitoring and managing therapies by evaluating physiological changes
- Limiting iatrogenic injury and complications to therapy
- Their vigilance and clinical judgment
- Integrating numerous services which are critical for optimal patient outcomes and abbreviated lengths of stay.
- Nurse–physician collaboration and positive interaction.

Patient–System Level Outcomes

Important patient'system outcome data include:
- *Recidivism*: Rehospitalization and readmission
- Costs/resource use.

In addition to patient and system factors, nurses can decrease the patient's length of stay through:
- Coordination of care
- Prevention of complications
- Timely discharge planning
- Referral to community resources.

CURRENT ENVIRONMENT

We have fewer nurses entering and staying within nursing. Creative strategies to recruit and retain experienced critical care nurses are a priority for the profession.

Nurses make a significant contribution:
- To the quality of patient care services
- Containment of costs
- Reducing mortality rates
- Length of stay and complications
- Increasing family satisfaction
- Readiness and ability to function upon discharge.

Issues/Challenges

Many of the challenges faced by nurses today are because:
- Most of them are females and by virtue of this fact they need to play multiple roles in the Indian context
- Poor training facilities and educational infrastructure
- Lack of respect from physicians
- Inadequate control over the content of nurses' work
- Poor working conditions
- Inadequate pay for what nurses consider to be professional responsibility
- Conflict with other healthcare providers
- Inadequate staffing patterns
- Unresponsive nursing leadership
- Lack of support in dealing with death and dying; dealing with families
- Intensity of emotions in interpersonal situations
- Rapidly changing technology
- Narrow patient care focus
- Great responsibility.

CONCLUSION

Hospitals need to provide autonomy for nurses, foster positive attitudes of physicians toward collaborative practice and enhance availability and quality of support services.

Constant training—a definite solution:
- Train, observe, and correct the new healthcare person in ICU
- Constant surveillance of subordinates for each of their activity
- Continue upgradation of knowledge to newer modalities available.

The critical care nurse is a product of the history of nursing, the struggles of women in our society, the modern ICU environment, and most importantly, the conflicts and positive relationships with other care providers.

The era where any person who knows only how to fill up the syringe will be taking care of critically ill patient has come to an end. There are few excuses for making mistake and jeopardizing the lives of those who entrusted to our care. A critical care nurse must do right on first time and then every time. The consequences of performance below standard of care can be disastrous.

Ability and opportunity to nurture and save a life of a patient at the nadir of his condition is a blessed thing for any human being. Respect it.

SUGGESTED READING

1. American Nurses Association. Nursing's social policy statement, Washington DC, 1995. American Nurses Foundation.
2. Curley MAQ, Moloney-Harmon PA (Eds). Critical Care Nursing of Infants and Children. Philadelphia: W.B. Saunders Co.; 2001.
3. French P. Social Skills for Nursing Practice. London: Croom Helm; 1987.
4. Fuhrman BP, Zimmerman J (Eds). Pediatric Critical Care, 3rd edition. US: Elsevier Health Sciences; 2006.
5. Jacques RW. Untheorized dimensions of caring work: caring as a structural practice and caring as a way of seeing. Nurse Admin Q. 1993;17:1-10.
6. Knaus WA, Draper EA, Wagner DP, et al. An evaluation of the outcome from intensive care in major medical centres. Ann Intern Med. 1986;104(3):410-8.
7. Kuruvilla J. Essentials of Critical Care Nursing. New Delhi: Jaypee Brothers Medical Publishers (P) Ltd; 2007.
8. Kuruvilla J. Stress among critical care nurses in Christian Medical College Hospital, Vellore. 1990. Unpublished.
9. McBride AB. How nursing looks today. Indiana University Alumni Magazine. 1994.
10. Proceeding of National Teaching Institute, American Association of Critical Care Nurses, 1992.
11. Singh S. Critical Care Nursing. New Delhi: Anmol Publications; 2006.
12. www.acnn.org
13. www.allnurse.org
14. www.rcn.org.uk
15. Zander K. Nursing case management: Strategic management of cost and quality outcomes. J Nurs Admin, 1988;18(5):23-30.

Extracorporeal Membrane Oxygenation

40

Amish Vora, Praveen Khilnani, Suneel K Pooboni

LEARNING OBJECTIVES

- To get an overview and understanding of the principles of extracorporeal membrane oxygenation (ECMO)
- To be able to take the next step toward applying this after further practical training.

DEFINITION

Extracorporeal membrane oxygenation (ECMO) is a technique of adaptation of conventional cardiopulmonary bypass to support the function of the lungs or heart or both for a prolonged period of time. It can be done in cases of reversible cardiopulmonary failure, for a period of days to weeks.

HISTORY

ECMO is a life-saving innovation that takes over the function of the lungs and to some extent the heart, in order to provide gas exchange. From 1944, when it was first recognized that oxygen could be diffused into the body from a semipermeable membrane to the first bypass in the 1950s, ECMO has come a long way. There are safe and less laborious methods used today.

EVIDENCE BASE FOR ECMO

In 1985 Bartlet et al. did a prospective study for newborns with respiratory failure where one patient was put on conventional ventilation which died and 11 were put on ECMO and all survived. Only 1 of 11 had intracerebral hemorrhage. So began the journey of ECMO.

In 1989 Oruke et al. did a randomized trial of 39 newborn infants with severe persistent pulmonary hypertension of the newborn (PPHN) and respiratory failure; met criteria for 85% likelihood of dying. In phase I, 4/10 conventional medical therapy (CMT) (conventional) group died, all ECMO babies survived. Randomization was halted after the fourth CMT death. Next

20 babies treated with ECMO (phase II), 19/20 survived. The overall survival of ECMO-treated infants was 97% (28 of 29) compared with 60% (6 of 10) in the CMT group P <0.05.

Babies with severe respiratory failure at birth exhibit a wide spectrum of impairment and disability at the age of 4 years. A policy of transfer for consideration for ECMO support reduced the number of children who die but this is not offset by an increase in severe disability in survivors. This was proven in 1996!

Similarly in adults, in 2009 Giles et al. did a randomized control trial "CESAR trial" of 180 adults showed not only significant survivor at discharge but also at 6 months.

INDICATIONS FOR ECMO

In disorders unresponsive to maximal conventional treatment, such as:

Neonates:
- Severe meconium aspiration syndrome
- Severe respiratory distress syndrome (RDS)
- Persistent pulmonary hypertension of the newborn
- Septic shock
- Severe bacterial/viral pneumonias
- Prolonged cardiopulmonary bypass.

Children:
- Severe bacterial/viral pneumonias
- Aspiration pneumonias
- Severe burns with acute respiratory distress syndrome (ARDS)
- Prolonged cardiopulmonary bypass
- Low cardiac output resulting from right, left, and biventricular failure following the repair of a congenital heart defect
- Pulmonary vasoactive crisis following repair of congenital heart defect leading to severe hypoxemia, low cardiac output, or both
- As a bridge to cardiac/lung transplant
- As a bridge to recovery in temporary cardiomyopathy secondary to renal failure, myocarditis, and severe burns with ARDS, myocarditis, etc.
- Poisonings needing temporary support.

Adults:
- Severe bacterial/viral pneumonias
- ARDS
- ARDS secondary lung contusion/polytrauma
- Septic shock
- Post cardiac surgery
- Poisonings needing temporary support.

ELIGIBILITY CRITERIA

Any of the following and underlying disease process which is likely to be:

Reversible: While the following criteria are guidelines, a rapidly worsening child with high, damaging ventilator settings and refractory hypoxemia that does not strictly have these numbers could also be considered a candidate for ECMO.

1. Oxygenation index (OI) more than or equal to 40 for 0.5–6 hours; OI = (MAP × FiO$_2$ ×100)/ PaO$_2$ (mm Hg)
   Standard criteria: OI more than or equal to 40 on maximal conventional ventilation
2. PaO$_2$ less than 5.3 kPa (40 mmHg) for more than 2 hours or PaO$_2$ less than 6.7–8.0 kPa (50–60 mm Hg) for 2–12 hours despite maximal ventilatory support.
3. Persisting acidosis and shock, pH less than 7.25 due to metabolic acidosis, raised lactate and intractable hypotension despite inotropic medications and correction of hypovolemia/preload.
4. *Murray score in adolescents/adults*: The Murray score uses the average score of 4 elements graded on a 0–4 scale to establish ARDS severity.
5. Individual assessment.

CONTRAINDICATIONS TO ECMO

Absolute contraindications:
- Intracerebral hemorrhage—In neonates, Grade 3 or 4 intraventricular hemorrhage (IVH)
- Severe and irreversible brain injury
- Severe and irreversible lung, liver or kidney disease
- Lethal malformations or congenital anomalies
- Significant non-treatable congenital heart disease.

Relative contraindications:
- Gestational age less than 34 weeks (difficulty in cannulation and possibility of IVH)
- Birth weight less than 2 kg (difficulty in cannulation)
- 10 to 14 days of mechanical ventilation (possibility of lung fibrosis)
- IVH Grade 1–2
- Disease states with a high probability of a poor prognosis.

ECMO MACHINERY AND TUBING (FIG. 1)

The blood pump is either a centrifugal pump or a roller pump. Most of the units have switched over to centrifugal pumps in the last decade. The size of these pumps have been miniaturized in comparison to the previous versions due to technological advances. The circuit tubing is made up of a special polymer, Tygon. A venous reservoir (Bladder) is used with the roller pump. The oxygenator does the work of exchanging both oxygen and carbon dioxide. Currently, most units use hollow-fiber, polymethoxy pentane (PMP) oxygenators, which are compact and very efficient. After successful gas exchange, the oxygenated blood is warmed to a required temperature in the heat exchanger, by a countercurrent mechanism of circulating warm water.

Safety Devices and Monitors

Pressure monitors at three different places yield vital information. Pre-pump pressure monitor indicates the preload status of the patient, as indicated by excessive negative pressures during hypolvolemia. Pre- and post-membrane pressure monitors and the resulting gradient indicate the health of the oxygenator and accumulation of the clots within the membrane. Air bubble detectors identify microscopic air bubbles in the returning arterialized blood and

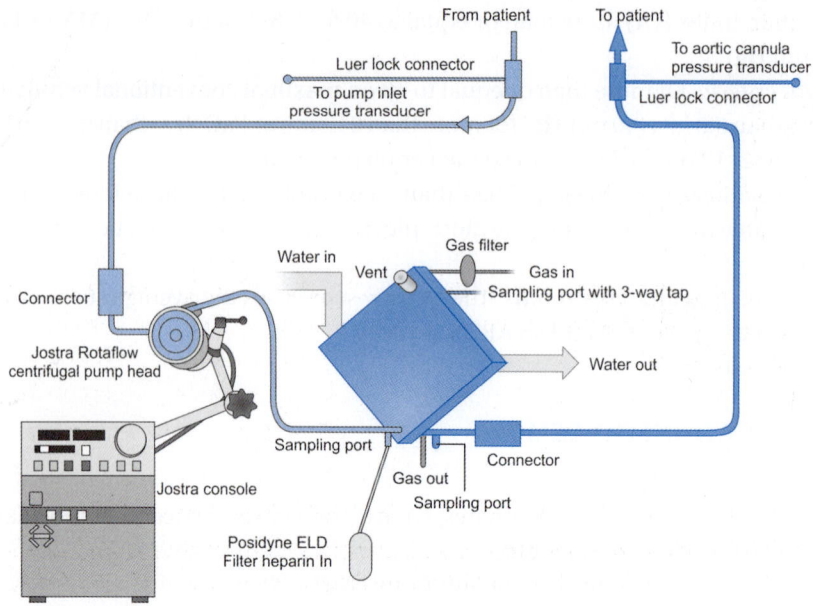

Fig. 1: Extracorporeal membrane oxygenation circuit diagram.

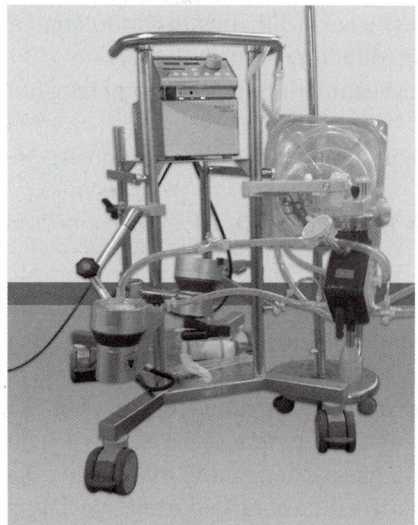

Fig. 2: Machine.
Courtesy: Maquet India.

automatically turn off the blood pump. Some membrane oxygenators are inbuilt with the integrated mechanism of air traps. Arterial line filters between the heat exchanger and the arterial cannula are used to trap air, thrombi, and other emboli. A continuous venous oxygen saturation monitor and temperature monitor are other important safety features (Fig. 2).

Types

There are two major types of ECMO:
1. Veno-venous or VV
2. Veno-arterial or VA

Mixed types:
- VVA
- VVVA

Veno-venous (VV-ECMO): Facilitates gas exchange; blood is removed from the venous side and then pumped back into it, but does not provide hemodynamic support and is used in hypoxemic respiratory failure when the cardiac function is good.

Veno-arterial ECMO (VA-ECMO): Allows gas exchange and hemodynamic support while blood is pumped out from a vein and returned into an artery.

Arterio-venous ECMO (AV-ECMO): Facilitates gas exchange by using the patient's own arterial pressure to pump blood from the arterial to the venous side.

Cannulation: Blood cannulae and sites of cannulation for good venous return are the lifelines for ECMO. The cannulae for vascular insertion are wide bore cannulae, preferably with wire reinforcement. Cannulation can be done by any intensivist or surgeon with prior experience of inserting ECMO cannulae under supervision. Various techniques such as semi-seldinger, open, and ultrasound-guided methods can be used for cannulation. Double lumen cannulae might need placement in a cardiac laboratory for facilities such as fluoroscopy or echo guidance. Cannulae might puncture the vessel or atrial wall resulting in a cardiac tamponade, which should be promptly recognized and treated. Hence, cardiac surgeons should be readily available. Usually, for veno-venous cannulation, double lumen Avalon cannulae are preferable, but, they are not available in India at this time and are expensive. In the absence of Avalon double lumen cannulae, Oregon double lumen cannulae can be used (less robust). In the age group beyond 2 years, the femoral vein can be used for draining the blood by keeping the tip of the cannula at the IVC/RA junction and return the cannula in the neck, via the right internal jugular vein. The right internal jugular vein is preferred as its course is straight unlike the left one. In case of thrombosis or tying the internal jugular vein during de-cannulation thereby do not attempt accessing both internal jugular veins for cannulation. The opposite side jugular vein should be fully functional to take over the venous flow from the head. Nomograms are available for deciding the right size cannulae for any age/weight. At the time of cannulation, 75–100 units/kg heparin is given as a stat dose, depending on the clotting profile of the patient.

Antibiotic cover: We should treat the infections but should not abuse antibiotics as the emergence of drug-resistant bacteria would be a real problem. In India, multidrug resistant infections are responsible for reduction in our survival rates by at least 20%. We give one dose of antibiotic to cover for the skin flora at the time of cannulation and decannulation.

GOLDEN RULES OF SUCCESS

- *Asepsis*: Be very meticulous with asepsis. Early recognition of infection and treating with appropriate antibiotics is important.

- *Position of cannulae*: Cannulae tend to migrate in mobile patients when the sutures become loose, especially in long-term ECMO. Hence, one should be extremely cautious in safe guarding the position of cannulae, as cannulae are the lifeline for ECMO.
- *Dry body weight*: Once the patient is stable on ECMO, we should diuresis the patient to the dry body weight either by means of using diuretics or by placing them on continuous veno-venous hemofiltration (CVVH), which is very easy on ECMO as you do not need to put any special cannulae into the patient. CVVH circuit can be connected to the ECMO circuit. Right time for initiation and right time to come off: One should not delay in initiating ECMO support if the patient fulfils ECMO criteria. Similarly, when the lungs are better (ventilate with moderate settings associated with improvement in the general condition of the patient), one should give trial off for patient off the ECMO support.

MANAGEMENT

Ventilator settings: The reason for ECMO is to bypass the lungs at least partially and let them "rest". Universally, it has been accepted to keep the patients while they are on ECMO on "rest" ventilator settings. Peak inspiratory pressure (PIP) of 20 cm H_2O, positive end expiratory pressure (PEEP) of 10 cm H_2O, rate of 10/min, and inspiratory time of 1 second with FiO_2 30%. If you do not ventilate the lungs, they go into a state of collapse due to non-recruitment of alveoli. It is also agreed to minimize the pressures following severe barotrauma involving multiple pneumothoraces. High PEEP and very low tidal volumes are used to prevent atelectasis. There are times, we oscillated patients on minimal oscillatory settings to recruit lungs, especially while they are on long-term respiratory ECMO support. By minimizing the sedation on patients, we can extubate them while they are breathing for themselves. Randomized controlled trials (RCTs) are on-going at this stage to decide on the best ventilator strategies.

Initial period of lung rest: It has been recommended to use an initial period of lung rest as it gives time for the lung to recover. Suctioning and draining big pleural effusions may be necessary during this period. Effective diuresis might help too.

Recruitment of lung: After an initial period of 4–5 days of lung rest, we try to recruit the lung by physiotherapy, postural therapy, and appropriate suctioning means (conventional versus sterile fibre-optic bronchoscopy as needed).

Anticoagulation: This is one of the most crucial problems. Heparin acts by inhibiting antithrombin 3 and is the most commonly used drug for anticoagulation on ECMO. The levels of anticoagulation can be measured in terms of activated clotting time (ACT) which is a practical bed side tool. Other ways of monitoring anticoagulation are measuring heparin levels, Factor X assay, and thrombo-elastograms for the functional element. Heparin levels have to be maintained within a tight range as measured by ACTs of 160–180 for venovenous ECMO and 180–200 for venoarterial ECMO. Usually continuous heparin infusion of 10–15 (10–40) units/kg/h will suffice to maintain the target ACTs, though it might vary from time to time. Hence, heparin infusion rate has to be altered to maintain the desired ACTs from time to time. In case of deficiency of anti-thrombin 3, heparin requirement will increase significantly. Antithrombin levels can be measured and supplemented in case of deficiency. The newer anticoagulants are also used but will not be discussed here.

Sedation: Keeping the patient appropriately sedated to avoid over-sedation and onset of critical care myopathy is important to balance out the problems due to excessive mobility leading to the displacement of ECMO cannulae. Adequate analgesia, avoiding cumulative toxicity of the sedatives by stopping and restarting sedatives/paralytic agents and being conscious about renal clearance versus augmented renal clearance would be useful for optimal recovery.

Feeding: In the absence of circumstances leading to intestinal ischemia, early enteral feeding is recommended.

Ventilator-associated pneumonia (VAP): Prevention of VAP is very important to minimize the duration spent on ECMO.

Tracheostomy/ETT: If the duration is ECMO is expected to be long, early tracheostomy might be useful. Tracheostomy is also useful for clearing secretions. The timing of tracheostomy decision will differ from children to adults.

Surgical procedures: Emergency surgical procedures are not ideal. If emergency procedures are required, they should be done right in time, taking precautions to secure hemostasis.

Renal support: After initial stabilization on ECMO, attempts should be made to take fluid off either by using diuretics or by instituting continuous venovenous hemofiltration.

CNS: Constant observation of the wakeful status of the patient besides regular neurological assessment would be required. Investigations such as EEG, cerebral functioning analysing monitoring (CFAM), cranial ultrasonography, CT scan of the brain, and near-infrared spectroscopy (NIRS) are helpful.

Complications: Patient-related and machine-related complications can happen while on ECMO. Examples of patient-related complications are: bleeding versus clotting, hemolysis, renal failure, hypertension, cardiac dysfunction, arrhythmias, neurological complications, infections, etc. Mechanical complications could be due to oxygenator failure, tube rupture (on roller pump), pump failure, heat exchanger fault, clots in the circuit, cracked connectors, cannula-related problems such as kinking and displacement of cannulae.

Family: As it is going to be very stressful emotionally for patient as well as the families, we inform the family about the progress and expectations from time to time.

Weaning: Once the blood gases start to improve, simultaneously associated with improvement in chest X-ray findings and clinical improvement. When there is continuous satisfactory improvement in the general condition of the patient, we tend to recruit the lungs and try to take them off ECMO through a procedure called trial off. It the trial off is successful, cannulae can be removed/repaired for reverting back to ventilator support.

POST-ECMO CARE

Looking after the patient in the stabilization period is very essential for treating these critically ill children successfully.

OUTCOMES

In neonatal respiratory ECMO, 94% of patients will get better. In pediatric and adult respiratory ECMOs, successful outcomes are close to 60–70% in experienced centers. In cardiac ECMO, positive outcomes are to the tune of around 60%. Invariably, outcomes will depend upon the age group, indication for ECMO, the complications during the course of ECMO, and the experience of the center.

As per the INSPIRED (Indian Network of Specialist Pediatric intensivists for research Education and Data) Indian data therapy from Jan 2011—Jan 2017 for children under 16-years of age is: Total of 84 cases of ECMO were reported. Fifty children underwent respiratory ECMO from 9 institutions with a 42% survival. Total of 34 children underwent cardiac ECMO from 8 centers with 73.5% survival.

Extracorporeal membrane oxygenation continues to represent an important support option in select critically ill newborns infants and children. With increased experience, this procedure has become safer, more effective alternative to many less efficacious conventional therapies.

According to the sale of ECMO equipment from 2017 India has done 700 plus ECMO/year. This number will keep on increasing and the rate as which use of ECMO is increasing in India we may be doing highest number of ECMO/year by 2030.

KEY MESSAGES

- ECMO is a life-saving albeit labor and cost-intensive procedure.
- It can be appleied to a variety of serious conditions.
- It is an important arm of pediatric critical care.
- The procedure should be taught in tertiary and quaternary care units and not undertaken by inexperienced hands.

SUGGESTED READING

1. Bartlett RH, Roloff DW, Cornell RG, et al. Extracorporeal circulation in neonatal respiratory failure: a prospective randomized study. Pediatrics. 1985;76(4):479-87.
2. Khilnani P. Anticoagulation on extraxcorporeal membrane oxygenation (ECMO). QMJ. 2017;2017.
3. Khilnani P, Oza P, Pooboni S, et al. ECMO Indian Scenario. J Ped Crit Care. 2014;I:24-33.
4. Mittal S, Saroha V, Vora A, et al. Centrifugal versus roller pump for neonatal extraxcorporeal membrane oxygenation—outcome and complication rates. Ped Crit Care Med. 2014;15:28-29.
5. Mittal S, Saroha V, Vora A, et al. Centrifugal versus roller pump for pediatric extraxcorporeal membrane oxygenation—outcome and complication rates. Ped Crit Care Med. 2014;15:109-10.
6. O'Rourke PP, et al. Extracorporeal membrane oxygenation and conventional medical therapy in neonates with persistent pulmonary hypertension of the newborn: a prospective randomized study. 1989;84:6;957-63.
7. Peek GJ, Mugford M, Tiruvoipati R, et al. Efficacy and economic assessment of conventional ventilatory support versus extracorporeal membrane oxygenation for severe adult respiratory failure (CESAR): a multicentre randomised controlled trial Lancet. 2009;37:1351-63.
8. The Red book: ELSO : Extracorporeal Cardiopulmonary Support in Critical Care, 4th edition.
9. UK collaborative randomised trial of neonatal extracorporeal membrane oxygenation. UK Collaborative ECMO Trail Group. Lancet. 1996;348:75-82.

Pediatric Organ Donation and Donor Maintenance

41

Manish Sharma

LEARNING OBJECTIVES

- To understand the concepts surrounding Pediatric Brain Death
- To understand the basic laws that govern the declaration of brain death for organ transplant
- To carry out appropriate tests required.

CONCEPT AND HISTORY

"Organ donation is when an individual permits an organ of theirs to be removed, legally, either by consent while the donor is alive or after death with the consent of the next of kin."

Historically, death was defined by the presence of putrefaction or decapitation, failure to respond to painful stimuli, or the apparent loss of observable cardiorespiratory action. However, with development in resuscitation measures and invention of mechanical ventilators, respiratory arrest was prevented. Vital functions can currently be maintained artificially when the brain has ceased to function.

HISTORICAL PERSPECTIVE

- Prior to the arrival of mechanical respiration, death was defined as the cessation of circulation and breathing.
- 1959—Coma de'passe' by Mollaret and Goulon
- 1968—Irreversible Coma/Brain Death by Harvard Medical School—Ad Hoc Committee
- 1981—Uniform Determination of Death Act—President's Commission for the Study of Moral Issues in Medication
- 1994—American Academy of Neurology guidelines for the determination of brain death
- 2005—pointers for determining brain death.

Figures 1 and 2 show the status of organ donation worldwide (including India) and the organs donated, respectively.

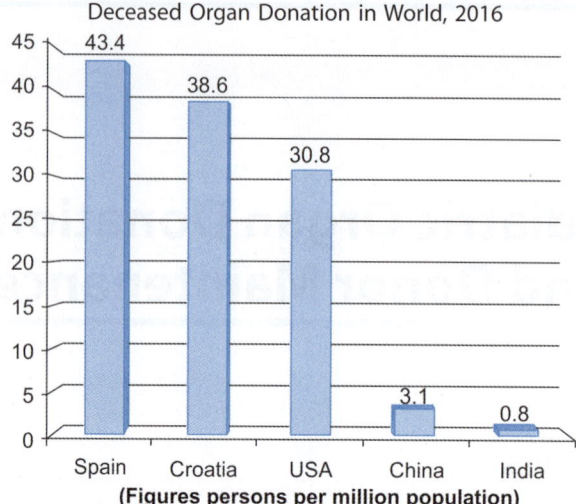

Fig. 1: Organ donation statistic in India and World.
Source: International Registry in Organ Donation and Transplantation. (2016). Deceased Organ Donation in World—2016. [online] Available from http://www.irodat.org. [Last Accessed April, 2019].

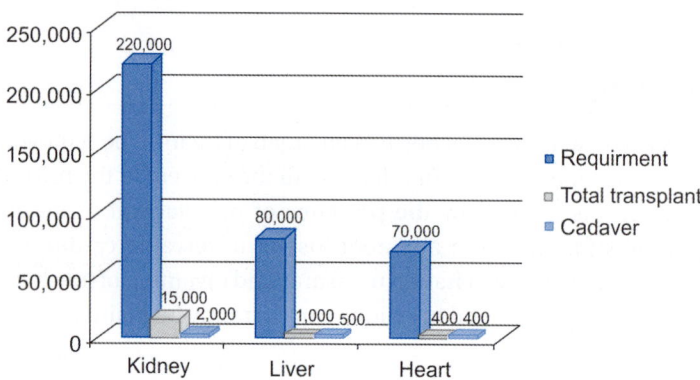

Fig. 2: Organs donated.

BRAIN DEATH CURRENT CONSENSUS

- Absent cerebral function
- Absent brainstem function
- Apnea.

At present, there is no clear moral framework for donation from children and it seems that there is a wide range of views regarding what constitutes best practice in this area. For an adult donor, decisions regarding organ donation are generally created on behalf of an individual on the basis of that person's known needs and beliefs. Organ donation made on behalf of children differs owing to these important factors:

- Children have differing abilities to form decisions depending on their age or maturity and many are unable to make any decisions at all.

- Very often there is very little or no proof of a child's wishes or beliefs on which to base a call about donation.

  The nature of care in pediatric medicine is more family-centered than in adults, this implies that working within the limits of the child's interests, pediatricians encourage families to reach a decision about a child's care that is right for the family as a whole and which therefore takes under consideration the interests of a wider group of individuals than only the child who is the patient.

  The number of children who will become organ donors is restricted by several factors. Brain death in childhood is relatively uncommon, and lots of children who die will have received aggressive medical therapies, or suffer from diseases that preclude successful transplantation of their organs. Additionally, organ donation is only possible once a child dies in hospital.

  It is necessary that families considering organ donation perceive that the organs given by their child might not go to another child. The potential to help others will be seen as a welcome chance by some families. Involving families in decision-making is a powerful manner of helping them feel in control—this will have a big impact on how the experience is remembered.

Criteria for CNS determination of brain death:
- Irreversible coma
- Absence of cortical function
- Absence of brain stem function
- Apnea
- Two examinations at defined intervals for age.

TESTING FOR BRAINSTEM DEATH (BOXES 1 AND 2)

A person is dead once he has irreversibly lost the capacity for consciousness and breathing, this implies loss of brainstem function. In patients who have suffered cardiopulmonary arrest (including failed resuscitation), loss of brainstem function occurs as a consequence of catastrophic brain injury. In these patients, for the purpose of organ donation, death is diagnosed after confirming simultaneous onset of apnea and unconsciousness, the absence of circulation for a minimum of 5 minutes (central pulse on palpation and heart sounds on auscultation) and the absence of neurological reflexes (pupillary responses, corneal reflex, and motor response to supraorbital pressure), any contributing causes for the arrest should have been reversed.

Irreversible brainstem damage also happens in patients with other causes of coma.

In patients with coma, testing brainstem reflexes is used for assessing brainstem function, whereas the capability for breathing is tested using apnea testing. Irreversible loss of both functions is mandatory to confirm brainstem death, unlike in persistent vegetative state where the ability to breathe is preserved.

Box 1: Appropriate terminology.
- Say "dead", not "brain dead"
- Say "artificial or mechanical ventilation", not "life support"
- Time of death = time of second examination, including apnea and/or ancillary test completion
- When a patient meets all criteria for brain death, they are legally dead. NOT when ventilator removed, NOT when heart beat ceases.
- State law and local institutional policies should be reviewed and followed
- Ask staff, not talk to the patient as if he is still alive.

Brainstem testing involves three distinct stages:
1. Identifying the cause and excluding potentially reversible causes
2. Testing brainstem reflexes
3. Apnea testing.

In India, the legal framework for organ donation is in place according to the Transplantation of Human Organ Act (THOA—1994) legislation, this law was amended in 2014 and most of the states follow the amended law.

The following should be reversed before the tests are undertaken:

> **Box 2: Who can certify brain death?**
>
> Personnel authorized to perform apnea testing as per THOA-2014 Act:
> - RMP—incharge of the hospital in which brainstem death has occurred
> - RMP—nominated from the panel of names sent by the hospitals and approved by the appropriate authority
> - Neurologist/neurosurgeon
> - RMP—treating the aforesaid deceased person.
>
> *(Where neurologist/neurosurgeon is not available, any surgeon or physician and anesthetist or intensivist, nominated by medical administrator incharge from the panel of names sent by the hospital and approved by the appropriate authority shall be included)*

- *Shock or persistent hypotension based on normal systolic or mean blood pressure values for the patient's age*: Systolic blood pressure or mean arterial pressure ought to be in a suitable range (systolic blood pressure not 92 SDS below age-appropriate norm) based on age
- Hypothermia
- Severe metabolic disturbances are capable of inflicting a potentially reversible coma, together with electrolyte/glucose abnormalities
- Recent administration of neuromuscular-blocking agents
- Drug intoxications, together with but not restricted to barbiturates, opioids, sedative and anesthetic agents, antiepileptic agents, and alcohols.

Pharmacological agents that might have an effect on the results of testing should be discontinued and levels determined as clinically indicated. Low-to-mid therapeutic levels of barbiturates should not preclude the utilization of EEG testing.

All the following reflexes should be absent:
- Pupillary reactions should be fixed and dilated
- Corneal reflex
- Pharyngeal and tracheal gag reflex using tongue depressor or suction catheter
- Pain response by applying pressure to temporomandibular joint or supraorbital ridges
- Vestibulo-ocular reflexes using caloric testing (canal should be unobstructed).

There may also be difficulties in patients with high-cervical spine injuries when respiratory drive may not be reflected by respiratory effort. Such patients may require ancillary testing.

Cold Caloric Test

Patient's head is positioned at 30° from horizontal, so that the external auditory meatus and outer canthus are vertically aligned. 50 mL of ice cold water is injected into the ear over 1 minute, while observing the eyes for movement. A normal response is ipsilateral movement of both eyes and horizontal nystagmus to the contralateral side, but this is absent in patients with brainstem death. The second ear should be irrigated after an interval of several minutes.

Apnea Testing

This test is the final confirmatory test. The aim is to confirm the effect of raise in the arterial CO_2 when the ventilator is disconnected to assess respiratory function. In a patient with normally functioning brainstem, hypercarbia and subsequent metabolic acidosis should stimulate respiration by stimulating the medullary centers. Loss of respiratory drive reflects severe brainstem damage and loss of capacity for independent breathing.

Testing

The patient should be disconnected from ventilator and 100% oxygen should be given through the endotracheal tube at a flow rate of not more than 5 L/min, so as to avoid ventilator autocycling and CO_2 washout by a Venturi effect. It may cause some serious complications including pneumothorax, severe hypoxemia, hemodynamic instability, and even cardiac arrest.

Apnea test:
- *Monitor at least with HR and peripheral capillary oxygen saturation (SpO_2)*
- *Preoxygenate with fraction of inspired oxygen (FiO_2)*
- *Do not allow hypocarbia*
- *Disconnect the ventilator and give O_2 at less than 5 L/min via a catheter into the ET tube (J-R circuit can be used)*
- *Search for respiratory movements for 10 minutes*
- *Repeat blood gas to see rise of CO_2 more than 60 mm Hg*
- *Abandon test, if desaturation, hemodynamic instability, or arrhythmias.*

Another attempt to check for apnea is also performed at a later time or an ancillary study is pursued to assist with determination of brain death.

Continuous positive airway pressure ventilation has been used during apnea testing. It should also be kept in mind that several current ventilators automatically change from a continuous positive airway sure mode to mandatory ventilation and deliver a breath when apnea is detected.

Brainstem Death

Brainstem death is confirmed after the second set of apnea tests and the time of death is recorded as the time of completion of the second set. Documentation is done on a checklist with at least two doctors signing at every stage of the process.

Those carrying out the tests should not have, or be perceived to have, any clinical conflict of interest and neither doctor should be a member of the transplant team. Every transplant center ought to have a transplant coordinator for organ donation whose role is to approach the family and obtain consent.

The patient should be placed back on ventilator support and medical management should be continued till the second neurological examination and apnea test confirming the brain death is completed.

Ancillary Studies

Ancillary studies are not required to establish brain death and should not be viewed as a substitute for thorough neurological examination. These may be used to assist doctors and family in making the diagnosis of brain death:
- When apnea testing cannot be completed safely
- If there is uncertainty regarding the results of the neurological examination
- If a medications residual impact may be present
- To reduce the inter-examination observation period.

For social reasons, allowing members of the family to better comprehend the diagnosis of brain death.

Four-vessel cerebral angiography is the gold standard for determining the absence of cerebral blood flow. This test can be difficult to perform infants and small children, may not be readily available at all institutions, and requires moving the patient to the angiography laboratory.

Electroencephalographic documentation of electrocerebral silence (ECS) and use of radionuclide cerebral blood flow determinations to document the absence of cerebral blood flow stay the most widely used methods to support the clinical diagnosis of brain death in infants and children. Interpretation of ancillary studies needs the expertise of appropriately trained and qualified people.

The physician caring for critically unwell infants and children should remember the potential impact of therapeutic modalities such as hypothermia on the diagnosis of brain death. Efforts to adequately rewarm before performing any neurological examination and maintain temperature throughout the observation period are essential. A core body temperature of 35°C (95°F) ought to be achieved and maintained throughout examination and testing. This temperature is consistent with current adult guidelines and is comparatively simple to attain and maintain in children. Severe metabolic disturbances can cause reversible coma and interfere with the clinical evaluation to determine brain death. Reversible conditions such as severe electrolyte imbalances, hyper- or hyponatremia, hyper- or hypoglycemia, severe pH disturbances, severe hepatic or renal dysfunction, or inborn errors of metabolism might cause coma in a newborn, infant, or child. These conditions ought to be known and treated before analysis for brain death.

Drug intoxications, including barbiturates, opioids, sedatives, intravenous and inhalation anesthetics, antiepileptic agents, and alcohols, can cause severe central nervous system depression and alter the clinical examination to the point where they can mimic brain death. Testing for these drugs should be performed, if there is concern regarding recent ingestion or administration. Once available, specific serum levels of medicines with sedative properties or side effects should be obtained and documented to be in a low-to-mid therapeutic range before neurological examination for brain death testing. Longer-acting or continuous infusion of sedative agents may also interfere with the neurological analysis. These medications should be discontinued. Adequate clearance (based on the age of the child, presence of organ dysfunction, total quantity of medication administered, elimination half-life of the drug, and any active metabolites) should be allowed before the neurological examination. In some instances, this might require waiting many half-lives and rechecking serum levels of the medication before conducting the brain death examination.

If neuromuscular-blocking agents are used, they ought to be stopped.

Other uncommon causes of coma such as neurotoxins and chemical exposure, i.e. organophosphates and carbamates, should be thought about in rare cases within which an etiology for coma has not been established. Clinical criteria for determining brain death might not be present on admission and may evolve during hospitalization.

Assessment of neurological function is also unreliable after resuscitation after cardiopulmonary arrest. It is reasonable to defer neurological examination to determine brain death for 24 hours. If there are issues concerning the validity of the examination (e.g. flaccid tone or absent movements in a patient with high spinal cord injury or severe neuromuscular disease) or if specific examination components cannot be performed as a result of medical contraindications, an ancillary study can be pursued to help with the diagnosis of brain death.

Number of Examinations and Examiners

Nakagawa TA, Ashwal S, Mathur M, et al. Crit Care Med. 2011;39(9):2139-55.

Endorsed by:
- Society of Critical Care Medicine
- Section on Critical Care, AAP
- Section on Neurology, AAP
- Child Neurology Society
- Many others.

Recommended observation periods between brain death examinations based on age and also the results of neurodiagnostic testing:
- Two examinations and EEGs separated by a minimum of 48 hours were recommended for infants of 7 days to 2 months.
- Two examinations and EEGs separated by a minimum of 24 hours were recommended for children 2 months to 1 year. A repeat EEG was not necessary, if a cerebral radionuclide scan or cerebral angiography demonstrated no flow or visualization of the cerebral arteries.
- For children 1 year and above, an observation period of 12 hours was recommended and ancillary testing was not required when an irreversible cause existed.

The observation period during this age bracket could be decreased, if there was documentation of ECS or absent CBF.

The general consensus was the younger the child, the longer the waiting period unless ancillary studies supported the clinical diagnosis of brain death and if, therefore, the observation period could be shortened. The consensus recommendation is that these examinations be performed by cancel physicians concerned in the care.

BRAIN DEATH IN TERM NEWBORNS

The ability to diagnose brain death in newborns continues to be viewed with some uncertainty primarily as a result of the small range of brain-dead neonates reported within the literature and whether or not there are intrinsic biologic variations in neonatal brain metabolism, blood flow, and response to injury.

Clinical Examination

Limited data are offered regarding brain death in newborns as criteria may be difficult as a result of the possibility that some of the brainstem reflexes might not be fully developed and that it is also difficult to assess the extent of consciousness in a critically ill, sedated, and intubated neonate.

Brain death can be diagnosed in term newborns (37 weeks gestation) and older, provided the physician is conscious of the limitations of the clinical examination and ancillary studies in this age bracket.

It is vital to carefully and repeatedly examine term newborns with particular attention to examination of brainstem reflexes and apnea testing. Like with older children, assessment of neurological function in the term newborn may be unreliable immediately after an acute catastrophic neurological injury or cardiopulmonary arrest. A period of 24 hours is usually recommended before evaluating the term newborn for brain death.

Apnea Testing

Neonatal studies reviewing $PaCO_2$ thresholds for apnea are limited. However, information from neonates who were ultimately determined to be brain dead revealed a mean $PaCO_2$ of 64 mm Hg suggesting that the threshold of 60 mm Hg is also valid within the newborn.

Apnea testing in the term newborn is also complicated by the following:

Treatment with 100% oxygen might inhibit the potential recovery of respiratory effort and profound bradycardia might precede hypercarbia and limit this test in neonates. A thorough neurological examination should be performed in conjunction with the apnea test to make the determination of death in any patient. If the apnea test cannot be completed as previously described, the examination and apnea test are often tried at a later time or an ancillary study may be performed to help with determination of death. Ancillary studies in newborns are less sensitive than in older children.

Observation Periods in Term Newborns

Based on information extracted from available literature and clinical expertise, the committee recommends the observation period between examinations should be 24 hours for term newborns (37 weeks) to 30 days of age.

Ancillary studies performed in the newborn 30 days of age are limited. The available information suggests that ancillary studies in newborns are less sensitive than in older children. Awareness of this limitation would suggest that longer periods of observation and repeated neurological examinations are required before making the diagnosis of brain death and also that like in older infants and children, the diagnosis should be made clinically and based on repeated examinations instead of relying solely on ancillary studies.

The Transplantation of Human Organs and Tissues Act: Revised 2014 (THOA-1994)

Brainstem Death

"Brainstem death" means the stage at which all functions of the brainstem have permanently and irreversibly ceased and is so certified.

No organ can be removed until the certification and authorization process is complete.

The cost for maintenance of cadaver or retrieval or transportation or preservation of organs or tissue is not be borne by the donor family and may be borne by the recipient or institution or government or non-government organization or society.

A hospital has to be accredited by the competent authority to certify brain death for organ transplant. The criteria for this and committee formation are available in the rules of the THOA guidelines and there are state and regional rules that need to be followed.

The coordinator is the key person who handles all paper work on standardized forms that are available.

MANAGEMENT OF A BRAIN-DEAD PATIENT (TABLES 1 AND 2)

Following the diagnosis of brain death, a race against the clock starts. The method of counseling the relatives and getting consent for organ donation progress whereas the intensivist tries to keep the donor's organ system viable for donation. This process can be extremely difficult, since a variety of physiological changes that occur within the brain-dead patient proceed inexorably to hypoperfusion of the various organs that are intended for harvesting. The intensive care

Table 1: Management of potential organ donors.

Basic monitoring		Routine investigation		Special management	
Management	Goal	Investigation	Goal	Management	Goal
Continuous monitoring of core temperature	Body temperature <35°C	Serum sodium	135–145 mEq/L	Peripheral warning (and core warning, if required)	Body temperature >35°C
Urine output	Urinary output ≥1.0 mL/kg/h	Left ventricular ejection fraction	>45%	Electrolytes and IV fluids	Appropriate IV fluid choice (preferably crystalloid balance salt fluid) >60 mm Hg
Oxygen saturation	>95%			• Mean arterial pressure • Central venous pressure • Arterial pH • Nutritional support antibiotics	7.35–7.45 as per ICU protocol note required routinely should be given based on culture Gram-staining results

Table 2: Changes that occur following brain death.		
Derangement	Cause	Approximate incidence
Hematological	Disseminated intravascular coagulation (DIC)	
Hypothermia	• Hypothalamic damage • Reduced metabolic rate • Vasodilation and heat loss • Invariable, if not prevented	Invariable, if not prevented
Hypotension	Vasoplegia, hypovolemia, reduced coronary blood flow, myocardial dysfunction	81–97%
Diabetes insipidus	Posterior pituitary damage	46–78%
DIC	Tissue factor releases coagulopathy	29–55%
Arrhythmias	Catecholamine storm, myocardial damage, reduced coronary blood flow	25–32%
Pulmonary edema	Acute blood volume diversion, capillary damage	13–18%

team has to counteract these changes and optimize the perfusion of those organs for as long as it takes for consent to be obtained for organ donation. The guideline that follows commits to provide a road map to allow for the largest potential yield of organs. It should be recognized that, even when everything is done perfectly, conversion from recognition of brain death to actual organ donation is painfully low in our country.

PATHOPHYSIOLOGY

- *Cardiovascular issues*: Raised pressure inflicting brain death leads to Cushing's reflex, which stimulates a release of epinephrine upon a thousand times normal. This can result in subendocardial ischemia, arrhythmias, pulmonary edema, and a resultant decrease in cardiac output together with hypertension. As the reflex subsides, the epinephrine levels reduce to subnormal and the underlying decrease in ejection fraction becomes unmasked inflicting severe hypotension. Soon, the posterior pituitary stops secreting vasopressin and the urine output increases, which, if not matched by intravenous fluids and corrected with vasopressin or its analogs, can result in hypovolemia aggravating the hypotension and systematic hypoperfusion. If hypotension is not corrected, it can result in available organs being rendered unusable.
- *Endocrine changes*: The main emphasis is on replacing vasopressin secreted by the posterior pituitary.

Methylprednisolone in supraphysiological doses has been associated with decreased extravascular lung water, decreased level of inflammatory markers, and increased organ retrieval; and hydrocortisone in low doses has been shown to reduce vasopressor requirement.

There is some evidence that routine intravenous triiodothyronine (T3) leads to improvement in catecholamine responsiveness and consequently, higher organ perfusion, though this impact seems less important than appropriate fluid and vasopressor management. Additionally, a low-dose insulin infusion aids within the avoidance of hyperglycemia.

SPECIFIC MANAGEMENT

Communication Issues

It is important to state to the relatives without ambiguity and equivocation the fact of the patient's brain death. Following this, time should be given for the families to adjust the fact of the patient's death only then should the process of counselling the next of kin begin. Hierarchy of the family of the donor should be ascertained, so that the person responsible for giving consent for organ donation is established. The member of ICU team, who has conveyed the news of brain death, should not be involved in counseling the relatives.

General Nursing Care

It should continue in every manner.

Monitoring

The brain-dead donor needs extremely close monitoring to detect decomposition and treat it urgently (Box 3). The following monitors are desirable:
- Core temperature (either nasopharyngeal, esophageal, rectal, or indwelling bladder catheter)
- Electrocardiography (ECG)
- Invasive blood pressure (arterial catheter)
- Central venous pressure (CVP) (subclavian or IJV)
- Peripheral capillary oxygen saturation
- End-tidal CO_2
- Hourly urine output.
  These should be initiated as soon as possible when death is established.

> **Box 3: Routine investigations—the subsequent investigations ought to be performed.**
> - CBC
> - Blood grouping and cross-matching
> - Coagulation profile—PT/PTTK
> - RFT-BUN, creatinine
> - Complete LFT
> - Serum electrolytes—Ca, Mg, Na, K, phosphate
> - Blood sugar
> - Urine analysis
> - ABG with lactate.
> - *Cardiac evaluation*:
>   - ECG
> - *Radiology*:
>   - Chest X-ray and cardiac echocardiography
>   - USG for abdominal organs—liver, kidney, pancreas
> - Microbiology
> - Surveillance cultures of ET Asp, blood, urine, any other fluid, e.g. ascitic fluid viral markers
> - HBsAg
> - Anti-HCV
> - HIV-1 and -2

Fluid Management of the Brain-dead Organ Donor

Maintenance Fluid

Fluid therapy is aimed to preserve organ function whereby they can be transplanted in the patient. If the serum sodium rises above 150 mEq (as often happens once diabetes insipidus supervenes), the fluid can be shifted to 5% dextrose. In either instance, it is critical not to fall behind the urine output, and it is extremely important to watch urine output on an hourly basis, an increases fluids whenever needed.

KEY MESSAGES

- Organ donation should be encouraged by all concerned when there is a potential donor.
- Local and National Guidelines should be strictly followed.
- Correct terminology should be employed by all concerned to avoid confusion in the family.
- Brain-dead examinations and guidelines should be followed.
- Hospital policy should be made and a committee formed.

SUGGESTED READING

1. Kostch K, Ulrich F, Reutzel-Selke A, et al. Methylprednisolone therapy in deceased donors reduces inflammation in the donor liver and improves outcome after liver transplantation: a prospective randomized controlled trial. Ann Surg. 2008;248(6):1042-50. [online] available from http://www.ncbi.nlm.nih.gov/pubmed/19092349. [Last accessed April, 2019].
2. McKeown DW, Bonser RS, Kellum JA. Management of the heartbeating brain-dead organ donor. Br J Anaesth. 2012;108 (Suppl 1):i96-107.
3. Nakagawa TA, Ashwal S, Mathur M, et al. Guidelines for the determination of brain death in infants and children: An update of the 1987 Task Force Recommendations. Crit Care Med. 2011;39(9): 2139-55.
4. Schemic SD, Ross H, Pagliarello J, et al. Organ donor management in Canada: recommendation of the forum on medical management to optimize donor organ potential. CMAJ. 2006;174(6): S13-32. [online] Available from http://www.pubmedcentral.nih.gov/articlerender.fcgi?artid=1402396&tool=pmcentrez&rendertype=abstract. [Last accessed April, 2019]
5. THOA-1994. The Transplantation of Human Organs and Tissues Act. Revised 2014. New Delhi: Professional Book Publishers; 2018.

Index

Page numbers followed by *b* refer to box, *f* refer to figure, *fc* refer to flow chart, and *t* refer to table.

A

ABC *See* Airway breathing circulation
ABCD *See* Airway, breathing, circulation, disability
Abdomen 222
Abdominal compartment syndrome 377
  treatment of 377
Abdominal distension 312, 387
Abdominal ultrasound in trauma, focused 388
Abdominal wall 265
ABO
  and Rh compatibility 481
  incompatible transplant 354
ABP *See* Arterial blood pressure
Abrasions 387
Absorbed toxin, elimination of 401
Absorption atelectasis 59
Abundant secretions 92
Acalculous cholecystitis 366
Accelerated protocol 272
Accidents 392
ACE *See* Angiotensin converting enzyme
Acetaminophen poisoning 336
Acetyl salicylic acid toxicity, severity of 406*b*
Acid peptic disease 314
Acid-base
  analysis, steps in 132
  disorders 132
Acidemia 129
Acidosis 9, 132, 235, 244, 274, 363
  persistent 295
  severe 192, 293
Acinetobacter
  baumannii 528
  calcoaceticus 494
  species 498
ACLS *See* Advanced cardiac life support
Acorus calamus 397
Acquired immunodeficiency syndrome 40
ACTH *See* Adrenocorticotropic hormone
Activated charcoal 397, 403, 410
  administration 412

Activated partial thromboplastin time 330
Acute respiratory distress syndrome 59, 91, 92, 136, 137, 137*b*, 138*b*, 230, 296, 332, 430*f*, 487, 543, 556
  clinical features 143
  epidemiology 139
  history of 143
  incidence 139
  investigations 143
  management of 143
  pathophysiology 140
  pediatric 149
  phases of disease 141
  risk factors for 138*b*
Adenosine 199
  triphosphate consumption 275
Adjunctive drugs 274
Adrenal hyperplasia, congenital 235
Adrenal insufficiency, risk of absolute 235
Adrenal pituitary axis failure 235
Adrenergic agent 180
Adrenergic alpha-2-agonists 539
Adrenergic receptors 206
Adrenocorticotropic hormone 278
Adsorption 300
Advanced airway 28
  considerations 28
  in place 26*t*
Advanced cardiac life support 404
Advanced life support 4
  pediatric 1, 19
AED *See* Automated external defibrillator
Aedes aegypti 363
Aedes albopictus 363
Aerodigestive colonization 500
Agents causing seizure 400
Agitation 413
AIDS *See* Acquired immunodeficiency syndrome
Air-entrainment in venturi mask 55*f*
Airway 6, 9, 10, 21, 27, 243, 383, 470
  and breathing 12, 230

and respiratory issues 437
breathing circulation 200
   disability 314
   disability assessment 314
cartilage formation 137
disease 77, 82
driving pressure 70
inability to protect 92
injury 434
management 435
obstruction 91, 434
opening 22
parts of 83f
pressure 90f
   release ventilation 81
resistance 137
trauma 89
Alagille syndrome 343, 344, 350
Alanine
   aminotransferase 366
   transaminase 166
Albumin 347, 481
   infusion 349
Alcohol 409, 568
Alcohol poisoning 427
   clinical features 427
   differential diagnosis 428
   laboratory investigations 428
   management 428
   source 427
   toxic levels 428
Aldicarb (temik) 427
Aldosterone antagonist 175
ALF *See* Acute liver failure
ALI *See* Acute lung injury
Alimemazine 534
Alkalemia 129
Alkali denaturation test 312
Alkalosis 45
Alloimmune hepatitis, congenital 330
Allopurinol inhibits 466
ALT *See* Alanine aminotransferase
Alveolar capillary
   barrier dysfunction 141
   membrane 59
Alveolar disease, diffuse 145
Alveolar fluid clearance, impaired 142
Alveolar gas equation 130
Alveolar maturation 137
Amanita phalloides 327

Amenable lesions, surgically 255
American College of Cardiology 202
American College of Critical Care Medicine 159, 227
American Epilepsy Society 269, 278
American European Consensus Conference 136
American Heart Association 20, 122, 164, 202
Aminoglycosides 45, 335
Amiodarone 200
Amlodipine 224
Ammonia serum levels 328
Amrinone 180
ANA *See* Antinuclear antibody
Analgesia 536
Analgesic
   agents 537t
   drugs 539
Ancillary studies 8, 568
Andom blood sugar 39
Anemia 166, 171, 187
   severe 174
Angiotensin 208, 224, 227
Angiotensin converting enzyme 181, 224
   inhibitors 176, 181
Anion gap
   acidosis
      high 295
      normal 295
   estimation 294
Anomalous left coronary artery 166
Anterograde amnesia 534
Anti liver, kidney microsome 330
Antiarrhythmic drugs 193
Antiasphyxia valve 100, 100f
Antibiotic 230, 234, 314, 517, 523
   class of 524
   cycling 524
   inhaled 504
   selection of 522
   stewardship 530
   Stewardship Program 522, 530
   use, transparent monitoring of 523
Antibiotic therapy
   administration of 523
   de-escalation of 523
   management 522
   prolonged 510
Antibody and complement 493
Anticholinergic effects 412
Anticoagulant 314
   balance disturbance 227

Anticonvulsant overdose, clinical manifestation of 446t
Anti-D globulins 481
Antidiuretic hormone 33
   in critical illness, causes of increased 39t
Antidotes 248, 402
Antiepileptic agents 568
Antihistamines 412
   management 412
   source 412
Antihypertensive drugs 224t
Anti-inflammatory response syndrome, compensatory 327
Anti-LKM *See* Anti liver, kidney microsome
Antimicrobial resistance 521
Antimicrobial therapy initiation 523
Antinuclear antibody 330, 247
Antipsychotic drugs 422
   clinical manifestations 422
   management 422
Antipsychotics, spectrum of 422
Antipyretics 411
Antiseizure medication 225
Antiseptic cleaning of meatus 518
Antismooth muscle antibody 330
Antisnake venom 248, 453, 454t
   doses of 455
Antitrypsin deficiency, alpha-1 350
Antitubercular drugs isoniazid 327
Antivenom 453
Anti-voltage gated potassium channel 275
Anxiety 34
Aortic arch, interrupted 166
Aortic blood flow 158
Aortic dissection 225
Aortic regurgitation 169, 171
Aortic valve, bicuspid 171
Aplastic anemia 483
Apnea 392
   testing 567
APTT *See* Activated partial thromboplastin time
AR *See* Aortic regurgitation
Arachidonic acid 538
ARDS *See* Acute respiratory distress syndrome
ARF *See* Acute renal failure
Arrhythmia 44, 183, 184, 190, 375, 572
   cause of 198
   diagnosis of 197
   management of 197
   reentrant 185

Arterial blood 128
Arterial blood gas 8, 117, 129, 172
   analysis 128
      basic concepts 129
      systematic analysis of 129, 130
Arterial blood pressure 157f, 278
Arterial hypoxemia 50
Arterial ischemic stroke 242
Arterial lactate 8
Arterial oxygen gradient 130
Arterial pressure monitoring, systolic pressure for 155
Arterial pulse
   contour methods 161
   pressure variation 158
Arterial saturation 122
Arteriovenous
   fistula 303
   graft 303
Artesunate 247
Ascites 349
Aseptic technique 518
ASMA *See* Antismooth muscle antibody
Aspartate aminotransferase 366
Aspartate transaminase 166
Aspergillus 494
Asphyxia 19
Aspirin 134
AST *See* Aspartate aminotransferase
Asthma 12, 91
Asymptomatic bacteriuria 515
Asynchrony 79
   termination 79
Ataxia 413
Atelectasis 58, 91
Atelectrauma 144
Atenolol 181
Atracurium 542
Atrial fibrillation 183, 187, 187f
Atrial flutter 187, 187f, 190
Atrial tachycardia 184
   ectopic 184, 188, 188f, 190
   multifocal 184, 188
Atrioventricular block
   first degree 195, 195f
   third degree 196f
Atrioventricular canal, common 166
Atrioventricular nodal reentry tachycardia 189, 186
Atrioventricular reciprocating tachycardia 185, 186, 189

Atrioventricular tachycardias 184
  reentrant 184
Atrium, right 157
Atropine 426
  test 426
Auditory canal, external 439
Autoimmune 327
  hemolytic anemia 327
  hepatitis 327, 330, 349
Automated external defibrillator 201
Auto-trigger 109
AVNRT *See* Atrioventricular nodal reentry tachycardia
AVRT *See* Atrioventricular reciprocating tachycardia
Axonal injury, diffuse 242, 249

B

Bacillus Calmette-Guérin 352
Bacillus species 513
Bacteremia 509
Bacterial meningitis 242
Bacterial pneumonias, severe 556
Bag-mask
  one rescuer using 23
  rescuers using 24
  technique 23
  ventilation 243, 253
Balloon atrial septostomy 177
Barbiturates 263, 409, 536, 568
Barium swallows 318
Barotrauma 68
Basic life support 19, 201
Basilar skull fractures 266
Battery support 101
BCG *See* Bacillus Calmette-Guérin
Bendiocarb (Ficam) 427
Benzodiazepine 230, 413, 534, 535
Beriberi 166
Beta adrenergic 206
Beta-agonist therapy 44
Beta-blocker 178, 181, 224, 225, 416
  management 416
  nonselective 316, 320
  source 416
Bicarbonate 294
  loss of 294
Bicycle injury 381

Bile duct
  excretory pump defects 349
  paucity syndrome 344
Biliary atresia 342, 350
Bilirubin 347
Biological pacemakers 179
Bispectral index 541
Bladder, full 265
Bleeding 308, 466
  active 314
  control of 387
  diathesis 313
  management of 374
  severe 369, 374
  tendency 431
  ulcers 322
Blood
  ammonia levels 247
  beta-hydroxybutyrate 294
  components, availability of 480
  gas and electrolytes 172
  group compatibility 353*t*
  ketones 294
  mimicking substance 311
  products 476
  substance 311
  sugar 8, 573
  transfusion 45, 149, 177, 440
Blood flow 215*f*
  increase in 258
  manipulation of 319
  rate 304
Blood glucose 290, 294
  by glucometer 398
  levels 289
Blood pressure 9, 154, 173, 205, 215*f*, 216, 220, 385, 386, 458, 460
  diastolic 153
  elevated 220
  four-limb 223
  in head injury 253
  increases 260
  measurement of 223
  monitoring, noninvasive 154
  normal 220, 232
  systolic 229
Blood urea nitrogen 432
  high 316
  levels 303
Blood vessels 260
  change in resistances of 260*f*

Blood volume loss 385
    estimation of 314
Blood-brain barrier 249, 303
Blood-gas analyzer 494
Blood-stained vomiting 387
Blow-by oxygen 52
BLS *See* Basic life support
Body
    antioxidant defense mechanisms 59
    compartments in children, water content of 33*t*
    homeostatic mechanisms 464
    surface area 159
    water distribution in children 32
Bowel infarction 318
Bowel irrigation, whole 403, 446
BP *See* Blood pressure
Bradyarrhythmias 194
    treatable causes for 197*t*
    treatment of 197
Bradycardia 183, 197, 392, 399, 411, 424
    cause of 9, 202
    child with 9
    mechanisms of 194
Bradypnea 400
Brain
    abscess 242
    compliant 258
    malformation, congenital 270
    parenchyma 258
    tissue 262
    tumors 270
Brain death 572*t*
    current consensus 564
    diagnosis of 568, 569, 571
    examination 568
    in term newborns 569
        apnea testing 570
        clinical examination 570
    mimic 568
Brain injury
    prevent secondary 248
    primary 249
    secondary 249
Brain-dead
    donor 573
    organ donor 573
    patient, management of 571
Brainstem
    death 567, 571
        testing for 565

    dysfunction 248
    function 242
        examination of 244
    severe 254
    testing 566
Breath
    exhaled 505
    types of 79, 80*f*, 80*t*
Breathing 6, 9, 10, 21, 22, 27, 243
    decreasing patient's work of 87
    pattern 88
    rescue 22, 27
    work of 5
Bronchial asthma 58, 132
Bronchiolitis 91
    acute 57
Bronchodilator medications 413
Bronchopneumonia 430*f*
Bronchoscopes 494
Bronchospasm 424
Budd-Chiari syndrome 327, 344
Bufencarb 427
BUN *See* Blood urea nitrogen
Burkholderia
    cepacia 494
    cereus 494
Burkitt's lymphoma 465
Burns, severe 138
Button battery ingestion 436
    clinical manifestation 437
    complications 439
    differential diagnosis 437
    investigations 437
    management 437
    prevention 439
    source 436
Butyrophenones 534
Byler disease 344

C

Calcium 45, 235
    and phosphorus in blood, normal ranges for 46*t*
    concentration 235
    sensitizers 208
Calcium channel blocker 223, 224
    poisoning 417
Calcium level 216
    routine 235

Candida 498, 512, 513
  species 511, 512
Candiduria 517
  persistent 517
Cannula 53*f*
Capillary blanch test 385
Capillary filling time 173, 229, 386
Capnogram
  differential diagnosis of abnormal 124, 125*t*
  normal 123*f*
Capnography 122
  indications for 126
Captopril 181
Carbamazepine 403, 409, 446
Carbaryl (Sevin) 427
Carbofuran (Furadan) 427
Carbon dioxide
  displaces 130
  end-tidal 8, 123, 125, 384
  monitors
    clinical applications of 124
    mainstream 123
    side stream 124
    types of 123
Carbon monoxide poisoning 440
  clinical features 441
  differential diagnosis 442
  laboratory tests 442
  management 442
  prevention 443
  sources 440
Cardiac arrest, primary nature of 19
Cardiac arrhythmias 183, 444
Cardiac catheterization 174
Cardiac complications 429
Cardiac dysfunction 244
Cardiac evaluation 573
Cardiac failure 36, 305, 361
Cardiac injury 191
Cardiac lesion 172
Cardiac manifestations 366
Cardiac output 161
  assessment of 159
  effect on 88
  factors affecting 165
  terms of 205
Cardiac resynchronization therapy 205
Cardiac rhythm disorders 392
Cardiac sodium, blocks 202
Cardiac tamponade 386

Cardiac tumors 191, 192, 196
Cardiogenic pulmonary edema 96
Cardiogenic shock 38, 191, 374, 445
Cardiomyopathy 191
Cardiopulmonary
  arrest 4
  bypass, prolonged 556
  resuscitation 9, 19, 21, 28, 122, 200, 201, 269
    two-rescuer 24*t*
  status, assessment of 350
Cardiorespiratory
  arrests, pediatric 197
  problems 117
  status 282
Cardiotoxicity 444
Cardiotoxins 450
Cardiovascular
  effects 412
  function, effects on 142
  illness 217
  issues 572
  side effects 422
  system 345, 397
Carnitine 181
Caroli's disease 344
Carvedilol 181, 320
Catalase 59
Catastrophic illness, cases of 324
Catecholamine 191, 207*f*, 227
  resistant shock 232
Catheter
  management 517
  material 510
Catheter-associated urinary tract infection 515
  clinical presentation 516
  laboratory findings 516
Catheter-related bloodstream infection 509-511
  diagnostic criteria 511
  etiological agents 511
  management 512
  prevent 513*b*
  risk factors for 510, 510*b*
Cationic detergents 434
Causing injury, highest risk of 533
CBC *See* Complete blood count
CCF *See* Congestive cardiac failure
Cefepime 502
Ceftazidime 502
Cellular dysfunction 361
Central diabetes insipidus 42

Central nervous system 40, 213, 242, 330, 345, 366, 381, 397, 400, 446, 485
    depression 400
    disorders 132
    effects 412
    severe 568
    symptoms 406, 476
Central sleep apnea 111
Central venous
    line, long-term 513
    oxygen saturation 161, 162
        interpreting 162
    pressure 165, 278, 573
        monitoring 156
    saturation 161
Centres for Disease Control 524
Cephalhematoma 266
Cerebral blood 260
    flow 249
        autoregulation of 221f
Cerebral cortex, intact 241
Cerebral cortical function, loss of 242
Cerebral disease 41
Cerebral edema 290, 296, 324, 328, 333, 337
Cerebral herniation syndrome, evolving 265
Cerebral hypoperfusion 296
Cerebral malaria 242
Cerebral metabolic rate 275
Cerebral monitoring 266b
Cerebral perfusion pressure 259
Cerebral salt wasting 41, 41t
Cerebral vessels, severe constriction of 262
Cerebrospinal fluid 246
Cerebrovascular accidents 398
Cerebrovascular event 270
Cervical spine
    immobilization 254
    injury 254
    protection 384f
CFT See Capillary filling time
Channelopathy 193
Chelation in iron poisoning, indications for 415b
Chelation therapy 415
Chennai declaration, goals of 529b
Chest
    compression 21, 24, 27, 197
        and ventilation ratio 25t
    pain 312
    radiograph 469

Chest wall
    compliance 137
        reduced 144
    elastance 144
CHF See Congestive heart failure
Child
    abuse 392
    chest rise 22
    receiving desferrioxamine 414f
    with encephalopathy, transport of 331
    with polytrauma, management of 380, 382
    with toxin ingestion, management 398b
Children and infants, relief of choking in 29
Children, reference charts for 238
Chin-lift maneuvers 253
Chloral hydrate 536
    triclofos 534
Chloride 294
    containing fluids 294
Chlorpromazine 534
Chlorpropamide 418
Chlorthiazide 180
Cholestasis 358
Cholestatic diseases 344
Cholinergic (nicotinic) 401
Cholinergic symptoms 444
Chronic dialysis 303
Ciprofloxacin 502
Cisatracurium 542
Citrate intoxication 308
Citrobacter 498
Clonidine 224, 225, 534, 539, 544
    side effects 544
Clostridioides difficile
    colitis 313
    infection 236, 524
CMPA See Cow's milk protein allergy
CMV See Cytomegalovirus
CNS See Central nervous system
Coagulation disturbances 324
Coarctation of aorta 225
Cobra toxin 450
Cobratoxin 450
Codextrin 301
Coexistent pneumonia 172
Cold caloric test 566
Cold shock 227
Cold water causes, immersion in 391
Colloid 38
Colonic polyps 313

Colonoscopy 322
Coma 241, 400
    etiology of 242t, 248
    inducing agents 272t
    level of 251
    phase 278
      repeat 278
Comatose child 241
    evaluation of 243
    management of 247
Comorbid conditions 314
Compassionate family support 284
Complete blood count 278, 315, 367
Compression 9
    ventilation ratio 24
Computerized tomography scans 388t
Condom catheters 515
Conduction abnormalities 195
Confusion 413
Confusional migraine, acute 242
Congenital heart disease, postoperative 168
Congestive cardiac failure 57, 458, 459
Congestive heart failure 40, 219
    signs of 196
Conjugated pneumococcal 352
Consciousness 241
    level of 244, 398, 426
    loss of 250, 381
Continuous positive airway pressure 58, 86, 93f, 96, 138
    circuit 58f
    mode 93
Convection 300
Conventional medical therapy 555
Conventional pulse oximetry 122
Conventional ventilators 98f
Convulsive status epilepticus 535
Corticosteroids 148
Counterregulatory hormones 288
Cow's milk protein allergy 313
CPAP *See* Continuous positive airway pressure
CPK *See* Creatine phosphokinase
CPR *See* Cardiopulmonary resuscitation
Cranial nerves, examination of 244
Craniofacial trauma 92
C-reactive protein 359
Creatine phosphokinase 272
Crepitations 171
Crigler-Najjar syndrome 344
Critical aortic stenosis 177
Critical care, association of 546
Critical illness neuromyopathy 236
Critically ill children 4, 358, 510
    colloids in 38
    crystalloid in 38
    energy expenditure in 357
Critically ill state 4
Crohn's disease 314
Croup 12
CRT *See* Cardiac resynchronization therapy
Cryoprecipitate 481
Crystalloid 11
    fluid normal saline 228
Cushing's triad 243, 254, 262
CVP *See* Central venous pressure
CVS *See* Cardiovascular system
CVVHDF *See* Continuous venovenous hemodiafiltration
Cyanide poisoning 50
Cyanosis 244, 400
Cyanotic heart disease 140
Cyclic adenosine monophosphate 540
Cyclooxygenase, inhibition of 538
Cyclosporin 342
Cytomegalovirus 330
Cytopenia, effect of 480
Cytosolic calcium 208

D

Death, predictors of 394
Decerebrate posturing 262
Decompensation, signs of 349
Decompressive craniectomy 265
Decontamination procedures 415, 432
De-escalation phase 235
Dehydration 296, 335
    assessment of 291
    treat 43
Dengue 244, 246, 363
    case classification 366t
    diagnosis 368
    hemorrhagic shock 38
    illness, course of 364f
    in pediatric intensive care unit 362
    infection 363
    management of 370fc, 371fc
    severe 363, 369
    shock 36
      syndrome 38

syndrome, expanded 366
treatment of 378
vasculitis 375
virus 375
with hypotensive shock 372*fc*
Dental hygiene, assessment of 351
Deoxyribonucleic acid 275
Dexmedetomidine 539, 540, 544
Diabetes 359
    insipidus 42, 572
        treatment of 43
    mellitus 132
        type 1 290, 297
Diabetic ketoacidosis 42, 43, 246, 288, 290, 297, 406, 459
    diagnostic criteria for 288*b*
    in children 288
    severity of 289*t*
Dialysate flow rate 304
Dialysis disequilibrium syndrome 303
Diamond-Blackfan syndrome 483
Diaphoresis 400, 444
Diarrhea 132, 424, 444, 466
Diastolic dysfunction 166, 374
    accounts 166
Diastolic function 205
Diastolic relaxation 211
Diazoxide 224
DIC *See* Disseminated intravascular coagulation
Dichlorvos 424
Diffusion 300
    defects 51
Digeorge syndrome 45
Digoxin 175, 180, 191, 202, 403
Dimethoate 424
Diphtheria 196, 352
Diphtheria/pertussis/tetanus 242
Disability 6, 12, 243, 385
Discharge planning 111
Disclosure to family 282
Disease, unilateral 139
Disseminated encephalomyelitis, acute 242, 247, 366
Disseminated intravascular coagulation 244, 459, 485
Diuretics 180, 466
Dizziness 466
DKA *See* Diabetic ketoacidosis
DNA *See* Deoxyribonucleic acid
Dobutamine 175, 180, 208, 214

Domestic accidents, result of 249
Donor evaluation 353
Donor selection 353
Donor's organ system 571
Dopamine 175, 180, 207, 208, 214
Downey test 312
Doxorubicin 166
Doxycycline 247
DPT *See* Diphtheria/pertussis/tetanus
Driving pressure 144
Drowning 138, 269, 391
    hospital management 393
    management 392
    prehospital care 392
Drowsiness 413
Drug
    blocking renin 224
    cycling 536
    intoxications 568
    overdose 138
    removal, altered 308
    toxicities 191, 192
Dual-lobe transplant 354
Dudenal ulcer 314
Dynamic respiratory mechanics, measurement of 66
Dysconjugate gaze 245
Dyserythropoietic anemia, congenital 483
Dysfunction, surfactant 142
Dysphagia 321
Dyspnea 171
Dysrhythmias 183

E

Early goal directed therapy 233, 234*b*
Ebstein's anomaly 172, 188, 195, 198
EBV *See* Epstein-Barr virus
ECG *See* Electrocardiography
Echocardiogram 198
Echocardiography 2
ECMO *See* Extracorporeal membrane oxygenation
Ecstasy 327
ECT *See* Extracorporeal treatment
Edema
    formation 141
    forming states 40
EEG *See* Electroencephalogram
Ejection fraction 165

Elapids 449, 451
Electrocardiography 278
Electrocerebral silence 568
Electroconvulsive therapy 276
Electroencephalogram 246, 278
    burst suppression on 273f
Electroencephalography 330
Electrolyte 360
    abnormality 192
    and sugar 331
    disorders 38
    imbalance 191, 284, 293
    in critically ill child 32
Electrophysiological
    monitoring 266
    testing 197
Emergency care, pediatric 395
Emergency management 12
Emergency response system 27
Emergency room
    pediatric 13
    steps of stabilization in 291
Emesis 424
Enalapril 181
Enalaprilat 224
Encephalitis 269, 366
Encephalopathy 41, 327, 469
End-expiratory
    occlusion maneuver 65
    positive pressure 89
    volume 88
End-inspiratory occlusion maneuver 65
Endocrine changes 572
End-of-life care 280, 281, 286
    guidelines for providing 281
Endogenous colonization 492f
End-organ
    damage 223
    perfusion 154
Endoscopic sclerotherapy 321
Endoscopic therapy techniques 320t
Endoscopic variceal band ligation 321
Endoscopy 320
    upper 321
Endothelial cells, non-fenestrated 301
Endothelial dysfunction 363
Endothelin 227
Endotoxin production 227
Endotracheal intubation 147
Endotracheal tube 58, 75, 87, 122, 493

Enteral nutrition, hurdles in establishing 359
Enteric fever 242, 244
Enterobacter 498
Enterococcus species 516
Envenomation 397, 398, 449
    stage of 461
    treatment of 248
Environmental stimulation 265
Eosinophilia 360
Eosinophilic gastroenteritis 314
EPAP *See* Expiratory positive airway pressure
Epidural empyema 242
Epidural hematoma 255, 266
Epigastric pain, history of 312
Epilepsy 392
    surgery 276
Epinephrine 175, 180, 197, 209, 214, 231
    injection, diluted 320
Epithelium and mucous, ciliated 493
Epstein-Barr virus 330, 344
Equation of motion, elements of 64f
Erabutoxins 450
Erythrocyte sedimentation rate 247
Escherichia coli 498, 511, 516
Esmolol 181, 224, 225
Esomeprazole 319
Esophageal Doppler 160
Esophageal perforation 321, 439
Esophageal stricture 321
Esophagitis 314
Estimated creatinine clearance 237
Estimation of weight 7
Ethylene glycol 429
Etiology-specific treatment 336
Etomidate 536
Eucalyptus oil 397
Euphoria 427
Exhaled tidal volume 68
Expiratory asynchrony 79, 109
Expiratory port 100, 100f
Expiratory positive airway pressure 90, 94-96, 139
Extracellular fluid 42
    volume 41
Extracorporeal life support organization 149
Extracorporeal membrane oxygenation 2, 149, 179, 209, 216, 482, 555, 560
    arterio-venous 559
    care, post 561
    circuit 558f
    contraindications to 557

eligibility criteria 556
evidence base for 555
history 555
indications for 556
journey of 555
machinery and tubing 557
management 560
neonatal respiratory 561
role of 149
veno-arterial 559
veno-venous 559
Extracorporeal treatment 403, 404, 404b
algorithm for 404fc
Extrahepatic biliary atresia 342, 344
Extrahepatic manifestations 343
Exudates 219
Eye 222, 434
conjugate lateral deviation of 245
examination 244

F

Fab fragment antivenom 453
Facemask
full 104f
simple 53, 53f
total 104f
Facial nerve paralysis 439
Familial adenomatous polyposis 322
Familial hemophagocytic lymphohistiocytosis 477
Fanconi's anemia 483
Fatal arrhythmias 203
Fatty acid
long-chain 360
oxidation defect 330
Febrile neutropenia 468
clinical evaluation 469
core concepts 468
laboratory evaluation 469
management of 470, 471fc
patients
high-risk 469
low-risk 469
risk stratification 469
Febrile nonhemolytic transfusion reaction 482
Fecal occult blood test 317
Feeding
difficulty 171
in special situations 358
poor 516

Fenitrothion 424
Fenoldopam 225
Fentanyl 181, 537, 538
bolus 544
Fenthion 424
Fever 187, 244, 265, 468, 516
FFP See Fresh frozen plasma
Fiber optic cable 261
Filtered red cells 481
FIO_2 See Fraction of inspired oxygen
Firstline initial therapy phase 271
Fixed-concentration devices 52, 54
Flail chest 387
Flaviviridae 363
Flecainide 202
Fluconazole 512
Fluid 229, 332
administration, principles of 230b
balance 234
calculation 291
correction, rate of 292
in critically ill child 32
management 147, 573
overload 299, 376, 377
treatment of 377
refractory shock 231
replacement 37
resuscitation, guidelines basic tenets of 229b
type of 292
Fluid therapy 291
in hemorrhagic shock 386
in intensive care unit 36
rationale 291
Fluoroquinolones 512
FOBT See Fecal occult blood test
Focal alveolar consolidation 145
Forced expiratory volume 127
Forced vital capacity 127
Formetanate (carzol) 427
Fosphenytoin 264
Frank-Starling
curve 156, 157f, 206f
principle 165
Free fatty acid 459
Fresh frozen plasma 234, 386, 433, 480, 481, 489
Frozen cells 488
Fulminant colitis 322
Fungal infection 478
risk of 470
Fungemia 509

Furosemide 174, 180, 224, 225, 466
Futility, recognition of 282
FVC *See* Forced vital capacity

G

G6PD *See* Glucose 6-phosphate dehydrogenase
GABA *See* Gamma aminobutyric acid
Galactosemia 326, 330
Gallop sounds 171
Gamma aminobutyric acid 446
Gamma globulins 481
Gamma irradiation 488
Gamma-aminobutyric acid 269, 273, 275
Gas
    chromatography mass spectroscopy 247
    exchange, alterations in 142
    generators, types of 113
    source 74
Gastric contents, aspiration of 138
Gastric lavage 401, 410, 423
Gastritis 314
Gastroenteritis 43
    with systemic toxicity 444
Gastroesophageal reflux 312
Gastrointestinal bleeding 335
Gastrointestinal hemorrhage 335
Gastrointestinal irritation 406
Gastrointestinal symptoms, nonspecific 516
Gastrointestinal tract 34, 40, 312-314, 436*t*
Gastrointestinal tract bleed 310, 314*b*
    acute 311
        overt 317*fc*
    causes
        of lower 312
        of occult 314*b*
    child with 315*t*
    chronic 311
        occult 317*fc*
    epidemiology 310
    etiology of 311
    in children 313
    initial evaluation 314
    management 315
    obscure 311, 318*fc*
Gaze palsy, lateral 245
Genitourinary trauma 389
GER *See* Gastroesophageal reflux
Germ cell tumor 466, 471
GIT *See* Gastrointestinal tract

Glasgow coma scale 40, 243, 251, 384
Glimepiride 418
Glipizide 418
Globular cardiomegaly 172
Glomerular filtration rate 33
Glucose 235
    6-phosphate dehydrogenase 397, 440
    delivery rates 235
    homeostasis 327
Glutamate 269
Glutaminergic drive 275
Glutathione 59
Glyburide 418
Glycopyrrolate 426
Graft availability, innovations to increase 354
Graft versus host disease 482, 487
Gram's stain 497
Gram-negative bacilli 511
Granulocytes 487
Great arteries 172, 196
Great vessels 470

H

Haemoglobin, deoxygenated 119
Haemophilus influenzae 352
Hallucinations 413
Haloperidol 534
Hand hygiene 518
Handling extubation failure 91
HAP *See* Hospital-acquired pneumonia
Harris benedict formula 358
Hashimoto's encephalopathy 247
HAV *See* Hepatitis A virus
Hb *See* Hemoglobin
HBSAG *See* Hepatitis B surface antigen
HBV *See* Hepatitis B virus
Head injured patients, triage of 253*fc*
Head injury 9
    in children 249
    minor 252
    moderate 251
    radiological criteria for minor 252
    severe 251
Heart 219
    burn 312
    disorders, congenital 192
    transplant study, pediatric 180
    transplantation 180
Heart block 202, 366

complete 196, 197
third-degree 195
Heart disease
    acquired 192
    congenital 188, 191, 195
    structural 178
Heart failure
    acute 164, 167t, 168, 181
    based on pathophysiology, etiology of acute 166
    classification of acute 170
    etiology of acute 166
    management in acute 173t
    mild 190
    pathophysiology of acute 171t
    pediatric 179
    severity of acute 170t
    symptoms in acute 165
Heart rate 8, 165, 200, 205, 386, 460
    abnormal 244
    normal range of 184t
    particularly 5
Heat moisture exchanger 74
Heimlich maneuver, role of 392
Heimlich's maneuver 29
Helmet mask 105f
Hemangioendothelioma 344
Hematemesis, cause of 312
Hematocrit 367
Hematoma 249
Hemodialysis 404
    indication of 408
    intermittent 299, 302
Hemodynamic considerations 332
Hemodynamic monitoring 153
    clinical examination 153
    preload assessment 156
Hemodynamic variables, common 160
Hemodynamics instability 92
Hemoglobin 120
    concentration 8
Hemolysis 308, 360
Hemolytic uremic syndrome 485, 489
Hemophagocytic lymphohistiocytosis 377, 476, 477, 478fc
    acquired 478
    classification of 477
    clinical features 476
    laboratory abnormalities 477
    management 478
    pathophysiology 476
Hemorrhage 219, 434
    control of 385
    stigmata of recent 322
    with exudates, flame-shaped 244
Hemorrhagic enteritis 414
Hemorrhagic shock, classification of 385t
Hemorrhagins 450
Hemothorax 387
Henoch-Schönlein purpura 312, 313
Heparin 45
Hepatic artery 331
Hepatic decompensation
    assessment of 349
    management of 349
Hepatic dysfunction 238, 411
    severe 568
Hepatic encephalopathy 324
    advancing 334
    stages of 329t
Hepatic enzymes 166
Hepatic failure 132, 342
Hepatic fibrosis, congenital 350
Hepatic malignancy, primary 343
Hepatic vein occlusion 327
Hepatitis 244, 336, 366
    A 325, 326, 352
        infection 330
        virus 330, 344
    B 352
        acute 336
        infection 330
        surface antigen 330
        virus 344
    C infection 330
    D infection 330
Hepatoblastoma 343, 344, 466
Hepatocellular carcinoma 342, 344
Hepatocellular injury 327
Hepatotoxic drug, dose-related 327
Herniation syndromes 245, 245t
Herpes simplex encephalitis 246
HHV-6 *See* Human herpes virus 6
High frequency
    oscillator ventilation 82, 83t, 84, 145
    ventilation 145
Histotoxic hypoxia 50
Hodgkin lymphoma 471
Home mechanical ventilation 109

Home noninvasive ventilation
  machine 97f
  ventilator 96
Home ventilation
  long-term 112
  via tracheostomy 110
Hospital antibiotic stewardship programs 524, 525t, 526t
Hospital treatment, out of 270
Hospital-acquired
  infection 509
  pneumonia 491, 492, 499b, 503
Host genetic factors 140
Host's deleterious 227
HR *See* Heart rate
HSP *See* Henoch-Schönlein purpura
Human coronavirus 494
Human herpes virus 6 326
Human immunodeficiency virus 353
Human Organ Act, transplantation of 566
Human Organ Transplantation Act 342
Human Organs and Tissues Act, transplantation of 571
Human papillomavirus 352
Human T-cell lymphotropic virus 487
Humidification 99
  devices 99f
  system 74
HUS *See* Hemolytic uremic syndrome
Hybrid therapy 304
Hydralazine 224, 225
Hydration, aggressive 475
Hydrocarbon ingestion 429
Hydrocephalus 242, 243
Hydrocortisone 235
Hydrophidae 449
Hyperaldosteronism 349
Hyperammonemia 336, 358
Hyperbaric oxygen 442
Hypercalcemia 46, 235
  causes 46
  clinical features 46
  treatment 47
Hypercapnic respiratory failure 91
Hypercarbia 249, 253, 270, 392, 570
Hyperemia 258
Hyperglycemia 235, 288, 358, 400
Hyperglycemic hyperosmolar state 290
  diagnostic criteria for 290b
Hyperkalemia 9, 44, 45f, 174, 192, 197, 299, 464, 467

Hyperleukocytosis 474
  clinical features 474
  differential diagnosis 474
  etiology 474
  management of 475, 475fc
  pathophysiology 474
Hypermagnesemia 48
  causes 48
  clinical features 48
  management 48
Hypernatremia 41
  approach to 42fc
Hypernatremic dehydration 43
Hyperoxaluria, primary 344, 350
Hyperphosphatemia 47, 432, 467
  causes 47
  clinical features 47
  treatment 47
Hypersplenism 486
Hypertension 219, 220, 254, 303, 349, 399
  acute severe 219
  alpha-mediated 224
  applied physiology 220
  bradycardia 254
  clinical features 222t
  etiology of 221, 221t
  initial stabilization 223
  malignant 220
  management 223
  noncirrhotic portal 344
  portal 349
  severe 225
  stage I 220
  stage II 219
Hypertensive crises 219
Hypertensive emergency 219
  and urgency 219
Hypertensive encephalopathy 219
Hypertensive urgency 219
Hyperthermia 399, 400
Hypertonic saline 263, 333
Hypertriglyceridemia 477, 535
Hyperuricemia 174, 464
  management of 466
Hyperventilation 262
Hypoalbuminemia 349
Hypocalcemia 45, 192, 196, 243, 308, 432, 464, 467
Hypocapnia 262
Hypofibrinogenemia 477
Hypoglycemia 174, 243, 246, 248, 269, 274, 296, 331, 400

Hypokalemia 9, 43, 45f, 174, 192, 193, 197, 293, 308, 432
   severe 293
Hypomagnesemia 48, 308
  causes 48
  clinical features 48
  treatment 48
Hyponatremia 38, 39, 174, 263, 270
  causes of 40t
  degrees of 34
  dilutional 41
Hyponatremic dehydration 41
Hyponatremic encephalopathy 40
Hyponatremic seizure 41
Hypoperfusion 249
Hypophosphatemia 47, 294, 308
   clinical features 47
   treatment 47
Hypoplastic left heart syndrome 177
Hypotension 132, 227, 269, 270, 399, 422, 469, 572
  persistent 334, 566
Hypotensive shock 243, 371
Hypothermia 197, 243, 264, 275, 308, 393, 399, 566, 572
  prolonged 264
Hypotonic intravenous solutions 34
Hypotonic solutions as maintenance fluids 37
Hypoventilation 254
  reflection of 130
Hypovolemia 9, 187, 197
Hypovolemic shock 37
Hypoxemia 50, 129, 132, 197
  mechanisms of 50
Hypoxemic respiratory failure 91
Hypoxia 12, 50, 187, 191, 192, 249, 363, 392, 429
Hypoxic ischemic
  encephalopathy 244
  insult, acute 269

I

IBD *See* Inflammatory bowel disease
Ibuprofen 537
ICP *See* Intracranial pressure
Icterus 327
IDA *See* Iron deficiency anemia
Idiogenic osmoles 296
Idiopathic neonatal hepatitis 344
Idiopathic thrombocytopenic purpura 486
IEM *See* Inborn errors of metabolism

Illness, severe 512
Imipenem 502
Immune
  deficiencies 324
  function 148
Immunization status, assessment of 351
Immunocompromised children 91
Immunodeficiency 140
Immunonutrition 360
Immunosuppressants 327
Immunosuppression 342, 510
In situ urinary catheter 516
Inborn errors of metabolism 242, 269
Indian Academy of Paediatrics 4, 529
Indolent infection 243
Indomethacin 43
Infant's airway 29
Infection 290, 326, 478
  bacteria 478
  control, effective 494
  parasites 478
  prevention of 517
  severity of underlying 510
  treatment of 247
  virus 478
Infectious disease consideration 334
Infectious Disease Society of America 521
Infective endocarditis 171
Inflammatory bowel disease 313, 314
Inflammatory cytokine mediated multiorgan 464
Inflammatory disorders 196
Influenza 352
  A 494
  vaccine 528
INH *See* Isonicotinic acid hydrazide
Inhalation anesthetics 568
Inhalational injury 138
Inherited disorders 270
Injury leads to secondary injury, primary 250fc
Injury, unidentified 398
Inotropes 180
Inspiratory
  asynchrony 108
  cycling 109
  hold maneuver 65f
  positive airway pressure 88, 90, 94, 95
  pressures 68
  trigger, ineffective 108
Inspired oxygen, fraction of 56, 137, 138
Insulin 288

administration of 293
requirements 235
therapy 293
  rationale 293
type and route of 293
Intensive care
  issues, other 376
  practice, blood components in 480
  unit 1, 20, 87
Intensive chemotherapy, after 463
Interfaces 101
  components of 102f
  full facemask 103
  helmet 105
  nasal 101
    masks 103
    pillows 102
    prongs 102
  total facemask 104
  types of 101f
Intermediate syndrome 425
International league against epilepsy 268
Interstitium 301
Intestinal duplication 313
Intoxication, stages of 414t
Intra-aortic balloon pump 179
Intracellular fluid 32
Intracerebral hemorrhage 555
Intracranial bleed 396
Intracranial hypertension 333
Intracranial injury, severity of 252t
Intracranial malformation 244
Intracranial pressure 223, 257, 257f, 330
  patients with raised 36
  raised 12, 74, 243
  wave forms 258f
Intrahepatic cholestasis 342
  progressive familial 344
Intranasal catheter 52, 53, 53f
Intraparenchymal injury 266
Intraparenchymal pressure transducers 261
Intrathecal perfusion, analgesic in 540
Intravascular hemolysis 440
Intravenous anesthesia-inducing agents 536
Intravenous calcium chloride 44
Intravenous hydration, aggressive 466
Intravenous immunoglobulin 354
Intubation and ventilation 333
Invasive blood pressure 573
Invasive hemodynamic monitoring 154

Invasive monitoring 128
  indications for 261
IPAP *See* Inspiratory positive airway pressure
Iron
  deficiency anemia 317
  preparations 413
Irritability 171, 516
Ischemia 249, 262
Ischemia-related cerebral injury 296
Ischemic heart disease 19
Ischemic stroke 375
Isoniazid 419
  clinical manifestations 420
  management 420
  source 419
Isonicotinic acid hydrazide 409, 420
Isoprenaline 211
Isoproterenol 175, 180
Isotonic saline 292

J

Jaundice 244
  absence of 327
  worsens 328
Jugular vein, internal 303
Jugular venous oxygen saturation 262
Jumpstart pediatric multiple casualty incidents triage 17fc
Junctional ectopic tachycardia 188

K

Kaliuretic action 175
Kawasaki disease 196
Kayser-Fleischer rings 329
Kerosene 429, 430f
  clinical features 430
  management 430
  source 429
Ketamine 230, 539
Ketoacidosis 294
Ketonemia 288
Ketones 134
Ketonuria, mild 290
Ketosis 400
Ketotic hypoglycemia 327
Kidney 219
  disease, chronic 223
  functions 360

injury 238, 464
    acute 219, 292, 296, 299, 335
Klebsiella 511
    pneumonia 494, 528
    species 498

L

Labetalol 224, 225
Lacosamide 275
Lacrimation, excess 424
Lactic acidosis 327, 432, 535
Lansoprazole 319
Laryngeal edema 434
Laryngeal mask airway 28
Laundry detergent packets 434
Left ventricle failure 165
Left ventricular dysfunction 140
Leg raising, passive 158, 158f
Legionella pneumophila 494
Leptospira serology 246
Leptospirosis 244, 326
Leucodepleted blood components 487
Leucodepletion 487
    methods of 487
Leukemia 465, 473
Leukemoid reaction 474
Leukopheresis 475
Levetiracetam 264
Levofloxacin 502
Levosimendan 178, 208, 210
Lidocaine 202
Life support
    discontinuation of 30
    withdrawal of 283
Life-threatening
    organ ischemia 220
    problems, immediate 434
    symptoms, case of 223
Light-emitting diodes 119
Linezolid 512
Lithium dilution 161
Live donor liver transplant 342, 352
Liver
    functions 315, 360
    support systems 337
    tests 331
Liver disease
    end-stage 346, 349, 351
    pediatric end-stage 347
    primary 343

Liver enzymes 328
    elevated 432
Liver failure
    acute 324, 328, 336, 336t, 344-345, 400, 414
    causes of acute 326, 327
    chronic 328
    etiology of acute 330t
    management of acute 331
    pathogenesis of acute 327
    pediatric acute 324
    subacute 328
    subdivisions of acute 325t
Liver transplant
    evolution of 341
    indication of 411
        pediatric 342, 344b
    patients listed for 334
Loop diuretics 45
Lorazepam 535
Low blood pressure 233
Low efficiency dialysis, sustained 299, 304, 404
Lower gastrointestinal tract bleed 311, 316fc
    causes of 313t
    endoscopy 322
    in children 312
Lower respiratory tract 497
    infection 117, 483
Low-middle income countries 297
Low-platelet count 363
LRT *See* Lower respiratory tract
LSD *See* Lysergic acid diethylamide
Lumbar puncture 246
Lung
    collapsed 90
    normal 82
    recruitment of 560
    rest, initial period of 560
    restrictive 96
    tissue 498
    ultrasound 505
    virtues of monitoring 62
Lung disease
    chronic 91, 140
    restrictive 110
    type of 145
Lung injury
    acute 136, 137, 144
    causes of direct 141
    direct 59
    transfusion-related acute 138

Lung mechanics
    from chest wall, dissociation of 66
    mathematics of 68t
    monitoring of 67
    with ventilation 62
Lychee fruit consumption 444
Lyme disease 195, 196
Lymphocyte 480, 488, 493
Lymphohistiocytosis 330
Lymphoma 473
Lysergic acid diethylamide 400

M

Machine with nasal cannula 113f
Magnesium 47, 278
    depletion 45
Magnetic resonance imaging 278
Magnetoencephalography 278
Maintenance fluid 36, 573
    calculation 292
Malaria 244, 246, 359
Malathion 424
Male sex 392
Malnutrition, severe 345
Management skills 171
Mandatory ventilation, intermittent 80
Mannitol 263
MAO *See* Monoamine oxidase
Masimo pulse oximetry 122
Mask hypovolemia 254
Maternal blood ingestion 314
Maternal lupus 196
Mature cells 474
Mean arterial pressure 9, 153, 155, 259
Measles 352
Mechanical ventilation 74, 86, 122, 157f, 332
    basics of 73
    control variables in 77
    controlled 83
    indications 73
    physiology 74
Mechanical ventilatory cycle 79f
Meckel's diverticulum 312, 313, 314, 322
Meckel's scan 318, 319f
Meconium aspiration syndrome, severe 556
Mediastinal mass 472f
    anterior 471
    posterior 471

Mediastinal syndrome
    management of superior 473fc
    superior 470
        etiology 471
        laboratory evaluation 472
        management 473
        pathophysiology 470
Mediastinitis 321
Medical management, supportive 324
Mefenamic acid 411
MEG *See* Magnetoencephalography
Membrane's effectiveness 300
Meningitis 269
Mental status 385
    altered 444
Meperidine 537
Meropenem 502
Mesothelium 301
Metabolic abnormalities 192
    management of individual 467
Metabolic acidosis 288, 289, 406, 407
    cause of 419
Metabolic activity of brain 263
Metabolic alkalosis 132, 174, 308
Metabolic cause 246
Metabolic derangements 457, 459fc
Metabolic disease 269, 326, 344
Metabolic disorder 343
Metabolic liver disease 330
Metabolic requirements 137
Metamizole 538
Methemoglobinemia 445
    causes 447
    clinical features 447
    investigations 447
    management 448
Methiocarb (mesurol) 427
Methomyl (lannate) 427
Methylene blue 448
Methylprednisolone 572
Metolazone 180
Metoprolol 181
Microcentrifuge 367f
Micrococcus 513
Micronutrients 360
Microstream technology 126
    advantages 127
Midazolam 272, 534, 541
    infusion syndrome 535
Midbrain 244

Milk bank pasteurizer 494
Milk protein allergy 312
Milrinone 180, 214
Mimic common diseases 400*t*
Mineral 360
    deficiency 359
Minoxidil 224
Miosis 424
Mitochondrial
    cardiomyopathies 174
    dysfunction 275
    hepatopathies 330
Mitral regurgitation 169
Mitral stenosis 166
Mivacurium 542
Mixed venous
    blood 161
    oxygen saturation 162, 215, 231
Molecular adsorbent recirculating system 404
Monitoring devices 261
Monoamine oxidase 326
Monro-Kellie doctrine 257*f*
Morphine 181, 537, 543
    side effects 543
Mortality and morbidity, cause of 249
Mortality in trauma 380
Mosquito repellent poisoning 439
    clinical manifestations 439
    management 440
    source 439
Motion, equation of 63
Motor system examination 245
Motor vehicle occupant injury 381
Mouthwash 494
MR *See* Mitral regurgitation
MRI *See* Magnetic resonance imaging
MRSA *See* Methicillin-resistant *Staphylococcus aureus*
Mucosal edema 434
Mucosal irritation and swelling 444
Multidrug-resistant 506
    pathogens, risk factors for 499*b*
Multiorgan dysfunction 337
    syndrome 326
Multiple-dose activated charcoal 403
Mumps 352
Muscarinic antagonist 426
Muscarinic effects 424
Muscle
    relaxants 253, 392, 543
    twitching 303

Muscular dystrophies 196
Mushroom poisoning 327, 336
Mycobacterial infection 478, 513
Mycobacterium tuberculosis 494
Myeloid leukemia, acute 471
Myocardial contractility 165
Myocardial contraction 165
Myocardial contusion 386
Myocardial dysfunction 46, 73
Myocardial ischemia 187, 196
Myocardial necrosis, less 203
Myocardial oxygen 175
Myocardial performance, increase 175
Myocardial relaxation 178
Myocarditis 191, 192, 366, 375, 556
Myocardium 165
Myoclonic epilepsy, progressive 270

N

N-acetyl cysteine, role of 337
N-acetylcysteine infusion 410
    oral route 411
    side effects 411
Naloxone 248
Narcotics 34
Nasal cannula 53, 56
    heated-humidified high-flow 57
    high-flow 113*f*, 147
    oxygen
        delivery 57*f*
        therapy, high-flow 112
Nasal masks 103*f*
Nasal pillows 102, 102*f*
Nasal prongs 52, 53, 53*f*, 102, 102*f*
Nasal septum perforation 439
National Antimicrobial Resistance Surveillance System 529
National Policy for Containment of Antimicrobial Resistance 529
Natriuretic peptide 178
Natural killer 330
NAVA *See* Neurally adjusted ventilatory assist
NCS *See* Nonconvulsive status
Near-infrared spectroscopy 162, 262
Nebulized medication 494
NEC *See* Necrotizing enterocolitis
Necrotizing enterocolitis 313, 318
Neem oil 397
Neisseria meningitides 352

Neonatal and childhood illness, management of 528
Neonatal hemochromatosis 330, 336
Neoplasm 242
Nephroblastoma 466
Nephrotoxic drugs 335
Nerium oleander 443
Nesiritide 178
Neural mechanism 110f
Neuroblastoma 466, 471
Neuroimaging 276
Neuroleptic malignant syndrome 422
Neurological complications 375
Neurological deficit 250
Neurological disorder 251
Neurological examination 244, 252
Neurological function 398
Neurological status, assessment of 350
Neurological survey, quick 385
Neurology 222
Neuromuscular blockade 149
    context of 541
Neuromuscular blocking agents 542, 542t
Neuromuscular disease 110
    severe 110
Neuromuscular disorders 74
Neuromuscular excitability 46
Neuromuscular weakness 58
Neuronal death, severe global 260
Neuronal injury, reducing 263
Neuroparalytic snakebite 248
Neurophysiological methods 541
Neurosurgeon 265
Neurotoxins 450
Neutropenia 468, 512
    profound 468
    prolonged 468
Neutrophil count, absolute 471
New York Heart Association 170
Newer agents 213
    angiotensin II 213
    istaroxime 213
    methylene blue 213
    omecamtiv mecarbi 213
Nicardipine 224
Nifedipine 223, 224, 225
Nitric oxide 148, 332
    inhaled 148
Nitroglycerine 176, 181, 212, 214, 460
Nitroprusside 212

NIV *See* Noninvasive ventilation
NK *See* Natural killer
NMDA *See* N-methy-d-asparate
N-methyl-d-aspartate 269, 275
Nodalol 320
Nonbleeding visible vessels 322
Noncardiogenic pulmonary edema 296
Nonconvulsive status 272
    epilepticus 398
Nonhemolytic febrile transfusion reactions 487
Non-Hodgkin lymphoma 471
Noninvasive measures 262
Noninvasive respiratory monitoring 118
Noninvasive respiratory support 147
Noninvasive ventilation 86, 87, 98, 373
    acute 106
    advantages of 89
    contraindications for 91, 92f
    data monitoring 106
    disadvantages of 89
    goals of 89
    indications for 90
    machines
        components of 98
        of action of 88
    mode of 92, 93f
    monitoring 106
    physiology of 87
    specific hospital-based ventilator 97f
    steps of initiating 105
    terminologies in 90
    troubleshooting 107
Nonionic detergents 434
Nonketotic hypoglycaemia 400
Nonmalignant causes 471
Non-neurological injuries, management of 388
Non-pharmacological treatment 533
Nonpulmonary sepsis 138
Nonrebreathing mask 52, 55, 56, 56f
Nonresolving inflammatory 227
Nonsteroidal anti-inflammatory drugs 312, 365, 537, 538
Nontraumatic cardiac arrests 19
Nontraumatic coma 251
Nontuberculous mycobacteria 494
Nonvariceal bleed 321
Noradrenergic neurons, hyperpolarization of 540
Norepinephrine 180, 209, 214, 232
Normocarbia, maintain 332

Nosocomial
    infection 491
    pneumonia 491
Novel therapies 275
NSAIDs *See* Nonsteroidal anti-inflammatory drugs
NSBB *See* Nonselective beta blocker
Nucleic acid metabolism, product of 464
Numbness 444
Nurse competencies 548
    advocacy/moral agency 548
    caring practices 548
    clinical judgment 548
    collaboration 549
    facilitator of learning 549
    systems thinking 549
Nursing care 213
    general 573
Nutrition 336
    assessment of 359
    enteral 359
    goals of 357
    in critically ill children 357
    parenteral 359
Nutritional assessment 359
    clinical examination 359
    laboratory examination 359
Nutritional status, assessment of 350
Nutritional support 149

O

Obesity hypoventilation 110
Obstructive lung disease 111
Obstructive sleep apnea 86, 96, 111
Occasionally colloid 11
Odor 400
Oleander poisoning 443
    clinical features 443
    differential diagnosis 444
    laboratory investigations 445
    management 445
    source 443
Oliguria, child with 238
Ominous sign 289
Oncologic emergencies, common pediatric 463*t*
Oncological emergencies 463
ONSD *See* Optic nerve sheath diameter
OPC *See* Organophosphate
Ophitoxemia 451

Opioid 535, 538, 568
    derivatives 537
Optic nerve sheath diameter 330
Optiflow system 113
Oral fluids, intravenous to 373
Oral hypoglycemic agents 418
    clinical features 418
    management 419
    source 418
    sulfonylurea compounds 418
Oral intubation 332
Oral mucosa 118
Oral rehydration solution 42
Organ allocation and prioritization 347
Organ donation statistic 564*f*
Organ dysfunction 369, 568
Organ function assessment, tests for 368
Organ hypoperfusion, denoting 228
Organic acidemia 344, 358
Organocarbamate poisoning 426
Organophosphate 420
    compounds 424
        induced delayed polyneuropathy 425
Organs donated 564*f*
Ornithine aspartate 333
Ornithine transcarbamy 330
ORS *See* Oral rehydration solution
Orthogonal polarization spectral 161
OSA *See* Obstructive sleep apnea
Osmotherapy 243
Osmotic agent 301
Osmotic compensatory mechanisms 328
Osmotic diuretics 263
Osmotic therapy 333
Osteomyelitis 513
Ototoxicity 174
Overfeeding 358
Oxamyl (vydate) 427
Oxidative stress 59
Oxygen 50, 101, 120, 177, 442
    and face tents 52
    consumption 162, 263
    content 120
    facemask 56
    hazards of 59
    hood (oxyhood) 52, 55, 56*f*
    humidification of 51
    masks, simple 52
    utilization 275
Oxygen delivery 120, 162
    and consumption 51

Oxygen delivery devices 11, 56t
   low-flow 53f
      and high-flow 52t
Oxygen dissociation curve 120f
   with left shift 120f
Oxygen extraction
   indicator of 262
   ratio 162
Oxygen saturation 571
   index 139, 140
   of arterial blood 120
Oxygen therapy 50
   administration of 52
   monitoring of 58
   weaning from 59
Oxygenation 130, 197
   determining 130
   index 140
      common 162

P

Packed red blood cells 303, 482, 483b
   indications 483
Paget's disease, advanced 166
Pain 34, 532
   abdominal 516
   assessment of 540
Painless rectal bleeding, causes of 313b
Pancreatitis 138, 366
Pancuronium 542
Pantoprazole 319
PAO_2 See Partial pressure of arterial oxygen
Papilledema 219, 244
Paracetamol poisoning 408
   management of 409
Paracetamol toxicity, stages of 409b
Paracetamol-induced hepatotoxicity, mechanism of 408
Paraoxysmal neurological disorder 242
Parasympathetic stimulation 457
Parenchymal disease 76
Parenchymal lung disease 82
Parenteral fluids 34
   maintenance 35t
Parenteral nutrition 510
   induced liver injury 344
   total 360
Paresthesias 444

Partial pressure
   of arterial oxygen 131, 137, 138, 172
   of carbon dioxide 126, 131
   of oxygen 50
      in alveolus 131
Patent ductus arteriosus 166, 169
Pathology, type of 96t
Patient level outcomes 552
Patient population 546
Patient's brain death 573
Patient-nurse level outcomes 552
PAWP See Pulmonary arterial wedge pressure
PCV See Pressure control ventilation
PDA See Patent ductus arteriosus
PDE See Phosphodiesterase
Peak end expiratory pressure 76
Peak inspiratory pressure 68, 144
Pedestrian injury 381
Pediatric arrhythmias, treatment of 198
Pediatric assessment triangle 5
Pediatric bradycardia algorithm 200fc
Pediatric cardiac arrest 26fc
   algorithm 20fc
Pediatric injury severity, measurement of 381
Pediatric intensive care 1
   unit 117, 211, 254, 280, 423, 480, 491, 532
Pediatric liver transplant, contraindications to 345, 345b
Pediatric oncology 483
Pediatric organ donation and donor maintenance 563
Pediatric population 184
Pediatric rifle criteria, modified 237t
Pediatric trauma 382
   score 381t
   unique aspects of 382
PEEP See Positive end-expiratory pressure
Peptic ulcer 314, 365
Perforation 434
Pericardial effusion 375
Pericarditis 321, 366
Peripheral capillary oxygen saturation 573
Peripheral vein 511
Peritoneal dialysis 299, 301
   advantages of 301b
   mechanisms 301
   prescription 302
Peritonitis 321
Pertussis 352
Petechiae 244

Phenobarbitone 446
Phenomena, transient 253
Phenoxybenzamine 224
Phenylephrine 212, 214
Phenytoin 446
Phosphate 294, 464
    enema 294
Phosphodiesterase 181
    III inhibitors 211
Phosphorus 47, 278
Physical examination 314
Physiology, pediatric and adult 137t
PICU *See* Pediatric intensive care unit
Piggy backing 232
Pimobendan 208
Piperacillin-tazobactam 502
Pirimicarb (pirimor) 427
Plant toxidrome 444t
Plasma 480
    exchange and oxygen 440
    leakage, severe 369, 373
    proteins 481
Plateau pressure 66, 68, 144
Plateau waves 259f
Platelet 480, 481
    aggregation 148
    destruction, increased 486
    dysfunction 363, 486
    increased consumption of 485
    production, decreased 485
    random donor 484
    single donor 484
    types of 484
Platelet transfusion 374, 484
    criteria to transfuse 484
    efficacy 486
    indications 485
Platinum half hour or golden hour 382
PMN *See* Polymorphonuclear neutrophils
Pneumonia 57, 58, 91, 132, 138, 228, 263, 332, 429
    characterization of 496
    development of 491
    healthcare-associated 491, 499b
Pneumothorax 387, 439
Point-of-care ultrasound 2
Poison
    categorization of 396
    classification of 396
    indicated 402
    individual 405

Poisoning 395
    acute single dose 408
    anticholinergic 244
    antidepressant 244
    childhood 395
    epidemiology of 395
    general management 396
    in children 395
        and adults 396t
    management of 405
    treatment of 248
    unrecognized 397, 398
Poisonous and nonpoisonous sting, phases of 459fc
Poisonous snakes, common 453
Poisonous sting 458
Polio virus, inactivated 352
Polymorphic ventricular tachycardia 202
Polymorphonuclear
    leukocytes 493
    neutrophils 497
Polyp 314
Polysaccharide pneumococcal 352
Polytrauma, child with 383f
Pontine lesions 244
Porphobilinogen 247
Porphyria 247
Positive end-expiratory pressure 65, 71, 87, 138, 145, 177, 230, 332, 460
Positive pressure ventilation 34, 87f, 143, 177
Postcardiac arrest care 30
Post-concussion syndromes 252
Postprandial hyperglycemia 289
Post-pyloric feeding 359
Post-traumatic seizures, immediate 265
Potassium 43, 464
    correction 293
Potential organ donors, management of 571t
PPI *See* Proton pump inhibitor
Pralidoxime 402, 426
Prazosin 181
Precordial activity, increased 171
Predigested formulae 360
Pressure control ventilation 96
    mode 94
Pressure support 90
    ventilation 81
Pressure ventilation, negative 74, 86, 87f
Pressure versus flow 155
Pressure-regulated volume control ventilation 81

Pressure-volume
  curve relationship 128
  loop 69
PRIS See Propofol infusion syndrome
Probable tests 246
Promethazine 534
Prophylactic medication 264
Prophylactic platelet 485
  transfusion 484
Propionibacterium 513
Propofol 272, 535, 541
  infusion syndrome 272, 535
Propoxur (baygon) 427
Propranolol 320
Propylene glycol 535
Prostaglandin 181
Protein 360
  C deficiency 344
  energy malnutrition 359
  metabolism 358
Prothrombin time 278
  altered 315
Proton pump inhibitor 316
Pseudohyponatremia 40
Pseudomonas 511, 524
  aeruginosa 494, 498, 500, 512, 513, 528
  species 516
Psychosocial assessment 352
PTT See Partial thromboplastin time
Pulmonary arterial wedge pressure 137
Pulmonary artery 166
  catheters 138
Pulmonary contusion 138
Pulmonary edema 58, 91, 299, 572
Pulmonary function tests 127
  clinically relevant 127
  research 127
Pulmonary hypertension 166, 168
  acute 168
  persistent 556
Pulmonary mechanics, alteration of 142
Pulmonary metastasis 343
Pulmonary pressures, reduces 211
Pulmonary vascular
  remodelling, risk of 137
  resistance 142
  tone, systemic and 205
Pulmonary vasculitis 138
Pulse
  amplification, distal 155
  check 24, 27
  oximeter work 119
  poor 173
  rate 8, 385
Pulse oximetry 118, 172
  critical discussion on 119
  limitations of 119
Pulse pressure 229
  maximal 157
  minimal 157
  narrow 229
  variation 157
  wide 229
Pulseless
  arrest algorithm 201*fc*
  electrical activity 197
  ventricular tachycardia 28, 193
Pulsus paradoxus 171
Pupil
  constricted 399
  dilated 399
  unequal 243
Pupillary size and reaction 398
Purious hyperkalemia 44
Pyrazinamide 327
Pyrexia 400

Q

QRS complexes 187
QT syndrome, long 191, 193
QTC prolongation 422, 432
Quinine 247

R

RAAS See Renin-angiotensin-aldosterone system
Rabies 242, 352
Rabiprazole 319
Ramsay sedation scale 541*b*
Rat killer poisoning 431
  clinical manifestations 431
  laboratory investigations 432
  prevention 433
  prognosis 433
  source 431
Rebreathing mask, partial 52, 54, 56
Rectal diazepam 270
Red blood cells 361, 480
Refeeding syndrome 361

Refractory metabolic acidosis 299
Refractory seizures 536
Refractory status epilepticus 243, 278
Remifentanil 537, 538
Remote symptomatic epilepsy 270
Renal disease 43
Renal disorders 132
Renal dysfunction 568
Renal failure 36, 46, 376
    acute 40
    chronic 483
    indices, classification using 237t
    transient 263
Renal function 33
    assessment of 350
Renal insufficiency, physiological 33
Renal replacement therapy 299, 468
    basics of 299
    continuous 299, 305, 336
    modes of 301
Renal stones 274
Renal support 237, 561
Renal tubular acidosis 44
Renal tubules 464
Renin-angiotensin-aldosterone system 178, 220, 224
    blockade 225
    stimulation of 167
Residual capacity, functional 88, 137
Residual pyloric stenosis 414
Respiration 426
    accessory muscles of 118
Respiratory
    alkalosis 406
    depression 413
    distress and shock 377
    distress/failure 373
    endoscopy 535
    mechanics, physiology of 63
    monitoring 117
    muscle reserve 137
    syncytial virus 494
    therapy equipment, contaminated 500
Respiratory failure 10, 73, 555
    acute 91, 96
    anticipate 10
    pathology causing 96
    severe 92
Respiratory rate 9, 244, 385
    by age, normal 239
    normal 118t

Respiratory syndrome
    pediatric acute 140t
    severe acute 494, 501
Respiratory system 66
    and ventilation 332
    compliance 144
    mechanical properties of 63
Resuscitation 19, 407
    fluid 37
    monitoring of 386
Retinal hemorrhage 244
Reye's syndrome 327, 333
Rh negative 482
Rh positive 482
Rhabdomyosarcoma 471
Rheumatic fever 195, 196
Rib injuries 387
Ribonucleic acid 275, 363
Rickettsial infections 247
Rickettsial meningoencephalitis 242
Rifampicin 327, 409
Ringer's lactate 362
RNA *See* Ribonucleic acid
Rocuronium 542
Ross classification 170, 170t
Rotavirus 352
RSE *See* Refractory status epilepticus
Rubella 352
Rumack-Matthew nomogram 410, 410f

S

Safety devices and monitors 557
Salicylate 403
    poisoning 405
Saline, volumes of normal 292
Sarcoma 471
Sarin 424
SARS *See* Severe acute respiratory syndrome
Schizophrenia, drugs in 534
Schofield's equations 358
Schwartz formula 237
Sclerosant injection 320, 321
Sclerosing cholangitis 344
    primary 342, 349
Scorpion 457
    venom, pathogenesis of 458fc
Scorpion envenomation 457
    clinical features 458
    diagnosis 460

incidence 457
pathogenesis 458
prognosis 461
treatment 460
Scorpion sting 449
    envenomation 459fc
Sea snakes 452
Second therapy phase 271
Sedation 532, 533
    and analgesia 264
        protocol for 540fc
    assessment of 540
    goals of 533
    holidays 536
    sedative drugs 534
Sedative agents 534t
Sedative drugs 539
Seizures 242, 250, 264, 270, 400
    aggressive treatment of 264
    unrecognized 265
Senning operation 168
Sensorium 292
    altered 303
Sepsis 226, 227, 263
    syndrome 228
    with organ dysfunction 228
Septic shock 38, 74, 226, 235, 556
    compensatory mechanisms 227
    management of 229t
    microcirculatory changes 226
    pathophysiology 226
    pediatric and neonatal 233fc
    symptoms for 231
    therapy of 226, 235
Septicemia 132, 335
Sequential organ failure assessment 228t
Serotonin and noradrenaline reuptake inhibitors 423
Serotonin reuptake inhibitors, selective 423
Serotonin syndrome, risk of 423
Serratia 511
Serum
    ache 426
    alpha fetoprotein 346
    bicarbonate 290
    electrolytes 466, 573
    glutamic pyruvic transaminase 314
    glutamic-oxaloacetic transaminase 314
    osmolality 292
        effective 295
    salicylate level 406

Severity assessment, quick 426t
Shigella encephalopathy 242
Shock 132, 187, 244, 363, 369, 377, 566
    anaphylactic 38
    clinical parameters for 227b
    cold hypotensive 362
    compensated 369, 371fc
    delayed 414
    management 205
        of snake bite 455
    neurogenic 386
    non-cardiogenic 138
    recognition of 227
    resolution, signs of 369
    severe 215
    steps in management of 205b
    types of 216fc
Shunt 51
Sick-day rules 297
Sickle cell disease 483
Sideroblastic anemia 483
Sieving coefficient 300
Silverman-Anderson index 118t
Sinus
    bradycardia 195
        treatment of 195
    nodal dysfunction 197
    tachycardia 8, 183, 184, 187, 422
        treatment of 188
    venous thrombosis 242
SIRS *See* Systemic inflammatory response syndrome
Skin 222
    burns 203
    dry 400
    integrity, loss of 510
    necrosis 439
Skull fractures 266
SLED *See* Sustained low-efficiency dialysis
Snake
    poisonous 453
        cobra 453
        krait 453
        russell's viper 453
        saw-scaled viper 453
Snake bite 455
    renal failure 456
Snake envenomation 449
    clinical features 451
    epidemiology 449

first aid 452
local signs of envenomation 451
severity of 454t
treatment 452
  inside hospital 453
Snake venom 450
enzymes 450
nonenzyme
  polypeptides 450
  proteins 450
SNP *See* Sodium nitroprusside
Sodium 38
benzoate 333
corrected 292
loss of 39, 40
nitroprusside 176, 181, 214, 216, 224, 225, 460
overload 42
valproate 446
Solute and fluid removal, mechanisms of 300
Solvent-induced encephalopathy, chronic 276
Spironolactone 175, 180, 224
Spontaneous eye opening 241
Staphylococcus 510
  coagulase negative 498
Staphylococcus aureus 510, 512, 516, 524
  methicillin-resistant 494, 498, 503
  methicillin-sensitive 503
Static preload measurements 156
Static respiratory mechanics 64
Status asthmaticus 539
Status epilepticus 242, 268, 444
etiology 269
pathophysiology 269
protocol 277t
systemic effects during 270
Stem-cell therapy 179
Stenotrophomonas maltophilia 494
Sterile equipment 518
Steroid 262, 327
administration 235
and immunotherapy 275
therapy 235
Stomach contents, aspiration of 321
Storage and shelf life 481
Stroke volume 165
variation 157
Subarachnoid hemorrhage, particularly 41
Subcutaneous catheter 513
Subcutaneous emphysema 438*f*
Subcutaneous insulin, transition to 295

Subdural
empyema 242
hematoma 255, 266
Subfalcine herniation 245
Subgaleal hematomas 266
Subglottic secretion drainage 505*f*
Submersion 391
Succinylcholine 542
Sulpha 409
Superoxide dismutase 59
Supratherapeutic ingestion, repeated 408
Supraventricular tachyarrhythmia 184, 188
Supraventricular tachycardia 8, 183, 189*fc*
management of 189
Surfactant therapy 147
SVR *See* Systemic vascular resistance
Swap transplant 354
Sweating 171
Swimming skills, inadequate 392
Sympathetic storm 457
Sympathetic tone, increase in 167
Sympatholytic agents 224
Sympathomimetic poisoning 244
Symptomatic hyponatremia 39
Synchronization 79
Synchronized intermittent mandatory ventilation 80
Syndrome of inappropriate antidiuretic hormone secretion 34, 40, 41*t*
treatment 41
Syndromic epilepsies 270
Systemic endogenous vasodilators, levels of 332
Systemic inflammatory response syndrome 216, 227, 327, 334
Systemic toxicity 451
Systemic vascular resistance 153, 224, 229
Systemic ventricular failure 168
Systolic dysfunction 166, 374
Systolic pressure variation 157

T

Tabun 424
Tachyarrhythmias 184, 199*fc*
management of 198*t*
Tachycardia 171, 173, 184, 186, 375, 399, 422, 444
child with 8
narrow complex 185*f*
reentrant 186*f*
type of 188

Tachypnea 171, 399, 400
Talbot formula 358
Tamponade (cardiac) 9
Tandem mass spectrometry 247
TAPVC *See* Total anomalous pulmonary venous connection
TCA *See* Tricyclic antidepressant
Tension pneumothorax 9
Teratoma 471
Terlipressin 319, 320
Tetanus 352
Tetralogy of Fallot 211
Thalassemia 483
Theophylline 45, 403, 413
Thermodilution 159
Thiazides 174
Thioridazine 422
Third therapy phase 272
Thoracic disorders, restrictive 110
Thoracic electrical bioimpedance 159
Thoracic fluid index 160
Thoracic trauma 388
Thrombocytopenia 315, 360
    dilutional 486
    with absent radius syndrome 485
Thromboplastin time, partial 278
Thrombosis 308, 327
Thrombotic thrombocytopenic purpura 485, 489
Thymic tumor 471
Thyrotoxicosis 166
Tidal volume 143
TIPSS *See* Transjugular intrahepatic portosystemic shunt
Tissue
    capnometry 161
    engineered vessels 179
    oxygenation 161
        assessment of 161
        monitoring 161
Tolerance development, causes for 275*b*
Tongue, cyanosis of 118
Tonic downgaze 245
Tonic upwardgaze 245
Tonic-clonic seizures 419
Tonsillar herniation 245
Topiramate 275
Torsemide 224
Total anomalous pulmonary venous connection 169
Total blood volume 303

Tourniquet test 364
Toxic
    dose 405
    encephalopathy 242
    ingestion 244
    level 441
    symptoms 420
Toxicity
    acute 424
    mechanism of 405, 416, 418, 419, 421-424, 427, 429, 436, 439, 443
    of chemicals, mechanism of 431*t*
Toxidromes 395, 400, 401*t*
Toxins 9
    and specific antidote 402*t*
    cause of 444
TR *See* Tricuspid regurgitation
Tracheal intubation 253
Tracheobronchial obstruction 472
Tracheostomy 561
Tramadol 537, 539
Transcatheter interventions 178
Transitory state, type of 241
Transjugular intrahepatic portosystemic shunt 316, 321
Transplant recipients, vaccination in 352*t*
Transpulmonary pressure 66, 70, 88
Transpulmonary thermodilution 161
Transverse myelitis 375
Trauma 9, 138
    abdominal 388
    score, revised 381*t*
Traumatic brain injury 270, 535
    severe 249
Tricuspid regurgitation 169
Tricyclic antidepressant 402, 420, 421
    clinical manifestations 421
    management 421
    source 421
Trigger asynchrony 79
Triglycerides 272, 360
Trimethoprim-sulfamethoxazole 326
TTP *See* Thrombotic thrombocytopenic purpura
Tubercular meningitis 242
Tubular necrosis, acute 43
Tumor burden, large 465
Tumor lysis syndrome 46, 464
    clinical evaluation 466
    laboratory evaluation 466
    management 466

pathophysiology 464
risk factors 465
risk stratification 465
Tympanic membrane, perforation of 439
Tyrosinemia 326, 330

U

Ultrafiltration 300
Ultrasonography abdomen 388
Uncal herniation 245
Uncertain compensation 134
Underfeeding 358
Upper gastrointestinal
    endoscopy 437
        role of 435
        series 318
Urea cycle defect 330, 344
Uremia 299
Urethral catheter, indwelling 515
Uric acid 464
Urinalysis 466
Urinary alkalinisation 467
Urinary catheter 518
    in-dwelling 543
Urinary retention 422
Urinary tract infection 515
Urination 424
Urine
    analysis 573
    osmolality 237
    output 229, 385
        reduced 171
    sediment 237
    sodium 237

V

Vagal maneuvers 190
Valproate 264
Valve stenosis 166
Vancomycin intermediate staphylococci 528
VAP *See* Ventilator-associated pneumonia
Variable-concentration devices 52
Variceal bleed 321
Varicella 352
Varicella-zoster virus 326
Vascular malformation 313, 314
Vasculotoxins 450
Vasoactive agents 205, 207*t*
    classification of 206

effects of 215*f*
individual 208
Vasoactive drugs 232
    titration of 232
Vasoactive therapy, goals of 215
Vasodilators, direct 224
Vasopressin 210, 214, 227, 232
    receptors 208
Vecuronium 181, 542, 543
Venom 457
Venomous snakes, species of 449*b*
Veno-occlusive disease 327, 330
Venous blood gas 8
Venous oxygen saturation 161
Venous reservoir 557
Venous system, intracranial to extracranial 258
Venovenous hemodiafiltration, continuous 306, 307*f*, 404
Venovenous hemodialysis, continuous 306, 307*f*
Venovenous hemofiltration, continuous 306, 306*f*, 560
Ventilation 21, 197
    adaptive support 81
    assist-control mode 81
    assisted modes 81
    control mode of 78*f*, 80
    dual mode 81
    duration of 84
    hybrid modes 81
    machines, types of noninvasive 95
    modes of 80
    newer mode 81
    noninvasive 86
        contraindications 90
        indications 90
    phases of 77
    proportional assist 81
Ventilator
    hardware 74
    settings 560
    settings, initial 82
Ventilator-associated pneumonia 491, 492, 494*t*, 496-498, 499*b*, 501*t*, 506, 561
    diagnosis 495
    management of 504
    pathogenesis 492
    prevention 499
    probable 496
    risk factors 493
    treatment 501
Ventilator-induced lung injury 62
Ventricle failure, right 166

Ventricular arrhythmias 48, 202, 375
Ventricular assist device 179
Ventricular contractions, premature 191, 191*f*
Ventricular fibrillation 19, 193, 193*f*, 200, 201
Ventricular septal defect 166, 169
Ventricular tachyarrhythmias 191
Ventricular tachycardia 19, 185, 192, 200, 201
    wide complex 192*f*
Venturi mask 52, 54, 55*f*, 56
VF *See* Ventricular fibrillation
Viperidae 449
Vipers 451
Viral
    infections, transmission of 487
    meningoencephalitis 242
    pneumonias 556
Virtual anesthesia 533
Vital signs, interpreting abnormal 8
Vitamin
    deficiencies 349, 359
    essential 360
    K 343, 433
        administration 238
Volatile agents 541
Volatile organic compounds, analysis of 505
Vomiting 132, 444, 466
    and gastric bleeding 92
VSD *See* Ventricular septal defect
VT *See* Ventricular tachycardia

W

Warfarin compounds 431
Warm shock 205

Warning signs 369
Washed cells 488
Water
    gain 39
    homeostasis 33
    intake, excessive 40
    loss into cells 42
    losses, unreplaced 42
Weakness 444
Weaning from invasive ventilation 91
Weaning phase 278
Wenckebach phenomena 195
Wheezing 171
White blood cell 480
    filter 488
Whole blood 482
    indications 482
    unit of 480
Wilson's disease 327, 328, 330, 344
Withdrawal syndrome 543
Wolff-Parkinson-White syndrome 186, 188, 198
Worsening hypoxemia 59

Y

Yellow phosphorus 432

Z

Zidovudine 409
Ziprasidone 422
Zygomycetes 494